Advance Acclaim for

PSYCHOTROPIC DRUGS AND THE ELDERLY: FAST FACTS

"This is the most comprehensive geriatric psychopharmacology text ever. Contains extensive information, some of which is difficult to find in any text."

—Sanford Finkel, M.D., Professor of Clinical Psychiatry, University of Chicago Medical School

"Sadavoy provides a remarkably comprehensive and practical treatment of psychotropic drug use in the elderly. *Psychotropic Drugs and the Elderly: Fast Facts* delivers an in-depth overview of all the major classes of psychotropic drugs prescribed to older patients and informs the physician about efficacy, application, and safety issues. This book will be an outstanding addition to one's clinical management guides."

—Gene D. Cohen, M.D., Ph.D., Director, Center on Aging, Health & Humanities, George Washington University

"This is a practical and user-friendly desk reference on the use of psychotropic drugs with elderly clients. Sadavoy tells you everything you wanted to know about psychotropic drugs with this client population and he provides it all in the form of a clear outline in which much of the material is presented in tabular format. *Psychotropic Drugs and the Elderly: Fast Facts* is destined to become the standard reference in the field of psychopharmacology and aging. Dr. Sadavoy's wisdom, clarity and clinical focus are embedded throughout this text."

—George T. Grossberg, M.D., Samuel W. Fordyce Professor and Director of Geriatric Psychiatry, St. Louis University School of Medicine

PSYCHOTROPIC DRUGS AND THE ELDERLY FAST FACTS

OTHER BOOKS IN THE *FAST FACTS* SERIES

Psychotropic Drugs: Fast Facts, Third Edition
by Jerrold S. Maxmen, M.D., Nicholas G. Ward, M.D.
with Steven L Dubovsky, M.D., as special advisor

Sexual Pharmacology: Fast Facts
by Robert Taylor Segraves, M.D., Ph.D., and Richard Balon, M.D.

Psychotropic Drugs and Women: Fast Facts
by Victoria Hendrick, M.D., and Michael Gitlin, M.D.

A NORTON PROFESSIONAL BOOK

PSYCHOTROPIC DRUGS AND THE ELDERLY FAST FACTS

Joel Sadavoy, M.D., FRCP (C)

W. W. Norton & Company
New York • London

NOTICE

We have made every attempt to summarize accurately and concisely a multitude of references. However, the reader is reminded that times and medical knowledge change, transcription or understanding error is always possible, and crucial details are omitted whenever such a comprehensive distillation as this is attempted in limited space. We cannot, therefore, guarantee that every bit of information is absolutely accurate or complete. The reader should affirm that cited recommendations are still appropriate by reading the original articles and checking other sources, including local consultants and recent literature.

DRUG DOSAGE

The author and publisher have exerted every effort to ensure that drug selection and dosage set forth in this text are in accord with current recommendations and practice at the time of publication. However, in view of ongoing research, changes in government regulations, and the constant flow of information relating to drug therapy and drug reactions, the reader is urged to check the package insert for each drug for any change in indications and dosage and for added warnings and precautions. This is particularly important when the recommended agent is a new and/or infrequently used drug.

Printed in the United States of America
First Edition

Production Manager: Leeann Graham
Manufacturing by Quebecor World Fairfield

Library of Congress Cataloging-in-Publication Data

Sadavoy, Joel, 1945–
Psychotropic drugs and the elderly / Joel Sadavoy.
p. cm. – (Fast facts)
"A Norton professional book."
Includes bibliographical references and index.
ISBN 0-393-70375-4
1. Psychotropic drugs. 2. Pharmacokinetics. 3. Geriatric psychopharmacology.
I. Title. II. Fast facts (New York, N.Y.)
[DNLM: 1. Psychotropic Drugs—pharmacology—Aged. 2. Psychotropic Drugs—therapeutic use—Aged. QV 77.2 S124p 2004]

RM315.S197 2004
615'.788—dc22 2003070180

W. W. Norton & Company, Inc., 500 Fifth Avenue, New York, N.Y. 10110
www.wwnorton.com

W. W. Norton & Company Ltd., Castle House, 75/76 Wells St.,
London W1T 3QT

1 3 5 7 9 0 8 6 4 2

Dedication

For Sharian

Contents

Abbreviations xiii

Acknowledgments xix

Introduction 3

Structure and Goals of the Book 4

Research and Sources of Data 6

Challenges Posed by the Data 7

Dosing Challenges 8

Side-Effect Challenges 9

The Importance of Basic Pharmacology 10

Indications and Contraindications 10

Overview of General Pharmacokinetics and Pharmacodynamics 11

1. Antidepressants 23

Overview 23

Depressive Disorders in Elders 24

Non-Depressive Disorders for which Antidepressants Are Used 38

Geriatric Antidepressant Pharmacotherapy Issues 45

Choosing and Using Specific Antidepressants 49

Phases of Antidepressant Treatment 53

Prognosis of Depression with Treatment 55

Nonresponse to Antidepressant Treatment 58

Depression Therapy Decision Pathways 65

Side Effects of Antidepressants 70
Receptor Affinity–Side-Effect Relationship 89
Drug–Drug Interactions 90
Family and Caregivers 96
Heterocyclic Antidepressants 97
Irreversible MAOIs 111
Selective Serotonin Reuptake Inhibitors (SSRIs) 123
Individual Antidepressant Drug Profiles 135
Buproprion (BUP) 135
Citalopram 144
Clomipramine 151
Desipramine 155
Duloxetine 157
Escitalopram 158
Fluoxetine 158
Mirtazapine 166
Moclobemide 174
Nefazodone 179
Nortriptyline 186
Paroxetine 191
Phenelzine 200
Sertraline 202
St. John's Wort 209
Trazodone 210
Venlafaxine 217

2 Antipsychotic Agents 229
Overview 229
Atypical Antipsychotics 231
Typical Antipsychotics 232
Clinical Conditions Treated with Antipsychotic Agents 236
Principles of Treatment with Antipsychotics 262
Neuropharmacology of Neuroleptics 266
Choosing an Antipsychotic Drug 266

Administration and Dosing 273
Side Effects of Antipsychotics 279
Side Effects of Antipsychotic Drug Class 281
Antiparkinsonian Agents 303
Drug-Drug Interactions 306
Overdose with Typical Antipsychotics 307
Overdose with Atypical Antipsychotics 308
Individual Antipsychotic Drug Profiles 308
Aripiprazole 308
Clozapine 308
Fluphenazine 322
Haloperidol 325
Loxapine 332
Olanzapine 334
Perphenazine 342
Quetiapine 345
Risperidone 350
Thioridazine 359
Thiothixene 363
Ziprasidone 366

3 Antianxiety Drugs and Sedative/Hypnotics 371
Overview 371
Benzodiazepines 372
Pharmacology 376
Geriatric Issues 386
Anxiety Disorders 394
Other Conditions Where Benzodiazepines May be Used 400
Side Effects 401
Drug–Drug Interactions 410
Sleep Disorders 411
Alcohol Abuse and Alcoholism 423
Discontinuation/Withdrawal and Rebound Syndromes 426

Overdose 429
Individual Anti-Anxiety and Sedative/Hypnotic Drug Profiles 430
Alprazolam 430
Buspirone 436
Chloral Hydrate 441
Clonazepam 444
Diazepam 446
Estazolam 448
Lorazepam 449
Midazolam 453
Oxazepam 455
Temazepam 457
Triazolam 459
Zaleplon 462
Zolpidem 465
Zopiclone 471
Herbal Remedies 474

4 Mood Stabilizers 479
Overview 479
Pharmacology 482
Indications for Mood Stabilizers 485
Bipolar Disorder 485
Treatment of Bipolar Disorder 492
Individual Mood Stabilizer Drug Profiles 502
Carbamazepine 502
Gabapentin 509
Lamotrigine 513
Lithium 516
Topiramate 538
Valproic Acid, Valproate, Divalproex 541

5 Cognitive Enhancers 551
Overview 551
Pharmacology 553

Clinical Indications: Dementia 554
Treatment of Dementia 564
Cautions and Contraindications 571
Donepezil 574
Galantamine 582
Rivastigmine 587
Tacrine 592

Appendix A: Newly Approved Drugs 597
Aripiprazole 597
Escitalopram 599

Appendix B: Profile of Psychotropic Drugs 605
Antidepressants 605
Antipsychotics 617
Anxiolytics/Hypnotics 628
Mood Stabilizers 634
Cognitive Enhancers 638

References 641

Index 727

Abbreviations

AAG	alpha-1 acid glycoprotein
AChE(I)	acetylcholinesterase (inhibitor)
ACE	angiotensin converting enzyme
ACH	acetylcholine
AD	antidepressant
ADH	antidiuretic hormone
ADL	activities of daily living
AGP	alpha-1 acid glycoprotein
AIMS	adult involuntary movement scale
ALT	alanine aminotransferase
ALS	amyotrophic lateral sclerosis
AMPA	alpha-amino-3-hydroxy-5-methyl-4-isoxazole propionic acid
AP	antipsychotic
ASA	acetylsalicylic acid
AST	aspartate aminotransferase
ATP	adenosine triphosphate
AV	atrioventricular
BBB	bundle branch block
BChE	butyrylcholinesterase
bid	twice a day
BP	blood pressure
BPD	bipolar disorder
BPRS	Brief Psychiatric Rating Scale
BPSD	behavioral and psychological symptoms of dementia
BS	
BSE	bovine spongiform encephalitis
BUP	bupropion
Ca	calcium
cAMP	cyclic adenosine monophosphate

CBC complete blood count
CBS Charles Bonnet syndrome
CBT cognitive–behavioral therapy
ChE cholinesterase
CHF congestive heart failure
CIBIC+ clinician interview-based impression of change (with caregiver input)
Cmax maximum plasma concentration of a drug with therapeutic dosing
CNS central nervous system
COPD chronic obstructive pulmonary disease
CPS Compendium of Pharmaceutical Specialties
CR controlled release
C_{ss} mean steady-state concentration
CT computerized tomography
CVA cerebrovascular accident
CYP cytochrome P

DAT dementia of the Alzheimer's type
D/C discontinue
DLB dementia with Lewy bodies; diffuse Lewy body (disease)
DOPA dihydroxyphenylalanine

EB erythrohydroxybupropion
ECA epidemiologic catchment area
ECG electrocardiogram
ECT electroconvulsive therapy
EEG electroencephalogram
EO early onset
EM extensive metabolizers
EOS early onset symptoms
EPS extrapyramidal syndrome
ER extended release

FBS fasting blood sugar
FDA Food and Drug Administration (U.S.)
FMO flavin-containing mono-oxygenase

g gram
GABA gamma-aminobutyric acid
GAD generalized anxiety disorder
GDS Geriatric Depression Scale
GFR glomerular filtration rate
GI gastrointestinal

GLD glutamate dehydrogenase
GM grand mal
GU genitourinary

HAM-D Hamilton Rating Scale for Depression
HB hydroxybupropion
HCA heterocyclic antidepressant
HCl hydrochloride
hg hemoglobin
Hg mercury
HIV human immunodeficiency virus
HPA hypothalamic–pituitary axis
HPB Health Protection Branch (Canada)
hs hors somnium (at bedtime)
HVA homovanillic acid
5HT 5-hydroxytriptamine (serotonin)

IADL instrumental activities of daily living
IBS irritable bowel syndrome
ICU intensive care unit
IM intramuscular
IPT Interpersonal Psychotherapy
IP3 inisitol triphosphate
IR immediate release
IU international unit
IV intravenous

kg kilogram

LFT liver function test
l/kg liters per kilogram
LOS length of stay
LTC long-term care

MADRS Montgomery–Asberg Depression Rating Scale
MAO-A monoamine oxidase A
MAO-B monoamine oxidase B
MAOIs monoamine oxidase inhibitors
mCPP m-chlorophenylpiperazine
mEq milliequivalents
M/F male/female
mg milligram
Mg magnesium
MI myocardial infarction
min minutes

ml	milliliter
mm Hg	millimeters of mercury
mm	millimeter
mmol/l	millimoles per liter
MMSE	Mini Mental State Examination
MRI	magnetic resonance imaging
MS	multiple sclerosis
NA	noradrenergic
NaRI	noradrenaline reuptake inhibitor
NE	norepinephrine
NMDA	N-methyl-D-aspartate
NMS	neuroleptic malignant syndrome
NPI	neuropsychiatry inventory
NPO	nil per os (nothing by mouth)
NSAID	nonsteroidal anti-inflammatory drug
NaSSA	noradrenergic and specific serotonergic antidepressant
OBRA	Omnibus Budget Reconciliation Act
OCD	obsessive–compulsive disorder
OD	overdose
ODV	O-desmethylvenafaxine
OTC	over the counter
PD	personality disorder
PDA	panic disorder with agoraphobia
PDR	Physicians' Desk Reference
PO	per os (by mouth)
PO_4	phosphate
prn	as needed
PSD	poststroke depression
PSP	progressive supranuclear palsy
PTSD	posttraumatic stress disorder
PVC	premature ventricular contraction
q	every
qd	everyday
QEEG	quantitative EEG
qid	four times a day
qhs	every evening before bed (hors somnium)
QRS	refers to a component complex of the ECG
qod	every other day
QTc	corrected QT interval on ECG
RBC	red blood cell
RCT	randomized controlled trial

REM	rapid eye movement
RIMA	reversible inhibitor of monoamine oxidase-A
SAM-E	
SDAT	senile dementia Alzheimer's type
SIADH	syndrome of inappropriate antidiuretic hormone
SLE	systemic lupus erythematosus
SNRI	serotonin noradrenergic reuptake inhibitor
SOB	
SPECT	single photon emission computerized tomography
SPF	sun protective factor
SRI	serotonin reuptake inhibitor
SSRI	selective serotonin reuptake inhibitor
ST	
STD	sexually transmitted disease
T½	Hours required to eliminate 50% of a drug from the body
TB	threohydroxybupropion
TCA	tricyclic antidepressant
TD	tardive dyskinesia
TIA	transient ischemic attack
tid	three times a day
Tmax	time to peak plasma levels
TMS	transcranial magnetic stimulation
TRH	thyrotropin-releasing hormone
TSHs	thyroid stimulating hormone (sensitive)—refers to screening test for thyroid function
μg	microgram
UTI	urinary tract infection
UVA	ultraviolet A
UVB	ultraviolet B
VA	Veterans Administration
VaD	vascular dementia
Vd	volume of distribution
VPBs	ventricular premature beats
VPC	ventricular premature contractions
WBC	white blood cell
XR	extended release

ABBREVIATIONS

Acknowledgments

This book was a team effort. Anne Marie Metelsky-Vico, Senior Administrative Coordinator in the Department of Psychiatry at Mount Sinai Hospital, Toronto, coordinated this project and produced the detailed tables of drug descriptions, availability, and cost. James Prochaska initiated the computer database and library searches for the background material. Beth Sadavoy developed the structure for tracking references, conducted searches, and coordinated the team of researchers who tracked down the many hundreds of references and articles used in the book. I want to thank my research assistants Elissa Press, Aliza Weinrib, Ivana Miletic, Daniel Sadavoy, Ari Lesk, Michael Sadavoy, and Annie Simpson. I want to express my deep thanks to Drs. Sanford Finkel and Anne Hildebrand for their generosity of time and their invaluable assistance in providing a close reading of parts of this manuscript. Needless to say, any errors or ommissions are my responsibility. I am also deeply indebted to Margaret Ryan for her outstanding editorial work, and A. Deborah Malmud, Michael J. McGandy, and Andrea Costella of W.W. Norton for their professionalism, expertise, and sensitivity.

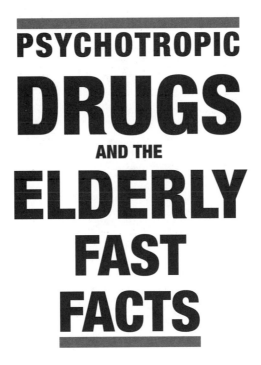

PSYCHOTROPIC DRUGS AND THE ELDERLY FAST FACTS

Introduction

The study of psychotropic drugs for elders is an increasingly complex field. These classes of drugs are in wide use among this population. A cursory review of the field will reassure the unwary practitioner that we now have a new generation of drugs that is easy to use, effective, and possess low side-effect risk. However, a closer examination reveals just how complex and difficult the management of psychiatric disorders in elders really is, including the complexity of effectively using the array of new psychotropics now available.

The scope of this issue is evident from studies of drug use in various settings: 8% of elderly women seen in general practice settings receive a psychotropic drug prescription, compared to 5% of men. Factors increasing the rate of prescription include

- Caucasian race
- Increasing age
  - √ Rate in those >85 years old is 1.5 times that for 65–69-year-olds
- Location of treatment
  - √ In nursing homes upward of two-thirds of patients receive psychotropic drugs
    - □ Most are getting antidepressants and substantial numbers antipsychotics
- Inappropriate drug prescription (including type of drug and excessive dose and duration of therapy)
  - √ In elders, 14–23% in the community and 12–40% in nursing homes

Table I.1. Drugs not Usually Recommended for Elders

antispasmodic GI agents—dicyclomine, hyoscyamine, propantheline, belladonna alkaloids
anxiolytics/sedative hypnotics—flurazepam, meprobamate, chlordiazepoxide, diazepam, all barbiturates, high-dose prescriptions of lorazepam (3 mg), oxazepam (60 mg), prazolam (2 mg), triazolam (0.25 mg)
chlorpropamide
digoxin (0.125 mg)
dipyridamole—orthostatic hypotension
disopyramide
ergot mesyloids—ineffective
first-generation antihistamines—chlorpheniramine, diphenhydramine, hydroxyzine, cyproheptadine, promethazine, dexchlorpheniramine—anticholinergic effects
indomethacin—CNS side effects
iron supplements (>325 mg)
meperidine
methyldopa
muscle relaxants—methocarbamol, carisoprodol, oxybutynin, metaxalone, cyclobenzaprine—anticholinergic, sedation, weakness
pentazocine
phenylbutazone—blood dyscrasias
propoxyphene
reserpine—depression, hypotension, sedation
ticlopidine
tricyclic antidepressants—amitriptyline, doxepin, amoxapine, maprotiline, protriptyline, imipramine, trimipramine
trimethobenzamide—EPS

Prescribing patterns are changing. The last decade has seen the introduction of more than a dozen new-generation psychotropic agents, which have transformed the prescribing patterns of practitioners.

- √ More than one-third of all antipsychotic drug prescriptions are now atypicals
- √ More than one-half of antidepressants are SSRIs

STRUCTURE AND GOALS OF THE BOOK

Psychotropic Drugs and the Elderly: Fast Facts is drug-focused, not disease-focused. In contrast to geriatric texts that start from the perspective of treatment, this book is focused on the drugs. I have not attempted to include comprehensive clinical descriptions of disorders or the nonpharmacological aspects of management, although the basics of diagnosis are included when relevant to drug use. Hence in reading the chapter on antidepressants, for example, the reader will need to turn to other texts for more comprehensive discussions of depressive disorders in elders.

The goal is to provide a comprehensive and authoritative guide to the use of drug classes, specific agents and, when appropriate, their combinations. I have kept narrative to a minimum, presenting the material in tabular and outline format. The purpose is to provide rapid access to very thorough information without having to plow through a lot of extraneous detail.

For each class of agents such as antidepressants, I have begun each section with general summary information. Although some of this information may be repeated in the sections on individual drugs, as far as possible I have kept repetition to a minimum. When consulting this text with a question about drug treatment, read the general sections along with the specific drug information in order to get the whole picture.

Practical Drug Use

Practitioners can turn directly to the specific drug profile for answers to questions such as: How does a specific drug interact with the drug profile of the patient?, What are the specific side effects of the drug in question?, What is the best dose and how should I titrate the dose increases? Yet keep in mind that, for the sake of minimizing repetition, the pharmacological qualities common to a class of drugs will be contained in the general introduction to the class of drugs and usually will not be repeated in the case of each specific drug in that class. Individual drug profiles are cross-referenced to ease finding this information; the index will also aid in tracking down specific information. I recommend that the reader begin by looking up the specific drug and then proceed by adding in the general components as needed. One caution: Some of the lists of drug-drug interactions and side effects rely on the integration of the general information with the data on the specific drug; looking at both sections is advisable for completeness. If the reader needs to know the various dosages forms (e.g., tablet versus capsule versus extended release forms, liquid, injectable), appearance, and cost range for a given drug, please consult Appendix B: Profile of Psychotropic Drugs.

Academic Study

If using the book for study purposes, the best approach is to begin with the general introductions to the individual chapters. Each class of drugs is introduced with an authoritative and detailed summary of the members of the class, their labeled and off-label uses, general modes of utilization of the class, specific details on pharmacology, side effects and toxicology, as well as other pertinent data. This information will provide a solid base for study regarding psychotropic drug-use in the elderly. Chapter introductions also contain summary descriptions of the disorders for which the class of drug is to be used and specifics about ways in which to use the class with these disorders. Note: The descriptions are not intended to be exhaustive discussions of the disorders themselves. All the information regarding disorders is data based (or indicated otherwise where necessary) and it can be used for preparation for examinations or tests. Once again the specific drug profiles will offer additional details when relevant.

RESEARCH AND SOURCES OF DATA

Data for this book are derived from general adult and geriatric evidence-based, peer-reviewed sources wherever possible, with an obvious special emphasis on geriatric data. Sources include a thorough review of the literature based on comprehensive searches of the major medical electronic databases (1980–2003) for every drug and condition, major geriatric psychopharmacology texts and other publications, occasional reliable Internet resources, Cochrane databases of evidence-based trials, and clinical case descriptions (including the best letters to the editors, clinical case descriptions, and the occasional opinion of esteemed experienced clinicians).

Naturally, for completeness, I have consulted the familiar, pharmaceutically-produced drug information sources such as the *PDR* and *CPS*. My approach was to review all literature on a drug or class through Medline and other searches first, incorporating it into the appropriate chapter. Only then did I add material from the pharmaceutical company sources in publications such as the *PDR* or *CPS*. However, I have made no attempt to repeat the overinclusive lists of information, especially side effects, in these sources. Rather, I have tried to extract those items that are most clinically relevant and reflect the experience of investigators and clinicians. The lists of side effects in this book, therefore, contain those effects which are likely to be drug-related, in contrast to incidental findings in large premarketing studies. In taking this approach, I may have inadvertently missed the occasional adverse effect that clinicians will encounter or included some that I should have omitted. Although I have tried to be thorough, I welcome feedback from readers so that future editions will be as accurate as possible regarding our psychotropic treatment of geriatric patients.

I have critically evaluated all clinical information and used case reports at times. Where geriatric data are sparse or the data are drawn from general adult studies, I have tried to note it in the text. Specific geriatric drug information based on empirical, controlled studies is often unavailable. There is ample clinical information on the treatment of the elderly which has been included, but readers may nonetheless share my frustration at the lack of reliable, evidence-based data to guide clinical usage in regard to elders, especially for older agents. I have kept personal experience in mind throughout, but only as it relates to empirical data.

The greatest challenge in writing this text has been the need to track down reliable sources of information that are not contaminated by the myriad of biasing factors, marketing strategies disguised as scientific data, and so on. I have read most of the references listed, rather than relying on secondary sources, and evaluated the information. However, necessarily I have unwittingly repeated information and clinical lore that may turn out to be erroneous as studies emerge in the future. Additionally, computer searches, though a boon to research, are not always exhaustive in the results they produce. Sometimes relevant articles do not show up, despite attempts to use a variety of search terms. Additional articles were identified from other reference sources such as review articles. Sometimes I tracked these down, but at other times I used a secondary analysis when it was corroborated by alternative sources.

CHALLENGES POSED BY THE DATA

In many cases the practice patterns are far in advance of the evidence, especially because results of studies with new agents are skewed by (1) publication bias in favor of positive results, (2) uncontrolled studies that far outnumber controlled studies, and (3) pharmaceutically sponsored studies and publications. A lot of data come from marketing studies (i.e., required by licensing bodies). They follow an accepted format and design, which is adequate for efficacy and general safety studies, but in no way can be seen as the final word on general effectiveness nor as a guide to clinical practice in specific clinical situations. Indeed, recent data on antidepressant trials clearly show the efficacy results from studies of selected populations often are not relevant to unselected naturalistic patient populations. Similarly, a substantial amount of published material in the pharmacological literature comes in the form of supplements to journals. Although the information in these reports is generally written by very reputable investigators and clinicians, it is also true that the standard of review and peer criticism is not the same as for regular peer-reviewed articles that would appear in general issues of the same journal. I have tried to take this factor into account in evaluating the validity of the material.

Despite these biases and problems, however, the clinician is faced with the need to treat. I have tried to interpret the data with this need in mind and to indicate the nature of the evidence behind recommendations whenever appropriate—that is, general adult data extrapolated to pertain to elders (as is very common), practice based on clinical trials and experience, case-report data, and so on.

Unfortunately, lack of empirical data forces us, as clinicians, to use trial and error. Geriatric drug therapy remains an art. Although the body of empirical data is growing rapidly, it is still true that each patient is his or her own clinical trail. In this book the reader will find all-too-frequent notices that geriatric data are few or that information is based on general adult data. I had to make a basic decision about whether or not to use general adult data. I decided to include this data because clinical experience suggests that many actions and drug effects are similar in elders and general adults. The book should be more useful for day-to-day prescribing with the complete data picture included. However, it is crucial to bear in mind that although there are many similarities between geriatric and general adult patients, there are also many significant differences.

DOSING CHALLENGES

For most drugs the dose range is often very wide. This range is the result of the wide variation in metabolic efficiency in elders, the array of medical comorbidities encountered, the often unpredictable sensitivity of the brain to medication effect, frequency of concurrent medication use and drug interactions, uncertain compliance, and family and social complexities. It is also the consequence of inadequate data due to few geriatric dose-finding studies, a problem with most medications and especially the newer drugs. For older medications, we have the advantage of long years of clinical experience. We have less experience with some newer drugs, so the absence of clinical trials that focus on optimal dosing in elders is more problematic. I have tried to combine what is known about the pharmacology of new agents, the general adult data, and clinical experience to date. When the data are unclear, the best advice is to use reduced doses initially, increase doses slowly, use combination therapies very cautiously, and watch patients, especially frail elders, carefully.

With regard to dose selection, I should declare a bias up front. In my clinical experience one of the commonest problems in starting a patient on a new medication regimen is the induction of side effects because the initial dose is too aggressive. Patients then become alarmed or are truly intolerant of the drug and give up. Because many side effects are time-limited and dose-dependent, I have taken to starting at very low doses to test patients' tolerances. However, I also know that there is a significant danger of underdosing in geriatric practice, so I am not reluctant to push the dose of a drug to its maximum tolerated level within the clinical guidelines of the drug I am using. The key issue is timing. Slowly increased increments can improve success. These philosophies are reflected in the recommendations and guidelines for drug use. Note that doses contained in tables and elsewhere in this book should be used as guidelines, rather than recommendations, and individualized for each patient. This is especially true for the higher dose ranges, which may be associated with significant side effects. Genetic phenotyping may make dosing decisions more accurate as it becomes widely available.

Note: Before prescribing any agent, check side effects (especially "black box" warnings), drug–drug and drug–illness interactions, and appropriateness of dosing recommendations.

SIDE-EFFECT CHALLENGES

Safety and side-effect profiles of drugs are generally based on large pooled data sets. Although these reports are often reassuring with regard to safety, individual patients need to be monitored for infrequent but significant events. I have indicated the most salient of these in the side-effect sections, under serious events. In the introductory section for each class, tables summarize comparative side effects for some agents. Such comparisons, although useful as a quick reference, are limited in completeness and sometimes by the nature of available data. They should be used with these cautions in mind. Special side-effect concerns for individual drugs are outlined in the section dealing with the individual drug.

Most medication-induced problems can be caught and dealt with early if the patient is being closely monitored. Many problems arise because prescriptions are given and renewed without speaking to patients or families and caregivers about what to watch for. This failing occurs in both home and institutional settings. For example, the extrapyramidal side effects of many agents may be subtle and go unobserved unless specifically watched for, producing instability of gait and increased risk of falls.

Tracking patients' responses to drugs presents many problems, including the cost of appointments and the logistics of elderly patients getting to appointments. However, iatrogenically-induced morbidity is very common, especially in elders, and is responsible for patient suffering and even greater costs. So monitoring is not only good medical practice, it is cost-efficient, preventive medicine as well.

Wide variations in prescribing patterns are present between general practitioners and specialists, and practice varies from setting to setting. For example, some data suggest that general psychiatrists use higher drug doses than geriatric psychiatry specialists and that general physicians use lower doses for shorter trial periods. General working knowledge of the pharmacology of the drugs used and a diagnosis-based working plan are often lacking in the treatment of medically ill elders in hospital. Race and culture also influence prescribing patterns. For example, African American elders are three times less likely to receive antidepressants, especially SSRIs, than Caucasian elders, and atypical antipsychotics are more likely to be prescribed to white, middle-class patients. One implication of this data is that members of visible minorities communties are not receiving optimal pharmacological intervention for mental disorders.

THE IMPORTANCE OF BASIC PHARMACOLOGY

In order to avoid aversive drug interactions and anticipate side effects, the clinician is best prepared by having a good working knowledge of the metabolic properties of drugs. With the exception of those clear-cut situations where the concurrent use of agents is absolutely contraindicated, clinicians are frequently in the position of combining drugs, despite theoretical concerns about possible interactions. In these situations the keys to success are (1) knowledge of the potential for side effects, (2) vigilance and careful monitoring, and (3) education of patients and families on what to watch for and when to contact the physician.

Physiological data may seem dull and sometimes irrelevant to clinicians. However, I have included such information whenever it is available to increase the depth of information provided and to allow the clinician the opportunity of working from first principles to sort out a difficult clinical situation (e.g., can this combination of drugs be used and what might be the potential dangers, side effects, etc?)

The reader should keep in mind that management of geriatric patients requires a comprehensive and integrated approach to therapy. For every disorder and situation, psychotherapy, family interventions, marital work, social supportive intervention, collaboration with other clinicians, communication with community agencies, and so on, should be presumed to be part of the management. Detailing these issues is beyond the scope of this book and the reader is directed to other texts of geriatric psychiatry and neuropsychiatry for such discussions.

INDICATIONS AND CONTRAINDICATIONS

Indications for the use of a given class of drugs or specific agent include the approved indications (so-called labelled indications) and unapproved (off-label) use. Off-label indications include an array of applications for which the drug has been tried and found useful, although it may not have been put through the studies necessary for FDA or HPB approval. For example, some SSRIs are approved for panic and anxiety disorders, whereas others are not; however, there is likely little clinical difference in efficacy between the approved versus unapproved drugs.

Some general contraindications apply to all drugs and are not included in the lists of contraindications for each agent. These include

- History of sensitivity or allergic reaction to a given drug or class
- General cautions about sedative side effects; cautions about using machinery and driving are assumed
  - √ Drugs that may be of special concern with regard to motor function in vulnerable individuals, especially driving, include benzodiazepines, other hypnotics/anxiolytics, cyclic/sedating antidepressants, sedating typical (especially low-potency) and atypical antipsychotics (e.g., clozapine and olanzapine), opioids, and sedating antihistamines.

Contraindications relevant to a specific class of drugs are noted in the introduction section for each class of agents—for example, the contraindication of using HCAs concurrently with MAOIs; dangers associated with the interaction of drugs and physical conditions; cardiac disease and HCAs; or dementia and anticholinergics.

For each agent, I indicate the various interacting factors (i.e., drug–drug and drug–illness interactions) that will help the clinician decide whether to use a given drug for a specific patient. However, in most instances the cautionary concerns are relative, not absolute, and clinical judgment, rather than reliance on rules, is necessary.

OVERVIEW OF GENERAL PHARMACOKINETICS AND PHARMACODYNAMICS

The term *pharmacokinetics* refers to the effect of the body on drug concentrations in various tissue components over time (i.e., the result of liver metabolism, absorption, excretion, and so on).

The term *pharmacodynamics* refers to the effect of the drug (and its interactions) on the body at specific drug concentrations (in plasma and/or tissue).

- Adverse reactions are 7 times more frequent in those aged 70–79 than in those 20–29.

- One-sixth of all hospital admissions of those over 70 have been attributed to adverse drug effects (compared to 1 in 35 in the rest of the population).
- Despite potential factors altering drug tolerance, many patients tolerate medications remarkably well.

Basic pharmacokinetic data are not always easy to use. Often one element of the metabolic pathway is compensated for, or otherwise influenced by, other elements. Moreover, the interaction of parent compounds with their metabolites is often crucial in determining the net effectiveness of a medication and the side-effect profile. Hence, the array of interacting variables may bewilder the clinician. A practical strategy is to administer drugs with caution and based on the best available evidence for efficacy, major drug interactions, and side-effect profile in elders, watching closely for emergent adverse effects. If these arise, it is then useful to examine metabolic pathways, drug–drug interactions, effects of metabolites versus parent drug, interaction of medical problems (e.g., reduced liver perfusion), end organ vulnerabilities, such as dementia, and so on.

Pharmacokinetic data are included for every drug in its appropriate section. For the reader's convenience, these data are usually tabulated in comparative form in the general introduction to the class of drugs.

Pharmacokinetic effects have important clinical relevance, although the precise implication of the research cannot always be determined from the raw data alone. For example, metabolic pathways in the liver may explain only part of the story of how a drug is cleared from the system.

Age-Related Factors

Age-related changes in the organs and systems that metabolize drugs begin to accelerate at about age 40 and lead to (1) gradually increasing variability of drug disposition and response, (2) gradual diminution in the rate of drug elimination, and (3) compromised homeostatic reserve. Numbers of some receptor sites diminish with age—for example, dopamine and acetylcholine—thereby increasing sensitivity to drug action. Reduction in homeostatic mechanisms that increase side effects include postural control, orthostatic circulatory response, thermoregulation, visceral muscle function, laryngeal reflexes, hypoxic responses, and cognitive function.

Metabolism and elimination of drugs does not decline uniformly with age. There is wide variability and less predictability in elders; some eliminate drugs as efficiently as younger patients, whereas others

Table I.2. Definitions of Basic Pharmacological Terms

Pharmacokinetic Parameter	Clinical Relevance
Clearance	Refers to overall elimination rate of a drug from the body; volume of blood from which the drug is removed per unit of time. This parameter is dependent on intrinsic physiological functions such as hepatic metabolism (biotransformation) and renal efficiency. Reduced clearance leads to prolonged half-life and accumulation of the drug under situations of chronic dosing.
Volume of distribution (*Vd*)	Extent to which a drug is distributed throughout the body; a reflection of body size, lipid solubility, and extent of lean versus nonlean body mass, as well as the drug's chemical properties (i.e., solubility and protein binding).
Time to peak plasma levels (Tmax)	Time to reach maximum plasma concentrations of the drug. The shorter the Tmax, the more rapid the onset of acute effects. Fast Tmax and associated high peak plasma concentrations may be associated with adverse effects (e.g., cardiac arrhythmias with HCAs, seizures with buproplon). Dangers can be reduced by using divided doses in vulnerable individuals (e.g., cardiac patients, frail elders).
Active metabolite	Product of metabolism of a drug that has active pharmacological properties, sometimes therapeutic and sometimes toxic. Activity of a metabolite may differ substantially from the parent compound regarding duration of half-life, degree of efficacy, cause of side effects, and drug–drug interactions (e.g., HB metabolite of bupropion or ODV metabolite of venlafaxine).
Linear versus nonlinear pharmacokinetics	*Linear:* Dose change produces proportional increase or decrease in plasma concentration of the drug. *Nonlinear:* Dose change produces disproportionate change in plasma concentration, usually due to saturation of mechanisms mediating biotransformation/elimination of the drug. *Relevance:* Dose titration may be difficult and less predictable with non-linear drugs.
Half-life ($T_{1/2}$)	The number of hours it takes for 50% of a drug to be eliminated from the body. It is a derived value (dependant variable) based on the relationship between the volume of distribution (direct relationship) and the clearance rate (inverse relationship). Mathematical equation is $0.639 \times \text{Vd/clearance}$ $T_{1/2}$ determines the frequency with which a drug must be given. Short half-life of a few hours often means that a drug must be given more than once a day to maintain therapeutic plasma levels—a disadvantage for many elders who often have trouble organizing more complex dosage regimens. Long half-life may mean the drug/metabolites will accumulate with the potential for delayed, increased adverse effects (e.g., diazepam or fluoxetine); longer half-life reduces the impact of noncompliance.
Mean steady state or plasma concentration (C_{ss})	Concentrations achieved after repeat administration when amount of drug excreted balances amount of entering plasma. At a given dosage rate, Css increases if clearance decreases; usually achieved after *5–6 half-lives* of repeated administration. Because of slow metabolism of some drugs in elders, the time to reach steady-state drug concentrations is often markedly prolonged in elderly. Example: For an antidepressant with half-life of 48 hours, age-related prolongation of half-life by 100% means an increase from 9 to 18 days to reach a steady state. Example: Fluoxetine may not reach steady state for weeks.
CYP 450 metabolic pathways	Made up of several liver enzymes responsible for metabolizing drugs. A given drug (protagonist) may induce or inhibit these enzymes and thereby induce or inhibit the metabolism of another coadministered drug(s) (target), by altering a given enzyme's capacity to metabolize the target. Result: higher/lower plasma levels of the target/metabolites, with increased/decreased efficacy and side effects.

Table I.3. Age-Related Changes Affecting Pharmacokinetics

Organ System	Change	Pharmacokinetic Considerations
Gastrointestinal tract	Decreased • Intestinal and splanchnic blood flow • Gastric acid output (increased pH) • Gastric motility • Absorption surface	• Decreased rate of absorption and possibly bioavailability of lipid soluble chemicals, such as vitamins and minerals. √ Less effect on lipid soluble drugs √ Water soluble substances unaffected by age • Increased gastric pH improves absorption of basic drugs (e.g., antidepressants) and reduces absorption of acid drugs.
Circulatory system	• Decreased synthesis and concentration of plasma albumin. • Increased alpha1acid glycoprotein.	• Increased or decreased free concentration of drugs in plasma.
Kidney	• Function declines progressively and inversely with age at a rate of 1–1.9% per year. • Decreased glomerular filtration rate (about 35% between 20 and 90 years of age) and blood flow. • Loss of glomeruli.	• Decreased renal clearance and increased plasma concentration; especially important when metabolites cleared by the kidney are psychoactive (e.g., benzodiazepines, lithium). • Decreased creatinine clearance. √ Serum creatinine may not be a reliable measure of creatinine clearance (e.g., declines with decreased body mass). √ Calculated creatinine clearance by formula is a better measure. Creatinine clearance $= \frac{(140 - \text{age in years}) \times \text{body weight}}{72 \times \text{plasma creatinine}}$
Liver	Two pathways of metabolism: • *Phase I:* Oxidative (involves P-450 enzymes, cytochrome b5, nicotinamide-dyphosphonucleotide hydrogenase (NADPH)-cytochrome-C-reductase)-age-related decrease in activity/amount of oxidative drug metabolism (especially over age 70). √ CYP3A4 and possibly 1A2 decline with age. √ 2D6 is unchanged. • *Phase II:* Conjugation and acetylation-unaffected by age. • Decreased hepatic blood flow.	• Decreased hepatic clearance of drugs leads to increased plasma concentration. √ Considerable interindividual variation
Muscle and water	• Decreased lean body mass (7% decrease). • Increased adipose tissue (12% increase in women and 18% in men), especially in frail and very old (over 85). • Body water decreases by 8%.	• Increased volume of distribution of lipid soluble drugs, leading to slower elimination (e.g., some antidepressants), or • Increased concentration of drugs distributed in body fluids (e.g., lithium).

Adapted from DeVane and Pollock.

have significantly reduced capacities. Many elderly patients require full adult doses to achieve therapeutic effect, despite the fact that side effects may be more evident.

Pharmacokinetics may be altered by

- Lifestyle habits (e.g., diet, alcohol consumption, smoking)
- Concurrent drugs
- Genetic polymorphisms of hepatic enzymes
- Diseases

Although age alone is not an indication for lower drug doses, elders frequently require lower doses. Reductions in starting dose are especially important for those patients over the age of 70.

Drugs differ in their pharmacokinetic linearity. Nonlinear pharmacokinetics may magnify effects of CYP enzyme inhibition and increase chance of deleterious drug–drug interactions.

Nonlinearity may be created in patients who are (1) genetically deficient in specific hepatic isoenzymes, (2) taking drugs that inhibit relevant isoenzymes, or (3) have concurrent medical (generally, hepatic or renal) disorders that substantially impair drug clearance.

Absorption is not altered by age alone, in the absence of gastrointestinal disease, but may be altered/prolonged by concurrent drugs commonly taken by elders, such as antacids, fiber supplements, or anticholinergics. IM or IV routes of administration bypass gastric absorption, resulting in faster absorption. Age, per se, has the least effect on absorption and metabolism.

Distribution of a drug is influenced by

- Tissue blood flow
- Plasma protein binding
- Lean/nonlean body mass (fat mass increases with age)
- Total body water (reduced with age)
- Extracellular volume
- Gender (i.e., women/men: increase in proportion of body fat from 33/18% [age 20] to 48/36% [over 70])

Clinical effects of distribution changes include accumulation of lipid soluble drugs in adipose tissues, with prolongation of action and plasma half-life, and increased side effects.

Drug plasma levels may not be reliable indicators of pharmacological activity in the body. Recent evidence suggests some drugs remain centrally active long after plasma levels decline (e.g., lithium).

Clearance is reduced with age, as a general rule. Renal clearance declines predictably with age, and hepatic clearance is not as predictable as renal. Hepatic clearance depends on 3 factors:

- Hepatic blood flow (difficult to measure)
- Phase I metabolism (P-450 and other enzymes)
    - √ Includes demethylation, ring hydroxylation, and sulphoxidation
    - √ May produce active or toxic metabolites
    - √ Strongly influenced by age, sex, and genetic factors
    - √ Demethylation becomes less efficient with age; may affect metabolism of some drugs (e.g., clozapine)
    - √ May be prolonged by age-specific declines in CYP3A enzyme activity
- Phase II metabolism (glucuronidation and conjugation)
    - √ Metabolites generally inactive and renally excreted
    - √ Glucuronidation not yet known to be affected by age

Clearance is also affected by

- Medical illness (e.g., hypothyroidism delays hepatic metabolism of some drugs)
- Concurrent medications
- Smoking
- Alcohol
- Nutritional status

Clearance data for specific drugs are often extrapolated to the elderly from data derived from studies of younger individuals. Therefore, the data cannot be taken as fully reliable. Despite some indications that, for some drugs, clearance may not decline in healthy elders (e.g., fluoxetine data), clinical caution is necessary because many older patients appear to have increased susceptibility to reduced clearance and subsequent drug accumulation.

Protein Binding

- Albumin levels decrease in elders, whereas alpha-1 acid glycoprotein (AAG) increases.
- AAG binds chlorpromazine, desipramine, and haloperidol, among other drugs.

The clinical relevance of the relationship between protein bound fraction and free (presumably clinically active) portions is not clear. Overall protein binding changes appear to have little pharmacodynamic effect. Reduced protein binding can reduce measured plasma ranges of some drugs in a given patient. Protein binding is reduced in old age for several drugs.

Overview of the Physiology of Neurotransmission by Transmitter Substances

To aid the reader in understanding use of psychotropic drugs, it is important to understand basic definitions and principles of pharmacodynamics and pharmacokinetics. What follows is a basic overview to introduce the concepts and relate them to elders, as necessary.

Presynaptic Activity

- Amino acids are synthesized into transmitter substances and stored in vesicles in the presynaptic nerve endings.
- Neuronal signal triggers release transmitter substance.
  - √ Transmitter released into synaptic cleft; release governed by
    - ▫ Extracellular calcium entering presynaptic nerve ending
    - ▫ Amount of transmitter in synapse
    - ▫ Activity of transmitter on presynaptic terminal (i.e., the autoreceptor).
    - ▫ Feedback system that regulates further release (transmitter inhibits its own release by acting on the presynaptic area autoreceptor like a thermostat).

Postsynaptic Activity

- Postsynaptic neurons contain protein molecules embedded in bulbous nerve terminals.
  - √ Each is a receptor that binds with one transmitter substance.
    - ▫ Binding is also influenced by other neurotransmitters (i.e., peptides or neuromodulators, hormones, and prostaglandins).
    - ▫ *Note:* Receptors can be located in the presynaptic as well as postsynaptic membranes.
  - √ A single neurotransmitter can have several receptor sites, each with a specific function.
    - ▫ Receptors can change in function, depending on the availability of neurotransmitters.
    - ▫ If neurotransmitter is in short supply, receptor sites increase in number (up-regulation) or decrease in number (down-regulation).
  - √ Psychotropics can secondarily cause up- or down-regulation, depending on their effect on the concentration of neurotransmitters.
  - √ Postsynaptic transmission can be simple or complex.
    - ▫ Simple direct transmission with GABA and ACH and some serotonin and dopamine paths.
    - ▫ Complex transmission along all norepinephrine and some serotonin and dopamine paths

Table I.4. Transmitter Substances and their Area of Impact

Transmitter Substance	Area of Impact
Dopamine	• Muscle movement • Psychosis • Mood
Norepinephrine	• Mood • Arousal • Memory
Serotonin	• Mood • Anxiety
Acetylcholine (ACH)	• Muscular coordination • REM sleep • Mood • Memory
Gamma-aminobutyric acid (GABA)	• Widely distributed √ Inhibitory neurotransmitter √ May be link between sets of neurons √ Anxiety association
Glutaminergic acid	• Excitatory amino acids

- √ Steps in neurotransmission
  - ▫ Presynaptic release of neurotransmitter (first messenger) binds at postsynaptic receptor site.
  - ▫ In complex transmission, receptor proteins stimulate or inhibit further synaptic events.
  - ▫ If stimulated, receptor protein activates an enzyme that produces second messenger molecules (e.g., adenylate cyclase leads to conversion of ATP to cAMP, which is a second messenger; other second messengers include inisotol triphosphate (IP3) and diacylglycerol (DAG, converted by phospholipase C).
  - ▫ The second messenger amplifies the signal by activating another enzyme, protein kinase, which then carries out the specific function of the neuron and continues transmission.
- √ After synaptic binding, neurotransmitter is taken back into the presynaptic terminal (reuptake) where a small proportion is metabolized; remaining portions not taken into the presynaptic nerve ending are metabolized and removed from further synaptic activity.
- √ ACH and GABA are metabolized by enzymes present in synapse or postsynaptic terminal.

P450 (CYP) Isoenzymes

Cytochrome P450 isoenzyme system (CYP450) is made up of an array of enzymes, or isoenzymes, that metabolize psychotropic and other drugs. These enzymes are located in the endoplasmic reticulum and expressed mainly in the liver. The enzymes that are relevant to drug metabolism belong to CYP families 1–4. Enzymes transform

Table I.5. Ethnoracial Differences in Drug Metabolism

Enzyme	% Poor Metabolizers by Ethnoracial Group
CYP2D6	Caucasian, 3–10% Asian/African American, 0–2%
CYP2C19	Caucasian/African American, 3–5% Asian, 18–23%
CYP1A2	Caucasian, African American, Asian, 12–13%

substances into more polar products that are eliminated in the urine.

The normal population is divided into phenotypes: extensive metabolizers (EM) and poor metabolizers (PM, inherited as autosomal recessive trait) based on genetic subtyping of CYP2D6 and CYP2C19; prediction of phenotype is 90–95% accurate.

- PM individuals show
  - √ Higher peak plasma concentrations
  - √ Longer plasma half-lives
  - √ Lower total and metabolic excretion rates

A subtype of ultrarapid metabolizers has also been identified (gene amplification of 2D6). PM individuals need to be treated with even lower doses of drugs and EM or ultrarapid metabolizers need higher doses.

Genetic polymorphisms produce enzymes that are functionally normal, abnormal, or inactive. These polymorphisms lead to ethnoracial differences in metabolism of drugs. However, although interracial differences have been demonstrated, there are virtually no studies involving elders. Genetic variability is only one important factor that produces the high interindividual differences in drug metabolism in elders.

Drugs are not only metabolized by these enzymes, they interact with them in other ways that may potentiate or inhibit their activity in relation to the metabolism of other drugs. A drug degraded by one isoenzyme can act as a competetive inhibitor to the degradation of another drug metabolized by the same isoenzyme.

CYP-450 Inhibition

Inhibiting the CYP-450 enzyme causes accumulation of the inhibiting drug or coadministered drugs ordinarily metabolized by that enzyme. Effects can be adverse or may enhance action of the coadministered drug.

- Example: Coadministration of SSRI with low doses of HCA may be therapeutic, but with higher doses of HCA can be toxic.

Note that data on drug metabolism by specific enzymes may be imprecise, since a given drug can be a substrate for many enzymes, or affect enzymes differentially, depending on dose.

- Example: Clomipramine is a substrate for seven CYPs. Sertraline at doses of 50 mg has weak interaction with TCAs, but at higher therapeutic doses may have greater effect on metabolism.

In addition, drug interactions show marked intersubject variability. For example, increases in desipramine vary between 30% and 1,000% when used concurrently with paroxetine, sertraline, or fluoxetine. Some isoenzymes (e.g., CYP1A2 and 3A4) are inducable (i.e., activity increased) by exogenous agents such as smoking and barbiturates. The clinician should take note of these interactions and proceed with appropriate caution, recognizing that it is difficult to develop precise guidelines in this regard. Hence, once again, start low, go slow, and monitor prudently if using combinations in the elderly.

Action of Specific Isoenzymes

CYP2D6

This enzyme comprises 1.5% of total P450 content but is responsible for 25% of all drug metabolism, including hydroxylation of many antidepressants (paroxetine, desipramine, imipramine, amitriptyline, clomipramine, nortriptyline, and venlafaxine) and antipsychotics (perphenazine, fluphenazine, thioridazine, clozapine, and risperidone). Data for healthy elders does not show marked decline in activity of 2D6 secondary to aging. However, 2D6 is especially susceptible to inhibition by quinidine and some SSRIs, especially paroxetine.

CYP2C19

This enzyme does show age-related decline in activity. Example: Citalopram and clomipramine are metabolized more slowly in the elderly.

CYP3A4

This enzyme comprises 30% of liver P450 enzymes. In combination with 2D6, it accounts for 80% of the metabolism of currently used drugs.

- Age-related decline in activity
- Action may be greater in young women than in men and postmenopausal women.
- Clinical effect may be relevant in some but not all.
  - √ Example: Nefazodone levels shown to be 50% higher in older women than in older men and younger subjects.
- Found in intestinal mucosa as well as liver.

CYP1A

- Possibly declines with age.
- Demethylates imipramine and metabolizes caffeine, theophylline, and probably propranalol, clomipramine, and amitriptyline.
- Induced by smoking.
- Inhibited by paroxetine (weakly).

Clinical Relevance of Pharmacodynamics and Pharmacokinetics

The clinical relevance is illustrated when considering combination/augmentation therapies, which may be associated with drug–drug or drug–illness interactions (e.g., Parkinson's disease and typical antipsychotics). Factors related to combination/augmentation therapies include the following:

- A lowering of the serum concentration of one of the drugs thereby worsening overall outcome.
- Increased serum concentration of one compound induced by the other could improve its action or cross the threshold for side effects (e.g., fluoxetine increases concentration of desipramine).
- Drugs can enhance or impede the pharmacodynamic action of one/another (e.g., an SSRI–risperidone or clozapine combination introduces the antagonism of 5HT2 by the antipsychotic, thereby possibly impeding the SSRI action; this example remains theoretical rather than clinically relevant at this time).
- Additive effects of pharmacological activity (e.g., anticholinergic or sedative effects).

Clinically, changes in bioavailability with aging are often more theoretical than actual. Changes lead to increased volume of distribution for lipid soluble drugs, which includes most psychotropics. Because half-life is directly proportional to volume of distribution, it increases. Clinicians should therefore anticipate the need for reduced dosage levels in the elderly. In addition, some drugs remain in the body for prolonged periods after discontinuation.

- Especially true for phenothiazines.
- Lorazepam (a short-acting benzodiazepine) can be detected in some elders as long as 6 weeks after discontinuation.

Furthermore, renal efficiency declines with age; this decline has particular relevance for drugs that are partially or completely cleared by the kidney (e.g., lithium, gabapentin).

1. Antidepressants

OVERVIEW

This chapter begins with a brief description of the key diagnostic indications for antidepressants when used for elders, including affective disorders, anxiety disorders, pain and behavioral disturbances (e.g., with dementia). It continues with general descriptions of pharmacological treatment, including factors that determine choice of drugs and general comparisons of the drug choices. Specific guidelines are offered for use of antidepressants during acute, continuation, and maintenance phases, and prognostic factors for relapse and recurrence are described. Strategies for determining and managing refractory responses to therapy are described, including substitution, combination, and augmentation. The chapter includes a decision-pathway model for treatment of elders, a comprehensive description of side effects and their management, and a detailed discussion of drug interactions and metabolic pathways.

Table 1.1. Classification of Antidepressants and Usual Doses

Drug Names	Usual Starting Dosage mg/day (minimum in frail elders)	Usual Maintenance Dosage mg/day (maximum dose)
SELECTIVE SEROTONIN REUPTAKE INHIBITORS (SSRIs)		
citalopram (Celexa) (liquid form available)	10–20 (3)	20–30 (40)
escitalopram (Lexapro)	10 mg	10 mg (20)
fluoxetine (Prozac) (liquid form available)	10 mg (5)	20 (50)
fluvoxamine (Luvox) (not indicated for depression in U.S.—OCD only)	25–50	50–150 (300)
paroxetine (Paxil) (liquid form available)	10–20 (5)	20–30 (40)
paroxetine CR	12.5	25–37.5 (50)
sertraline (Zoloft) (liquid form available)	25–50 (12.5)	50–100 (200)

(*cont.*)

Continued

Drug Names	Usual Starting Dosage mg/day (minimum in frail elders)	Usual Maintenance Dosage mg/day (maximum dose)
HETEROCYCLIC ANTIDEPRESSANTS		
Secondary Amines		
amoxapine (Asendin) (NR)	25	75
desipramine (Norpramin)	10–40	50–100 (100–150)
maprotiline (Ludiomil) (NR)	25	50–75
nortriptyline (Aventyl, Pamelor)	10–30	40–100 (150)
protriptyline (Vivactil) (NR)	5	10–20
Tertiary Amines		
amitriptyline (Elavil) (NR; IM form available)	10	50–200
clomipramine (Anafranil)	10–25	75–150
doxepin (Sinequan) (NR; topical form available for pruritis)	10	50–200
imipramine (Tofranil) (NR; IM form available)	10	50–200
trimipramine (Surmontil) (NR)	25	25–75
MONOAMINE OXIDASE INHIBITORS (MAOIs)		
Irreversible		
phenelzine (Nardil)	15	30–45 (75)
tranylcypromine (Parnate)	10	20–30
Reversible Inhibitor MAO-A (RIMA)		
moclobemide (not available in the U.S.)	150	300–450 (600)
ATYPICAL NORADRENALINE AND DOPAMINE REUPTAKE INHIBITOR		
bupropion (Wellbutrin)	37.5–75	75–300 (300)
bupropion SR	100	150–300 (400)
NORADRENERGIC AND SPECIFIC SEROTONERGIC ANTIDEPRESSANT (NaSSA)		
mirtazapine (Remeron, Remeron sol. tab.)	7.5–15	15–45 (45)
SEROTONIN AND NORADRENALINE REUPTAKE INHIBITOR (SNRI)		
venlafaxine (Effexor) venlafaxine XR	25–75 (smallest dose of XR form is 37.5)	37.5–200 (300)
SEROTONIN REUPTAKE AND 5HT2 RECEPTOR INHIBITION		
nefazodone (Serzone) (discontinued in Canada)	50–100	50–400 (500)
trazodone (Desyrel) (not generally recommended as antidepressant, but some restricted utility)	25–50	50–600 (600 rarely)

NR = Not recommended for routine use

DEPRESSIVE DISORDERS IN ELDERS

- Treatment of depression in the elderly is complex and involves the full array of biopsychosocial interventions.
- Effective therapy depends, in large part, on accurate diagnosis, since treatment strategies vary based on the type of depression.

Standard Classification of Depression

- Major depressive disorder
  - √ Single episode and recurrent
- Dysthymic disorder
- Adjustment disorder with depressed mood
- Psychotic depression
- Bipolar I disorder
  - √ One or more manic or mixed episodes, usually accompanied by major depressive episodes
- Bipolar II disorder
  - √ One or more major depressive episodes accompanied by at least one hypomanic episode
- Cyclothymic disorder
  - √ Presents at different phases as depressed or hypomanic mood
- Mood disorder (may be depressive or manic) due to
  - √ A general medical condition
  - √ Substance use
- Depressive disorder not otherwise specified
  - √ includes minor depressive disorder

Disorders may be of varying severity and include melancholia or associated psychotic symptoms. The presentation of depressions may be colored by comorbid conditions. These comorbid conditions can include personality disorder or PTSD.

Table 1.2. Symptoms of Major Depression

1. Depressed mood most of the day nearly every day.
2. Markedly diminished interest or pleasure in all, or almost all, activities, most of the day, nearly every day.
3. Significant weight loss or gain, or decrease or increase in appetite nearly every day.
4. Insomnia or hypersomnia nearly every day.
5. Psychomotor agitation or retardation nearly every day.
6. Fatigue or loss of energy nearly every day.
7. Feelings of worthlessness or excessive or inappropriate guilt nearly every day.
8. Diminished ability to think or concentrate, or indecisiveness, nearly every day.
   - √ Indecisiveness may resemble similar behavior associated with OCD and be considerably disabling.
9. Recurrent thoughts of death, or suicidal ideation or attempt.

Note: Major depression is defined as the presence of either or both symptoms 1 and 2, plus enough of symptoms 3–9 to make a total of 5 or more symptoms with a minimum duration of 2 weeks.
Minor depressive disorder is identical to major but involves fewer symptoms (2 required) and less impairment.

Characteristics of Depression in Late Life

Late-life depression is a multidimensional disorder affecting

- Mood
- Well-being
- Physical functioning

- Social functioning
- Cognitive functioning

It is a common disorder of older adults, often persistent and recurrent. Rates vary substantially in different settings and with different comorbid conditions.

- Studies vary in methodology and rates show wide ranges (Table 1.3).

It produces severe impairment in functioning, ≥ lung disease, arthritis, hypertension, or diabetes, and is associated with higher rates of

- Suicide
  - √ About 2 times the rate in the general population.
  - √ Highest risk in white males over age 80.
  - √ Commonest associated diagnosis is depressive disorder, usually first episode of major depression.
  - √ Three-fourths of those who commit suicide see their primary care physician in the preceding month.
- Mortality and morbidity
  - √ Recent data suggest that only severe depression accounts for increased mortality, usually due to cardiovascular causes.
  - √ Other data show excess mortality of 1.6–2.5 times reference population.
    - ▫ Males 3 times rate of excess mortality.
    - ▫ Females 2 times rate of excess mortality.
  - √ Increases likelihood of death in nursing home residents by 59%.
  - √ Independent risk factor for increased ischemic heart disease and post MI cardiac mortality.
- Cognitive impairment
  - √ May be significant and sometimes hard to distinguish from dementia.
    - ▫ Dementia syndrome of depression (previously called pseudodementia) usually the result of concurrent depression and dementia.
    - ▫ Pure pseudodementia uncommon.
    - ▫ Significant cognitive impairment associated with depression usually improves with treatment of depression but often does not remit completely.
    - ▫ Emerging data show that persistent depressive symptoms are markers for later cognitive decline at 4-year follow-up.
    - ▫ Episodic depression is not associated with cognitive decline.
- Increased utilization of outpatient health services, laboratory tests, imaging

Table 1.3. Rates of Depression in Various Settings and Disorders

Setting/Disorder	Rate of Depression (percentages reported in various studies)	Comments
General community	• Depressive symptoms 10–15%; major depression 1.4–5%	• Conservative rates for depressive symptoms but much higher rates in some studies (up to 30%).
Seniors centers	• > 33%	• Group of volunteers.
Primary care settings	• 17–37%	• Major depression 10% (but only 1% receive specialized care).
Nursing homes	• 20–40%	• Rate is for noncognitively impaired residents; mostly minor depression, but 10–20% meet criteria for current major depressive episode.
Hospitalized elders	• 5–13%	• Major depression; a further 25% had less severe but clinically significant depressive symptomatology.
Cerebrovascular disease patients	• 25%	
Poststroke patients	• 25–50%	• Two types of depression: major depression may be associated with left anterior ischemic lesions; minor depression may be associated with posterior lesions of the right hemisphere. When depression is severe, cognitive impairment may be significant. Treatment of depression often improves cognition, which often seems to be related to the mood disorder rather than the stroke per se.
Parkinson's disease patients	• 43%	• Range 25–70%
Coronary artery disease patients	• 15–25%	
Postmyocardial infarction patients	• 20–30% major depression; 25% minor depression	• Mortality increased 4–6-fold.
Dementia patients	• Major depression 17–31%; depressive symptoms 50%	
Alzheimer's disease patients	• Major depression 15%; 30–40% less severe depressive symptoms	• Often difficult to diagnose with certainty; antidepressant treatment (SSRIs, venlafaxine, bupropion, nefazodone, mirtazapine) effective in reducing symptoms of depression and increasing MMSE scores when diagnosis of depression is accurate, but not in absence of depression or if an inaccurate diagnosis is made. Differentiation may be difficult, resolved with a trial of therapy. Weight loss is often associated and is a predictor of increased disability and mortality.
Cancer patients	• 20–25%	
Diabetes patients	• 15–20%	• Associated with impaired glycemic control.
Arthritis patients		• Increased risk of depression is 40–50%.
Hypertension patients		• Three-fold increase in risk of depression; as depression severity increases, rates of stroke, MI and mortality increase.

Assessment of Depression

- Psychiatric history and examination
- Use of standardized scales (e.g., MMSE, HAM-D, Cornell Scale for Depression, GDS, Montgomery–Asberg Depression Rating Scale (MADRS)

Table 1.4. Assessment Checklist for Depression

Assessment Component	Comment
Full psychiatric history	Use corroborative sources as available and appropriate, determine reason for assessment at this time; examine cognitive function, somatic preoccupations and concerns, psychological components, premorbid personality, mood states, reality testing, and psychosis.
Anxiety assessment	Common comorbid feature of depression in elders.
Suicidality or risk of violence	Skillful inquiry sometimes necessary to elicit true intent, especially when culturally-determined shame leads patients to hide suicidality.
Examination of cognitive functions	Institute full dementia screen if findings of disorientation, memory deficits, apathy, impaired concentration, evidence of work impairment or reduced high-level functioning in complex daily tasks (e.g., driving, banking), disorganized personal care or environment; especially pertinent if deficits predated symptoms of depression.
Assessment of ADL/IADL	Activities of daily living and instrumental ADL.
Past psychiatric history	Prior episodes of depression may have emerged many years ago; bipolar history.
Social history	Includes assessment of adaptation to new roles, losses, conflicts, social supports abuse.
Medical history	Depending on presentation, assess for medical problems (e.g., cerebrovascular disease, metabolic problems); give special attention to possible causes of reversible dementia.
Physical and neurological examination	Specialty referral if medical or neurological conditions are suspected.
Laboratory screening	CBC Urinalysis Medication plasma levels Chemistry screen • $Ca/Mg/PO_4/Na/K$ • Fasting Blood Sugar • B_{12}, folate • Iron Serology-syphilis, HIV Renal function Liver function Thyroid function
Substance abuse screening for current substances and history of use	Includes alcohol, benzodiazepines, barbiturates, and opiates

(cont.)

Continued

Assessment Component	Comment
Concurrent medications	Evaluate for depressogenic properties or likelihood of interaction with antidepressant or other concurrent treatment; recently discontinued agents; OTC agents
Neuroimaging	If depression is associated with focal neurological signs or other atypicality that may be neurologically based (e.g., apathy), consider CT (with or without contrast), MRI, SPECT

Diagnosis of Depression in Elders

Accurate diagnosis in elders is sometimes complicated by differences in presentation and other factors.

- Diagnosis frequently missed (two-thirds to three-quarters of the time) in all settings—ambulatory, institutional, and especially medically ill hospitalized patients.
- When a diagnosis is made, drug treatment is generally (1) not instituted, (2) inadequate, or (3) inappropriate.
- Missed diagnosis leads to
  - √ Increased social dysfunction
  - √ Risk of suicide
  - √ Increased use of medical services
  - √ Polypharmacy
  - √ Risk of institutionalization

Table 1.5. Age-Specific Features of Depression

Feature	Comment
Medical comorbidity	Frequently associated
Vegetative symptoms	Increased, especially anorexia and weight loss; may be life threatening
Melancholia and rumination	Increased rate
Ideational symptoms	Fewer; suicidal ideation and guilt may be less common
Cognitive disturbances	More common; limited accuracy of symptom(s) and history reporting; confused clinical picture
Social withdrawal	Increased
Subjective dysphoria	Awareness of depression not voiced as much
Somatic concerns	Increased preoccupation; chronic pain may exacerbate depression
Fatigue; lack of drive and interest	Greater than in general adult patients
Underreporting of psychiatric symptoms	Elders (and caregivers) erroneously conclude it is a normal part of aging
Masking of depression	Due to medical/neurological comorbidities; diagnosis sometimes confirmed only after successful antidepressant trial

(*cont.*)

Continued

Feature	Comment
Family history	Similar rates for depressive disorders that began in adult years, but reduced familial patterns in late onset depression.
Secondary depression	Depressogenic medications taken more commonly by elders
Medication compliance	Increased nonadherence

Symptoms sometimes said to be more common in elders, although not necessarily supported by more recent studies, include

- Increased feelings of tension and irritability
- Dominance of somatic complaints
- Increased thoughts about death
- Loss of energy and interest
- Delusional (paranoid) thinking
- Neurovegetative features

Age and medical comorbidity-related physiological changes make somatic features of depression less reliable diagnostic criteria in elders. Greater reliance is placed on cognitive-affective symptoms of sad/downcast/depressed mood, suicidal ideation, sudden diminished interest in activities, a sense of hopelessness or worthlessness, avoidance of social interaction, psychomotor agitation/retardation, and difficulty with decision-making or initiating actions.

Severe Depression

Characteristics of severe depression include the following:

- Symptom picture
  - √ Symptoms are in excess of those required to make a diagnosis of depression.
    - ▫ Melancholia, psychotic depression, or depression associated with other risk factors for nonresponse such as physical illness, anxiety.
  - √ New-onset anxiety disorders are generally comorbid with depression in the elderly.
    - ▫ Anxious depression, in general, may respond less readily to treatment.
- Social and functional parameters impaired.
- Response to treatment
  - √ Poorer in the short term.
  - √ Results improve with increased duration of therapy and aggressive dosing (general adult data), and with concurrent psychotherapy.

- Medication response
  - √ Clinical experience and available data indicate that antidepressants are effective in, and tolerated by, this severely depressed population, although they are
    - More sensitive to side effects.
    - Require slower dose titration.
  - √ SSRIs may be less effective for severe depression than HCAs or SNRIs (general adult data).
    - Comparative studies in elders show mixed results.
    - Risk/benefits favor SSRIs over tertiary amine HCAs and MAOIs because of safer side effect/overdose/toxicity profiles.
  - √ Bipolar disorders may be less responsive to HCAs than unipolar forms of depression.
  - √ Overall, SSRIs are a good starting point for antidepressant pharmacotherapy for severely depressed elders, with some caveats:
    - Some potential advantage of venlafaxine or mirtazapine over SSRIs, with fewer side effects than the TCAs and MAOIs (emerging general adult data).
    - Bupropion may be more effective than SSRIs in melancholic depression, with more favorable side-effect profile (general adult data).
    - HCAs sometimes show modest superiority over SSRIs in reducing symptoms of depression in elders, but differences are not consistent.
    - Some recent studies show equal antidepressant effectiveness, with better tolerance for SSRI even when compared to secondary amine HCAs.
  - √ Head-to-head studies sometimes show greater efficacy of one drug over another in subpopulations.
    - Nortriptyline more effective in inducing remission than citalopram in severe depression.
    - SSRIs may be less effective in patients with dementia and depression, than in depression alone.

In the very old

- √ Data are especially lacking on use, efficacy, and side-effect profile of antidepressants, especially in severe depression with medical and cognitive comorbidity.
- √ Drug choice is made on a case-by-case basis, taking patient and drug characteristics into account.
- √ Medications have more limited effectiveness in community-dwelling elders because of poor compliance and resistance to treatment.
- √ Social service home care may improve outcome.

Late-Onset Depression

- May be a marker for onset of subsequent dementia.
  - √ Associated with mild cognitive deficits.
  - √ High incidence after stroke.
- Late onset depression correleted with higher rates of subcortical white matter intensities on MRI.
- Treatment responsive.
- Vascular lesions suggest possibility of a vascular depression subtype.

Depression with Dementia

- Prevalence of depression in dementia may decrease with increasing severity of the dementia.
  - √ This pattern is possibly associated with reduction in cholinergic function.
- Efficacy of antidepressants.
  - √ Significantly reduced in major depression associated with dementia (Alzheimer's disease or vascular dementia), especially in very old patients.
  - √ Those who respond show less total improvement than non-CNS-associated depressives.
- All classes of antidepressants may be effective for depression with dementia although data are lacking.
  - √ Based on overall data, SSRIs are much preferred.
  - √ Some studies suggest sertraline and citalopram may offer some advantage.
  - √ Positive responses have been demonstrated with fluoxetine and paroxetine, in modest doses.
- Side-effect profile often the limiting factor in treatment, especially with HCAs.
  - √ Recent data confirm that cardiac side effects are always a concern with HCAs (including secondary amines) and relegates them to third-line treatments.
  - √ Side effects that are especially problematic in this population include
    - ▫ Decreased cognitive efficiency
    - ▫ Postural hypotension
    - ▫ Daytime sedation
    - ▫ Falls
  - √ Many patients tolerate secondary amine HCAs remarkably well in most situations, if they are used cautiously, especially nortriptyline.

Dementia Syndrome of Depression (Pseudodementia)

- Depression associated with cognitive symptoms often heralds true dementia.
  - √ In the presence of significant cognitive impairment, a fully reversible dementia syndrome of depression (pseudodementia) is rare.
  - √ Episodic depression is less likely to herald dementia than persistent depressive symptoms.
- Often presents as a retarded and psychotic depressive syndrome.

Aberrant Grief Reactions

- 10–20% of those who experience spousal loss develop depression in first year after loss.
- Treatment
  - √ Psychosocial intervention alone.
  - √ Combination of drug and psychosocial intervention (especially in more severe depressions).
  - √ Nortriptyline improves depressive symptoms and ADL dysfunction associated with bereavement (mean dose about 50 mg/day).
  - √ Significant risk of relapse or recurrence after successful initial treatment.
- ADL functioning is impaired in most of those who develop depression after bereavement.

Secondary Depression

- Mood disorders are common as secondary or associated factors with medical conditions such as the following:
  - √ Stroke
  - √ Heart disease
  - √ Parkinson's disease
  - √ Thyroid and parathyroid abnormalities
  - √ Arthritis
  - √ Malignancies (lymphomas, pancreatic cancer)
  - √ Viral infections
- Possible causes include pharmacotherapeutic agents.
  - √ Antihypertensives
    - especially some Beta-blockers
  - √ Analgesics
  - √ Steroids
  - √ Antihistamines
  - √ Antiparkinsonian agents

Caregiver Depression

- Primary family caregivers of demented elders, especially spouses, are at significant risk of depression.
- Treatment requires full range of psychosocial and pharmacological interventions: Education; Environmental changes; Family therapy; Home care and support; Psychotherapy

Dysthymia and Minor Depression

- Common in elders.
  - √ Significant morbidity.
- Usually late onset.
- Risk of minor depression increased by medical illness or personality disorder.
- Often underdiagnosed.
  - √ Sometimes mistaken for demoralization and worry.
- Usually preceded by a triggering event.
  - √ Past history of depression infrequent.
  - √ Fewer physiological symptoms present.
- Associated with low testosterone levels in men (compared to normal levels in major depression).
- Best managed initially with education and careful observation for 2 weeks, followed with active intervention, as necessary.
  - ▫ Includes psychotherapy and antidepressants.
  - ▫ Psychosocial interventions are essential to recovery in some who do not respond to medication and may be the primary intervention.
  - ▫ Psychotherapy may be useful as an adjunct and sometimes as primary intervention.
- May respond to antidepressant therapies.
  - √ Generally underutilized in this population, especially by family and nonpsychiatric physicians in medical institutions, although recent data suggest that medication may be less effective in minor depressions than in other forms of late-life depression.
  - √ By consensus, drugs of choice are SSRIs (alternates: venlafaxine, bupropion).
    - ▫ Sertraline effective in elders.
    - ▫ MAOIs, while more challenging to employ in elders, have shown effectiveness in general adult studies.
    - ▫ Risk/benefit (i.e., side effects vs. improvement of mood disturbance) must be carefully considered in these elders.

Poststroke Depression

- Occurs in at least 30% of stroke survivors.
- Predicts poor response to rehabilitation, even with antidepressant therapy.
- Diagnosis frequently missed, and even fewer are treated.
- Antidepressants effective but some data suggest younger patients are more responsive than older.
  - √ SSRIs are agents of first choice.
  - √ New data suggest SSRIs (specifically sertraline) have antiplatelet-aggregation properties that protect against stroke and heart disease.

Psychotic Depression

- Occurs in 3.6% of depressed elders in the community and 20–45% of hospitalized depressed elders.
- May be associated with increased cognitive impairment.
  - √ Higher rates of vascular risk factors.
  - √ More frequent deep white matter lesions on MRI.
- Higher rates of relapse/recurrence and possibly lower rates of recovery and greater chronicity.
- Associated with violent suicide.

Treatment considerations include the following factors.

- All antidepressants effective, in combination with antipsychotic therapies, but overall response rate is modest at best (25–50% range).
  - √ Effective pharmacotherapy requires combination of antidepressant *and* antipsychotic medications, rather than either alone.
  - √ Note cautions re. combining drugs
    - ▫ Example: Increased HCA levels with some antipsychotic medications.
- Antidepressant choice.
  - √ Drug of choice not clearly demonstrated.
  - √ SSRIs, TCAs, and venlafaxine XR have shown effectiveness.
  - √ Dose and blood levels of HCAs are similar to nonpsychotic major depression.
  - √ Some data indicate that HCAs offer some efficacy advantage in severe depressions, but data conflict, for example:
    - ▫ Some newer data suggest SSRIs may offer advantage in managing the psychotic element and in prophylaxis during maintenance phase (data still emerging, and definitive geriatric evidence lacking at this time).

- Suggestive evidence that SSRIs may be more effective than HCAs in relapse prevention (but studies are flawed, and more geriatric data is necessary).
- Some case reports suggest HCA antidepressants may be associated with induction of delusions.

- Antipsychotic choice
  - √ There is now consensus that atypical antipsychotics are a more desirable treatment option than typicals.
    - Drugs of choice for this indication are risperidone, olanzapine, quetiapine, possibly ziprasidone.
    - Clozapine is often effective in patients refractory to first-line combination antipsychotic therapy, but use with caution.
    - aripiprazole is an emerging option but geriatric data are still limited.

Table 1.6. Dosing of Antipsychotics in Combination with Antidepressants for Psychotic Depression

Drug	Starting Dose (mg/day)	Target Dose Range (mg/day)	Maximum Dose (mg/day)
olanzapine	2.5–5	5–15	12–20
risperidone	0.25–0.5	1–2	4–6
quetiapine	12.5–25	50–250	325
clozapine	6.25–12.5	50–100	200–250
haloperidol	0.25–0.5	0.5–4	6
perphenazine	2–4	5–15	15–20

Note: Maximum dose ranges associated with high rates of side effects.

    - Emerging data on olanzapine suggest good efficacy when combined with citalopram or paroxetine (general adult data, open study).
  - √ Antipsychotic should be continued for 6–12 months.

- ECT
  - √ May be the best first-line therapy, especially in severe cases.
  - √ ECT alone far more effective than medication (30–70% medication vs. 80–90% ECT) (mixed age data).
  - √ Clinical data suggest that most antidepressants are safe in combination with ECT, but controlled data for the elderly are minimal. Fluoxetine, paroxetine, and trazodone may prolong seizures, but clinical significance is not clear.
  - √ Response to pharmacotherapy takes longer than to ECT and is not as effective or robust.
  - √ Longer acute treatment periods (> 8 weeks) necessary to evaluate responsiveness in a given patient.
  - √ Prognosis with treatment not clear.
    - ECT responders who are placed on maintenance antidepressant therapy have higher rates of relapse/recurrence than

those responding to antidepressants in the first place and then maintained on the medication.
- Maintenance ECT may be a more effective option for ECT responders, but data are few.
- Depression subtype (e.g., mood congruent vs. mood incongruent symptoms), does not discriminate outcome (general adult data).

Bipolar Disorder (BPD)

This section discusses antidepressant treatment of BPD. See Chapter 4, pp. 479–550, for discussion of mood stabilizers and BPD.

Treatment of bipolar depression includes the following considerations.

Table 1.7. Medication for Depression in Bipolar Subtypes

Subtypes of Bipolar Depression	MedicationTreatment: Mood Stabilizer Plus
Bipolar 1—severe, but otherwise uncomplicated	Antidepressant (with or without ECT)
Bipolar 1—with psychosis	Hospitalization usually necessary; antipsychotic plus antidepressant (+/− ECT)
Bipolar I—mild	Consider mood stabilizer alone
Bipolar II—major depression, psychotic	Antipsychotic plus antidepressant (+/− ECT)
Bipolar II—Major depression, nonpsychotic	Antidepressant
Bipolar II—mild depression	Antidepressant

- Recommendations vary with subtype.
  - √ A general rule with patients in a depressive episode of bipolar disorder who have frequent or rapid cycles:
    - Avoid antidepressants alone and use mood stabilizers alone, if possible, or in combination with antidepressants, if necessary.
    - However, most of the expression of bipolar disorder is depressive.
    - Newer data suggest that depressed bipolar patients who can be maintained on antidepressants, without inducing manic switch, have better long term stability.
  - √ Relapse prevention and maintenance therapy regimens have not been well established for elderly patients with bipolar disorder.
  - √ Important to avoid rapid switches from depression to hypomania/mania during antidepressant therapy of bipolar II patients. Antidepressants are sometimes necessary in the depressed phases, despite posing a high risk of switching to manic phase.
    - Risk factors (general adult data) for switching include
      1. History of mania
      2. Family history of mania

3. Premorbid cyclothymic tendency
4. Female gender
5. Early onset
6. Hypothyroidism
7. Frequent recurrences of depression
8. History of rapid cycling

▫ Reduced risk of manic switch in treatment of late-onset depression.

▫ Mood stabilizers reduce the risk of switching to manic states.

- Antidepressant drugs of choice (extrapolated from general adult data; few geriatric studies).
  - √ SSRIs and bupropion are best first-line antidepressants and have equal efficacy.
    - ▫ Both have a low rate of switch to manic phase.
  - √ Drugs that are more likely than SSRIs or bupropion to induce hypomanic switch include
    - ▫ Tricyclics, especially imipramine
    - ▫ Venlafaxine
    - ▫ MAOIs
  - √ Little clinical experience reported in treatment of bipolar depression with newer antidepressants, including venlafaxine and mirtazapine.
  - √ Nonresponse may require ECT, which is the single most effective intervention.
  - √ Transcranial magnetic stimulation (TMS) an emerging option.
    - ▫ Although not yet readily available, it shows some promise.
  - √ Psychotherapy and alliance-building approaches for patient and family caregivers are always useful adjuncts, especially to control caregiver burnout and rejection of the patient.

NON-DEPRESSIVE DISORDERS FOR WHICH ANTIDEPRESSANTS ARE USED

Antidepressants are used for many non-depression indications, often in conjunction with nonpharmacological therapies.

Obsessive–Compulsive Disorder (OCD)

See also page 396.

- Geriatric data very sparse.
- A chronic condition; onset most often in young adult life but also may begin in old age.
  - √ Annual incidence of new cases .64% (> 65 yrs.) in ECA study (few cases).

- 6-month prevalence of OCD (> 75 yrs.)
  - √ .2–1.2 % men
  - √ .3–1.3% women
- Symptoms may be
  - √ Standard form—contamination obsessions or washing compulsions.
  - √ Novel form—somatic symptoms, religiosity, or moral scrupulosity; compulsive paraphilias (e.g., fetishism).
- SSRIs may reduce symptoms by about half, but do not eliminate them (general adult data).
  - √ Effectiveness in elders not established, but clinical experience similar to younger groups.
- Treatments of choice for elders include serotonergic compounds such as fluoxetine, fluvoxamine, sertraline, paroxetine, citalopram, and clomipramine.
  - √ Clomipramine may be the most effective of these, although side effects are more limiting in some elders.
- Response to medication delayed 12–26 weeks (general adult data).
- Maintenance dose 2–3 times higher than for depression.

Panic Disorder

See also page 394.

Geriatric data are very sparse in this area. What we do know:

- Lifetime prevalence of 3.5%.
- Most cases are chronic, originating earlier in life.
- Clinical profile similar to younger patients.
- Patients may be especially sensitive to misinterpreting physical side effects of medication as anxiety symptoms.
  - √ Important to take time to educate patients and families about the side effects, course of treatment, and importance of staying on the therapy, if possible, given that many side effects remit with time.
- Many agents effective, some with formal licensing approval for this indication and some not.
  - √ Efficacy in elders has not been specifically established and is largely extrapolated from general adult data.
  - √ Not all effective agents are recommended for elders.
  - √ Panic symptoms often responsive to agents with serotonin reuptake inhibition properties, including
    - ▫ SSRIs
    - ▫ Venlafaxine XR
    - ▫ Trazodone
    - ▫ Nefazodone
    - ▫ Clomipramine

    - √ Target symptoms may worsen before improvement occurs.
    - √ Side-effect profile of drugs sometimes limits achievement of therapeutic dose (e.g., trazodone)
- Treatment may be effective years after the onset of the disorder.
- SSRIs and venlafaxine XR increasingly are the drugs of choice because of favorable side-effect profile.
    - √ But start slow, because this class can induce anxiety if dose titrated too quickly.
- MAOIs in elders are difficult to manage.
- HCAs
    - √ Clomipramine is the most effective HCA for treatment of panic (general adult data).
    - √ Utility limited in elders because of unfavorable side-effect profile.
        - Hypotensive, anticholinergic, and cardiac effects.
- Benzodiazepines are problematic in elders because of falls, sedation, and dependency (see Chapter 4).
- SSRI-responsive (fluoxetine) new-onset panic disorder, reported following thalamic stroke.

Social and Other Phobias

See also page 395.

- Common in elders.
    - √ Reported rates of 10–12%.
- May arise *de novo* in old age.
- Agoraphobia without panic most common subtype.
    - √ When associated with panic, pharmacological treatments of choice include SSRI antidepressants (but all classes are effective) and benzodiazepines.
    - √ Best treatment without panic not established; treatment focuses on CBT and behavioral strategies.

Generalized Anxiety Disorder

See also page 397.

- Little empirical data in elders.
- Reported rates of 3.7–4.7%.
- Does not arise commonly in old age, in pure form.
- Comorbid feature in up to 70% of major depression, including poststroke depression.
    - √ Anxiety and depression are distinct phenotypic entities, but may share underlying neurochemical (especially serotonin) imbalance.

- Antidepressants are treatment of choice when anxiety is comorbid with depression.
  - √ SSRIs or venlafaxine.
  - √ Nortriptyline not as effective.
- Concurrent anxiolytic in the early stages of treating anxious depression, or use of a sedating/anxiolytic antidepressant improves outcome.
- Anxiolytics are effective for management of primary GAD (without depression) but pose a dilemma in frailer elders (see Chapter 3, p. 371).
  - √ Buspirone is an alternative to benzodiazepines.
    - ▫ May not be as effective.

Posttraumatic Stress Disorder

- Common disorder in subgroups of elders exposed to severe or prolonged trauma.
  - √ Examples: Refugees and other immigrants, political prisoners, war veterans.
- Some evidence for efficacy of antidepressants of various classes, but
- SSRIs are the drugs of choice.
  - √ Paroxetine has an approved indication (trials include elders up to 78 years old).
  - √ May require higher dose ranges (general adult data).
    - ▫ Paroxetine 40–60 mg
    - ▫ Sertraline 150 mg
    - ▫ Fluoxetine 40–60 mg
    - ▫ Geriatric-specific doses not yet established
    - ▫ Some elders cannot tolerate these higher general adult levels
- Mirtazapine or venlafaxine may be useful.

Pathological Emotionalism

- Characterized by affective outbursts, such as weeping or laughing, in absence of depressive illness.
- Occurs in association with various neurological disorders, including poststroke, DAT, PSP, ALS, MS, traumatic brain injury, cerebral hypoxia, and brain tumors.
  - √ Occurs in up to 20% of poststroke cases.
  - √ Serotonergic mechanisms implicated.
- Treatment
  - √ SSRIs recommended.
  - √ Secondary amine TCAs also effective.
  - √ Clinical reports suggest that anticholinergic properties of TCAs may be useful in PSP.
    - ▫ Improves both depression and motor functioning.

- Nortriptyline may be best because of otherwise favorable side-effect profile.

Alcohol Abuse Treatment

- Antidepressants used as adjuncts to psychotherapy and other abstinence strategies.

Chronic Pain

- TCAs, especially amitriptyline, effective in chronic pain syndromes.
  - √ Analgesic effects of TCAs are independent of antidepressant effects.
  - √ Often used in doses considered subtherapeutic for depression (e.g., 10–50 mg).
- SSRIs also may be helpful but data conflicting.
  - √ Some evidence that idiopathic pain syndromes share common pathogenesis with depression.
    - Disturbance in the central serotonergic system.
    - Noradrenergic pathways also implicated.
    - Data include a few geriatric patients.
- Venlafaxine promising.
- Trazodone does not improve pain.
- Postherpetic neuralgia
  - √ More common in elders.
  - √ Diagnosis made 1–6 months after healing of lesions.
  - √ Most important risk factors for development are
    - Age—50% are > 65 yrs.
    - Possibly female gender.
  - √ Best therapeutic response: adrenergically active TCAs, including amitriptyline and desipramine.
    - Important to start drug therapy within 3–6 months of neuralgia onset for best pain relief results.
    - Usual cautions when using TCAs.
  - √ No data on SNRIs.
- Painful diabetic neuropathy occurs in about 4–5% of diabetic patients.
  - √ Often associated with sleep disturbance.
  - √ Treatment includes improved control of blood sugars, analgesics such as morphine, NMDA antagonists, and systemic local anesthetics.
    - Tricyclic antidepressants—nortriptyline 25 mg titrated to 150 mg max daily dose, as for depression.
    - Anticonvulsants s (see Chapter 4, p. 479).

Personality Disorders (PD)

- PD is comorbid with major depression in 33% of elders.
- Cluster B is especially associated with treatment resistance and excess disability after treatment of the depression.
  - √ SSRIs have shown effectiveness in borderlines and also may improve other trait-related behaviors.
  - √ MAOIs have been useful in younger patients with PD but are more problematic in the elderly.
  - √ Doses and protocols for both are those used for treatment of depression.

Other Conditions

Aggression in schizophrenia

- SSRIs have shown beneficial effects as adjuncts in decreasing aggression (general adult data).

Agitation (part of the BPSD picture) associated with dementia (see Chapter 2, p. 229, Antipsychotics).

Agitation in depression

- More common in severe depression.
- Characterized by mild forms (e.g., worry) or more severe forms (e.g., panic, somatic anxiety).
- Distinguish between anxiety, hypomanic agitation, and akathisia.
- Consider divalproex as part of management in doses sufficient to produce therapeutic levels (see p. 541).

Vocally disruptive behavior

- May be acute or chronic, continuous or intermittent.
- Usually associated with dementia; often with associated depression, psychosis, sleep disturbance.
- Occurs (less often) in nondemented patients with psychosis secondary to Parkinson's disease and depression.
- Sometimes correlated with communication difficulties and pain.
- Treatment is multifactorial, involving environmental change, behavioral reinforcement, interpersonal interaction.
  - √ SSRIs or trazodone may be helpful if depression is suspected, even in the absence of a formal diagnosis.
  - √ Patients on AChEIs may be less vocally disruptive.
- Reconsider drug regimen frequently to avoid creeping pharmacology—one drug added to another.
  - √ Often general physicians are reluctant to discontinue the drugs ordered by a specialist, who may follow the patient too infrequently to monitor the drug side effects.

Fronto-temporal dementia

- Associated personality and behavioral symptoms include agitation or apathy, loss of inhibition, compulsive behaviors, eating disorders or impairments of executive functioning; rarely develop parkinsonism.
  - √ Behavioral symptoms may respond to serotonergic drugs such as SSRIs or trazodone and cholinergic drugs such as AChEIs.
  - √ Paroxetine induced significant behavioral improvement over 14 months (small N study compared to piracetam).
  - √ AChEIs do not improve the cognitive impairment component.

Apathetic and avolitional depressed states

- May respond best to activating antidepressants.
  - √ Bupropion, derived from same chemical base as amphetamine, may be more effective.
  - √ Methylphenidate or other stimulants useful adjuncts especially in apathetic states associated with medical comorbidity.

Table 1.8. Uses of Antidepressants in the Elderly

Clinical Conditions	Effective Antidepressant Drugs	Drugs of Choice
Mood Disorder • Major depressive disorder • Minor depressive disorder • Bipolar disorders • Cyclothymic disorder • Dysthymic disorder • Substance–induced	All antidepressants; some indication that TCAs, MAOIs, venlafaxine, and mirtazapine may be more effective than SSRIs in severe and melancholic depression	*Unipolar psychotic major depressive disorder:* SSRI/venlafaxine XR *Minor depressive disorder:* SSRI
Subtypes of depression especially relevant to the elderly • Vascular depression • Late-onset depression • Minor depression • Depression with dementia √ Dementia syndrome of depression • Mood disorder secondary to other medical conditions √ Physical illness (e.g., stroke, Parkinson's) • Atypical: anxious/panic or masked depression with somatization • Depressive symptoms associated with aberrant grief reactions; traumatic grief • Depressions comorbid with personality disorders, posttraumatic stress disorder • Caregiver depression	All antidepressants; some suggestion that atypical depression responds better to SSRIs	*BBB* (*bundle branch block*): SSRI, bupropion SR, venlafaxine XR, mirtazapine *Coronary artery disease:* SSRIs, bupropion SR, mirtazapine, venlafaxine XR, possibly nefazodone *Dementia:* SSRIs, especially citalopram, venlafaxine XR, bupropion SR, possibly nefazodone, mirtazapine *Diabetes:* SSRIs, bupropion SR, venlafaxine XR, possibly mirtazapine or nefazodone *Hypertension:* SSRIs, mirtazapine, bupropion SR, possibly nefazodone, TCAs *Hypotension:* SSRIs, bupropion SR, venlafaxine XR, possibly mirtazapine

(*cont.*)

Continued

Clinical Conditions	Effective Antidepressant Drugs	Drugs of Choice
Anxiety Disorders • Panic disorder • Social phobia • Generalized anxiety disorder (GAD) • Posttraumatic stress disorder (PTSD) • Obsessive–compulsive disorder (OCD)	Panic: SSRIs, venlafaxine, TCAs Social phobia: SSRIs, MAOIs (reversible and irreversible) GAD: SSRIs, venlafaxine PTSD: SSRIs, nefazodone, mirtazapine, venlafaxine OCD: Serotonergic drugs (clomipramine most effective of the group); SSRIs (especially the less selective drugs, such as fluvoxamine and fluoxetine)	Panic: SSRIs, venlafaxine XR social phobia: SSRIs PTSD: SSRIs: sertraline, paroxetine, fluoxetine OCD: SSRI trial; clomipramine in severe cases if side effects are tolerated
Other Conditions • Pathological emotionalism • Alcohol abuse • Chronic pain • Personality disorder • Agitation (BPSD) in dementia, including fronto—temporal dementia, vocally disruptive behavior • Avolitional/amotivational states	Pathological emotionalism: SSRIs recommended, TCAs Alcohol abuse: SSRIs as adjunct Chronic pain: TCAs, SSRIs, possibly venlafaxine XR Personality disorder: MAOIs, SSRIs Agitation: Serotonergic agents: SSRIs, trazodone Avolitional states: Bupropion, stimulants	Pathological emotionalism: SSRIs; PSP (consider nortriptyline) Chronic pain: nortriptyline; consider amitriptyline for unresponsive cases Agitation: Citalopram, sertraline Avolitional states: methylphenidate

GERIATRIC ANTIDEPRESSANT PHARMACOTHERAPY ISSUES

The elderly are a highly heterogeneous group and each patient should be evaluated on his/her own merits. Goals of treatment include:

- Remission of symptoms of depression
- Relapse and recurrence prevention
- Improved quality of life
- Enhanced functional ability
- Improved general health status
- Reduced mortality
- Reduced health-care costs
- Reduced family/caregiver strain and burden

Elder-specific concerns include:

- Few elders receive the treatment they need.
  - √ Treatment is usually low-dose antidepressant therapy, often inadequate to needs.

- Elders often take longer to respond to antidepressant therapy.
  - √ Shown in meta-analytic study of response of fluoxetine
  - √ May be the result of the longer dose escalation schedules necessary in many elderly patients.
  - √ Therapeutic trials should be 6–12 weeks.
    - ▫ Chance of response is much lower if there is *no initial* response in first 2 weeks.
  - √ Even after improvement in first 6–8 weeks, additional improvement often occurs with continuing treatment.
    - ▫ Maximum improvement occurs between 8–16 weeks and sometimes longer.
- High incidence of drug noncompliance.
  - √ Estimated as high as 40–75%.

Factors Influencing Treatment and Drug Choice

Diagnostic features

- Type of depression (e.g., unipolar vs. bipolar).
- Severity of depression.
  - √ Consider merits of drug vs. ECT.
- Comorbid features (e.g., anxiety).
- Age-specific clinical presentations of disorders (e.g., differentiating depression from dementia or somatization).
- If present, type of anxiety disorder (e.g., GAD, panic, phobia, OCD).

Comorbid Physical Conditions

- Cardiovascular disorders.
  - √ Depression post MI associated with much higher risk of cardiac mortality; vigorous treatment indicated.
  - √ Use SSRIs or newer classes of antidepressant.
  - √ TCAs (e.g., nortriptyline) more effective but greater CVS side-effect risks.
- Neurological disorders (e.g., tremor, falls).
- GU disorders (e.g., prostatic hypertrophy).
- GI disorders (e.g., constipation).
- Visual impairment (e.g., glaucoma).

Age Effects on Pharmacodynamics/Kinetics

See page 12.

Concurrent Medications

- Both prescription and OTC drugs.

Prior Response to Drug Treatment

- Assess
  - √ Type/appropriateness of prior medication.
  - √ Adequacy of prior dose/duration of drug trial.
  - √ Prior family/compliance factors.
  - √ Factors that may have interfered with responsiveness that are no longer present.
  - √ Factors that have recently emerged that were not present before but may now interfere.

Compliance Factors

Follow elders carefully; compliance highly variable, especially in community dwellers.

- 70% of patients fail to take 25–50% of prescribed medication.

Non compliance factors in the elderly include:

- Complexity of multiple drug regimens for multiple illnesses.
- Adding a medication to an already complex daily regimen.
- Inadequate information about need for therapy and drug usage.
- Unclear prescribing instructions.
- Failure of physicians to follow-up on prescriptions.
- Communication difficulties caused by
  - √ Sensory impairment (e.g., cannot read labels)
  - √ Physical frailty
  - √ Cognitive impairment
  - √ Language and cultural differences
  - √ Patient disorganization
  - √ Caregiver and patient prejudices about psychiatric medication

To enhance compliance, assess and address:

- Cognition
- Sensory impairment
- Frailty
- Appropriate coordination of care and relationship with primary care physician.
- Patient understanding of importance of long-term therapy (i.e., getting well but also remaining well).
- Appropriate/effective monitoring and managing of side effects.
- Enhancing quality of life where possible (e.g., facilitating social interaction by referral to seniors clubs).
- Family involvement often crucial to compliance and successful treatment; educate families and enlist them as allies to participate in treatment decisions; maintain family therapeutic alliance by educating them, offering telephone contact and updates (with patient's permission as appropriate; beware of preempting the

competent patient's decision- making;); inquire about family members' feelings about psychiatric medication.
- Social factors (e.g., isolation, financial limitations).

Cognitive Factors

Assess and address:

- Influence on compliance.
- Drug-induced increased impairment.
  - √ Sedating effects produce greatest impairment.
  - √ Anticholinergic effects further impair cognitive performance.

Side Effect Profile

See pages 70–90.

Drug Efficacy

- Overall efficacy in elders.
- Unique spectrum of efficacy for specific patient.
  - √ Previous response to treatment
  - √ First-degree family member response to treatment
  - √ Record of the drug in relapse prevention

Cost/Cost Effectiveness

- Comparative cost-effectiveness for specific antidepressants in elders not well established.
- availability of insurance/formulary coverage

Tolerability

- Acute tolerability index:
  - √ Avoid amitriptyline, imipramine, and doxepin as first-line agents in elders.
- Late emergent intolerance:
  - √ SSRIs have lower rate of side-effect–induced discontinuation than TCAs during maintenance therapy.

Simplicity of Dosing Schedule

- Compliance improves with fewer doses/day.
- Determine availability of flexible dosage forms (small dose size or preparations easily split into smaller doses) especially for patients sensitive to side effects, and when increasing dose to therapeutic levels must be done more cautiously.

Need for Drug Monitoring

- Examples: lithium or TCA plasma levels, blood pressure monitoring during dose escalation with venlafaxine.

Need for Family Involvement

- Assess reliability of caregivers in administering drug according to instructions.
  - √ Commonest patient error is failure to take a prescribed dose, rather than inadvertent overdose.

CHOOSING AND USING SPECIFIC ANTIDEPRESSANTS

Comparison of Drugs

In general, *all antidepressants are equally effective for depression* but have differing side-effect profiles. There are insufficient data to strongly recommend one drug over another in terms of efficacy, although some head-to-head studies sometimes favor specific drugs. For example, mirtazapine was found to be more effective than paroxetine in a geriatric population. Some general adult data suggest that venlafaxine (and possibly mirtazapine) is more effective in severe depressions and may be more likely to induce remission (as opposed to partial improvement) than SSRIs. Studies indicate favorable results of antidepressant treatment in all forms of depression in elderly, regardless of agent used.

- Robust data support superiority of antidepressants over placebo to produce treatment response and remission.
  - √ *Treatment response* is generally defined as a decline of 50% on Hamilton Depression Rating Scale (HAM-D) scores.
  - √ *Remission* is defined as an 80% decline to a score of < 8–10.
    - ▫ This level is usually reached after the initial treatment period typically used in geriatric studies (8–12 weeks).
  - √ Advantage over placebo effect variable, but all antidepressants offer about a 25–40% advantage over placebo in the physically healthy elderly (about double the placebo effect), taking into account dropouts, partial responders, and treatment failures.
  - √ Some studies are more optimistic, reporting 80% response rates with vigorous persistent medication therapy.

Time to onset of action is one of the "Holy Grails" of antidepressant research and development. There are still no breakthroughs, although many have claimed a more rapid effect early in the life of the drug, only to be disproved later.

- All antidepressants have approximately the same lag time to onset of therapeutic action: 2 weeks or more.
  - √ Some drugs show more rapid action in specific studies, but none is consistently better than others.
    - ▫ Mitazapine may have a more rapid onset, but data are not robust.

        - Very limited data suggest combination of serotonergic and noradrenergic agents may enhance speed of action onset (e.g., fluoxetine and desipramine), but clinical utility in elders not established.
    - √ Response of depression to therapy often goes in a stepwise fashion, with cycles of improvement and decline.
        - Temporary return of symptoms is common and does not predict outcome of therapy.
        - Persist with a full trial of AD therapy before changing drugs.

Antidepressants improve both *symptoms* of depression and *quality-of-life measures* in elders.

- SSRIs, and other new-generation ADs, are better tolerated and safer than older tertiary TCAs because of more favorable side-effect and toxicity profiles.
    - √ Most head-to-head comparative studies of SSRIs have used older tertiary amines (especially imipramine and amitriptyline).
    - √ In head-to-head studies with secondary amines (especially nortriptyline), dropout rates and tolerability are comparable to SSRIs, regardless of age factors.
    - √ Frailty, per se, reduces tolerability to TCAs and may be a marker for increased mortality rates.
    - √ Many otherwise healthy elders tolerate TCAs such as nortriptyline, desipramine, and clomipramine well enough to be able to use these medications when necessary, with some important caveats:
        - Greater caution is necessary in medically impaired elders and those taking interactive concurrent medications, (e.g., antihypertensives or anticholinergic agents).
        - While acute tolerability may be adequate, long-term treatment may be problematic because:
            1. TCAs increase heart rate by 10% and may increase risk of cardiac mortality post MI or in ischemic heart disease due to type 1C antiarrhythmic action, a particular problem in patients with underlying ischemic or other heart disease.
            2. Chronic anticholinergic effects (present even with secondary amines) may lead to significant adverse effects with increasing age (e.g., central effects such as cognitive impairment, and peripheral effects such as *dry mouth and* denture problems, GI impairment, visual impairment, glaucoma, and urinary hesitancy/retention).

MAOIs are infrequently used for elders.

- Very few controlled studies or clinical reports.
- Few data available suggest robust response and good tolerability.

- Data indicate that MAOIs have been underutilized in elders.
  - √ New-generation drugs have now taken over so completely that the issue is no longer often raised clinically.

Characteristics of an ideal antidepressant for the elderly include:

- Effective and prevents relapse.
- Side-effect profile that is safe with coexisting medical illnesses (e.g., little effect on cardiovascular system).
- Minimal interactions with concurrent drugs.
  - √ Polypharmacy very common in elders.
- Half-life of primary compound and active metabolites < 24 hours to avoid accumulation and increased risk of side effects/toxicity.
- Once daily dose to minimize compliance problems e.g., due to cognitive problems.
- Safe in overdose.
- Low protein-binding capacity (reduces drug interaction).
- Satisfactory cost–benefit ratio.
- Does not disrupt cognitive and psychomotor performance (e.g., through anticholinergic or sedative effects).

Safety

The acute therapeutic index provides information on the degree of safety in overdose instances and the risk of lethality per drug overdose.

- HCAs
  - √ Lethality of HCAs is probably directly related to level of cardiac toxicity of a given drug.
  - √ Desipramine has highest lethality of HCAs: other HCAs likely to result in death are amitriptyline, doxepin, trimipramine, maprotiline.
    - ▫ Nortriptyline is less lethal than amitriptyline.
  - √ HCAs inhibit sodium fast channels and sodium–potassium pump. This action mediates adverse cardiac conduction effects at one order of magnitude above therapeutic plasma concentrations.
    - ▫ Hence OD of 10 times daily therapeutic dose (15–20 mg/kg; 750–1000 mg) can be fatal (general adult data).
    - ▫ Older TCAs carry a high risk.
- MAOIs
  - √ Lethality appears related to induction of severe serotonin syndrome.
- SSRIs, SNRIs, and NaSSAs
  - √ Very low risk of fatality in overdose.

Pharmacokinetic Interactions

See pages 11–21.

Pharmacodynamic Interactions

See pages 11–21.

- Identify pharmacotherapy risk factors, such as polypharmacy (norm in the elderly).
  - √ Average older American uses three prescription drugs and four OTC drugs/day.
  - √ Nursing home residents take seven prescription drugs/day.
- Inquire carefully about
  - √ OTC drugs.
    - ▫ Antihistamines
    - ▫ NSAIDs
    - ▫ Sleep preparations
    - ▫ GI remedies
    - ▫ Herbal medicines (e.g., St. John's Wort)
  - √ Alcohol or other drugs of misuse.

Note: Active inquiry is necessary. Patients may not spontaneously volunteer use of OTC drugs, alcohol, or other drugs of misuse, since they are not prescribed and hence may not be considered "medications." Patients are unlikely to respond to antidepressant therapy in presence of active substance abuse. Choice of antidepressant may depend on interaction with concurrent medication.

Table 1.9. Checklist for Selecting Antidepressant Drug

Factors	Action/Assessment
Safety	Acute therapeutic index
Pharmacodynamic interactions	P450 interaction
	Polypharmacy
	OTCs
	Substance abuse, especially alcohol
Pharmacokinetics	Plasma protein levels
	Liver and renal metabolism
	Body mass composition (muscle/fat ratio)
Medical comorbidity	
Tolerability profile	
Situational efficacy	Setting (nursing home, medical, community)
Cost	
Simplicity of dosing schedule	
Need for specific monitoring	Blood levels
Need for family involvement	

Antidepressant Dosing in the Elderly

- Dosing with antidepressants is far from an exact science.
- Geriatric dose ranges have not been well established for most antidepressants.
- Although ranges are based on the ¼–½ of general-adult-dose rule, some healthy elderly patients, especially if otherwise vigorous, require doses closer to the general adult range.

- Lower dosage ranges are more the norm in debilitated and institutionalized elders, although sometimes full adult doses are necessary (e.g., sertraline response in dementia requires 100 mg range).
- With most antidepressants, steady states are achieved more slowly, so titrate more slowly in elders.
  - √ Severity of depressive condition may make long titration schedules undesirable.
- Side effects do not always correlate with plasma concentrations of some drugs (e.g., SSRIs).
  - √ More rapid dose escalation sometimes possible, especially for severe cases.
- Overall the decision of when to increase dose must be individualized.

Pharmacoeconomic Considerations

There is an increasing trend to utilize *more expensive newer agents* in elders. In some studies SSRIs, when compared to TCAs, were shown to be as cost-effective or better, despite much higher acquisition costs.

- Performance of SSRIs said to be enhanced by more favorable side-effect profile and therefore greater compliance, tolerability, and effectiveness, since course of therapy more likely to be completed.
- No data for other new-generation drugs.

Note: Pharmacoeconomic data should be interpreted cautiously. Cost-effectiveness data of SSRIs in general adult studies do not consistently support positive conclusions, and comparisons are somewhat biased against TCAs. Studies do not compare secondary amines, which have a more favorable side-effect profile and are used more commonly in the elderly than tertiary amines.

PHASES OF ANTIDEPRESSANT TREATMENT

Acute Phase

- Adequate trial of medication is 8–12 weeks.
  - √ Many drugs require 12–16 weeks to achieve optimum effect.
- In study populations about 60% improve but not necessarily to full remission.
  - √ Remission rates in naturalistic studies are often much lower.
- Improvement in sleep and energy may be earliest signs of effectiveness.
- Course of improvement may be uneven, with worsening after initial improvement, before becoming better again.
- Subjective sense of improvement may lag behind objective signs.

- Residual symptoms common in elderly.
  - √ Affects prognosis: e.g., high risk of recurrence/relapse in partially treated psychotic depression.
- Comorbid anxiety symptoms are very common and often require adjunctive antianxiety medication.
  - √ Some antidepressants, such as mirtazapine, have early anxiolytic effects that may reduce need for adjunctive anxiolytics.
    - ▫ Mirtazapine also may have an earlier onset of action, independent of its anxiolytic properties.
  - √ Anxiolytics generally not recommended in presence of comorbid dementia. Small doses of a typical antipsychotic is an alternative.

Continuation Phase

The *continuation phase* extends to the end of the remission period (i.e., prevention of relapse after index episode).

- Generally considered to be 6–12 months but, for many patients, treatment should not be stopped at this point, since risk of relapse remains high in elders.
  - √ Especially in patients with unusually prolonged or severe depressive episode or intense suicidality.
- If medication must be discontinued, risk of relapse may be reduced by tapering rather than abrupt discontinuation.
- CBT or IPT augmentation reduces risk of relapse.

Maintenance Phase

The maintenance phase continues after the remission phase has passed to prevent another new episode (i.e., recurrence).

- Almost all evaluated antidepressants have shown partial but significant prophylactic efficacy against new episodes of depression in long-term treatment (geriatric and general adult data).
  - √ Specific geriatric data available for phenelzine, nortriptyline, and paroxetine.
  - √ Data not yet sufficient to recommend one agent over another.
    - ▫ Sometimes data conflict (e.g., poor maintenance performance of nortriptyline in one study and similarly poor performance of nortriptyline compared to favorable performance of phenelzine).
  - √ Combination of nortriptyline and lithium shown to be more effective prophylaxis than nortriptyline alone (in a mixed general adult population that included geriatric patients).
- Most effective maintenance regimen appears to be a combination of pharmacotherapy with psychotherapy.

- √ Geriatric studies done specifically with nortriptyline and IPT; no similar geriatric data for other agents.
- High-risk patients should continue on maintenance for a prolonged time.
  - √ Precise recommendation is difficult.
  - √ Ranges from 2 years (for patients with two episodes of depression) to indefinitely (for patients with > two episodes).
  - √ Recommendation: Indefinite maintenance for high-risk patients who tolerate the medication well.
- Breakthrough relapse rates, despite maintenance of full-dose medication, range from 9–33% (general adult data).
  - √ Relapse early in the course of treatment often related to loss of placebo effect.
- Recommendations are similar for depression and dementia.
- Dose and plasma levels in continuation and maintenance phases are the same as effective dose in acute phase.
- Monitor patients carefully during long-term maintenance therapy.
  - √ Dose adjustments may be necessary as patient ages, develops new concurrent medical problems, or begins taking new concurrent drugs.
- ECT
  - √ Patients who are intolerant of antidepressants after adequate trials or who relapse on medication therapies alone may respond to maintenance ECT (q 4–6 wks).
  - √ Medications that were ineffective prior to ECT should not be used for maintenance.

PROGNOSIS OF DEPRESSION WITH TREATMENT

- Geriatric patients on placebo or no maintenance treatment relapse 90% of the time.
- Effectiveness data (general adult data) indicate that high percentages (40%) of patients discontinue antidepressants in the first 3 months of treatment in naturalistic settings.

Acute Episode

- Prognosis for recovery variable but generally positive.
- About 60% of selected patients in clinical trials show partial or complete remission from a particular episode within 6 months with treatment.
  - √ Some studies show 30% of patients (general adult data) fail to respond to initial course of therapy even with adequate dose and duration.
  - √ An additional 20–40% do not tolerate the initial drug.

- Recovery rate at 1 year is 59–72%; comparable in young and old.
  - √ But some studies in elders show a low overall response rate to antidepressant treatment of 35–40%.
- Initial response profile may predict ultimate recovery and relapse rates.
  - √ Rapid initial responders show lower recurrence rates and may be maintained on pharmacotherapy alone.
  - √ Delayed responders do better with combined pharmacotherapy and psychotherapy.
- Most patients (90%) will eventually respond to first-, second-, or third-line treatment, if they are compliant and can complete recommended antidepressant trials.
  - √ Response time to second-line therapy and beyond may be longer than to first-line therapy.
  - √ The clinical dilemma is managing a patient's depressive pain during prolonged drug trials.
  - √ Nonresponders to first- or second-line therapy have a poor prognosis for response to third-line therapy and beyond, possibly including ECT.
    - ▫ Of those who fail to respond, some will eventually improve with time, but may take months or years.
- Supportive psychotherapeutic care is essential to optimal management but may be restricted by third-party payor restrictions or other practical limitations.
- One-third of patients are left with significant residual depressive symptoms.
- Best results occur with aggressive treatment within the side-effect tolerance zone of the patient.

Relapse and Recurrence

Getting patients better is only the first step; *keeping* them better is the major therapeutic challenge.

- Long-term maintenance therapy with antidepressants is the current wisdom
  - √ Not all studies show positive outcomes.
    - ▫ Some earlier studies suggested that maintenance beyond 8 months after index episode does not confer greater protection from relapse than placebo, especially with nortriptyline.
- Longer-term prognosis is modest in elders; relapse and recurrence are high even if maintenance therapy is continued.
  - √ Estimates of relapse risk on maintenance medication alone range from 17% to 43% (and possibly higher in higher-risk populations).
  - √ Statistics vary because studies sometimes mix relapse and recurrence into single outcome groups.

- Risk of relapse is highest in the first 2 years after index episode.
- Relapse after discontinuing antidepressant is generally effectively treated by reintroducing original drug.

Table 1.10. Risk Factors for Relapse

- Age: Older age of patient inconsistently associated with poorer prognosis.
- History of prior episodes: Risk of recurrence is 10 times higher if there has been one prior episode, and 14–18 times higher if there has been more than one episode.
  - √ Risk of recurrence after first episode is estimated at 50–80% and increases to 80–90% after a second episode.
- Chronic index depression: more than 2 years.
- Longer time to respond to treatment during initial treatment.
- Suboptimal maintenance antidepressant dose.
- Residual anxiety: high levels after improvement of symptoms during treatment.
  - √ May be an indicator of incomplete treatment.
- Poor subjective sleep quality.
- Residual depressive symptoms after successful treatment.
  - √ Complete remission during treatment is very important to positive long-term outcome.
- Inadequate relapse prevention: full-dose maintenance treatment after remission reduces relapse rates.
  - √ Discontinuation of maintenance therapy increases risk of relapse.

- Efficacy of antidepressant therapy is significantly augmented when combined with psychotherapy.
  - √ IPT has been investigated for this purpose in elders and found effective.
  - √ Other psychotherapies may be effective but not formally investigated in elders.
  - √ The most effective maintenance regimen is antidepressant combined with psychotherapy.
- ECT or combined medication and psychotherapy produce response rates as high as 80%.
- Formal treatment protocols in controlled settings produce the best results; poorer outcomes in “naturalistic” treatment studies (i.e., no formal treatment protocols).
  - √ In general practice settings many patients are maintained on antidepressants with little follow-up; doses are often subtherapeutic and many patients relapse without the physician’s awareness.

Management of Relapse and Recurrence during Maintenance or after Discontinuation

- Reinitiate prior treatment promptly, titrating to full therapeutic doses.
- If no response in 2 weeks, manage based on decision tree (below).
- If patient relapses *during* treatment
  - √ Review compliance.
  - √ Examine for new comorbid condition (e.g., recently diagnosed hypertension).

- √ Examine for new life stress.
- √ Relapse sometimes occurs spontaneously, in the absence of other causes and even on adequate maintenance.
  - ▫ Consider possibility of therapeutic window effect, where lowering dose may be effective (e.g., nortriptyline or fluoxetine).
- If a patient plateaus suboptimally during therapy, increase dose of drug.

NONRESPONSE TO ANTIDEPRESSANT TREATMENT

Table 1.11. Risk Factors for Increased Rate of Nonresponse to Antidepressant Therapy

Age/frailty	• Effect of age of onset remains controversial. • Middle and old-old may be at greater risk of relapse than young-old. • Relapse rates may be higher and time to relapse faster in frail older geriatric patients.
History	• Two or more depressive episodes. • Higher number and duration of prior hospitalizations. • ECT treatment. • Nonresponse to previous antidepressant treatment.
Diagnosis	High relapse rates associated with • Dysthymia (limited data). • Bipolar disorder. • Premorbid personality disorder or trait disturbances. • Psychotic symptoms.
Duration of index episode	> 2 years
Clinical picture	• High severity of index episode. • Neurological signs and symptoms. √ Dementia √ Impaired executive brain function (initiation and perseveration measures) may predict greater risk of (1) residual symptoms after treatment and (2) relapse/recurrence. √ Frontal lobe syndrome √ EPS √ Subcortical hyperintensities (MRI T_2-weighted lesions best seen in flare view) in frontal deep white matter, basal ganglia, and pontine reticular formation. ▫ Data conflict; recent study shows no difference in outcome. √ Discordance on quantitative EEG • Presence of parasuicidal behavior. • Presence of anxiety symptoms. √ High level during index depressive episode ▫ Data conflict on association of index anxiety and outcomes √ Residual anxiety
Response to treatment	• Failure to show any response to therapy within first 6 weeks. • Placebo-type drug response √ Patients who have a true drug response pattern (i.e., response after more than 2 weeks of treatment) vs. a placebo response pattern (i.e., response before 2 weeks) are more likely to relapse when drug therapy is discontinued.

(cont.)

Continued

Psychosocial factors	• Poor social adaptation • Disability • Bereavement • Role transitions (e.g., retirement) • Loss of social supports (e.g., absence of a confidant; possibly living alone). • Occurrence of negative stressful life events in past 12 months.
Medical comorbidity	• Chronic illness/pain √ Control of pain is a crucial first step in treating depression in medically ill patients with painful disorders such as cancer. √ High physical illness rating increases nonresponse/relapse risk. □ Especially MI
Adequacy of drug treatment	• Inadequate √ Therapeutic dose √ Duration of drug trial √ Inappropriate drug choice • Concurrent augmenting therapies may decrease risk. √ Adding a psychotherapeutic modality (CBT, IPT, brief dynamic) may improve certain residual symptoms (e.g., sleep disturbance, interpersonal conflicts, inappropriate behaviors). √ Some evidence that mild exercise improves symptoms of depression.

Treatment Strategies for Nonresponse to Antidepressant Therapy

Nonresponse is often associated with an inadequate trial of antidepressant therapy. Optimize therapy by reviewing the following factors.

Table 1.12. Review Checklist to Optimize Drug Therapy

- Dosing
- Plasma levels, where appropriate
  - √ Elders more prone to nonadherence to instructions, so plasma levels may be more important than in younger patients.
  - √ Therapeutic levels in elders are similar to general adults.
  - √ Using and interpreting plasma levels are not always simple.
  - √ Guidelines for obtaining interpretable results:
    - □ Establish kidney/liver function.
    - □ Measure after steady state has been reached (i.e., 5–6 half-lives of drug).
    - □ Ensure patient compliance.
    - □ Take sample at standard time 10–12 hours after last doses.
    - □ Evaluate effects of concurrent medications (e.g., cimetidine, beta blockers).
    - □ Measure both parent compound and active metabolites.
- Duration of drug trial
- Compliance
- Motivation for therapy
- Pharmacodynamic/kinetic factors
- Lifestyle
- Stressors
  - √ Comorbid illness
  - √ Concurrent substance abuse (especially alcohol)

Substitution Strategies (switching from one AD medication to another)

- SSRI resistance
  - √ Little research in elders, so conclusive recommendation on this strategy is not possible at this time.
  - √ Treatment resistance due to intolerance of one drug in class might be effectively remedied by switching to another in same class.
  - √ SSRIs have differing pharmacodynamics from each other, and one may be less troublesome than another in a given patient.
  - √ Switch to another antidepressant, in rank order of preference: venlafaxine XR, bupropion SR, TCA (nortriptyline), mirtazapine, MAOI.
- TCA resistance
  - √ Switching among tricyclics yields low rate of response.
  - √ Better response if switch is to MAOI (note geriatric cautions), especially with comorbid anxiety symptoms (general adult data).
  - √ Switch to another family of antidepressant.
    - ▫ SSRIs may be effective but less likely to be so if there has been nonresponse to a TCA.
    - ▫ Utility of other classes for TCA resistance not yet determined for elders.

Augmentation and Combination Strategies

Augmentation: Addition of a second (or even third) compound to an antidepressant that has been partially or completely ineffective. *Combination:* Addition of a second antidepressant and/or other agents.

- Very few studies or clinical reports in elders.
  - √ Available geriatric data indicate that augmentation increases the overall rate of response to antidepressant therapy.
  - √ Augmentation/combination treatments are riskier in elders because of drug interactions and lower compliance rates due to a more complex treatment regimen.
  - √ When effective, augmentation tends to work within 2–3 weeks (occasionally earlier; general adult data).
    - ▫ Augmenting agent often has to be given in full therapeutic doses.
  - √ High risk of relapse if effective augmentation is discontinued.
    - ▫ If discontinuation of successful augmentation therapy is necessary, it should be tapered slowly, monitoring for relapse.

- Evidence base is very slim overall and particularly so for elders.
  - √ Best evidence is for lithium and T3.
  - √ Some support for use of atypical antipsychotics.
  - √ Other agents not well supported by empirical evidence.
    - ▫ Best used on a clinical trial basis in individual patients who fail other first- and second-line interventions.

Lithium

- Addition to antidepressant (see Chapter 4, p. 479).

Thyroid hormone

- T_3 in low doses of 25–50 μg (general adult data) (50 μg in one geriatric study and most general adults tolerate 20–25 μg well).
  - √ Studied mostly with TCAs.
  - √ Little data support for effectiveness of thyroid hormone augmentation with classes of antidepressants other than TCAs and possibly MAOIs.
  - √ A few general adult clinical reports with SSRIs.
  - √ Effectiveness uncertain; hence used as second-line aumentation.
    - ▫ Comparable efficacy to lithium has been demonstrated in some studies.
  - √ Generally well tolerated in low doses used.
  - √ Long-term effects not clear.
    - ▫ May be some danger of inducing hypothyroidism if used for prolonged periods of several months.
  - √ T_4 effective in high doses (500–800 μg/day) in a general adult study.
    - ▫ Not generally useful in elders.

Buspirone

- Little geriatric data available.
- Overall, a disappointing augmenting agent; not recommended for this indication.
- Action uncertain.
  - √ Thought to activate postsynaptic 5HT1A receptors.
- Enhances SSRI action at doses of 15–30 mg for up to 3 months; caution in elders at higher doses.
- Caution in augmentation with nefazodone, since increased dizziness, headaches and insomnia emerge.
  - √ If necessary, try smaller doses of 2.5 mg bid; risk induction of mania/hypomania.

Pindolol

Pindolol is not a recommended strategy; effectiveness remains controversial and unproved in augmenting effectiveness or improving speed of SSRI onset of action (and possibly other classes of antidepressants).

- Pindolol: a beta-1 and -2 adrenergic blocker and a 5HT1A receptor antagonist.
  - √ 5HT1A action decreases 5HT synthesis and firing of 5HT neurons.
- Use in elders very limited, to date.
- If used, dose is 1.5 mg tid (about 60% of the general adult dose of 2.5 mg tid).

In trials, pindolol was used to enhance antidepressant onset of action; in most ambulatory cases this is not a necessary strategy, unless patient is suicidal or suffering unduly. In these cases consider hospitalization. Increased speed of onset is important in treatment of hospitalized patients, where short lengths of stay are the norm.

Anxiolytics

- Little or no good geriatric data available.
- Buspirone and clonazepam studied (especially for OCD).
- Classical benzodiazepines (general adult data) show no primary antidepressant effect in major depression.
  - √ May be helpful in combination with antidepressant therapy during first 2 weeks in patients with significant anxiety and sleep disturbance, but no empirical evidence for utility thereafter.
  - √ Some patients obtain significant anxiolytic effect and appear to benefit from longer-term use (see p. 371).
- Triazolobenzodiazepines (general adult data), especially alprazolam, show AD effects when used in doses about twice the anxiolytic dose, but are inferior to tricyclics.
  - √ Probably effective only in mild forms of major depression, but not with more severe clinical pictures or melancholia.
  - √ Improve some core depressive symptoms.
    - ▫ Psychomotor retardation as well as anxiety and sleep.
- Not generally used in elders.

Psychostimulants

There is little controlled evaluation of methylphenidate or dextroamphetamine as augmenters. Preliminary uncontrolled data in elders suggest psychostimulants may accelerate onset of action (of citalopram).

- Dose (estimated geriatric)
  - √ Methylphenidate 5 mg tid
  - √ Dextroamphetamine 2.5 mg tid
  - √ Pemoline (no geriatric data)
  - √ Modafinil: Very limited geriatric clinical experience reported as augmenter in depression.
    - ▫ When used in young–old geriatric patients dose is 200 mg q A.M.
  - √ Methylphenidate increases the plasma levels of some psychotopic agents.
  - √ Risk of hypertensive and hyperthermic crisis with MAOIs.
  - √ Caution post MI

Estrogen supplementation

- Estrogen replacement therapy may enhance AD effectiveness, but data not strong.
- Dose 15–25 mg/day (general adult data).
- *Note:* Recent data on negative effects of HRT on various aspects of aging (i.e., breast cancer and heart disease; make definitive recommendation impossible.

Mood stabilizers

- No geriatric data (and few well-controlled, general adult data) available.
- Not as effective for unipolar depression as for bipolar forms.
- Clinical experience suggests that best choice of mood stabilizer is divalproex.
  - √ Sodium valproate augmentation of fluoxetine and fluvoxamine sometimes effective (clinical case reports only).
    - ▫ Note pharmacokinetic interactions. Sodium valproate is a hepatic enzyme inhibitor, increasing plasma concentrations of TCAs.
- Lamotrigine may augment antidepressants in refractory depression (general adult data).
  - √ Especially useful in bipolar disorder (general adult data).
  - √ Sometimes useful in maintenance therapy of unipolar depression.
- Carbamazepine augmentation of MAOI and clomipramine:
  - √ *Note:* Pharmacokinetic cautions with carbamazepine: Hepatic enzyme induction action lowers TCA plasma levels, and inhibitor action may increase hydroxymetabolites of TCAs.
  - √ Not recommended for routine use.

Atypical antipsychotics

See Chapter 3.

Atypical antipsychotics have shown utility as adjunctive medication in psychotic depression.

- Risperidone
  - ✓ In low doses is a 5HT2 receptor antagonist
    - ▫ Facilitates the action of serotonin at the 5HT1A receptor.
  - ✓ Clinical case of elder suggests 0.5–1 mg risperidone augments AD action of SSRI (paroxetine).
    - ▫ Rapid response within a few days.
    - ▫ Improved sleep and possibly sexual response.
- Olanzapine and fluoxetine synergistic effect (general adult data).

Nimodipine (and other calcium channel blockers)

- May be effective in augmenting AD effects in vascular dementia; data should be viewed as preliminary at this time.
- Nimodipine dose 30 mg tid
  - ✓ Greater caution in patients already taking antihypertensive medication.
- Generally well tolerated in young–old patient group.
- Preliminary data (general adult) suggest possible utility for dopamine agonists (direct and indirect) such as pergolide.

Alternative therapies

Little support for use of St. John's wort, SAM-E, or omega-3 fatty acids in elders at this time.

Nonpharmacological augmenting strategies

- IPT
  - ✓ Substantially improves effectiveness of drug therapy; efficacy empirically demonstrated in combination with nortriptyline.
  - ✓ CBT (with nefazodone, general adult data) shown to be effective adjunct.
  - ✓ Overall, most forms of psychotherapy are probably effective adjuncts for major depression and are the preferred intervention for minor depression in elders.
    - ▫ Intensive insight-oriented therapy is not indicated during acute phases of depression.
- High-intensity light therapy not studied in elders with refractory depression but some experienced clinicians endorse this strategy.

- Total sleep deprivation (36 hrs.)
  - √ May enhance therapeutic response to AD treatment; obviously not very practical for elders.

Combination Therapy

- Well-constructed studies of efficacy for this strategy in elders not available.
  - √ Example: SSRI–TCA combinations
    - ▫ Caution in elders because of drug–drug interactions (e.g., increased TCA levels if 2D6 is inhibited; see Table 1.32, p. 95).
    - ▫ Dose of TCA used much lower than monotherapy dose, especially with fluoxetine and paroxetine.
    - ▫ Recommend starting dose of 25 mg nortriptyline.
    - ▫ Monitor plasma levels and ECG.
- Successful combinations in general adult studies include:
  - √ Fluvoxamine and moclobemide
  - √ Bupropion and TCA
  - √ Fluoxetine and desipramine
  - √ Nortriptyline and sertraline
  - √ Nortriptyline and fluoxetine
  - √ Mirtazapine and paroxetine
  - √ Bupropion and venlafaxine
    - ▫ Theoretical risk of increasing hypertensive side effect of venlafaxine by increasing plasma venlafaxine (more hypertensive) and blocking formation of active metabolite ODV (less hypertensive).

DEPRESSION THERAPY DECISION PATHWAYS

Definitions

- *Refractory:* Unresponsive to adequate trial of full range of effective therapies (< 25% symptom reduction).
- *Responsive:* At least 50% improvement on the HAM-D; often reflects only a partial response, with significant residual symptoms that may continue to be emotionally painful and limiting.
- *Remission:* No longer depressed; in the nondepressed range of the HAM-D.

Refractoriness or Partial Response (25–75% symptom reduction)

- Often due to inadequate doses of medication.
  - √ This is a concern in treating elders, because there is always a problem deciding on the balance between provoking side effects and maximizing the drug's action (or combination of drugs).

- In partially responsive or refractory patients push therapy to maximum tolerated doses within the therapeutic range.
  - √ Side effects/toxic effects can be minimized with careful observation and patient follow-up.

Algorithms for Drug Therapy of Depression

- Not well established for geriatric depression.
- Guidelines for timing of decisions are approximate and often have to be extended or reduced for a given patient.
- An important principle: It generally takes longer to reach therapeutic dose levels in side-effect sensitive elders.
  - √ It is believed that the therapeutic response also may be delayed by weeks in elders compared to younger patients.
    - ▫ Hence the recommended extension of the therapeutic trial period from 8 to 12 weeks in geriatric depression drug studies.

Decision-making pathways are based on moving in an organized manner among drugs that influence different transmitter systems—e.g., SSRIs, dual/mixed action agents, noradrenergic drugs, dopaminergic agents, serotonin blockers, and so on. In practice, such a clearly defined rational approach is not always feasible, though it forms the best basis for decision making.

Stage 1: Drug Monotherapy (Nonbipolar Depression)

Institute first-line drug in geriatric doses with or without concurrent formal psychotherapy.

- Drug of first choice
  - √ Previously untreated patients:
    - ▫ With mild to moderate depression, first line is currently an SSRI.
    - ▫ Other first-line drugs include bupropion SR, an SNRI (venlafaxine XR), or an NaSSA (mirtazapine) (the latter two for more severe depressions).
    - ▫ Take into account family history of AD drug responsiveness.
  - √ Previously treated patients with recurrence:
    - ▫ Use a previously effective drug first, especially if it is one of the newer-generation antidepressants (SSRI or newer antidepressants).
    - ▫ Use secondary amine (e.g., nortriptyline) for patients previously responsive to TCAs who have a history of failed trials of other newer agents.

- Decision point: Increase dose to maximum tolerated therapeutic dose
  - √ At 3–6 weeks, if there is no response at all at initial target therapeutic dose.
  - √ At 4–7 weeks if significant partial response (> 50%) at initial target therapeutic dose. Continue to full 12-week trial.
- Decision point: at 3–8 weeks of *maximal therapeutic dose*
  - √ If no response at all, switch antidepressants.
  - √ If partial response, use one of the following augmentation strategies for 3-week trial:
    - Combine with a second antidepressant (e.g., add bupropion, venlafaxine, or mirtazapine to SSRI; caution with bupropion and venlafaxine combinations—monitor blood pressure).
    - Add lithium (plasma level target of 0.3–0.7 mmol/l), especially if there is some indication of bipolarity or cyclical pattern to the depression.
    - Add T_3 (25–50 μg).
    - Consider atypical antipsychotic, especially if there are intense or frankly psychotic depressive symptoms; *avoid risperidone in presence of comorbid EPS.*
    - Alternatively, go directly to stage 2 (see comment below).
    - Buspirone 15–30 and pindolol 1–5 mg tid have been used as augmenters, but are probably ineffective.

Stage 2: Monotherapy Trial of Second Antidepressant

Substitute an antidepressant with a different mode of action than that used in stage 1 and continue drug monotherapy. Drugs with similar action (e.g., SSRIs) may be substituted with no washout in otherwise healthy patients who metabolize drugs well. Agents with long half-lives (e.g., fluoxetine) require washout to avoid induction of serotonin syndrome in vulnerable patients, if another serotonergic agent is introduced in high doses. If discontinuing, be aware that some agents have withdrawal syndrome potential—most SSRIs (especially paroxetine but not fluoxetine), mirtazapine, venlafaxine, and sometimes TCAs.

Table 1.13. Drug Choices for Stage 2 Trial

From	To	Alternate Choice
bupropion SR	SSRI, venlafaxine XR	mirtazapine, nortriptyline
nefazodone	SSRI, venlafaxine XR	bupropion SR, mirtazapine, nortriptyline
SSRI	venlafaxine XR, bupropion SR	nortriptyline, mirtazapine, different SSRI
TCA	venlafaxine XR, SSRI	bupropion SR, mirtazapine
venlafaxine XR	SSRI	bupropion SR, mirtazapine, nortriptyline

Note: Role of duloxetine not well established for elders and not yet approved by licencing bodies.

- Decision point: At 3–8 weeks, if no/very partial response on full therapeutic dose.
  - √ Add augmentation, as in stage 1.
  - √ Consider combination therapy.
  - √ Or begin washout period—varies based on drug used—and go to stage 3.

Stage 3: Monotherapy Substitution

- Substitute drug and class not already tried: MAOI, SNRI, NaSSA, or secondary amine TCA.
- Decision point at 3–8 weeks if no/very partial response on full therapeutic dose.
  - √ Add augmentation, as in step 2.
  - √ Initiate combination therapies not yet tried, such as
    - ▫ Bupropion SR plus SSRI
    - ▫ TCA plus SSRI
    - ▫ Mirtazapine plus SSRI
  - √ Or go to next stage.

Stage 4: Substitution with Fourth-Line Interventions

These interventions include MAOIs, which require full washout (see p. 113).

Stage 5: Combinations and Aumentation Strategies Not Already Attempted

If still no response, consider hospitalization or, with great caution in expert hands, unconventional combinations and therapies, such as TCA plus MAOI, vagus nerve stimulation, or repetitive transcranial magnetic stimulation.

At any stage, hospitalization and ECT are considerations for states of extreme suffering, psychotic depression, suicidal potential, or declining physical state secondary to the depression. ECT is the most effective treatment available for depression, but generally not before a full trial of medication to the third or fourth stage; often not acceptable to patients and families.

There is no general agreement on the best way to proceed at each stage. Augmentation has the advantage of not requiring a period of AD discontinuance, with possible delays during washout periods and/or loss of partial effect. Response may be faster than in switching classes. Some regimens recommend switching medications and continuing monotherapy for one or two more stages before augmentation.

Concurrent IPT, CBT, or supportive dynamic psychotherapy is indicated for augmentation at each step; may be effective first-stage monotherapy for mild depression with strong psychosocial determinants.

Decision Points

Decision making is challenging with partially or nonresponsive patients. Time to each decision point may be extended or reduced, based on clinical judgment and experience with the patient. Treatment pathway recommendations should be used as guidelines, not gospel.

If at 2 weeks, of monotherapy, no response at all in any of the depressive symptoms being monitored (e.g., sleep improvement, reduction in anxiety, slight increase in energy, "brief moments" of relief of depression), there is little likelihood of response to the particular drug. Switch or augmentation should be considered; however, some advise waiting 4 weeks before deciding.

- Augmentation regimens usually show some effect at 2–4 weeks
  - √ Occasionally take up to 6 weeks.
- At each stage, if there is remission with primary therapy or augmentation, begin continuation phase, followed by maintenance phase as appropriate.
- Note the goal of treatment is full remission.
  - √ Residual symptoms of depression are a prognostic indicator for relapse.

Additional Concerns in Combination Therapies

- Use neuroleptics routinely in delusional depression (see p. 35).
- Anxiolytics/hypnotics useful in first 2 weeks of therapy to manage comorbid anxiety/sleep disorder (see Chapter 4, p. 371).
- In extreme cases of nonresponse, multiple drug combinations may be tried.
  - √ Examples of reported cases of successful, more extreme combination therapies include
    - ▫ Lithium, doxepin, and phenelzine
    - ▫ MAOI, TCA, and lithium
- Combination therapies are obviously more difficult to manage, especially in frail elders, and should be used with extreme caution and monitoring.
  - √ Note danger of serotonin syndrome in many combinations, including lithium, bupropion and SSRIs, and the MAOIs.
- Educate patient and/or substitute decision makers about hazards.

- Document decisions carefully, including reasons for unusual intervention strategies.
  - √ Patients should be hospitalized for these trials.
  - √ Danger of interacting side effects (e.g., cardiovascular, hypotensive, neurological, or anticholinergic).

Follow-up and Education

Patients and families should be kept closely involved in the decision-making process, provided with rationales for decisions at each step. Prolonged trials of medication is a long and often very difficult and painful experience for patients who are suffering; their hope must be maintained to prevent despair.

Many patients and families fear medications for various reasons, including bad past experiences, cultural beliefs, or drug myths. Education and open discussion about decision-making are very important.

Communication about side effects will improve compliance, as will moving therapy along at the patient's tolerated pace of dose increase or drug substitution. Strategies include offering the option of calling the physician at home (in appropriate cases) and frequent clinic visits every week during dose/drug change/increase phases. Once the patient stabilizes and the continuation phase begins, visits can be spread out to 2–4 weeks, depending on tolerance and compliance issues. When cognitive or frailty factors make decision-making by the patient inappropriate, close contact with family or primary caregiver is essential at every visit.

SIDE EFFECTS OF ANTIDEPRESSANTS

- Tolerance to AD side effects, especially those of SSRIs, may develop over time.
  - √ Patients should be encouraged to put up with minor side effects in the expectation that mild symptoms will remit spontaneously as treatment continues.
- Patients may acquire idiosyncratic hypersensitivity to a given drug. A history of such is a contraindication to administration

Safety Concerns

- Caution advised when using the more toxic HCA and MAOI antidepressants.
- Special caution regarding safety concerns with patients
  - √ Who have a history of impulsivity.
  - √ Who are not communicative about thoughts and conflicts.

√ Who are not well known to the therapist.
√ Who fail to form effective treatment alliance.
√ Who are in a high-risk group (i.e., alcohol or other drug abuse, chronic pain, newly diagnosed severe illness, recent loss or unresolved grief reaction, family or personal history of suicidality, isolation and lack of confidants, high intensity of anxiety, intense preoccupation with suicidal ideation, recent disclosure of suicidal intent and availability of a method).

Anticholinergic Side Effects

Result from muscarinic cholinergic receptor blockade.

- Especially evident with HCA antidepressants (especially amitriptyline, clomipramine, doxepin, and protriptyline) low-potency antipsychotics, and drugs used therapeutically for their anticholinergic effects (e.g., benztropine, and oxybutinin).
  √ Reported anticholinergic effects with some SSRIs (e.g., acute angle closure glaucoma with fluoxetine and paroxetine).
  √ Uncommon with MAOIs.

Table 1.14. Anticholinergic Drugs

Drugs with Potentially Dangerous Anticholinergic Effects When Either Used alone or in Combination with Other Anticholinergic Agents	Common Indications
atropine solution, cyclopentolate, homatropine, tropicamide	Mydriatrics
atropine solution, *ipratropium*	Bronchodilators
atropine sulphate	Diarrhea
Brompheniramine, cetirizine, *diphenhydramine,* chlorpheniramine, clemastine, cyproheptadine, hydroxyzine, methdilazine, mepyramine, promethazine, trimeprazine	Antihistamines
codeine, *meperidine*	Analgesics
colchicines, furosemide, isosorbide dinitrate, prednisolone, theophylline	Possible anticholinergic agents
coumadin	Anticoagulant
cyclobenzaprine, orphenadrine	Skeletal muscle relaxants

(*cont.*)

Continued

Drugs with Potentially Dangerous Anticholinergic Effects When Either Used alone or in Combination with Other Anticholinergic Agents	Common Indications
dipyridamole, isosorbide, nifedipine	Antianginal/antihypertensive
donnatal (hyoscynamine + atropine + scopolamine)	GI spasm
hyoscine, cyclizine, dimenhydrinate, meclozine, trimethobenzamide, *promethazine,* prochlorperazine	Antiemetics
hyoscynamine, belladonna alkaloids, clindinium bromide, dicycloverine, glycopyrrolate, isopropamide, propantheline, ranitidine, methscopolamine bromide	Peptic ulcer, GI spasm
hyoscynamine, methenamine, oxybutinin, flavoxate, dicyclomine, propantheline	GU antispasmodics
procainamide, quinidine, disopyramide, digoxin	Antiarrhythmic
tolterodine	GU urgency/incontinence
trihexyphenidyl, benztropine, procyclidine, biperiden, ethopropazine, amantadine	Antiparkinsonian agents, antiviral agents, treatment of neuroleptic side effects
All TCAs—especially amitriptyline, imipramine doxepin, trimipramine, nortriptyline, protriptyline, amoxapine, maprotiline, clomipramine, trazodone SSRIs–paroxetine Atypical antidepressants venlafaxine	Antidepressants
Antipsychotics—most typicals (especially chlorpromazine, thioridazine, fluphenazine, prochlorperazine, thiothixene); clozapine; olanzapine (at higher doses)	Neuroleptics

Note: Reference sources for information in table: Salzman (2001) and Mintzer et al. (2000), Maxmen and Ward (2002).
Most potent anticholinergies are italicized.

- May be dose-responsive (but not always).
  - √ Begin with low doses and increase slowly to reduce intensity.
- *Note:* Dangers of anticholinergic toxicity increase greatly when anticholinergic drugs are used concurrently; *avoid combinations.*
- Bethanechol (cholinergic agent) is sometimes helpful for management of some symptoms.
  - √ Observe patient for cholinergic side effects (e.g., diarrhea, abdominal cramps, increased tearing).

Table 1.15. Anticholinergic Potency of Drugs

atropine
trihexyphenidyl
benztropine
amitriptyline
protriptyline
doxepin
imipramine
nortriptyline
desipramine
maprotiline
amoxapine
trazodone
phenelzine

Listed in descending rank order.

Table 1.16. Anticholinergic Symptoms

System Affected	Symptoms	Comments
Cardiovascular	• Tachycardia √ May worsen angina. √ Induce CHF. √ Induce supraventricular tachyarrhythmia. √ Orthostatic hypotension	Reduce dose or discontinue drug.
Central nervous system	Central anticholinergic effects include • Mild memory/ concentration impairment • Confusion/disorientation • Impaired recent memory • Gait impairment • Tremor • Frank delirium √ In 6% of patients treated with TCAs √ Agitation √ Hallucinations (visual) √ Delusions √ Assaultiveness	• CNS effects correlated with TCA concentration. > 450 ng/L. √ May be prolonged • Impaired recent memory, especially in patients with comorbid depression and dementia. • Delirium affects 15–38% of elderly medical inpatients; often associated with elevated serum anticholinergic activity (see table of anticholinergic drugs), infection, and elevated white count. √ agitation may be misdiagnosed and lead to neuroleptic that aggravates the problem.
Eye	• Blurred vision • Glaucoma • Eye irritation with contact lenses • Reduced lacrimation • Corneal damage secondary to reduced lacrimation.	Pupillary dilatation/inability to accommodate • Manage with √ bethanechol 10–30 mg tid √ 1% pilocarpine drops qid √ magnifying glasses Glaucoma • Narrow-angle glaucoma contraindication for anticholinergic agents. • Open-angle glaucoma a relative contraindication, with close follow-up. √ In very unusual circumstances (e.g., unresponsiveness to any other medication regimen), anticholinergic antidepressants may be used if patient is well controlled with eye drops. √ Monitor intraocular pressures very closely.

(cont.)

Continued

System Affected	Symptoms	Comments

Gastrointestinal	• Dry mouth (xerostomia)
	• Constipation
		Dry mouth
		• May interfere with appetite and nutrition (e.g., specific food avoidance and involuntary weight loss).
		• Increased water intake
		  √ May produce water intoxication.
		  √ Dilutional hyponatremia may be confused with SIADH.
		• Dryness can cause dentures to irritate or become ill-fitting.
		• Mouth ulceration, candida infection.
		• Loss of porcelain fillings.
		• Impaired perception of taste.
		• Increased dental cavities
		• Pain may be very distressing and cause agitation.
		• Management
		  √ Stimulation of salivary flow via sugarless gum, candies, artificial salivary fluid, (1% pilocarpine solution rinse, bethanechol 5–10 mg sublingually or 10–30 mg p.o. once/twice daily) chewing carrots or celery.
		
		Constipation
		• May be associated with
		  √ Stomatitis
		  √ Fecal impaction
		• May progress to paralytic ileus, especially if other anticholinergic drugs coadministered.
		• Prevent with
		  √ Increased liquids and bulk in diet
		    □ Bulk laxatives (e.g., Metamucil or docusate sodium)
		• Manage more serious constipation with cathartic laxatives, enemas, glycerine suppositories.
		  √ Consider bethanechol 10 mg/day to 30 mg bid.
		    □ Take 1 hour before or 2 hours after meals to avoid nausea

Psychiatric	• Anxiety • Worsening of depression	Reduce or discontinue drug.
Skin and appendages	• Inhibition of sweating • Dry skin • May rarely induce severe hyperthermia	• Reduce drug dose. • Apply hydrating skin lotion. • Discontinue drug in severe cases. • Caution in hot-weather outdoor activities.

Urinary	• Hesitancy, dribbling
	• Atonic bladder
	• Urinary retention
		• Retention may lead to urinary obstruction, necessitating catheterization.
		  √ Especially in men with prostatism, but may also occur in women.
		  √ Predisposes to urinary tract infection.
		  √ In the extreme, renal failure.
		
		• Management of retention
		  √ Physical workup for other causes of obstruction (e.g., prostatism).
		  √ Discontinue anticholinergic drug.
		  √ Consider bethanechol 10–30 mg tid (if no out-flow obstruction).
		  √ Emergency catheterization for acute obstruction.

Some symptoms exacerbated by even modestly anticholinergic agents

- Glaucoma
- Xerostomia
- Constipation
- Urinary retention
- Tachycardia in patients with preexisting myocardial ischemia

Symptoms of extreme cases of anticholinergic toxicity include

- Ataxia
- Hyperreflexia
- Seizures
- Coma
- Circulatory collapse

Illnesses in which symptoms may be worsened by anticholinergic agents include

- Dementia
- Angina
- CHF
- Diabetes mellitus
- Glaucoma
- Urinary dysfunction

Note: Although memory impairment is a side-effect risk with some anticholinergic antidepressants, the net effect of treating depression in elders is to improve cognitive performance overall.

Management of Anticholinergic Side Effects

Some side effects, remit spontaneously over time e.g., nausea, while others do not (e.g., tachycardia).

Prevent anticholinergic side effects by

- Minimizing dose of anticholinergic agents.
- Avoiding coadministration of drugs with anticholinergic properties.
  - √ If there is already a high anticholinergic burden of medication, even mildly anticholinergic drugs (e.g., paroxetine, venlafaxine) may precipitate side effects.
- Preventing anticholinergic rebound by slowly tapering doses.
- Being alert to potential anticholinergic side effects.
- Informing patients and caregivers about warning signs and dangers of anticholinergic side effects.
- Managing mild symptoms and encouraging patients to continue with effective therapies.
- Suggesting switching agents rather than using bethanechol, to avoid side effects.

Management of Delirium

- Treat as an emergency.
  - √ Marker for increased mortality and morbidity.
- Review medications, stop potentially offending drugs.
- Trial of physostigmine for most urgent cases.
  - √ Caution with heart disease, asthma, diabetes, peptic ulcer, bladder/bowel obstruction.
  - √ Be very cautious in elders and watch for
    - ▫ Vomiting, diaphoresis, abdominal pain, seizures, cardiac arrhythmia (sinus arrest, bradycardia)
  - √ Monitor BP, pulse
  - √ Dose—0.1 mg sub cutaneously, or by very slow IV drip (i.e., 1 mg over at least 2 minutes)
  - √ Observe clinical state—improvement occurs within 20 minutes
  - √ Repeat dose after 1/2–1 hour if no improvement
  - √ Administer with ECG monitoring, preferably by anesthetist or cardiologist
  - √ Manage severe agitation

See page 254 for full management of delirium

Extrapyramidal Side Effects

- Data from controlled clinical studies scarce.
- Most associated with amoxapine.
- May occur in elders treated with SSRIs.
  - √ Risk may be less with sertraline than fluoxetine (data not robust).
  - √ Increased risk at high doses and if combined with neuroleptic.
- Reactions include
  - √ Dystonic reactions
  - √ Akathisia
  - √ Exacerbation of parkinsonian symptoms such as tremor
- Manage by reducing dose or switching drugs.

Seizure Potential

- Seizure risk not reliably determined for elders.
- Rates for TCAs based on methodologically suspect studies.
- Possible risk factor for seizure induction include:
  - √ Advanced age
  - √ Major depression (above the increased risk associated with treatments and concurrent illnesses)
  - √ Prior ECT
  - √ High doses/peak plasma concentrations of drugs that lower seizure threshold

√ Concurrent use of drugs that inhibit metabolizing enzymes, especially CYP2D6 with HCAs
√ Concurrent use of drugs that lower seizure threshold (e.g., neuroleptics)

Table 1.17. Estimates of Seizure Potential by Drug

Drug	Seizure Incidence
bupropion IR	0.4%
bupropion SR	0.1%
TCAs	0.4–1.0% (data unreliable)
fluoxetine	0.2%
paroxetine	0.1%
sertraline	< 0.1%
venlafaxine	0.26%

Note: General adult data.

Cardiovascular Side Effects

Frequency and severity vary widely among antidepressant classes and drugs within classes. Most common in patients with preexisting cardiac pathology

- Cardiac side effects of TCAs (see p. 102).
- Avoid all TCAs or review planned use with a cardiologist in presence of preexisting conduction disorders.
- Discontinue if arrhythmia emerges during therapy.

Cardiac conduction disorders

- Nonspecific ST and T wave changes
- Prolonged PR interval
- Widened QRS complex
- QTc > 450 μ sec may be contraindication to use of TCA
- Avoid TCAs in patients with preexisting BBB

Congestive heart failure

- Decreased cardiac output, myocardial depression.
- Pedal edema—avoid trazodone and tertiary amines.

Blood pressure disturbance

- Hypotension or hypertension.
- MAOIs cause more hypotension than TCAs.

Heart rate disturbance

- Tachycardia, especially with anticholinergic drugs.

Head-to-head studies of cardiac side effects are still few in number.

- As a class, SSRIs have more favorable cardiac side-effect profile.

  - √ Do not induce clinically relevant cardiac side effects in elders (although sporadic case reports of postural hypotension, cardiac arrhythmias and unstable angina emerge from time to time).
- Hypotension: May be associated with mirtazapine, venlafaxine.
- Hypertension: Mild forms associated with venlafaxine.

Falls

Safest to assume that all antidepressants are associated with increased danger of falls (as are drugs from other classes, including antipsychotics, sedative hypnotics, and antianxiety drugs).

- *Note:* Depression, anxiety disorders, and agitation probably are independent risk factors for falling in elders
- SSRIs about equal to nortriptyline; no data on newer antidepressants.
- Falls may be caused by syncope (i.e., sudden transient loss of consciousness).
  - √ Both HCAs and nontricyclics (e.g. fluoxetine) implicated in syncope in elders.
- Concurrent medications also may be associated with increased risk of falls.
  - √ Sedatives, tranquillizers, cardiac drugs, antiparkinsonian drugs, thyroid replacement drugs, anticonvulsants, insulin, oral hypoglycemic agents, oral glucocorticoids, estrogen.
- Pathophysiology of falls probably multidetermined.
  - √ CVS instability most common—hypotension or cardiac arrhythmia
  - √ Primary gait instability (evidenced by increased postural sway tests)
  - √ Primary neurological effect suspected in some patients reporting sudden loss of muscle tone in legs
  - √ General weakness and debility
  - √ Sedation
- Incorporate gait evaluation and preventive measures when prescribing antidepressants.
  - √ Risk of falls not contraindication for antidepressants
  - √ Preventive strategies include program of muscle strengthening and balance training, Tai Chi group exercise, professional home hazard assessment and modification, limitation of concurrent psychotropic medications.
- May lead to hip fractures and other injuries in elders.
- Risk is greatest in early phases of therapy and diminishes with time (except with MAOIs).

Table 1.18. Relative Frequency of HCA versus SSRI Side Effects

SSRI > TCA	TCA > SSRI
Nausea	Dry mouth
Insomnia, vivid dreaming	Somnolence
Nervousness, agitation	Dizziness, hypotension
GI disturbances (anorexia, diarrhea, flatulence, constipation)	Constipation
Sexual dysfunction	Urinary obstruction
Headache	Palpitations
Weight loss	Glaucoma

Serotonin Syndrome

Serotonin syndrome is a potentially fatal syndrome produced by increased serotonin activity. It is thought to require almost complete inhibition of the degradation and elimination of serotonin from the synaptic cleft—that is, > 85% blockade of MAO-A and MAO-B and inhibition of serotonin reuptake.

- Other contributing factors include
  - √ Increased and/or decreased functioning of the cholinergic and dopaminergic systems.
  - √ Possible deficits in the peripheral serotonin metabolism, stimulating release of serotonin.
- Incidence is not well studied.
  - √ Full syndrome is rare.
  - √ Incidence of milder syndromes is not known but may be common.
- Most cases reported with combination of SSRIs and MAOIs, but also occurs with SSRIs alone.
  - √ May occur with combination of HCAs with SSRIs or MAOIs, possibly including selegiline.
- Syndrome may also occur with any of the SSRI or dual-action antidepressants, including SNRIs, NaSSAs, MAOIs, HCAs, and possibly buspirone, when
  - √ Combined with other serotonergic compounds, such as other antidepressants, l-tryptophan, selegiline, tramadol, possibly lithium carbonate, and carbamazepine.
  - √ Used in high doses.
- Onset abrupt.
  - √ Usually hours, but sometimes days after addition of serotomimetic agent.
- Duration
  - √ In younger patients remits within 24 hours of discontinuing agents, but may be much longer in elderly.
- Diagnosis: Coincidental use of a known serotonergic agent and at least three of the following:

- √ *Mental status changes:* restlessness (45%), confusion (42%), hypomania/agitation (21%), coma
- √ *Motor system changes:* myoclonus (34%), hyperreflexia, incoordination, rigidity, tremor
    - ▫ Myoclonus may be very significant in the full syndrome
- √ *Autonomic instability:* nausea, diarrhea, vomiting, shivering, tachycardia, postural hypotension, fever, mydriasis
- √ *Other symptoms of serotonin syndrome:* dizziness and risk of falls, delirium with delusions and hallucinations, seizure, diaphoresis, tachypnea, cardiac arrhythmia, mutism, trismus

- Severity
    - √ Ranges from mild to life threatening.
        - ▫ Possible that common SSRI side effects such as mild tremor, agitation, or diaphoresis are related to mild serotonin syndrome.
- Rule out
    - √ Other causes of symptoms, such as infection (including CNS infection such as meningitis or encephalitis), metabolic disturbance, substance abuse/withdrawal.
    - √ Neuroleptic malignant syndrome (neuroleptic agent begun or dose increased prior to onset of signs and symptoms).

Prevention: washout periods are not well documented for elders. A washout is not recommended when switching from SSRI or SNRI to SNRI, bupropion, nefazodone, mirtazapine or TCA in younger patients, however greater caution is necessary in geriatric patients when switching from one serotonergic compound to another, especially when the first drug has a long or prolonged half-life. There is special risk of serotonin syndrome when switching from SSRI, TCA, nefazodone or from SNRI to RIMA; if switching to clomipramine from SSRI, a washout of 2–3 weeks is necessary.

- Keep in mind extended half-life of drugs in some elderly patients (especially if accompanied by liver or kidney impairment) when calculating washout time from prior therapy.
- Wait at least 2+ weeks in healthy patient before switching from MAOI to SSRI or TCA, and longer in frail, impaired patient.
    - √ Exception is fluoxetine, which requires a washout of 5 weeks, or longer, in susceptible patients.
    - √ Paroxetine, sertraline, citalopram, and fluvoxamine require shorter washout of 14 days.
    - √ Note danger of withdrawal syndromes, especially with paroxetine and venlafaxine.
- Educate caregivers and patient about need for cautions.

Table 1.19. Drugs That Increase Serotonergic Activity

Inhibitors of Serotonin Uptake	Inhibitors of Serotonin Metabolism	Increase Serotonin Synthesis	Increase Serotonin Release	Serotonin Receptor Agonists	Increase Serotonin Activity	Other
amitriptyline	isocarboxazid	L-tryptophan	3,4 methylenedioxy-methamphetamine (ecstasy)	buspirone	lithium (nonspecific)	Electroconvulsive therapy
amphetamine	moclobemide		amphetamines	dihydroergotamine		
citalopram*	phenelzine		cocaine	sumatriptan*		
clomipramine	selegiline		fenfluramine			
cocaine	tranylcypromine		mirtazapine			
dextromethorphan						
escitalopram						
fluoxetine						
fluvoxamine						
imipramine						
meperidine						
nefazodone						
paroxetine						
sertraline						
tramadol						
trazodone						
venlafaxine						

* Sumatriptan has been safely coadministered with SSRIs but caution recommended in elders; case report of serotonin syndrome in monotherapy with citalopram.

Treatment of serotonin syndrome:

- Promptly discontinue offending agent(s).
  - √ In younger patients with mild symptoms, syndrome may remit spontaneously with continued treatment, but this is not an advisable strategy for elders.
- Supportive care
  - √ Fever reduction (although fever is usually mild)
  - √ Fluids
  - √ Mechanical ventilation, if necessary
  - √ Sedation with benzodiazepines (IV route, when indicated by severity)
  - √ Environmental support in cases of delirium
  - √ In more severe cases
    - ▫ Administer postsynaptic serotonin antagonist such as methysergide or cyproheptadine (4–12mg/day in divided doses) or use beta-blocker such as propranolol.

Syndrome of Inappropriate Antidiuretic Hormone Secretion (SIADH)

- Onset may be abrupt, within first few days of beginning treatment, although risk is greatest in first 2–3 weeks after beginning treatment (range 3–120 days).
- Depression has been associated with hyponatremic states.
- Symptoms include:
  - √ Weakness
  - √ Lethargy
  - √ Headache
  - √ Anorexia, nausea
  - √ Muscle cramps
  - √ Confusion, disorientation
  - √ Severe hyponatremia
    - ▫ Hyponatremia (serum Na < 130 mmol/L), low serum osmolarity, less than maximally diluted urine with inappropriately elevated urine osmolarity (> 200 mmol/L), urine sodium excretion too high (> 20mmol/l) for serum sodium concentrations
  - √ Other laboratory tests (renal, adrenal, thyroid) within normal limits (unless another comorbid condition present).
  - √ Convulsions, stupor, coma, death
- Course: Condition usually spontaneously returns to normal within 2–28 days of discontinuing SSRI or other drug.
- Differential diagnoses
  - √ Diuretic use (thiazide or loop diuretics)
  - √ Hyper- or hypovolemia
  - √ GI losses (vomiting, diarrhea, bleeding, intestinal obstruction)

- √ Skin losses (burns, cystic fibrosis)
- √ Edematous states (heart failure, hepatic cirrhosis, nephrotic syndrome with marked hypoalbuminemia)
- √ Renal dysfunction (hypoaldosteronism, Na-wasting nephropathy, renal failure)
- √ Endocrine dysfunction (cortisol deficiency, hypothyroidism)
- √ ADH producing tumors (e.g., small cell lung carcinoma)
- √ Pulmonary disease
- √ Polydipsia (e.g., in dry mouth secondary to anticholinergic medications, or in psychotic disorders)
- √ Reset osmostat syndrome

- Reported risk factors include:
  - √ Age > 65
  - √ Female gender (data unclear)
  - √ Low body weight
  - √ SSRI therapy; also reported (rarely) with tricyclics, MAOIs, and venlafaxine.
    - ▫ There may be crossover effect between SSRI and tricyclic in producing the syndrome (clinical report).
  - √ Concomitant SSRI and carbamazepine, diuretic (especially thiazide), ACE inhibitor, or NSAID
  - √ Possible dose response (i.e., increased risk at higher doses, but also idiosyncratic responses)
  - √ Increased risk if prior hyponatremia with diuretic therapy
  - √ Low sodium diet
  - √ Smoking
- Management
  - √ Prevention includes warning patient about possibility of this complication, monitoring clinical condition, and monitoring serum sodium in first 2–4 weeks in patients most at risk.
  - √ Measure serum sodium levels and urine osmolarity if symptoms emerge.
  - √ Discontinue causal agent (usually the only step necessary if syndrome is not severe).
  - √ Restrict water intake.
  - √ Administer intravenous sodium chloride (3% solution at 0.5ml/min) in more severe cases but avoid too rapid infusion (risk of secondary central pontine myelinolysis)
  - √ Avoid rechallenging patient with offending class of agents.

Weight Side Effects

- Weight gain may be a significant side-effect problem with many antidepressants
- Weight gain during treatment associated with
  - √ Improvement in depression

- √ Pretreatment weight loss (i.e., the greater the weight loss before treatment, the greater the weight gain with treatment)
- √ Specific antidepressant drug
  - ▫ Preliminary data suggest no difference in weight effect between TCA (nortriptyline) and SSRI (paroxetine).
  - ▫ Treatment of depression with TCAs not associated with weight gain in elders.

- Weight loss in elders is an important therapeutic factor, since it is associated with increased frailty and nutritional deficiencies.
- Significant weight gain increases vulnerability to cardiovascular pathology and diabetes, but may be welcomed in frail, poorly-nourished elders.
- May limit acceptance of and compliance with treatment.
- Management
  - √ Recommend weighing patients prior to treatment to assess weight changes.
  - √ Exercise
  - √ Reduce caloric intake
  - √ Switch class of drug

Risks of Breast Cancer

Data conflict on the incidence of breast cancer associated with antidepressants. A recent large study shows *no risk;* another shows *risk with some TCAs and SSRIs* 11–15 years later. Drugs at risk are listed below, but evidence is uncertain, and there are no geriatric-specific data.

- Possible increased risk
  - √ TCAs
    - ▫ Amoxapine
    - ▫ Clomipramine
    - ▫ Desipramine
    - ▫ Trimipramine
    - ▫ None of these is now routinely used for long-term therapy with elders.
  - √ SSRIs
    - ▫ Paroxetine
- No increased risk identified to date
  - √ HCAs
    - ▫ Amitriptyline
    - ▫ Maprotiline
    - ▫ Nortriptyline
    - ▫ Protriptyline
  - √ SSRIs
    - ▫ Sertraline
    - ▫ Fluoxetine

- Increased prolactin levels associated with increased tumor gowth.
  - √ SSRIs (especially paroxetine)

Sexual Side Effects

- High incidence of sexual side effects with most antidepressants but not well studied in elders.
- Do not assume sexuality is unimportant to elders purely on the basis of age.
- Evaluate each case individually.
  - √ Although many elders remain sexually active and/or concerned about sexuality, many also do not care.
- Continuing interest in sexuality in elders depends on many factors:
  - √ Availability of a desirable partner
  - √ Physiological capacity
  - √ Physical health—cardiovascular disorders, renal/urological disorders, liver disease, pulmonary disorders, neurological disorders, past surgical procedures, nutritional deficiencies, endocrine disorders all may impair sexual desire and performance.
  - √ Cognitive capacities
  - √ Depressive disorder—incidence of reduced sexual desire 31–72% (general adult data)
  - √ Preservation of libido
  - √ Reaction to perceived social stigma
  - √ Cultural norms
  - √ Practical considerations such as living arrangements (e.g., LTC facility)

The physiology of sexual function is highly complex, affected by a myriad of internal and external factors. Hypotheses re. neurotransmitters and sexual function include:

- Libido mediated by limbic system.
  - √ Increased by dopamine.
  - √ Inhibited by serotonin.
- Erection/vaginal lubrication.
  - √ D2 and adrenergic stimulation facilitate erection.
  - √ Alpha 1-adrenoreceptors' tonic action necessary to maintain penis in flaccid state.
    - ▫ Priapism caused by alpha-adrenergic antagonism (e.g., induced by trazodone).
- Orgasm/ejaculation.
  - √ Alpha 1-adrenoreceptor activation facilitates emission phase of fluid secretion and closes urethral sphincter.
    - ▫ Requires cholinergic action to facilitate opening.
    - ▫ Parasympathetic system influences ejaculation.

- √ Alpha1 blockade may produce contraction of smooth muscle, leading to painful ejaculation.
  - ▫ Anticholinergic drugs block parasympathetic action.
  - ▫ Cholinergic blockade and increased serotonin activity inhibit orgasm/ejaculation.
- Antidepressants less associated with sexual side effects
  - √ Nefazodone
  - √ Bupropion
  - √ Mirtazapine
  - √ Moclobemide

Table 1.20. Psychotropic Medications Associated with Sexual Impairment

SSRIs
- Widely varying reports from 2% to 43%
  - √ Geriatric data and relevance to elders not available
- Bupropion and nefazodone lowest rates—about 25%
- Paroxetine and mirtazapine highest rates—about 42%

Irreversible MAOIs
- M/F—80/57%

TCAs
- M/F—50/27–92%

Trazodone
- Especially within first month
  - √ May occur up to 18 months

SNRI
- Venlafaxine

Benzodiazepines
- Alprazolam
- Diazepam
- Clonazepam

Mood stabilizers
- Lithium
- Carbamazepine

Note: Examples of incidence are from general adult data.

Sexual side-effect symptoms include:

- √ Delayed orgasm
- √ Delayed ejaculation
- √ Loss or blunting of sexual interest
- √ Loss of sexual sensation
- √ Painful ejaculation
- √ Priapism
- Requires rapid intervention; may be irreversible after 6–8 hours.
- Prevention
  - √ Use agents with low incidence of sexual side-effects.

Clinical management strategies include:

- √ Pretreatment detailed evaluation of sexual concerns, habits, and responsiveness.
- √ Sexual counseling re side effects of drugs.
- √ Active sex inquiry.
  - Minority of patients, especially elders, spontaneously report problems.
- √ Behavioral interventions and coaching
- √ Investigation of symptoms via diagnostic tests.

Pharmacological management strategies (general adult data) include:

- √ Reduce dosage.
  - Risk relapse of depressive symptoms.
- √ Wait: mild symptoms occasionally, but not usually, remit spontaneously.
- √ Switch agents (usually necessary).
  - Try bupropion, nefazodone, moclobemide, mirtazapine.
  - Sometimes switching to another drug in the same family (e.g., another SSRI), alleviates problem.
- √ Consider 3-day drug holidays.
  - Not recommended.
  - Difficult to manage and risks discontinuation reactions or fostering of noncompliance.
- √ Adjunctive therapy appropriate in selected cases (doses adjusted to about half of recommended adult dose).
  - Caution recommended for elders because of side-effect potential; very little data.
  - Sildenafil
    1. Caution in patients with preexisting cardiovascular disease.
    2. Dose in elders not specifically determined.
    3. Try 25 mg 1 hour before intercourse; if ineffective but tolerated, increase to 50–100 mg.
    4. Special caution in patients taking drugs that inhibit CYP3A4 (see Table 1.32, p. 95).
    5. Do not combine with trazodone in males (risk of priapism).
  - Methylphenidate 5–15 mg/d
  - Bupropion 75–100 mg/d
    1. Caution with fluoxetine: Increases serum concentration of bupropion and lowers seizure threshold.
  - Buspirone 15–30 mg/day
  - Mirtazapine 15 mg HS
  - Bethanechol 5–10 mg 30 min. prior to sexual activity

- 5-HT2 / 3 antagonists
  1. Cyproheptadine 2–4 mg before coitus
     - Causes sedation/drowsiness on the day following use.
     - Theoretical danger of reversal of antidepressant effect of SRIs because of 5HT2 antagonism.
     - Not recommended for elders.
  2. Nefazodone—no geriatric data for this indication.
- Yohimbine 2.2–5.4 mg/day
  1. Alpha-2 adrenergic antagonist.
  2. Causes agitation/anxiety/panic.
  3. Not recommended for elders.
- Dopaminergic agents
  1. Amantadine 50–200 mg/day
  2. Pramipexole

Cognitive Effects

Table 1.21. Effect of Classes of Antidepressants on Cognitive Function

Antidepressant Class	Effect on Cognition
MAOIs	Little effect
NaSSA, SNRI	No data, but generally well tolerated
SSRIs	Little objective effect; subjective complaints of reduced concentration common
HCAs	Secondary memory retrieval

Table 1.22. Effect of Specific Antidepressants on Cognition

Drug	Effect on Cognitive Performance
Amitriptyline	Impaired concentration, reaction time, secondary memory
Trazodone	Impaired concentration
Sertraline	No effect on memory, or may improve memory
Moclobemide	May improve memory slightly
Nortriptyline (higher plasma levels)	Impaired verbal memory and free recall

Sleep Effects

Table 1.23. Effects of Antidepressants on Sleep

Effect	Drugs
Decreased sleep latency	Most antidepressants, except fluoxetine, sertraline, paroxetine
Total sleep time increased	Amitriptyline, nefazodone, trimipramine
Total sleep time decreased	Fluoxetine, venlafaxine
Sleep time unaffected	Mirtazapine, paroxetine, trazodone
Deceased REM activity	Most antidepressants, except bupropion, nefazodone, trimipramine
Increased REM latency	Most antidepressants, except bupropion, nefazodone, phenelzine, tranylcypromine

Note: General adult data.

RECEPTOR AFFINITY–SIDE-EFFECT RELATIONSHIP

Table 1.24. Effects of Neuroreceptor Antagonism or Stimulation

Action on Neuroreceptors	Associated Clinical Effects
Alpha adrenergic receptor antagonism	Reflex tachycardia Postural hypotension Dizziness Impaired ejaculation, decreased libido, priapism, anorgasmia Sedation
Muscarinic cholinergic antagonism	Dry mouth Blurred vision Constipation Urinary retention Sinus tachycardia Cognitive impairment
H1 histamine antagonism	Sedation Hypertension Weight gain
5HT2 stimulation	Agitation Akathisia Anxiety Panic attacks Insomnia: 5HT2A/2C involved in regulation of slow wave sleep Sexual dysfunction
5HT3 stimulation	Nausea GI distress Diarrhea Headache

Table 1.25. Choosing Antidepressant Drugs to Address Interaction of Side Effect and Clinical Condition

Therapeutic Concerns	Drug Choice
Intolerance of anticholinergic side effects	Avoid HCA use.
Post MI, cardiovascular effects (especially orthostatic hypotension), severe ischemic heart disease, some conduction abnormalities	SSRIs drugs of choice; HCAs contraindicated post MI and with ischemic heart disease; in general, avoid TCAs in presence of other CVS problems but still necessary in severe comorbid depression unresponsive to other antidepressants and in depression associated with pain; increased tachycardia with TCAs but less with SSRIs.
Hypertension	Avoid bupropion and possibly venlafaxine.
Severe depression (melancholia)	Secondary amine or SNRI may be more effective; SSRIs may be less effective.
Concerns about safety in overdose	Avoid HCAs; use SSRIs, NaSSA, bupropion, SNRI.

(cont.)

Continued

Therapeutic Concerns	Drug Choice
Comorbid anxiety	Use SSRIs, SNRI, NaSSA. Management *in absence of dementia* includes increasing antidepressant (non-TCA) to maximum dose; adding an anxiolytic (e.g., lorazepam, oxazepam, buspirone); switching to more anxiolytic antidepressant (e.g., mirtazapine). *In presence of dementia* use greater caution in increasing medication or adding anxiolytic; consider AChEI or atypical antipsychotic.
Oversedation	Use bupropion, some SSRIs, venlafaxine.
Comorbid cognitive deficits or medical illness	Avoid TCAs.
Concerns over drug–drug interactions	Avoid strong inhibitors of P-450 system (e.g., paroxetine, fluoxetine, fluvoxamine, bupropion).
Extrapyramidal comorbidities	First choice: SNRI, NaSSA; second choice: TCAs (secondary amines).
Seizures	Avoid bupropion IR in higher doses; most antidepressants lower seizure threshold.

Table 1.26. Linear versus Nonlinear Pharmacokinetics

Linear Pharmacokinetics	Nonlinear Pharmacokinetics
citalopram escitalopram fluoxetine mCPP (active metabolite of nefazodone) Most TCAs (tertiary and secondary amines) may increase in nonlinear fashion at higher doses • Imipramine (primary compound) linear but metabolite (desipramine) increases in nonlinear fashion with dose increases mirtazapine paroxetine trazodone venlafaxine	bupropion (unclear) clomipramine (at doses > 150mg/day) desipramine fluvoxamine moclobemide nefazodone phenelzine sertraline

DRUG–DRUG INTERACTIONS

There are two forms of interaction:

- *Pharmacodynamic:* One drug affects another mechanism of action.
  - √ Example: SSRI–MAOI combination may produce synergistic effects causing serotonin syndrome.
- *Pharmacokinetic:* One drug affects the metabolism of another.
  - √ Example: Fluoxetine increases plasma level of TCAs by inhibiting P450 enzymes.

Table 1.27. Pharmacokinetic Baselines of Antidepressants

	Bupropion	Citalopram	Fluoxetine	Fluvoxamine	Mirtazapine
Steady state in elders	25% higher		Data sparse. Manufacturer data show no difference to younger. Other data show plasma concentration twice as high in elders.	Clearance may be reduced by up to 50% in elderly.	3–5 days (general adult data)
Elimination half-life (elders vs. general adults)	34 vs. 14 hrs.	36–90 hrs.	Fluoxetine 70 hrs.; norfluoxetine 330 hrs.	25 vs. 22 hrs.	31 hrs. (men), 39 hrs. (women); no significant difference in elders.
Clinical implications	Increased side-effect risk, diminished efficacy, increased toxicity. Reduce starting dose by 25%.	Start at 10 mg dose (half of younger patients).	Proceed cautiously. Start at half adult dose and titrate to therapeutic levels.	Reduce starting dose.	

	Nefazodone	Paroxetine	Sertraline	Venlafaxine
Steady state in elders	50% higher	79 vs. 49 ng/mL	Some increase in concentration.	16% higher
Elimination half-life in elders				13 vs. 10 hrs.
Clinical implications	Reduce adult dose by 50% to start. Much clinical variability, so titrate to optimum dose—may be in same range as general adult population.	Begin at 10 mg (half adult dose) and increase cautiously, since steady-state concentration may increase faster than anticipated.	No strong evidence for dosage adjustments based on age alone.	Dose adjustments may not be necessary based on age effects alone, but comorbidity, physical frailty, warrant caution.

- Most SSRIs are CYP enzyme inhibitors.
  - √ Plasma concentrations of drugs metabolized by these enzymes may be increased.
  - √ Requires increased alertness to possible side effects from coadministered medications.

Table 1.28. Effect of Enzymes on Metabolism of Specific Antidepressants

Drug	Mild/Minimal	Moderate	Substantial
citalopram	2D6		3A4, 2C19
escitalopram			3A4, 2C19
fluoxetine	3A3/4	2C19	2D6, 2C9/10
fluvoxamine	2D6, 1A1	3A3/4	1A2, 2C19
nefazodone			3A3/4
paroxetine			2D6
sertraline	2D6	(n-desmethylsertraline) 3A4	
venlafaxine	2D6, 3A3/4 (n-desmethylvenlafine)		
mirtazapine	1A2, 3A,		2D6
bupropion			2B6 (metabolite HB by 2D6)

Note: Adapted from Preskorn 1997

Table 1.29. Enzyme-Inhibition by Antidepressants

Drug	CYP Enzyme Inhibited*	Examples of *Potential* Drug Interaction Caused by Enzyme Inhibition**
citalopram	No significant CYP inhibition	
escitalopram	little significant CYP inhibition	
†fluoxetine/ norfluoxetine	**2D6, 2C9, 2C19,** 1A2, 3A4/2D6, 3A4, 1A2	alprazolam, amphetamine, analgesics, carbamazepine, clozapine, codeine, dextromethorphan, diazepam, diclofenac, diphenhydramine, donepezil, galantamine, haloperidol, ibuprofen, naproxen, ondansetron, phenytoin, secondary amine TCAs, type IC antiarrhythmics, vinblastin, warfarin
†fluvoxamine	**1A2, 2C19, 3A4** 2D6, 1A1	*Contraindicated with terfenadine, astemizole, cisapride;* caffeine, clozapine, diazepam, mefenamic acid, olanzapine, omeprazol, phenacetin, piroxicam, propranolol, some TCAs, S- and R-warfarin, s-mephenytoin, tacrine, theophylline, thioridazine, tolbutamide
mirtazapine	Minimal effects	
nefazodone	**3A4**	*Contraindicated with terfenadine, astemizole, and cisapride;* alprazolam, antidepressants (sertraline, TCAs, venlafaxine), carbamazepine, cisapride, clonazepam, dexamethasone, dextromethorphan, diazepam, diltiazem, donepezil, erythromycin, estradiol, galantamine, lidocaine, loratadine, midazolam, nifedipine, propafenone, quinidine, R-warfarin, testosterone, triazolam, verapamil, zolpidem

(*cont.*)

Continued

Drug	CYP Enzyme Inhibited*	Examples of *Potential* Drug Interaction Caused by Enzyme Inhibition**
†paroxetine	**2D6, 2C9, 2C19**	amphetamine, analgesics, antiarrhythmics, antipsychotics, dextromethorphan, diphenhydramine, donepezil, galantamine, ondansetron, procyclidine, TCAs, warfarin; *Note:* clozapine and metabolite norclozapine may be increased by 40% with several SSRIs. *Bioavailability of paroxetine increased by cimetidine and decreased by phenytoin.*
sertraline/n-des-methylsertraline	2C9, 2D6, 1A2, 3A4	
venlafaxine	Minimal 2D6 in vitro but possible relevant effects in vivo	Increased anticholinergic effects with TCAs reported

Note: Clinical caution means: introducing concurrent medications at the low end of the therapeutic dosage range; monitoring impact of newly introduced psychotropic on side effects of concurrent medications or determining their blood levels until a steady state of antidepressant therapy is reached.

* Most relevant noted in bold. Require clinical caution

** Potentially increases plasma concentration of these drugs.

† Greatest likelihood to cause clinically significant pharmacokinetic drug-drug interactions.

Table 1.30. Nonpsychotropic Enzyme Inhibitors

CYP1A2	cimetidine, ketoconazole, grapefruit juice
CYP2D6	amiodarone, propafenone, quinidine, cimetidine
CYP3A4	grapefruit juice††

†† Grapefruit juice contains potent inhibitors (furanocoumarin 6, 7′-dihydroxybergamottin and flavenoid naringen) of the P450 system (especially CYP3A4 in the small bowel wall epithelium).

- Probable mechanism is to block action of 3A4 in the gut, thereby increasing plasma concentration of the drug (i.e., inhibits first pass metabolism but does not affect liver metabolism).
- Action occurs with one glass of juice and lasts 24 hours.
- Not always clinically relevant but in elders caution is necessary because of potentially greater sensitivity to increased plasma levels of drugs.

Table 1.31. Drug–Drug Interactions

Drug	Possible Effect of Interaction with SSRIs
AChEIs (donepezil, galantamine)	Cholinergic syndrome
Anticonvulsants (phenytoin, carbamazepine)	Increased levels of anticonvulsant
1C antiarrhythmics	Increased levels of antiarrhythmic
diuretics	SIADH
lithium	Possible SIADH
L-tryptophan	Serotonin syndrome
MAOIs	Serotonin syndrome
Oral anticoagulants	Increased risk of bleeding (especially GI)
Oral hypoglycemics	Hypoglycemia (with fluoxetine)
TCAs	Increase TCA plasma levels; possible increased side effects
Terfenadine, astemizole, and cisapride	Possible serious/fatal ventricular cardiac arrythmia; torsades de pointes (especially fluvoxamine)
Theophylline	Increased theophylline levels with fluvoxamine; coma and seizure risk
Typical antipsychotics	May increase half-life of antipsychotic

(*cont.*)

Continued

Drug	Possible Effect of Interaction with TCAs
IV adrenaline/NA, clonidine, guanethidine	Increased blood pressure (blocks action of centrally active antihypertensives)
Alcohol	Sedation, confusion, decreased reaction time
alprazolam cimetidine disulfiram erythromycin isoniazid methadone methylphenidate SSRIs terbinafine thiazide diuretics verapamil	All increase TCA levels; may enhance both antidepressant effect and TCA toxicity; diuretics enhance hypotensive effect; anxiolytics increase sedation
Amphetamines	Hypertension, arrhythmia, increased plasma concentration of TCA, enhanced tricyclic effect
Anticholinergics	Increased anticholinergic effects, toxic delirium, confusion, visual hallucinations
Anticoagulants	Enhanced anticoagulant effects
Antihistamines	Increased sedation and anticholinergic effects
Antipsychotics (usually typicals but some atypical interactions; e.g., clozapine)	Increased HCA levels; interacting additive side effects (e.g., anticholinergic effect, hypotension, sedation)
Barbiturates	Enhanced sedation, reduced blood levels of TCAs, respiratory depression
Beta blockers	Antagonism of antihypertensive effect
Chloral hydrate	Decreased TCA levels
Doxycycline	Decreased TCA levels
Estrogen	Increased TCA levels; possible lethargy, headache, akathisia, hypotension
Lithium	Increased tremor, myoclonus
MAOIs	*Fatal toxicity*
Methyldopa, l-dopa	Agitation, tremor, tachycardia; enhanced hypotensive effect of methyldopa
Narcotics	Mutual enhancement
Phenytoin	Decreased TCA levels
Procainamide	Prolonged cardiac conduction
Quinidine	Additive antiarrhythmic effects; prolonged cardiac conduction; increased TCA levels
Testosterone	Psychosis reported
Trihexyphenidyl	Decreased TCA levels
Vitamin C	Enhanced excretion of tricyclics

Drug	Possible Effect of Interaction with MAOIs

See Table 1.38, page 121.

Table 1.32. Enzyme Substrates: Inhibitors and Inducers

Enzyme (CYP)	Drugs Metabolized by Enzyme (substrates)	Inhibitors*	Inducers†
2D6	*Analgesics/opiates:* codeine, dextromethorphan, fentanyl, hydrocodone, meperidine, methadone, morphine sulphate, oxycodone *Antiarrhythmics:* flecainide acetate, encainide, mexiletine, propafenone HCL *Antidepressants:* amitriptyline, clomipramine, desipramine, fluoxetine, fluvoxamine, imipramine, maprotiline, mirtazapine, n-desmethylcitalopram, nortriptyline, paroxetine, trazodone, trimipramine, venlafaxine, *Antipsychotics*: aripiprazole chlorpromazine, clozapine, haloperidol, perphenazine, risperidone, thioridazine, zuclopenthixol *Beta blockers:* bisoprolol fumarate, metoprolol, pindolol, propranolol, timolol *AChEIs:* donepezil, galantamine	*Potent inhibitors:* fluoxetine paroxetine, quinidine, possibly bupropion *Other inhibitors:* amiodarone, chlorpheniramine, cimetidine, citalopram, clomipramine, haloperidol, indinavir, methadone, perphenazine, propafenone, ritonavir, sertraline, terbinafine	Not inducible
1A2	*Antidepressants:* amitriptyline, clomipramine, desipramine, imipramine, mirtazapine *Antipsychotics:* clozapine, haloperidol, phenothiazines *Benzodiazepines:* chlordiazepoxide, diazepam *Other:* acetaminophen, tacrine, theophylline, propranolol, warfarin, caffeine, phenacetin	Cimetidine, fluvoxamine, grapefruit juice, ketoconazole	aromatic compounds (smoking), carbamazepine, omeprazole, phenytoin, polycyclic, rifampin,
3A3/4	*AChEIs:* donepezil, galantamine *Analgesics:* acetaminophen, alfentanil, codeine, dextromethorphan *Antiarrhythmics:* quinidine *Anticonvulsants:* carbamazepine, ethosuximide *Antidepressants:* citalopram, escitalopram, mirtazapine, nefazodone, sertraline, TCAs, trazodone, venlafaxine *Antipsychotics:* aripiprazole, haloperidol *Antifungal agents*: itraconazole, ketoconazole *Antihistamines:* loratadine, astemizole, terfenadine *Benzodiazepines:* alprazolam, clonazepam, diazepam, midazolam, triazolam *Calcium channel blockers:* amlodipine, felodipine, isradipine, mibefradil, nifedipine, verapamil *Chemotherapeutic agents:* busulfan, doxorubicin, etoposide, paclitaxil, tamoxifen, vinblastin, vincristine *Cholesterol lowering agents:* statins *Immunosuppressants:* cyclosporine *Antibiotics:* clarithromycin, erythromycin, troleandomycin *Hormones:* cortisol, testosterone, estradiol, prednisone	Amiodarone, cimetidine, clarithromycin, erythromycin, fluconazole, fluoxetine, fluvoxamine, grapefruit juice inhibition of enzyme in the gut wall, indinavir, itraconazole, ketoconazole, metronidazole, nefazodone, nelfinavir, norfloxacin, quinidine, ritonavir, saquinavir, troleandomycin	Barbiturates, carbamazepine, dexamethasone, oxybutynin, phenytoin, rifampin, ritonavir, St. John's wort

(*cont.*)

Continued

Enzyme (CYP)	Drugs Metabolized by Enzyme (substrates)	Inhibitors*	Inducers†
2C9	*Antidepressants:* amitriptyline clomipramine, citalopram, imipramine, moclobemide *Benzodiazepines:* diazepam *Other:* hexobarbitol, losartan, mephobarbitol, omeprazole, phenytoin, proguanil, tolbutamide, warfarin *β-blockers:* propranolol	Amiodarone, chloramphenicol, fluconazole, fluvastatin, isoniazid, metronidazole, SSRIs (fluoxetine, fluvoxamine, paroxetine) omeprazole, zafirlukast	Chloral hydrate, phenobarbital, rifampin
2C19	*Antidepressants:* amitriptyline, citalopram, clomipramine, escitalopram, imipramine *Benzodiazepines:* diazepam *Other:* lansoprazole, mephenytoin, omeprazole, propranolol	Fluconazole, ketoconazole, lansoprazole, omeprazole, cimetidine, SSRIs (fluoxetine, fluvoxamine, paroxetine, sertraline), topiramate	Rifampin, carbamazepine, phenobarbital

* Drugs that inhibit action of the enzyme and may *increase* plasma concentration of substrates.
† Drugs that activate enzyme and may *reduce* plasma concentration of substrates.

FAMILY AND CAREGIVERS

Principles of management at home include the following:

- Establish effective therapeutic rapport with patient and, when appropriate, family members and other caregivers.
- Educate patient and significant others about the expected outcome of treatment, common and serious side effects, and course of action if concerned about adverse treatment effects.
- Frequent sessions during initial phases of treatment—q 1–2 weeks.
- Follow-up visits during continuation and maintenance phases.
- Monitor compliance.
  √ Home nursing services are helpful.
- Educate patients about potential for drug–drug interactions, and instruct them to notify physician about all concurrent medications.
- Institute appropriate collaboration and contact between physicians, social service agencies, pharmacist or other caregivers.
  √ Often practical for a nonphysician member of the team to coordinate.
- Conduct home visits, as practical and necessary.

Written summaries for the patient are helpful.

- Keep summaries as simple as possible.

- Give copy to the patient and to family member/caregiver, with patient's permission.

Table 1.33. Checklist of Written Instructions for Antidepressants

- Name of drug
- Dose and schedule of administration (generally ok with food, except trazodone, when absorption significantly increased by food)
- Warnings about side effects (e.g., driving, falls)
- Management of specific problems (e.g., constipation, hypotension)
- Caution to take only as prescribed
- What to do if a dose is missed (do not double up dose, especially certain drugs, e.g., bupropion)
- Caution about withdrawal syndromes with sudden discontinuation (e.g., paroxetine); how long to continue cautions after a drug is discontinued (e.g., prolonged action of fluoxetine)
- Warnings about interaction with concurrent drugs and OTC drug list to be avoided especially with MAOIs
- Brief description of delay to be expected before effects are felt
- Instructions on how, when, and why to contact prescriber
- *For MAOI:* Review diet, substance, and food restrictions (see p. 118)
- Reminder to notify doctors, dentists, and pharmacists

HETEROCYCLIC ANTIDEPRESSANTS

This class includes tricyclics (TCAs) and tetracyclics maprotiline and amoxapine (see Table 1.1, page 24). (As a class TCAs are among the best studied antidepressants in elders.) While secondary amines are the TCA drugs of choice in elders exceptions are the more anticholinergic secondary amines protriptyline and amoxapine. When used with appropriate cautions and monitoring, some members of this class especially nortriptyline (for depression) clomipramine (for OCD), trazodone (for sleep) and even low dose amitriptyline (for pain syndromes) remain important members of the arsenal used for treatment of the elderly. Medical conditions may limit tolerance to HCA antidepressants. Some members of the class are useful for anxiety disorders—e.g., clomipramine for OCD—while others are appropriate for non-psychiatric disorders i.e., chronic pain, fibromyalgia, arthritis pain, control of incontinence and bladder instability.

Mode of Therapeutic Action

- Mixed and non-specific inhibition of reuptake of neurotransmitters including serotonin, noradrenaline and (to a much lesser extent) dopamine, with affinity for muscarinic cholinergic, histaminic and adrenoreceptors (accounting for side effect profile)
  - √ Inhibition of NA reuptake
    - □ Imipramine, nortriptyline
  - √ Inhibition of 5-HT reuptake
    - □ Amitriptyline, clomipramine, desipramine

Table 1.34. Pharmacokinetic Parameters for Heterocyclic Antidepressants

Drug	Amine Subclass	Bioavailability*	Tmax (Hrs)	Volume of Distribution (L/Kg)	Protein Binding	Clearance†	Half-Life (Hrs)	Therapeutic Plasma Level	Metabolic Pathway
amitriptyline	tertiary	0.4–0.6	2–4	15.5	96%	700–1000 [<5] Reduced in elders compared to young	21–37	120–250	P-450 2D6, 1A2, 2C19, 3A4
amoxapine (general adult data)	Atypical secondary		1–2		90%		Parent (8 hrs in general adult data) 8-hyroxyamoxapine-prolonged-30 hrs (general adult data) 7-hydroxyamoxapine-6.5 hrs	Unknown	
clomipramine	tertiary	0.2–0.8	1.5–4	7–20	97%		20 (Parent compound) 36 (Demethyl-clomipramine)	160–400	P-450 1A2, 2C9/19
desipramine	secondary	0.5	4–6	15–37	90%	1600–2000 [<20]	12–31 (up to 46 reported)	60–160	P-450 2D6, 1A2
doxepin	tertiary	0.2–0.4	0.5–1	20	80%	75–110 [<1] reduced clearance with age	12–23 (parent) 51 (Active metabolite)	120–250	P-450 2D6, 2C19
imipramine	tertiary	0.8–1.0	1–2	21	89%	750–1300 [<1] reduced clearance with age	23–27	120–250	P-450 2D6, 1A2 2C19, 3A4
maprotiline	Tetracyclic; Structural analogue with properties of secondary amine	>0.9	8–24	22–52	88%	1060 [<10]	66 (29–113)	150–250	P-450 2D6
nortriptyline	secondary	0.6	7–8.5	21–27	93%	375–625 [<2]	18–45	50–150	P-450 2D6

* Fraction of dose to reach systemic circulation as active drug.
** Plasma concentration ng/mL.
† Volume of Plasma cleared in mL/min [% renal].
Compiled from various sources, particularly Preskorn (1993)

Note: The pharmacology of the parent compound often differs from metabolites (e.g., clomipramine metabolite [desmethylclomipramine] which inhibits NA reuptake).

Pharmacokinetics of HCAs

As a class HCAs have multiple mechanisms of action occurring over a relatively narrow range of concentration

- Very large interindividual variation in pharmacokinetic behavior is the rule with HCA metabolism.
- While lower doses are often required, the size of the dose reduction required is the result of many interacting factors beyond age per se
  - √ dose is often reduced too far based on age factors alone
  - √ therapeutic drug monitoring is a better method to adjust dosages (see p. 108).

Absorption

- Rapid and generally complete for most HCA antidepressants except maprotiline
- Unaffected by age or disease states

Oral Bioavailability

Generally low (20–80%) due to strong first pass effect-generally unaffected by food; increased by acute alcohol ingestion (reduces first pass effect)

Distribution

Rapidly and widely distributed

Protein binding

70–90% of metabolites are protein bound

- In general, highly protein bound to α_1-acid glycoprotein and to lesser extent albumin; wide interindividual variation using current techniques;
- Factors that increase concentration of α_1-acid glycoprotein are age and inflammatory conditions
  - √ Despite changes there is no increase in protein binding in elders
  - √ No clinically relevant effects from alterations in protein levels in inflammatory conditions such as rheumatoid arthritis or MI
- Protein binding is of much lesser clinical relevance than the variability in metabolism of HCAs

Clearance

- Decline in renal clearance in elders slows elimination of some HCAs and hydroxymetabolites
  - √ Clearance of imipramine and amitriptyline declines with age
  - √ Nortriptyline and desipramine clearance is unaffected by age
- Chronic alcohol intake increases clearance (decreases plasma concentrations)

Metabolism

Metabolism of HCAs often unpredictable in a given individual regardless of age—10–30-fold variability in serum HCA levels in younger healthy individuals

- Wide interindividual variability in age-related changes in p-450 system; hence wide variability in plasma levels of HCAs
- Plasma levels of imipramine, desipramine, amitriptyline and nortriptyline are higher in elders than younger patients at any given dose
- 50–60% of HCA enters systemic circulation after first pass metabolism
  - √ After first pass metabolism, the remaining parent compound is demethylated/hydroxylated in the liver and excreted into the gut where much is reabsorbed as either active or inactive metabolites (enterohepatic metabolism)
  - √ Efficiency of first pass metabolism decreases with age
  - √ Amount of tertiary amine demethylated at first pass decreases with age
  - √ First pass metabolism affected by
    - ▫ Individual variation
    - ▫ Illness—liver disease (e.g., cirrhosis or impaired right ventricular cardiac function causing reduced liver perfusion)
    - ▫ Concurrent other substances (e.g., cimetidine, alcohol, fluoxetine, fluvoxamine)
    - ▫ Altered first pass metabolism can alter Tmax and Cmax
  - √ GI bacteria may contribute to HCA metabolism by demethylation
    - ▫ May account in part for some of the wide interindividual variation in plasma concentrations
  - √ Metabolites are water soluble
    - ▫ Clearance depends on efficiency of kidneys which declines with age
    - ▫ Elders more likely to accumulate hydroxymetabolites which are cardiotoxic; marked by prolonged PR, QRS, QT intervals, and T wave flattening or inversion
  - √ Hemodialysis-does not significantly affect nortriptyline and doxepin metabolism

Half life

- Of parent compounds of tertiary amines is shorter than secondary amines but they are hydroxylated to secondary amines so, for practical purposes, their clinical effects are more prolonged.
  - √ Clinical relevance: tertiary amines are more sedating and toxic than secondary amines.
  - √ Metabolism from tertiary to secondary amine may be slowed in elders. The resultant higher proportion of plasma tertiary amine may predispose elders to greater incidence and intensity of sedation.
- Secondary amines are converted to water soluble hydroxymetabolites that are excreted by the kidneys. Renal clearance decreases with age so hydroxymetabolites may accumulate.

Side Effect Profile of HCAs

Over age 70, 25–35% of patients are withdrawn from therapy because of adverse side effects. Most important adverse effects are CNS and CVS.

Orthostatic Hypotension

- Danger of syncope/falls/stroke/MI
  - √ common in elders
  - √ Often very significant, sometimes impairing capacity to walk
  - √ Accommodation does not occur over time
- Associated with reflex tachycardia
  - √ Although hypotensive effect may be exacerbated in elders who often do not have the ability to produce compensatory increase in heart rate or have a low sodium balance
  - √ Especially prevalent if there is preexisting orthostatic hypotension or heart failure
  - √ Varies according to which HCA is used
- Most frequent CVS effect
  - √ Overall prevalence 10%; with preexisting cardiac disease 25–50%
- Not correlated with plasma concentrations
  - √ May occur at low doses
- Onset early in treatment
- Least frequent with nortriptyline
  - √ Produces hypotension above its therapeutic window
- Monitor BP carefully when using concurrent antihypertensives
  - √ Use lowest effective dose of antihypertensive
- During cardiac surgical procedures hypotension may be significantly exacerbated and hard to manage in the presence of long term HCA therapy
  - √ Discontinue HCA prior to surgery

- Management
  - √ Pretreatment and periodic evaluation for comorbid conditions predisposing to hypotension
  - √ Consider reducing or D/Cing concurrent drugs that may cause hypotension
  - √ Start antidepressant at low doses increasing more slowly in presence of hypotension
  - √ Use divided doses for nocturnal hypotension
  - √ Monitor BP lying and standing especially during first week and when increasing dose
  - √ Educate patients and families to dangers with instructions on rising slowly from sitting/lying to standing
    - Wait about 1 minute before standing and another 30 seconds before walking if at all light-headed
    - Hold onto a stable support
    - Climb stairs slowly
  - √ Consider elastic stockings during first few weeks of therapy while patient is accommodating to the drug
  - √ In unusual circumstances may use fludrocortisone (0.1–0.3 mg/day i.m. in divided doses) for 1–2 weeks
  - √ Salt tablets 0.6–1.8 g/day sometimes useful
  - √ Avoid epinephrine
  - √ Other agents that have been used include metaraminol, phenylephrine, norepinephrine, yohimbine, metoclopramide

Cardiac Conduction and Myocardial Effects

- Most commonly mild but sometimes persistent
- As severity of ischemic heart disease increases so does the risk of sudden death from HCA
- Tachycardia is usually supraventricular but may be ventricular;
- PVCs
- Impaired cardiac efficiency (reduced cardiac inotropy) may lead to heart failure
  - √ Induced by primary myocardial effect—i.e., myocardial depression, decreased cardiac output
  - √ Pedal edema relatively common
- Intracardiac conduction defects
  - √ Prolongation of QT, PR, and QRS intervals
  - √ BBB
  - √ Use ECGs to monitor cardiac side effects
    - Watch for widening of QRS complex or QTc interval beyond 450 μ secs
    - Prolonged QTc also predicted independently by age alone
- Flattening or inversion of T waves (because of slowing of atrial and ventricular depolarization)
  - √ Slowing may lead to AV block, BBB or PVCs

- Most commonly occurs in patients with preexisting cardiac problems including hypertension
- Class 1 antiarrhythmics (which include HCAs) increase post MI mortality risk (mechanism unknown)
- More common with amitriptyline and less common with maprotiline and amoxapine
- Monitoring
  - √ Monitoring serial ECGs is best way to manage patients at high risk of cardiotoxicity
    - ▫ If prolonged PR or QRS interval occurs may continue medication under supervision by a cardiologist
  - √ ECGs weekly during first 4 weeks of HCA treatment is indicated if there is preexisting cardiac vulnerability
  - √ ECG changes persist throughout duration of therapy
- Management
  - √ Consider beta blocker
  - √ Switch to another class of antidepressant.

Weight Gain

- Craving for sweets
  - √ See page 83

Oversedation/Drowsiness

- Varies according to HCA used
- Especially with amoxapine, maprotiline doxepin, trimipramine, amitriptyline, and imipramine
  - √ Nortriptyline and protriptyline are less sedating although sedation is still clinically relevant for elders with these drugs
- Tolerance may develop with time
- Management
  - √ If problematic prescribe at HS or switch to less sedating agent

Impaired Psychomotor Function

- Especially with tertiary amines
- Impairment in open road driving is comparable to 0.1% blood alcohol level

GI Symptoms

- Dry mouth
- Anorexia
- Nausea
- Vomiting
- Dyspepsia
- Diarrhea
- Bad taste (metallic or disgusting and rarely can be very severe and disturbing)

- Black tongue
- Glossitis
- Constipation

Weakness, Lethargy, Fatigue, Stuttering, and Depersonalization

- More common with clomipramine and imipramine
- Reduce dose; change drug

Induction of excitement restlessness, mania or hypomania, anxiety

- Danger with all antidepressants in treating depression especially if prior history of or strong family history of bipolar disorder
- Discontinue medication

Peripheral Anticholinergic Effects

See page 71.

Serotonin Syndrome

See page 79.

- Discontinue drug

Aggravation/Precipitation of Psychosis in Schizophrenia

- Danger of all HCAs may occur with both general adult patients and with elders
- Change drug

Sexual Dysfunction

Excitement, Restlessness, Mania or Hypomania, Anxiety

- Danger with all antidepressants, especially if prior history or family history of bipolar disorder
- Discontinue medication

Movement Disorders (EPS)

- May present pseudoparkinsonism, akathisia, acute dystonia, myoclonus
- Dyskinesia
  - √ Uncommon, but may arise with reduced dose
  - √ May spontaneously and rapidly disappear
- NMS (with amoxapine only)
- Tremor
- Especially with amoxapine
  - √ Occasionally reported with imipramine, amitriptyline, nortriptyline, clomipramine, trazodone
- Onset usually days to 2 months after initiating antidepressant
- Serum levels generally are within therapeutic range

- TD usually associated with
  - √ Concurrent neuroleptic
  - √ More highly anticholinergic antidepressant agents
  - √ Concurrent alcohol abuse
  - √ Stimulant use (e.g., dextroamphetamine)
  - √ Depression
  - √ More common in women
- Myoclonus infrequent at therapeutic doses but common in overdose and when combined with lithium

Seizures

- Rare
- Associated with
  - √ HCA overdose (multiple seizures and status epilepticus)
  - √ History of seizures
  - √ Concurrent organic brain disease
  - √ Chronically high plasma levels cause single or rarely fatal grand mal seizure.
- Related to dose and rate of dose escalation
- Usually occurs early in treatment
- Especially evident with clomipramine in doses over 225 mg

Sleep Disturbance

- Insomnia
- Vivid dreams
- Nightmares
- Hypnogogic phenomena
- Usually occurs when single HS dose used
  - √ Spread dose throughout the day; but symptoms can be very distressing and persistent requiring drug change

Impaired Glycemic Control

- Primary hyperglycemic action independent of weight gain
- Case report of hypoglycemia in combination with sulfonylurea
- Monitor and adjust hypoglycemic agent

Skin Rashes

- Most commonly exanthematous eruptions and urticaria as well as erythema multiforme
- Photosensitivity
- Skin flushing
- Diagnosis primarily on basis of history
  - √ Beginning drug for the first time within 1 week of skin eruptions

- If already sensitized to the drug i.e., allergic, eruption occurs almost immediately when the patient is rechallenged with the drug
- In patients who have asthma or aspirin allergy—consider allegic reaction to yellow dye 5 (tartrazine)
- Management
  - √ Discontinue suspected drug and substitute another class of drug
  - √ Avoid maprotiline (high incidence of rash)
  - √ If patient can be carefully followed, the rash is mild and the specific drug is required may sometimes elect to continue treatment cautiously.
  - √ Photosensitivity—avoid sunlight and use maximal strength sunscreens
  - √ Pruritis—consider antihistamines (caution re sedation in elders)
  - √ Tartrazine allergy—switch to drug without yellow dye number 5
  - √ Recommend patient have dermatologic consultation for more severe reactions
  - √ In severe cases glucocorticoids are necessary

Abnormal Taste

- Bitter taste from HCAs common but they also may produce loss of taste sensation or increased perception of other tastes.
  - √ Very occasionally this side effect can be severe and lead to marked discomfort and sensations of disgust with accompanying loss appetite

Dental Caries

- With prolonged HCA treatment
- Management
  - √ Dental hygiene
  - √ Regular dental examination

Infrequent Risk Of

- Hematological reactions
- elevation of liver enzymes/hepatitis
- Monitor blood and liver function indices during therapy with HCAs

Contraindications

- Ischemic heart disease
- Preexisting conduction defects especially BBB where conduction complications occur in 20%

Precautions for all HCAs include

- Sedation/CNS-related precautions (e.g., warnings about instability when getting up at night, avoiding driving or other hazardous activities until the response to the drug has stabilized)
- Cardiovascular disease—conduction defects, arrhythmias, acute MI
- History of urinary retention
- Glaucoma
- Thyroid disease/thyroid medication
- History of seizure disorder
- Avoid caffeine and narcotics
- Co-prescribing of some SSRIs (inhibitors of P-450 enzymes) with HCAs (e.g., reports of toxicity with combinations of fluoxetine and imipramine, desipramine, nortriptyline and clomipramine)
- TCAs have differing side effect profiles (e.g., maprotiline has a strong antiarrhythmic effect while doxepin does not prolong the conduction time)

Toxicity of HCAs

- Common cause of suicide by overdose in younger adults.
- Overdose less common method in elders but HCAs are dangerous regardless of age and should be prescribed with this factor in mind.
- Death from HCA overdose is usually due to cardiac arrest.
- Lethal dose is 10–15 times therapeutic dose.
  - √ Lethality is increased because of high lipid solubility; resulting wide distribution in the body tissues makes removal difficult in presence of toxicity
- Management of overdose includes
  - √ Full supportive measures including cardiac monitoring
  - √ Gastric lavage
    - ▫ Dialysis ineffective
  - √ Airway maintenance—intubation as necessary
  - √ Use of sodium bicarbonate is recommended for treatment of cardiotoxicity
    - ▫ Sodium reverses cyclic-induced sodium channel blockade and alkalinizes the patient
    - ▫ Strictly monitor: pH (therapeutic range 7.45–7.6 but not higher) and electrolytes
    - ▫ Avoid hyperventilation in combination with sodium bicarbonate: can produce dangerous alkalemia (pH>7.6) in some cases and may be fatal; unintentional hyperventilation may occur if ventilator rate is increased or patient spontaneously hyperventilates from anxiety upon awakening- decrease bicarbonate in such cases.

√ Ventricular arrhythmia: use lidocaine, phenytoin, or propranolol
√ Cardiac failure: use digoxin

Plasma Level Monitoring

- Monitoring plasma levels
  - √ Wait until steady state has been achieved at a given therapeutic dose (5–6 half-lives)
  - √ Draw blood sample in morning about 10–12 hours after last evening dose
- Plasma concentration monitoring of HCAs is clinically useful
  - √ Clinical response within the therapeutic range is 2–3 times the response rate outside the range
  - √ Some elders respond to lower levels
  - √ Monitoring of hydroxylated metabolites is not routinely available

Therapeutic Drug Monitoring (TDM)

Beyond plasma level determinations a rough measure of clearance rate for HCAs can be determined using this method of TDM.

1. Divide plasma HCA level by daily dose; this yields clearance rate estimate in nanograms per milliliter per milligram of daily dose.
2. Patients genetically or otherwise deficient in isoenzyme 2D6 activity will have clearance rate much higher than 1 ng/ml/mg (based on general adult data but useful for elders).
   - Normal metabolizer—0.5–1.5 ng/ml/mg
   - Rapid metabolizer or non compliance—<0.5 ng/ml/mg
   - Slow metabolizer—in range of 4+ ng/ml/mg

Guidelines for Use of Blood Levels

- Establish hepatic and renal function
- Ensure patient compliance
- Take into account concurrent medications
- Draw blood samples after steady state has been reached—about 5–6 half-lives of drug
- Measure both parent compound and metabolites when appropriate

Table 1.35. Therapeutically Useful Plasma Levels

amitriptyline	120–250 ng/ml
desipramine	115–200 ng/ml
imipramine (plus desipramine metabolite)	180–250 ng/ml
nortriptyline	50–150 ng/ml
clomipramine	160–400 ng/ml

When assessing therapeutically useful blood level for these drugs note the following:

- Data conflict on best therapeutic blood levels; ranges are approximations at best.
- Some data suggest no therapeutic benefit from plasma levels of imipramine higher than 200 ng/ml.
- Data on effective plasma levels of desipramine conflict. Some suggest *no benefit* from plasma levels *higher* than 115 ng/ml while other data indicate that response *requires* a level higher than 115ng/ml. The latter is probably correct. The best clinical approach is to start low and increase dose based on monitoring as described below, using clinical response, side effect monitoring and tolerance as the best guides.
- Keep in mind that most (90%) patients who are going to respond to therapy do so within 2–4 weeks after achieving a *therapeutic* level, so dose escalation schedule may determine speed of response to some extent.
- Clinical goal is to increase dose fast enough to reduce therapeutic response time as much as possible while not precipitating intolerable side effects.
- Many patients can achieve therapeutic levels within 2 weeks.

Dosing

Table 1.36. Doses

Drug	Common Daily Dosage Range in mg
	low high
amitriptyline (Elavil)	(10) 50–100 (200)
amoxapine (Asendin)	(10) 75–125 (300)
clomipramine (Anafranil)	(10) 50–100 (250)
desipramine (Norpramin)	(10) 50–100 (200)
doxepin (Sinequan)	(10) 75–150 (225)
imipramine (Tofranil)	(10) 50–100 (200)
maprotiline (Ludiomil)	(10) 50–150 (200)
nortriptyline (Pamelor, Aventyl)	(10) 50–100 (150)
protriptyline (Vivactil)	(5) 10–20 (40)
trazodone (Desyrel)	(25) 50–150 (300)
trimipramine (Surmontil)	(10) 50–100 (200)

Note: Low doses are starting but may also be therapeutic dose in some highly sensitive patients or slow metabolizers. *High dose* is maximum used in more aggressive regimens when medication is tolerated and side effects are not limiting. However these dose levels are not often achieved especially in frail elders and not recommended in routine geriatric practice.

- The doses above are on the conservative side at the low end
- Start at low doses and titrate slowly to therapeutic level
- Therapeutic dose varies considerably and there is little agreement on precise doses; ranges also vary and are gross approximations to guide the clinician

- √ Some patients may require full therapeutic dose to achieve blood level
- √ Doses for pain relief may be lower than antidepressant doses but not always; titrate to optimal response

- Correct dose level attained by monitoring and responding to
  - √ Therapeutic response
  - √ Adverse effects
  - √ Plasma levels
  - √ Serial ECG changes
- Once-daily dosing is generally used but some patients are very sensitive to cardiac effects of HCAs
  - √ Single dose may produce high maximum concentration (Cmax) of drug impairing cardiac conduction in vulnerable patients
  - √ Consider divided doses for
    - ▫ Patients on high doses of HCA medication
    - ▫ Severe liver or left ventricular cardiac impairment
    - ▫ Likelihood of concomitant significant acute alcohol intake
    - ▫ Concurrent use of drugs with similar cardiac effects (e.g., type 1 antiarrhythmics)
    - ▫ Use with drugs that inhibit first pass metabolism (thereby increasing Cmax)—e.g., fluoxetine, paroxetine, neuroleptics, quinidine
- Caution in discontinuing enzyme-inducing or inhibiting drugs since this will increase or decrease concentrations of HCAs accordingly

Washout Periods for HCAs

- Difficult to determine in the individual patient
- Steady state is achieved in about 5 days in healthy adults but is longer in elders
- HCAs washout in 5 days in healthy subjects but take considerably longer in some elders, those taking isoenzyme inhibitors or those who have concurrent diseases that impair metabolism
- Caution advised when washout is critical to care (e.g., switching from HCA to another interacting drug—MAOI or SSRI)

Withdrawal Syndrome

- May arise from peripheral cholinergic overdrive
- Withdraw HCA gradually over several days–weeks
- Rapid withdrawal can produce
  - √ Nausea, vomiting
  - √ General somatic distress—flu-like symptoms
  - √ Anxiety, agitation, panic
  - √ Sleep disturbance—dreaming, nightmares

- √ Abnormal movements
- √ Activation or hypomania
- √ Hyperthermia
- √ Tachycardia
- √ Onset: within 2–7 days after abrupt discontinuation
- √ Duration: 7–14 days

IRREVERSIBLE MAOIs

Irreversible class of MAOIs

- Hydrazines
  - √ Phenelzine
  - √ Isocarboxazid
- Non-hydrazines
  - √ Tranylcypromine
  - √ Note: Effects may begin and end faster than hydrazines
- Note for reversible MAOI (see Moclobemide, p. 174)

MAO

- Exists in 2 forms—MAO-A and MAO-B
  - √ MAO-A degrades serotonin and noradrenaline
  - √ MAO-B degrades dopamine and phenylalanine
  - √ In the intestine MAO-A and B metabolize tyramine
- Increases in concentration with aging
  - √ Provides theoretical rationale for use of MAOIs in depression of old age
- Platelet MAO (B) also increases with age, gender, and race
  - √ Highest in white females > black females > white males > black males

Irreversible MAOIs

- Bind irreversibly to MAO-A and B
- Duration of action is dependent on synthesis of new MAO rather than metabolic half-life of the drug itself
- MAO inhibition is prolonged for days beyond excretion of the drug, hence importance of a washout period before instituting other drugs which increase brain monoamines

Indications

- This class has been used successfully to treat depression in elders.
- Useful for patients intolerant of anticholinergic properties of other antidepressants and unresponsive to SSRI and newer agents.

- Response of some patients who are otherwise refractory to treatment means this class should not be completely abandoned.
- Some general adult data suggest MAOIs may be best suited for atypical forms of depression associated with hypersomnia, anergia, apathy, hyperphagia, hypochondriasis, inverse diurnal variation of mood, personality disorder (geriatric data not available).
- Effective in bipolar depression especially in patients with the anergic subtype but with significant risk of manic switch and hence should be used only with mood stabilizers (general adult data); such combination therapies are complex in elders.

Efficacy data for irreversible MAOIs

- Efficacy in the old-old not well studied or confirmed
- Overall comparable efficacy to other classes of antidepressants, including for treatment resistant depression
  - √ Some studies show phenelzine superior to HCAs in improving depressive symptoms but it is less well tolerated
    - ▫ Efficacy studies for major depression show mixed results possibly because of varying dose regimens
- No comparisons with SSRIs
- Phenelzine
  - √ Probably the safest MAOI for elders
  - √ Sexual dysfunction
  - √ Weight gain
  - √ Impaired glycemic control
- Tranylcypromine
  - √ Stimulant properties helpful in withdrawn apathetic patients
  - √ Less sedating and may be more rapidly reversible
  - √ Weight loss

Potentially severe side effects, especially in demented elders, require closely supervised or inpatient settings; however, well tolerated when

- Patients are carefully selected
- Optimal dosing and few dosing changes are used
- Unnecessary concurrent medication is eliminated

Pretreatment evaluation and patient selection are essential; factors to consider include

- Postural hypotension; instruct patient and caregivers on management (see p. 102)
- History of headaches which can mask premonitory signs of drug toxicity
- Concurrent drug regimen (see p. 119)
- Inability to comply with instructions—especially diet, monitoring of other medications (including OTC agents), substance abuse

- Contraindicated comorbid medical conditions (see p. 122)
- Food preferences and habits (see pp. 118–119)

Table 1.37. Pharmacokinetics of MAOIs

MAOI	Plasma Protein Binding	Elimination Half Life (Hrs)	T-max (Hrs)	Absorption	Metabolism
phenelzine	tight	1–4 (general adult data)	1–3 (general adult data)	GI-Rapid	acetylation
tranylcypromine	tight	1–4			

Note: General adult data; geriatric data not available.

- Clinical side effects (orthostatic hypotension, tachycardia) occur during Tmax
- Anticholinergic effects are weaker than TCAs but still may be significant especially phenelzine
- Metabolites of phenelzine- β-phenylethylamine and phenylacetic acid may be activating
- Linear dose response relationship (higher doses associated with better response)
- MAOI action and elevation of brain MAO ceases after about 3 weeks

Optimal dosing

- Established by convention and clinical experience for elders rather than formal dose finding studies
  - √ Modest doses are effective
  - √ But some require full adult dose for response (as with other antidepressants)
- Response does not correlate with plasma concentrations
- Dosing schedule
  - √ Short half-life requires BID administration
  - √ Insomnia
    - ▫ Give last dose earlier in the day
    - ▫ Tranylcypromine the most activating
  - √ Start with daytime dosing; occasional patients require night-time dosing because of daytime sedation
  - √ Phenelzine
    - ▫ Initial dose of 7.5–15 mg/day
    - ▫ Therapeutic dose range 7.5–30 mg/day
  - √ Tranylcypromine
    - ▫ Initial dose of 5 mg/day
    - ▫ Therapeutic dose range 5–30 mg/day

Augmentation

- Lithium
- Add T_3

Moving from MAOI to another agent or vice versa

- Allow minimum of 14–21 days for MAOI to clear before instituting one of the interacting drugs (clearance period of 10 days recommended for adults)
- Drugs with prolonged half lives (e.g., fluoxetine) should be washed out for 8–10 weeks in elders
- HCAs and many other antidepressants may require longer to clear from elders than younger patients

Loss of effectiveness

- Tolerance to AD effect may occur
  - √ Increase dose
  - √ Switch to another MAOI or back again later

Switching between MAOIs

Case reports of hypertensive crisis on abrupt switch from one MAOI to another especially phenelzine to tranylcypromine; wait 5–10 days before switching

Combination therapies

- In general avoid concurrent use of MAOI and other antidepressants (danger of serotonin syndrome or hypertensive crisis)
- Occasional indication for combination therapies but these are dangerous for elders and probably are best implemented by experienced therapists in hospital
- Guidelines for combination therapies
  - √ Patient selection
    - ▫ Refractory to other treatments with continuing severe depression
    - ▫ Good general physical health
    - ▫ Normal hepatic and cardiac function
    - ▫ Able to take medications responsibly
    - ▫ Do not take or can be weaned from multiple medications
    - ▫ Able to adhere to dietary restrictions
    - ▫ Do not abuse substances
  - √ These restrictions make combination therapy use in the elderly very limited
  - √ Avoid combinations with tranylcypromine (which is most often implicated in hypertensive crisis) and SSRIs, imipramine, clomipramine, desipramine, venlafaxine, mirtazepine, bupropion, nefazodone
  - √ Preferably use a sedating (rather than activating) HCA such as nortriptyline, amitriptylene, doxepin
  - √ Initiate both HCA and MAOI at the same time in small doses
    - ▫ MAOI is given in TID dose while the HCA is given in a single HS dose

- √ Begin at lowest dose of both HCA and MAOI
  - ▫ Titrate to therapeutic levels very slowly with careful monitoring of BP
  - ▫ Maximum dose of either medication is somewhat less than the full therapeutic dose of either one taken separately

Discontinuation

- If MAOI must be discontinued use extreme caution—taper very gradually to avoid
  - √ Sometimes severe hypertensive rebound effects
  - √ Cholinergic rebound which can include
    - ▫ Agitation
    - ▫ Vivid dreaming
    - ▫ Psychosis
- Withdraw about 1/3 of total daily dose every 4–5 days
- Tranylcypromine withdrawal occasionally resembles amphetamine withdrawal (tranylcypromine may be converted to amphetamine during metabolism) after long term use
  - √ Insomnia
  - √ Anxiety, agitation
  - √ Diarrhea
  - √ Headache
  - √ Delirium
  - √ Tremor

Monitoring

- Clinical monitoring
  - √ Routine BP
    - ▫ Continue to monitor for several months after stabilization on therapeutic dose for delayed onset orthostatic hypotension
    - ▫ Monitor supine, sitting and standing hypotension
    - ▫ Usual cautions re. orthostatic hypotension (see page 102)
    - ▫ MAOI may eliminate need for concurrent antihypertensive in some cases
  - √ Follow carefully for signs of palpitations or frequent headache during treatment—discontinue therapy if these symptoms emerge
- Plasma levels not clinically useful
- Monitor serum bilirubin and LFTs early in treatment and every 6 months thereafter
- Some research clinicians measure pretreatment platelet MAO as indicator of effective therapeutic levels for phenelzine but utility is controversial and the test is expensive (tranylcypromine inhibits platelet MAO at subtherapeutic doses, so monitoring is not clinically useful)
  - √ 80% inhibition of platelet MAO associated with positive antidepressant response

Toxic and Side Effects Profile

Side effects are especially troublesome in the old-old patient, but geriatric data are mostly from clinical reports. Commonest side effects include

- Orthostatic hypotension
  - √ By far the most common side effect
  - √ Monitor for the first month
  - √ Effects peak at 3–4 weeks
- Insomnia
  - √ Minimize by giving last daily dose no later than 4 pm
- Dizziness
- Mydriasis
- Piloerection
- Edema
- Tremor
- Anorgasmia
- Dry mouth
- Blurred vision
- Constipation

Table 1.38. Side Effects of MAOIs

Side Effects	Most Common	Most Serious and Less Common
Psychiatric disorders		Manic switch Anxiety Exacerbation of psychosis Paranoid outbursts Delusions
Central and peripheral nervous system disorders	Nervousness/agitation (tranylcypromine) Dizziness Headache Daytime sedation (phenelzine)—"nardil nod" afternoon sleepiness Tolerance usually develops after several weeks of treatment Sometimes improved with reduced dose Caution patients about hazards—i.e., falls, driving Anergia (phenelzine) Insomnia Initial insomnia with tranylcypromine Administer last daily dose no later than 4 pm Nightmares/vivid dreaming/hypnogogic phenomena Fatigue Delirium	Tremor Myoclonus Reduce or stop MAOI Exacerbation of impaired cognition Monitor cognition Peripheral neuropathy (secondary to B12 deficiency) Paresthesias and muscle weakness Prevent by coadministration of pyridoxine Responds to 100–300 mg/day of pyridoxine Manifests as gradual leg weakness and gait disturbance as well as stomatitis, anemia, ringing in the ears, irritability, carpal tunnel syndrome, hyperreflexia, rarely seizures or coma Lowers seizure threshold Insomnia May treat with benzodiazepine or low dose trazodone

(*cont.*)

Continued

Side Effects	Most Common	Most Serious and Less Common
Autonomic system	Sweating (tranylcypromine)	
GI disorders	Constipation Dry mucous mouth membranes	
Body as a whole disorders	Weight gain	
Respiratory disorders	Nasal congestion	
Skin and appendages		Rash, pruritis (infrequent)
Cardiovascular disorders	Hypotension by far the most common side effect (in >50% of patients-general adult data); often limits tolerance of dose increases and hence may limit effectiveness of the drug Onset gradual over several weeks; peaks at 3–4 weeks; may force discontinuation Common with CHF and preexisting hypertension Danger of falls Symptoms include dizziness, lightheadedness, coldness, headaches, fainting	Generalized edema (Phenelzine)
Special senses disorders		Blurred vision Increased intraocular pressure (narrow angle glaucoma) Dry eyes
Metabolic and nutritional	Weight gain (phenelzine)	Hypertensive crisis, Serotonin syndrome Temperature dyscontrol Possible hypoglycemia and potentiation of hypoglycemic agents Carbohydrate craving SIADH (case reports)
Urinary		Urinary hesitancy/retention
Reproductive		Impaired orgasm/ejaculation
Liver and biliary		Hepatotoxic reactions (rare; more often with hydrazines) Elevated AST/ALT- monitor LFTs Less common with tranylcypromine Symptoms include weakness, rash, nausea, jaundice, eosinophilia, elevated liver enzymes
Hematological		Blood dyscrasias (infrequent-rare) Anemia Leucopenia Agranulocytosis Thrombocytopenia

Note: MAOIs are weakly anticholinergic; no quinidine-like effects

Hypertensive crisis

- Occurs in about 5% of patients prescribed MAOIs despite education and instruction
- May induce potentially serious or fatal hypernoradrenergic syndrome
- Symptoms
  - √ Severe, exploding, headache—occipital radiating frontally
  - √ Hypertension—BP rise exceeds 20–30 points
  - √ Cardiac arrhythmia—palpitations, bradycardia,
  - √ Sweating
  - √ Mydriasis
  - √ Cold clammy skin
  - √ Pallor
  - √ Nausea, vomiting
  - √ Hyperpyrexia
  - √ Neck stiffness/soreness
  - √ Visual disturbances—e.g., photophobia
  - √ Constricting chest pain
  - √ May induce intracranial hemorrhage
- *Food or drug combinations that produce hypertensive crisis and should be avoided*
  - √ Tyramine (or tryptophan) rich foods
    - ▫ Raise blood pressure by releasing norepinephrine and epinephrine from either sympathetic nerve terminals and/or adrenal medulla
      - ◦ Normally tyramine is metabolized by MAO-A and B in the GI tract and never enters the circulation. If MAOs are inhibited, tyramine enters the circulation and causes release of greater than normal amounts of catecholamine
      - ◦ Tranylcypromine is most likely to cause this effect
  - √ Avoid protein foods that have been broken down by aging, fermentation, pickling, smoking, bacterial contamination
    - ▫ Smoked fish is ok (e.g., salmon, carp, white fish)
  - √ Prohibited food list for elders has been narrowed based on more recent data and now includes only
    - ▫ All decayed, spoiled, fermented, or aged foods even if not specifically on the list
    - ▫ Aged cheese—cheddar, stilton, gruyere, brie, emmenthal, camembert
      - ◦ Yogurt (moderate amounts), ricotta, cottage and cream cheese; processed cheese slices have insignificant amounts of tyramine
    - ▫ Avoid cheese-containing foods (e.g., pizza, fondue, many Italian dishes, salad dressings)

- √ Alcohol
  - ▫ Avoid beer and some red wines—e.g., Chianti, port
  - ▫ White wines such as Sauterne/Riesling have insignificant amounts of tyramine
  - ▫ Other alcoholic drinks (e.g., vodka, gin, whiskey) are safe if taken in true moderation
- √ fish—pickled herring, pickled herring brine
- √ Concentrated yeast extract especially marmite yeast itself and some products made with yeast; breads are safe
- √ Meat extracts—e.g., Bovril
  - ▫ Fermented (summer) sausage, salami, air-dried sausage, mortadella, and some other meats including aged beef, 5-day chicken liver and aged chicken, liver, liverwurst
  - ▫ Smoked sausage, fresh chicken liver, corned beef, smoked meat, pate, are all safe
- √ Vegatables and fruits
  - ▫ Italian, English, Chinese broad bean (fava) pods; the fava bean itself has no tyramine; similarly green bean pods
  - ▫ Fresh banana pulp has no tyramine but banana skins have significant concentrations as does rotten banana pulp
  - ▫ Avoid spoiled or dried fruit—e.g., bananas, figs, raisins
- √ Miscellaneous
  - ▫ Avoid Chinese food and oriental soup stocks (e.g., miso soup, Japanese soy sauce)
  - ▫ Avoid sour cream
  - ▫ Avoid excessive caffeine, aspartame
  - ▫ Extra caution re. eating spoiled protein rich foods; this is a particular problem with elders with reduced ADL capacity or cognitive impairment who often have spoiled food in the refrigerator

- Sympathomimetic drugs and hypertensive crisis
  - √ Caution patients about use of OTC drugs
  - √ OTC cold and sinus medications that contain sympathomimetic ephedrine
    - ▫ Nasal decongestants, including sprays (e.g., Dristan, Contac)
    - ▫ Hay-fever preparations
    - ▫ Sinus medications
    - ▫ Asthma inhalers
      - ◦ Use only pure steroid asthma inhaler beclomethasone, not isoproterenol or other β-adrenergic inhaler
    - ▫ Diet drugs/appetite suppressants
    - ▫ Safe agents include
      - ◦ ASA or Tylenol
      - ◦ Glycerin cough drops or plain Robitussin for cough—check labels

        - All antibiotics
        - If unsure patient should check with doctor
    - √ Certain anesthetics should be avoided such as pethidine
        - Withdraw MAOI antidepressants for 2–3 weeks prior to surgery or ECT and possibly longer in slow metabolizers of the drug such as frail elders and those with liver/kidney impairment
    - √ Avoid local dental anesthetics with epinephrine; if epinephrine is essential D/C MAOI 14–21 days prior if possible but be aware of dangers of depressive relapse
    - √ Sympathomimetics
        - Amphetamines
        - Cocaine
        - Ephedrine
        - Fenfluramine
        - Levodopa
        - Metaraminol
        - Methylphenidate
        - Phenylephrine
        - Phenylpropanolamine
        - Pseudoephedrine
    - √ Other drugs/substances to be avoided include
        - Alcohol
        - Catecholamines (e.g., dopamine, epinephrine, norepinephrine)
        - Catecholamine precursors (e.g., L–dopa, L-tryptophan, 5-hydroxytryptophan)
        - Cocaine
        - Dextromethorphan—possibly fatal reaction
        - L-tyrosine
        - Meperidine—serotonin crisis, possibly fatal hyperpyrexia
        - Methyldopa
        - Norepinephrine
        - Phenylalanine
        - Serotonergic drugs (e.g., dexfenfluramine, SSRIs)

Treatment of hypertensive crisis

- D/C MAOI
- Treat in the emergency department
- Treatment of choice is Phentolamine (5 mg IV) to lower BP
    - √ Administer slowly to avoid severe hypotensive action
- Sodium nitroprusside by slow iv has been used in severe cases (general adult data)
- Nifedipine 10 mg (sublingual preferred when used)
- Manage fever with external cooling

- If patient cannot get to an emergency department of a hospital, (e.g., lives in rural setting), consider as a last resort:
  - √ Supplying a few nifedipine for emergency use
    - Nifedipine 10 mg sublingually
    - Should reduce BP within 30 minutes or repeat dose
    - Caution patient about possible hypotension
      - Manage by lying down with feet elevated

Table 1.39. MAOI Drug Interactions

Drug	Interactive Effects
β-blockers	Bradycardia
alcohol (especially if high tyramine content (e.g., aged wine such as port))	Drowsiness, hypertensive crisis
amphetamines	Significantly increases BP (possible crisis)
β-blockers	Hypotension, bradycardia
barbiturates	CNS depression
benzodiazepines	Possible disinhibition
bupropion	Significantly increases BP
buspirone	Disorientation, confusion, amnesia, ataxia, myoclonus; possibly hypertension
caffeine	Cardiac arrhythmia; hypertension (possible crisis)
carbamazepine	Risk of seizures in predisposed patients (e.g., epileptics)
clonidine	MAOI potentiation
cocaine, crack	Hypertension
codeine	Hypertension, CNS depression
cyclobenzaprine	Fever, seizures
dextromethorphan	Significantly Increases BP, possible serotonin crisis; fatal toxicity
dopamine	Hypertensive effect
doxapram	CNS stimulation, hypertension
ephedrine	Significantly increases BP;
epinephrine	In local anesthetic may pose hypertensive risk; stop MAOI 2 weeks before procedure;
fenfluramine	Serotonin crisis
General anesthetics	CNS depression; Stop MAOI 2 weeks before surgery
guanadrel	Hypertension followed by hypotension
hydralazine	Tachycardia, possible hypertension
insulin, oral hypoglycemics	Increased, prolonged hypoglycemic episodes, hypotension
isoproterenol inhaler	Hypertensive (beclomethasone is better)
L-dopa, dopamine	Significantly Increases BP
levarterenol	Significantly Increases BP
lithium	Hypotension
L-tryptophan	Serotonin syndrome
meperidine	life-threatening reaction—fever, excitation, rigidity, hypertension, delirium
mephentermine	Significantly Increases BP
metaraminol	Significantly Increases BP
methylphenidate	Hypertensive crisis
other MAOIs	Hypertensive crisis, hyperpyrexia, hyperreflexia; wait minimum of 2 weeks before switching from one MAOI to another
phenothiazines	Hypotension; possible increase in EPS
phenylephrine	Significantly Increases BP (possible crisis)
phenylpropanolamine	Significantly Increases BP (possible crisis)

(cont.)

Continued

Drug	Interactive Effects
procaine HCl	Significantly Increases BP (possible crisis)
pseudoephedrine	Significantly Increases BP (possible crisis)
reserpine	Hypertension followed by hypotension
SSRIs/SRIs	Significant Serotonin Syndrome; may be fatal; special caution with long acting agent fluoxetine—high risk of hyperthermia
succinylcholine	Prolonged apnea (phenelzine)
sulphonylurea	Hypoglycemia (rarely)
	Hypotension
sympathomimetics	Fatal toxicity
TCAs and other heterocyclic antidepressants	Hypertensive crisis, fatal toxicity, hyperpyrexia, excitability, muscular rigidity, convulsions, coma; pharmacokinetic interaction
terfenadine	Increased MAOI plasma level and side effects
thiazide diuretics	Hypotension
tyramine	See food restrictions above

Contraindications to MAOIs

- Allergic reaction to MAOI
- CVA
- Hypertension
- CHF
- Food and drug combinations as above
- Pre-elective surgery patients—D/C MAOI 2 weeks before procedure
- Recurrent or severe headaches
- Hepatic disease
- Pheochromocytoma
- Discontinue before myelography

Use caution in administering MAOIs in cases of

- Parkinson's disease
- Angina
  - √ May mask pain
- Hyperthyroidism
  - √ Increased sensitivity to pressor amines
- Real impairment
- Seizure disorders
- Diabetes
  - √ May increase blood sugars

Overdose of MAOIs

- May be life threatening
- Hospitalize immediately
- Be alert to concurrent substances

- √ Other medications
- √ Alcohol

- Onset of symptoms within 6–12 hours but may be delayed by 24 hrs
- Resolves in 3–4 days but may be prolonged for a week or two-continue monitoring and observation during this time
- Early symptoms include drowsiness, severe dizziness, faintness, insomnia, anxiety, restlessness, irritability, flushing, severe headache, sweating, tachypnea, airway obstruction and snoring, tachycardia, tremor
- More serious symptoms include delirium (hallucinations, delusions, confusion, hyperactivity, incoherence), muscular hyperactivity, muscle rigidity, opisthotonus, hyperreflexia, coma, seizures, BP changes—profound hypotension, hypertension, tachycardia, cardiac arrhythmia, cardiac arrest, respiratory depression, fever or hypopyrexia, cool/clammy skin
- Treatment includes
  - √ Intensive supportive therapy
    - □ Start IV
    - □ Maintain electrolyte and fluid balance
    - □ Monitor vital signs and ECG
  - √ Emesis, activated charcoal and gastric lavage if overdose is caught early within a few hours of ingestion
  - √ Cardiopulmonary support
    - □ Protect airway from aspiration
    - □ Avoid adrenergic agents for hypotension
    - □ O_2 and ventilation as necessary
  - √ Control hyperpyrexia with external cooling as necessary
  - √ Hypotension is best managed with fluids
  - √ Monitor ECG
  - √ LFTs about a month after overdose

SELECTIVE SEROTONIN REUPTAKE INHIBITORS (SSRIs)

General Characteristics

- Fat soluble—easily penetrate blood brain barrier
- Eliminated by extensive hepatic biotransformation involving CYP450 system
- High volume of distribution
- Highly plasma-protein bound (except citalopram and fluvoxamine) especially to alpha 1-acid glycoprotein
- Little affinity for adrenergic, histaminic, cholinergic receptors
- May up-regulate β_1-adrenergic receptors after chronic treatment, and down-regulate 5-HT_{2a} receptors

Table 1.40. SSRIs and Pharmacokinetics

Drug	Plasma Protein Binding	Volume of Distribution	T_{max} (Hrs)	Elimination Half Life	Absorption	Clearance	Excretion	Metabolism	Linearity
citalopram	80% in general adult studies	12–16 L/kg (general adult data)	4 (1–6)	Elderly 1.5–3.75 days	Unaffected by food		Mostly by liver (85% general adult) but significant renal excretion of parent compound (6–23%)	Oxidative metabolism, n-demethylation mainly by CYP3A4 and CYP2C19 is the quantitatively most important step. Metabolite desmethylcitalopram-partially metabolized by CYP2D6—may be pharmacologically active. Other metabolites are didemethylcitalopram, citalopram-N-oxide—not likely clinically important	linear
escitalopram*									

fluoxetine	Extensive binding (95%) (general adult data)	26 L/kg (no difference in general adult data)	4–8	Fluoxetine 5 days; norfluoxetine 13 days; somewhat longer in women; steady state achieved in 2–4 weeks in general adults but longer in elders	Peak concentrations—6–8 hrs (general adult data). Administer with food (food slows rate but not extent of absorption)	30 L/hr	By kidney after hepatic metabolism	Demethylated to active metabolite norfluoxetine by CYP2D6; norfluoxetine is equipotent to parent compound	Fluoxetine Non-linear; norfluoxetine linear
fluvoxamine	Low- 77%	Estimated at 25 L/kg	2–8	25 (range 16–34) after multiple dosing; increases with increasing dose; modestly affected by age; increased with severe liver disease; steady state achieved in 10–14 days	Unaffected by food		94% in urine as metabolites	Unclear-probably metabolized by 1A2; Oxydative demethylation to 11 inactive metabolites	Non-linear

(*cont.*)

Continued

Drug	Plasma Protein Binding	Volume of Distribution	T_{max} (Hrs)	Elimination Half Life	Absorption	Clearance	Excretion	Metabolism	Linearity
paroxetine	99%	Extensive 3.1–12 L/Kg (general adult data). Steady state in 7–14 days in healthy adults but longer in elders.	3–8 (general adult data)	Increased in elders at 31 hrs (range 13–92 hrs); increases with dose due to saturation of the isoenzyme 2D6	Well absorbed. Unaffected by food or antacids.		62% kidneys 36% feces after hepatic metabolism	Metabolized by CYP2D6. Also inhibitor of 2D6. Glucuronide and sulphate metabolites inactive	Linear
sertraline	98%	20–25 L/kg	32 (only slightly higher in elders)	5–8 (general adult data)	Enhanced by food; peak plasma conc in 6–8 hrs (general adult data)		Significant biliary excretion; plasma clearance reduced by 40% in elders	Metabolized to inactive metabolite n-desmethyl-sertaline	Linear

* For data see Appendix A: Newly Approved Drugs

- SSRIs have 10-fold or more greater selectivity for blocking serotonin reuptake than norepinephrine reuptake

Indications

- Clinical experience in elders suggests overall comparable effectiveness and speed of onset of action among each drug and indications for their use are likely unchanged by age-related factors per se
- Depression with comorbid physical illness—SSRIs are effective and generally well tolerated but with a greater incidence of adverse effects than in otherwise healthy elders; best managed by caution with monitoring, dose size, and speed of dose increases
- SSRIs are first-line therapies in many disorders
  - √ Various forms of depression including comorbid depression in neurological conditions such as dementia or Parkinson's disease
    - ▫ Serotonergic, in addition to dopaminergic, dysfunction may be present in Parkinson's disease and associated with depression offering a rationale for SSRI use in this condition
  - √ Prophylaxis against relapse or recurrence of depression has been demonstrated with SSRIs
  - √ Anxiety, including panic disorders, phobias associated with panic disorder and, perhaps to a more limited extent, generalized anxiety disorder
    - ▫ SSRIs are often combined with anxiolytics in the early stages of treatment of anxiety disorders but combination should be used with appropriate caution in elders because of risk of over-sedation and gait instability (falls)
    - ▫ Anxiety disorders in elders associated with increased health service usage, increased mortality
  - √ Obsessive-compulsive disorders
    - ▫ Little geriatric data
    - ▫ General adult data suggests
      - ◦ SRIs most effective intervention (clomipramine and all SSRIs)
      - ◦ Trial of therapy is longer than in depression (up to 12 weeks)
      - ◦ Effective dose is higher in OCD than depression; generally maximum tolerated doses
      - ◦ Response in OCD is graded and partial in contrast to more complete response that may occur in depression
      - ◦ Relapse rate higher in OCD
      - ◦ Combination therapy such as fluoxetine with olanzapine, or risperidone, may improve effectiveness of therapy (general adult case report data)
  - √ Post-stroke depression

- Other uses (data not necessarily age specific) include
  - √ Emotional incontinence secondary to stroke and other neurological conditions including MS, traumatic brain injury, ALS, Huntington's disease, neoplasms, anoxia
  - √ May show primary effectiveness for dementia-related psychosis in elders (emerging studies)
  - √ Personality disorder (borderline)
    - ▫ May ameliorate personality trait disturbances such as aggressiveness, hostility, anxiety and anxious worrying (general adult data)
  - √ Hypochondriasis
  - √ Fibromyalgia
  - √ Adjuvant therapy for negative symptoms, alogia and affective blunting of schizophrenia (general adult data)
  - √ Some evidence for short term effectiveness in reducing alcohol intake and desire to drink; long term effect not demonstrated (general adult data)
  - √ Social phobia—SSRIs, MAOIs, HCAs and newer antidepressants have shown utility (general adult data) but data in elders limited for most agents
- Demonstrated efficacy of some SSRIs (citalopram, sertraline) for behavioral and psychological symptoms of dementia (BPSD) (may derive from finding of low serotonin levels and binding in Alzheimer's dementia and vascular dementia).
  - √ BPSD is a difficult syndrome to treat sometimes and no one medication class or drug has been shown to be specific for its management.
  - √ Inappropriate sexuality associated with dementia; no good geriatric data but has been used clinically with anecdotal evidence of positive effect.
- Recent data suggest that SSRIs ability to reduce platelet aggragation may make them useful in stroke prevention (data preliminary)

Table 1.41. Labeled Indications of SSRIs (Geriatric relevance)

	Depressive Disorders	OCD	Panic Disorder	Anxiety Disorders-Social Phobia	Anxiety Disorders-GAD	Anxiety Disorders-PTSD
citalopram	X					
fluoxetine*	X	X				
fluvoxamine	X (Canada only)	X				
paroxetine†	X	X	X	X	X	
sertraline**	X	X	X			X

* Fluoxetine also labeled for bulimia nervosa and is often used for panic disorder
** Sertraline also labeled for premenstrual dysphoric disorder
† Paroxetine also used for PTSD, neuropathic pain and headaches

Side Effect Profile of SSRIs

Side-effects of SSRIs, see pages 70–90.

- Selectivity for serotonin receptors makes SSRIs generally well tolerated as a class but far from side effect free in the elderly.
  - √ Very few studies in the nursing home population; little known about comparative efficacy of SSRIs in the very old.
- Generally SSRIs do not cause
  - √ Orthostatic hypotension or anticholinergic symptoms, but
    - ▫ Bradycardia/syncope reported with fluoxetine.
    - ▫ Acute angle closure glaucoma reported with fluoxetine and paroxetine.
    - ▫ Blurred vision caused by serotonin effects on innervation of the pupil.
  - √ Cardiac conduction effects or ECG changes.
  - √ Life-threatening effects in overdose; while toxicity in overdose is said to be a major benefit over heterocyclic antidepressants, overall incidence of suicide has not decreased–alternative methods have been used.
- Reported sporadic, generally insignificant association with increased blood pressure (non-geriatric).
- Tolerance to side effects often occurs, hence increase dose slowly to give patient time to accommodate.
  - √ Poor compliance or need to change medications because of side effects remains a significant issue with SSRIs, although not as great a problem as with TCAs.

Table 1.42. Relative Frequency of Side-Effects of TCAs vs. SSRIs

SSRI > TCA	TCA > SSRI
Nausea	Dry mouth
Insomnia/vivid dreaming	Somnolence
Nervousness/agitation	Dizziness/hypotension
GI disturbances—anorexia, diarrhea, flatulence, constipation	Constipation
Sexual dysfunction	Urinary obstruction
Headache	Palpitations
Weight loss	

Note: Some of these side effects (e.g., confusion/agitation, gait disturbance/falls, sleep disturbance, weight loss) are more troublesome or hazardous in the frail or institutionalized elderly. SSRIs often produce immediate side effects that will moderate over time. However, effects can be intense and cause patients and therapists to prematurely give up on the drug. Hence, for patients who have not had antidepressants before, start at the lowest available dose to test individual tolerance before increasing.

Overdose Safety

- Sufficient data for elderly not available.
- Fatal overdose with a single SSRI alone is rarely reported.

- Fatalities in overdose usually associated with concomitant substance ingestion—e.g., benzodiazepine, alcohol, HCAs, narcotic analgesics, diphenhydramine, MAOIs, beta-blockers, ASA, lithium.
- Concomitant CYP 450 inhibitor may be especially problematic.
- No significant age effects for fatal SSRI-related adverse drug effects identified.
- Symptoms associated with overdose are dose related (general adult data).
  - √ Moderate doses (up to 30 times common daily dose), associated with few or no symptoms.
  - √ Larger overdoses (50–75 times common daily dose) result in drowsiness, tremor, nausea, vomiting or more serious events.
  - √ Fatalities occur with exceptionally large overdoses (>150 times common daily doses). Elders are likely more susceptible and the amounts necessary for serious or fatal overdose may be less. Nevertheless SSRIs are much safer in overdose than first generation antidepressants.
- Main possible symptoms in overdose (general adult data).
  - √ Nausea, vomiting, sweating.
  - √ Agitation, restlessness, dizziness, lethargy, drowsiness.
  - √ Tachycardia, QT prolongation.
  - √ Hypomania, other signs of CNS excitation—e.g., tremor (very rarely seizures reported with very high serum levels).
- Treatment
  - √ Gastric lavage, activated charcoal, syrup of ipecac.
  - √ General supportive care.
  - √ Management of concurrent substances taken in overdose such as alcohol.
  - √ Suicide management—safety measures, psychotherapy, social environmental/interventions.

Selection of SSRI Antidepressant

There is no convincing between-drug differences in clinical effectiveness studies. In a given patient however, one SSRI drug may work when another has failed. Clinical consensus (not based on controlled clinical trials) among some experts is that citalopram is the SSRI of choice in elders with other first line choices including sertraline and paroxetine. Fluoxetine is a strong alternate choice while fluvoxamine is not favored for routine use in part because of propensity for drug-drug interactions.

- SSRIs are not identical.
  - √ Wide interindividual variability among SSRIs with regard to metabolism, pharmacogenetics, and pharmacokinetics in elders and patients suffering from somatic diseases.

  - √ Most SSRIs (except citalopram) bind to a large number of secondary receptors and enzymes that affect their clinical action
  - √ Aging increases half lives and steady state plasma concentrations of fluoxetine, paroxetine and, to a lesser extent, sertraline.
- Few comparative between-drug studies in elders.
  - √ Sertraline vs. fluoxetine.
    - ▫ Greater weight loss with fluoxetine.
    - ▫ Greater clinical improvement on sertraline (overall response rate was low for both drugs—sertraline 32% and fluoxetine 18%).
  - √ Paroxetine vs. fluoxetine.
    - ▫ Better response with paroxetine (but overall response was very low for both drugs—38% paroxetine, 17% fluoxetine).
- Base choice of SSRI on
  - √ History of prior response to a drug.
  - √ Tolerance of side effects.
    - ▫ Side effects vary among drugs—e.g., diarrhea may be more common with sertraline, constipation with paroxetine, activation with fluoxetine, sedation with paroxetine (but the evidence for specific differences between drugs is not strong).
  - √ Flexibility of dosage forms of the drug—greater flexibility is desirable.
  - √ Presence of concurrent medications that may be affected by the metabolism of the antidepressant (e.g., sensitivity to 2D6 inhibition or displacement of highly protein bound drugs such as warfarin leading to increased side effect of the displaced drug).
  - √ Clinical indication to switch class or drug (ineffectiveness/intolerance of a drug in another class of medication, or within same class).
  - √ Expense

Starting Doses

Minimum effective doses not established for SSRIs in elderly. Data conflict on need for titration of dose from lower starting dose to higher in elders.

- SSRIs demonstrate a flat dose response curve (i.e., increasing dose beyond maximum therapeutic level theoretically does not produce additional antidepressant action); hence SSRIs as a class do not require dose titration in general adults; clinically, increasing the dose is important to a complete clinical trial of these drugs.

- Because of side effects, for elders, start at half the recommended adult dose or lower if possible in vulnerable patients (e.g., with hepatic/renal impairment).
- Encourage the patient to tolerate mild early side effects to which they may accommodate.
- Increase dose gradually after patient has stabilized on starting dose.
  - √ Titrate to optimum effective dose—failure to achieve therapeutic dose a common cause of treatment failure.
  - √ Increase to a full adult dose if clinically indicated and patient tolerates side effects.
- Dosages and response times may vary for specific disorders (e.g., emotional incontinence associated with stroke may respond to standard doses within 2–3 days).
- Antidepressant effects continue to increase for several months after initial benefits become evident.

Discontinuation

- Taper SSRIs gradually
  - √ Communication among physicians is very important; often one doctor (usually non-psychiatrist treating another disorder) discontinues antidepressants, failing to realize the risks of abrupt discontinuation and of depressive relapse/recurrence.
- Tapering schedules are not defined yet for the elderly. Best to titrate to the tolerance of the patient. Some recommend a very conservative pace of about 10% per week, however, this may be too slow for patients whose clinical condition and distress require a more rapid changeover to another medication.
- May switch from one SSRI to another without a washout of a short acting drug in some patients but for longer acting drugs like fluoxetine, there is a risk of additive effects and induction of serotonin syndrome if there is no washout.
  - √ In general, for elders, best to taper previous drug before introducing another.
  - √ Reduced metabolism and excretion rates in some elders require longer washouts.
- Washout periods with MAOIs and HCAs
  - √ From SSRI to MAOI—2–5 weeks
    - ▫ Longer period is for fluoxetine
  - √ From MAOI to SSRI 2–3 weeks
  - √ From HCA to SSRI, taper slowly

Discontinuation syndrome

Rates of withdrawal syndrome are higher with shorter acting drugs (e.g., low with fluoxetine (14%) but high with sertraline (60%), paroxetine (60%), and fluvoxamine. The question as to whether discontinuation precipitates suicidal agitation is controversial. Some data conflict but recent studies do not support increased suicidality).

- Abrupt discontinuation of an SSRI often produces a syndrome that may include

Dizziness	Dysphoria
Sweating	Anxiety
Flu-like symptoms	Irritability
Nausea	Lightheadedness
Diarrhea	Paresthesias
Insomnia	Visual phenomena
Tremor	Confusion
Fatigue	Vivid dreams
Headache	Hot/cold flashes
Agitation	

There is a single general adult case report of new-onset compulsions and severe depression with discontinuation. There are also rare reports of hypomania.

- Onset soon after discontinuation (1–10 days)
- Duration of withdrawal symptoms varies but usually resolve spontaneously over time (although may take several days and in highly susceptible elderly patients a week or two)
- Discontinuation syndrome more intense with drugs with shorter half-lives such as paroxetine and less intense with drugs with longer half-lives, especially fluoxetine
- Prevention
  - √ Taper any patient who has been on a drug longer than 1 week
  - √ Taper by specified amount every 5–7 days (or longer intervals for elders who are likely to be slow metabolizers (e.g., hepatic impairment, frailty)
  - √ Special caution with paroxetine
  - √ Final dose may need to be lower than starting dose of a given medication

Table 1.43. Rate of Taper

Drug	Rate of Taper (q5-14 days)	Final Dose
fluoxetine	unnecessary	
fluvoxamine	25 mg	25–50 mg
paroxetine	5–10 mg	5–10 mg
sertraline	25 mg	25–50 mg
citalopram	10 mg	10 mg
venlafaxine	25 mg	25–50 mg

- Treatment
  - √ Reassure patient and family symptoms are generally short-lived and mild

- √ Reinstitute the SSRI and slow the rate of taper
- √ Introduce another SSRI
- √ Anticholinergic drug use
- √ If symptoms persist add an SSRI with a longer half life such as fluoxetine

- Reintroduce drug if withdrawal is severe before re-beginning a more gradual taper

INDIVIDUAL ANTIDEPRESSANT DRUG PROFILES

BUPROPRION (BUP)

Drug	Manufacturer	Chemical Class	Therapeutic Class
bupropion (Wellbutrin)	GlaxoSmithKline	propiophenone, phenylaminoketone	atypical AD

Indications: FDA/HPB

- Depression

Indications: Off label

- PTSD and depression
- May counter SSRI-induced sexual impairment (general adult data) when used as adjunct.
- Bipolar disorder—equal efficacy to SSRIs.
- Smoking cessation (under another proprietary label).

Pharmacology

- Metabolites TB and HB contribute to BUP's antidepressant action (by inhibition of NA uptake).
- Linear pharmacokinetics.
- Considerable interindividual variability in plasma concentrations of BUP.
- Use lower doses of BUP in elders.
- Effect of severe liver disease on metabolism not well studied.
  - √ Caution and lower doses to start are prudent measures.
- Reduce dose in significant renal disease (reduced creatinine clearance) and CHF.
- SR preparation:
  - √ Single dose—50% lower peak plasma concentration
  - √ Multiple doses—15% lower peak plasma concentrations

Mechanism of action

- Antidepressant mechanism of action not known but probably related to enhancement of noradrenergic function through inhibition of reuptake of NA.
  - √ Parent compound is relatively weak dopamine and noradrenaline reuptake inhibitor.
  - √ Metabolites, especially HB, contribute important antidepressant components of the drug's action by inhibiting NA reuptake.
- No serotonergic activity, no inhibition of MAO, and little affinity for muscarinic, histaminic, or alpha-adrenergic receptors.
- May block nicotinic receptors.
  - √ Hence relevance to smoking cessation.

Table 1.44. Pharmacokinetics of Buproprion

Bioavailability	Plasma Protein Binding	Volume of Distribution	Elimination Half Life	Tmax (hrs.)	Absorption	Excretion	Metabolized P450 System
> 0.8	82–88%	19–79 l/kg (reports vary)	30 hrs. (elders); steady state in 8 days; active metabolites accumulate to steady-state levels higher than BUP; they have longer half-lives and slower clearance than BUP: TB—38 hrs. EB—61 hrs. HB—34 hrs.	6	No significant food effect	Predominantly renal excretion of hydroxymetabolites; < 1% unchanged in urine	Metabolized by 2B6 to active metabolites: hydroxybupropion (HB), threohydroxybupropion (TB), erythrohydroxybupropion (EB). BUP not metabolized by 2D6, but inhibited 2D6 leads to accumulation of active metabolite HB.

Choosing a Drug

- *SR preparation is the form of choice for elders—reduces peak serum levels and seizure risk.*
- Apathetic, retarded geriatric depression—bupropion activating.
- No adverse sexual side effects.
  - √ Alternative antidepressant for patients with antidepressant-induced sexual dysfunction.
- General adult data indicate BUP has equal efficacy to other antidepressants.
  - √ May be superior in atypical and bipolar depression but somewhat less effective in typical depression.
  - √ Recommended as best for bipolar disorder.
    - ▫ Equal efficacy to SSRIs but some evidence it possesses less propensity for inducing manic switch (although geriatric data not available and general adult data sometimes conflict).
    - ▫ Best to use in combination with mood stabilizer in patients at high risk of mood switch.
- Requires bid (and, at times with IR form, tid) dosing.
- Seizure induction potential (little data for elders).
- Effective when used in combination with SSRIs for partially or unresponsive depressed patients.
  - √ Mechanisms of action may be complementary (general adult data; geriatric case reports only).
  - √ Use carefully in elders.
- Effective for depression associated with grief.
- Because of relatively sparse geriatric data, can only be considered a second-line antidepressant, although it is effective and probably well tolerated in many patients if cautions are kept in mind.

Quality of the data: Geriatric data are very sparse.

Dosing

- Daily dose regimen
  - √ Avoid hs doses to reduce activation and insomnia at night.
- Initiating therapy
  - √ Begin at lowest available dose.
    - ▫ Dosage flexibility can be enhanced—extended-release pill can be split without affecting release of bupropion.
  - √ Dosing should be about one-half the general adult dose to start and not exceed 75% of the adult dose.
    - ▫ Active metabolites are longer acting and increase in concentration with multiple dosing (to a steady state).
    - ▫ High plasma concentrations of BUP and hydroxymetabolites are associated with increased side effects and reduced antidepressant efficacy (possible therapeutic window

effect, but not confirmed; if so, elders at higher risk of exceeding the window).

- Initial dose
  - √ Bupropion SR (recommended): 50–100 mg once daily in the morning.
  - √ Bupropion IR: 37.5–75 mg daily in the morning.
  - √ Maximum single dose not established for elders.
    - ▫ In frail or otherwise compromised elders use 75 mg to avoid seizure risk.
- Increasing dose and reaching therapeutic levels:
  - √ bid doses (morning and evening)
    - ▫ At least 8 hrs or more apart (to avoid spikes in plasma concentrations associated with increased seizure risk).
  - √ Bupropion IR: Increase dose by 37.5–75 mg/day q 7 days, or more, to maximum tolerated dose.
  - √ Bupropion SR: Increase by 50–100 mg/day q 7 days, or more, to maximum tolerated dose.
  - √ Target therapeutic geriatric dose not determined.
    - ▫ Reasonable target is 100–200 mg/day; some healthy elders require and tolerate 300 mg/day.
    - ▫ Significant numbers of patients respond to 100–200 mg of SR form (general adult data).
    - ▫ There may be loss of efficacy if plasma levels of metabolites exceed optimal level.
- Dosing for off-label indications
  - √ Antidote to sexual impairment with other medications (especially SSRIs).
    - ▫ Dose 75–150 mg may be given 1–2 hours prior to anticipated sexual activity.
    - ▫ May be given on a scheduled basis in fuller therapeutic doses (100–200 mg).
    - ▫ May take 2+ weeks to achieve a response.

Combination Therapy

- Little geriatric data available.
- General adult data: Augmenting effects found by adding low–moderate doses of bupropion to
  - √ Venlafaxine
  - √ Paroxetine—case report (general adult data) of synergistic antidepressant action and reduced agitation; mechanism not clear.
  - √ Fluoxetine
  - √ Sertraline
  - √ Nortriptyline

- Caution in using combinations, since there are substantial interindividual differences in BUP plasma concentrations related to emergence of side effects.
  - √ Possible increased seizure risk when combined with TCA.

Side Effects

- Limited geriatric data available.
  - √ Some general adult studies contain geriatric patient subsamples.
  - √ Geriatric studies indicate side-effect profile and tolerability of BUP similar in general adult and geriatric samples.
- Overall, low rate—perhaps best tolerated of all available antidepressants.
- Fewer side effects with SR form.
- Many effects are dose related, and some are transient.

Table 1.45. Side Effects of Buproprion

Side Effects	Most Common*	Most Serious and Less Common
Body as a whole	• Weight loss—may be a problem in frail elders	
Cardiovascular	• Tachycardia • May induce hypertension. √ Sometimes severe, requiring treatment	• Ventricular arrhythmias √ Third-degree AV block
Central and peripheral nervous system	• Headache (20–25%) • Insomnia √ Shortens REM latency (general adult data) • Excitement/agitation (dose related; 12%) • Dizziness • Tremor • Sedation • Confusion	• Trigeminal neuralgia (general adult data) • Seizures √ *No geriatric data.* √ Risk greater with IR vs. SR forms (0.4% vs. 0.1%;) √ Strongly dose related. □ Higher doses rarely required in elders— > 450 mg of IR form/day √ Seizures not more common than with other antidepressants if SR preparation used in therapeutic doses (general adult data) √ Risk increases with low body weight and rapid dose escalation, so risk greater in frail elders • Delirium/toxic confusion —occasionally √ May occur in transient episodes mimicking TIA √ Visual/auditory hallucinations • Gait disturbance √ Geriatric case reports of falling backward (may be a dopamine perturbation) √ Dyskinesia (reversible)—case report

(cont.)

Continued

Side Effects	Most Common*	Most Serious and Less Common
Gastrointestinal	• Dry mouth (13%) • Constipation • Nausea (10–13%) • Vomiting • Abdominal pain • Anorexia	• Ileus (one case report)
Hematological		• Eosinophilia—case report
Metabolic and nutritional	• Sweating	• Serum sickness • Allergic reaction • Angioedema • Rare anaphylactic reactions
Musculoskeletal		• Arthralgia • Myalgia • Rhabdomyolysis
Psychiatric	• Agitation	• Switch into mania/rapid cycling—less likely than with other antidepressants • May induce psychosis if plasma levels of metabolites are too high (dopaminergic effect)
Skin and appendages		• Alopecia • Urticaria • Stevens–Johnson syndrome
Eye and ear	• Blurred vision • Tinnitus	• Conjunctivitis

* Percentages are examples from studies, not more precise figures from pooled data.

Monitoring

- Routine
  - √ Special review for any predisposition to seizures.
  - √ Routine screening laboratory workup, especially creatinine clearance.
  - √ Plasma levels not used routinely.

Drug Interactions

Bupropion may not be metabolized by 2D6, but metabolite hydroxybupropion (HB) probably is metabolized. Higher levels of HB associated with poorer antidepressant effect. Increased HB in elders and with coadministration of SSRI, valproate, or carbamazepine. Many interactions reported.

- Bupropion inhibits CYP2D6—decreased doses of some drugs may be necessary especially
  - √ Thioridazine—increased plasma levels and danger of ventricular arrhythmia
  - √ MAOIs—risk of hypertensive crisis; combination contraindicated
  - √ HCAs
  - √ SSRIs (paroxetine, sertraline, fluoxetine)
  - √ Antipsychotics (haloperidol, risperidone)

- √ Beta blocker (metoprolol)
- √ Antiarrhythmics (propafenone, flecainide)

- Monitor carefully all agents that lower seizure threshold:
  - √ Alcohol
  - √ Antipsychotics
  - √ Antidepressants
  - √ Antimalarials
  - √ Hypoglycemics/insulin
  - √ Theophylline
  - √ Tramadol
  - √ Systemic steroids
  - √ Lithium
  - √ Quinolone antibiotics
  - √ OTC stimulants/anorectic drugs
  - √ Ginkgo biloba
  - √ Drugs metabolized by CYP2D6 (see p. 95).
- Inhibitors of CYP2B6 may increase plasma levels of bupropion
  - √ Orphenadrine
  - √ Cyclophosphamide
  - √ Ifosfamide
  - √ Nelfinavir
  - √ Ritonavir
  - √ Efavirenz
  - √ Cimetidine
- Amantadine coadministration may lead to toxic confusional state with neurological symptoms (possible dopamine synergism).
  - √ Gross tremors, ataxia, gait disturbance, vertigo
- Inhibits demethylation of some tertiary amine tricyclics under clinical conditions.
  - √ E.g., doubles imipramine half-life, but no effect on desipramine
- Increased valproate levels—case report of psychosis with visual and auditory hallucinations.
- Fluoxetine—use caution.
  - √ Combination may produce agitation/anxiety/panic states in occasional patient (general adult data)
  - √ Single case reports of delirium, myoclonic jerks, mania, and seizures in combination with fluoxetine
- Caution with nicotine therapies (e.g., transdermal nicotine patch)—hypertension.
- Caution with levodopa—synergistic increase in dopamine levels.
- Warfarin—monitor INR, increased risk of bleeding.
- Hepatic enzyme induction may lower concentrations of BUP by
  - √ Barbiturates
  - √ Carbamazepine
  - √ Phenytoin
  - √ Rifampin

Effect on Laboratory Tests

Increase in serum liver enzymes (ALT, AST) infrequent, mild, and generally nonsignificant.

Special Precautions and Contraindications

Seizure precautions:

- Risk related to peak plasma levels of IR form as well as higher ranges of total dosage.
  - √ 450 mg range in general adult data, possibly lower in elders.
- Increase dosage slowly in elders.
- Do not use high single doses (i.e., no > 100–150 mg) or give drug doses close together (i.e., no less than 8 hrs apart).
- Contraindications
  - √ Predisposed to seizures
  - √ History of seizures
  - √ Organic brain disease (e.g., stroke)
  - √ Recent withdrawal from short-acting benzodiazepines, alcohol/substances of abuse
  - √ Concurrent use of drugs that lower seizure threshold (e.g., lithium, antipsychotics)
  - √ Fluoxetine concurrently may increase risk
  - √ Head trauma
  - √ Abnormal EEG
  - √ Poor metabolizers

Overdose, Toxicity, Suicide

No geriatric data available.

May be dangerous to elders in overdose.

- Acute overdose produces
  - √ Onset of symptoms 1–4 hours after ingestion (general adult data)
    - ▫ Seizures common (up to 20%; general adult data)
    - ▫ Status epilepticus (rare)
    - ▫ Persistent sinus tachycardia
    - ▫ Tremors
    - ▫ Cardiac conduction delays occasionally
- Rare fatalities with bupropion alone
  - √ Case report of fatality with bupropion and paroxetine combination (general adult data)

Management of overdose

- Recommend aggressive management—danger of occasional severe, perhaps life-threatening, toxic effects.

- Provide full supportive measures.
- Administer gastric lavage, activated charcoal.
- Monitor for
  - √ Cardiac dysrhythmias (uncommon but may occur with massive Bupropion overdose)
  - √ Acid-base and electrolyte imbalance
  - √ Cardiac arrest
- Administer anticonvulsant therapy, as necessary.

Caregiver Notes

- Monitoring and recognizing change
  - √ If the patient misses a dose, do not try to make up for it by increasing the next dose.
  - √ Follow prescribing instructions carefully.
  - √ Watch for side effects.
    - ▫ Excited, agitated behavior, insomnia
    - ▫ Unusual accusatory behavior, fearfulness, apparently responding to voices or visual images
    - ▫ New involuntary muscle movements, seizures
    - ▫ Loss of appetite and weight
    - ▫ Call physician when concerned or if adverse effects observed.

Clinical Tips

- Activation can be a limiting feature of this drug.
  - √ Not effective for comorbid anxiety/panic and may worsen symptoms (general adult data).
  - √ Address activating effects such as insomnia with brief concurrent course of benzodiazepine (with appropriate caution based on age and frailty).
  - √ Activating effect may be useful for frail depressed elders with reduced energy.
    - ▫ E.g., with comorbid medical conditions or "failure to thrive" conditions in nursing home populations.
    - ▫ Clinical impression, no supporting empirical data available.
- Some evidence for a therapeutic window, but plasma levels are not routinely monitored in clinical practice.
- Dopaminergic effects, although weak, could aggravate preexisting predisposition to psychosis in some patients.
  - √ Observe closely.
- Some weight loss sometimes associated with bupropion.
  - √ Caution in frail elders.
- In long-term therapy do periodic checks of renal function.

CITALOPRAM

Drug	Manufacturer	Chemical Class	Therapeutic Class
citalopram (Celexa)	Forest/Lundbeck	bicyclic phthalane	SSRI AD

Indications: FDA/HPB

- Depression

Indications: Off label

- Effectiveness demonstrated in elders for
  - √ Poststroke depression
  - √ Poststroke emotionalism
  - √ Depression comorbid with Parkinson's disease
  - √ Emotional/behavioral disturbances of dementia
- Acts as an emotional stabilizer in some patients.
  - √ Improved emotional bluntness, confusion, irritability, anxiety, fear, panic, depressed mood, restlessness, suspicion, delusions.
- A single trial shows it to be superior to both placebo and possibly also perphenazine in reducing neurobehavioral impairments, aggression/agitation, and affective lability/tension in nondepressed patients with dementia and psychosis.
- General adult data show effectiveness for
  - √ Panic disorder with/without agoraphobia
  - √ Social phobia
  - √ Obsessive–compulsive disorder, including unwanted repetitive behaviors
  - √ Alcohol abuse
  - √ Mixed data on effectiveness as adjunct for aggression in schizophrenia
  - √ Note: No benefit in fibromyalgia

Therapeutic actions by indication

- Effective in depression associated with dementia.
  - √ May improve cognition in treatment-responsive patients.
- BPSD associated with SDAT.
  - √ Often improves irritability, depressed mood, and may benefit emotional bluntness, psychosis, restlessness, confusion, anxiety, fear, panic.
- Effect on other forms of dementia not clear.
- Effective (65%) in poststroke depression (PSD) that begins after 7 weeks (earlier-onset mild depression more often remits spontaneously).
  - √ PSD effectiveness seems unrelated to whether stroke was left- or right-sided.

- Effective for depressive component of psychotic depression (case reports in general adults).
- May reduce aggressivity in schizophrenia (general adult data).
- In alcohol relapse prevention, may reduce alcohol craving and improve abstinence as adjunct to psychotherapy (general adult data).

Pharmacology

- See Table 1.40, page 124.
- Linear pharmacokinetics at therapeutic doses.
- Highly lipophilic.
- Steady-state plasma levels up to 4-fold higher in elders.
  - √ Significant interindividual variation in plasma levels.
  - √ Use lower doses of citalopram.
- Hepatic damage increases half-life (by 100% in general adults).
  - √ Use lower maximal doses not exceeding 20–30 mg.
  - √ Kidney function is less problematic.

Mechanism of action

Selectively inhibits uptake of 5HT. This action increases extracellular 5HT, which in turn activates the $5HT_{1A}$ autoreceptor. Resulting feedback loop leads to down-regulation of the inhibitory $5HT_{1A}$ autoreceptors and subsequent increase in serotonergic neurotransmission.

The most selective of the SSRIs

- Ten-fold more selective at blocking serotonin reuptake than paroxetine.
- Little affinity for postsynaptic 5HT, adrenergic, histaminergic, muscarinic, or dopaminergic receptors.
- No inhibition of MAO.

Choosing a Drug

A drug of first choice for elders.

- Usually well tolerated.
- Highly selective action of citalopram may reduce unwanted side effects.
- Not as effective as nortriptyline in head-to-head study in severely depressed elders, but somewhat better tolerated.
- Early response to treatment with citalopram (within first 4 weeks) reported.

Quality of the data

- Controlled data for efficacy in
  - √ Depressed elderly

- √ BPSD and SDAT
- √ PSD

Dosing

- Initial dose for patients > 65 years 10 mg/day in A.M.
  - √ May be given at night if daytime somnolence is a problem, but watch for sleep disturbances such as insomnia.
- Increasing dose and reaching therapeutic levels
  - √ Response rate varies in elderly.
    - ▫ Some elderly respond to 10 mg dose, whereas others may require full adult doses.
  - √ Increase dose to 20 mg (target dose for some patients) after 1 week if patient tolerates medication.
    - ▫ If not, wait longer for accommodation to occur.
  - √ If there is little or no clinical effect in 3–4 weeks, titrate to 30 and then to 40 mg (at 1–2-week intervals).
    - ▫ Higher dosage levels may improve response rate.
    - ▫ In younger adults 20 mg dose no better than placebo, so higher doses may be required, especially in otherwise healthy elders.
  - √ Therapeutic effect becomes most obvious at about 6 weeks in general adult studies but may take longer in elders, possibly because of longer titration schedules.
- Maintenance dose
  - √ Maintain at effective therapeutic dose (see general guidelines for antidepressant treatment maintenance, pp. 54–55).
  - √ Citalopram appears to be as effective as other SSRIs in preventing relapse.
  - √ Specific data for BPSD and PSD maintenance not available.
    - ▫ Clinical trial in individual patients is best method of evaluation.
  - √ Duration of maintenance therapy for social phobia not well determined.
    - ▫ Suggested guideline (general adult): 6–12 months after remission.
  - √ Phobia associated with panic disorder often improves after 3 months at 20–30 mg/day (general adult data, geriatric data not available).
    - ▫ Improvement of panic disorder symptoms may continue for several weeks after clinical effect begins.

Dosing for off-label indications

- BPSD 20–30 mg/day similar to general adult antidepressant dose.
  - √ BPSD in SDAT: Clinically significant response found after 4 weeks.

- OCD dose not established for elders; general adult dose is 20–60 mg and usually the higher dosage range (60 mg) is more effective (single general adult case report of successful treatment at 160 mg/day).
  - √ Geriatric dose should be titrated to highest tolerated level within the therapeutic range.
    - ▫ Therapeutic effect in OCD may be delayed for 4–6 weeks and possibly longer in elders.
    - ▫ Patients who benefit from treatment continue to improve for 4–6 months (general adult data).
  - √ Duration of therapy not established.
- Panic disorder: 10–30 mg/day; dose for elders not well established.
- Social phobia: 40 mg/day (general adult data).

Combination Therapy

See also page 60.

- Lithium: An effective adjunct in treatment-resistant elderly (pilot data supported by similar data from general adult studies).
  - √ Clinical effects within 1–2 weeks.
  - √ Monitor for side effects of combination.
- Methylphenidate: Augmentation may improve response rate and possibly accelerate the speed of onset of antidepressant effect (within 2 weeks).
  - √ Well tolerated (studied in a very old but small patient population).

Discontinuation and Withdrawal

- Discontinue slowly over 2–3 weeks to avoid withdrawal symptoms.
  - √ No strong withdrawal or rebound effects reported. As with other SSRIs, monitor for GI disturbance, anxiety, insomnia, dizziness, asthenia, impaired concentration, headache, migraine.

Side Effects

- Generally well tolerated by elders.
- Milder symptoms often transient and self-limited over 1–2 weeks.

Key side effects include agitation, anxiety, headache, dizziness, nausea, sweating, orthostatic hypotension.

Table 1.46. Side Effects of Citalopram

Side Effects	Most Common	Most Serious and Less Common
Autonomic system	• Dry mouth • Sweating	
Body as a whole	• Transient asthenia, emotional indifference, lassitude • Fatigue • Weight gain/loss	
Cardiovascular	• Possible bradycardia √ Caution in patients with preexisting vulnerability • In general, CVS effects are minimal • No evidence of effect on ECG other than slight decrease in heart rate	• Hypotension (including postural)
Central and peripheral nervous system	• Insomnia • Increased dreaming • Somnolence • Tremor • Headache (sometimes migrainous) • Dizziness	• Rare seizures • Myoclonus • EPS (rare) • Ataxia • Incoordination
Gastrointestinal	• Nausea or vomiting initially (but accommodation after about 1 week) (overall, nausea may be less common in elderly than general adult group, but occasionally can be severe enough to limit use of drug) • Anorexia	
Hematological		• Purpura • Epistaxis
Metabolic and nutritional	• Fever	• SIADH-induced hyponatremia
Psychiatric	• Agitation • Impaired concentration	• Induction of secondary mania (general adult case reports) • Confusion
Reproductive	• Ejaculatory dysfunction (especially delay), diminished sexual desire, orgastic dysfunction (dose-dependent effect)	

Monitoring (routine)

- No special precautions
- Routine baseline laboratory monitoring
- ECG at baseline and observe for bradycardia

Special monitoring: Serum sodium for hyponatremia

Drug Interactions

See also, Table 1.25 on page 89.

Citalopram metabolite desmethylcitalopram has affinity for CYP2D6 and inhibits its action. May inhibit metabolism of drugs metabolized by this enzyme, such as desipramine. Clinical significance is unknown in elders but caution advised in using combinations.

- Desipramine: Coadministration in elderly not advised; increased serum concentration of desipramine.
- No effect on blood level of amitriptyline or nortriptyline when citalopram was coadministered in one older patient, but there was synergistic therapeutic effect on depression.
- Increased levels of metoprolol reported.
- Clozapine—monitor.
- Cimetidine may increase concentration of citalopram.

Increased plasma levels of citalopram in combination with potent inhibitors of CYP3A4 (e.g., ketoconazole, itraconazole, fluconazole, erythromycin) or CYP2C19 (e.g., omeprazole).

Carbamazepine—may induce enzyme and reduce citalopram plasma levels, but little clinical significance noted to this point.

Anticoagualants and antiplatelet agents—may increase risk of bleeding.

Usual cautions with alcohol.

May aggravate antipsychotic-induced EPS.

Note danger of serotonin syndrome with coadministration of

- MAOIs—life-threatening complications; coadministration contraindicated.
- TCAs—possible, although combinations may be used with appropriate caution and monitoring.
- SRI drugs and serotonergic agents such as SSRIs, bupropion, lithium, clomipramine, mirtazapine, and nefazodone.
- Triptans—often used safely for younger patients.
- OTC/alternative medicines
  - √ Cold preparations (dextromethorphan)
  - √ SAMe
  - √ St. John's Wort
- Meperidine

Special Precautions and Contraindications

- Caution in coagulation disorders.
- General precautions with driving or hazardous machinery while taking citalopram.
- Monitor serum sodium and inquire periodically for signs of SIADH (see p. 82).
- History of adverse reaction to, or intolerance of, the drug is contraindicative.

Overdose, Toxicity, Suicide

Generally safe in overdose, unless taken with another serotonergic agent. Fatalities reported include concomitant serotonin agonists such as moclobemide, although some fatalities reported in general adults with citalopram alone at 100–200 times the therapeutic dose.

Symptoms of overdose are serotonin-related.

- At smaller doses (up to 600 mg in general adult patients), symptoms include
  - √ Dizziness
  - √ Sweating
  - √ Tachycardia
  - √ Nausea, vomiting
  - √ Tremor
  - √ Drowsiness/somnolence
- At higher doses (over 600 mg) more severe symptoms emerge, such as
  - √ Convulsions
  - √ ECG changes (nonspecific ST–T changes and widening of ECG complexes without arrhythmias), transient bundle branch block
  - √ Hyperventilation
  - √ Rhabdomyolysis
  - √ Confusion
  - √ Loss of consciousness
  - √ Coma

Management

- Provide general supportive care (e.g., airway, fluids).
- Administer gastric lavage and activated charcoal when indicated.
- Monitor vital signs and cardiac status (ECG).
- Diuresis, dialysis, hemoperfusion, and exchange transfusion are unlikely to be of benefit because of large volume of distribution.

Caregiver Notes

Side effects to watch for:

- For mild problems encourage patient to continue, since these often improve on their own.
- Agitation and sleep problems.
  - √ Can be addressed with temporary tranquillizing medication and reassurance.
- Increasing depressive symptoms, especially suicidal expressions.
  - √ *Take suicidal expressions seriously and contact physician or therapist.*
- *Do not* discontinue medication abruptly.
- Encourage patient to comply with physicians instructions

Clinical Tips

- Use of citalopram in BPSD is on a trial-and-error basis.
  - √ If depression is present, use depression guidelines for prescribing.
- May induce anxiety/agitation initially.
  - √ Usually transient, about a week or two, and patient may be encouraged to tolerate symptoms.
  - √ Concurrent anxiolytic may help to negotiate this period.
- Switching from tricyclic: Taper and discontinue before initiating citalopram.
- General adult guidelines suggest direct switch from paroxetine or sertraline to citalopram, but clinically this may lead to exacerbation of serotonin effects.
  - √ Best to discontinue one agent before starting the next.
  - √ Longer washout period with fluoxetine (up to 5–6 weeks) due to long half-life.
  - √ Discontinue fluvoxamine before switching.
  - √ Discontinue moclobemide several days before switching.
  - √ Minimum 14 days washout or longer when switching to irreversible MAOI.
- Monitor serum sodium levels especially in patients who have had hyponatremia associated with other treatment, such as diuretics.
- A parenteral form of citalopram is available, but no clear data that it is more effective than the oral.
  - √ Parenteral induction of treatment has been used in Europe, but utility is controversial.
  - √ May be useful for hospitalized patients who cannot swallow oral medications or refuse them.

CLOMIPRAMINE

Drug	Manufacturer	Chemical Class	Therapeutic Class
clomipramine (Anafranil)	Novartis	tertiary amine	TCA AD

Indications: FDA/HPB

- Depression
- OCD

Indications: Off label

- Chronic pain
- Social anxiety and phobia (general adult data)
- Panic disorder (general adult data)

Pharmacology

- Nonlinear pharmacokinetics at doses >150 mg/day.
- Steady state achieved over 2–3 weeks.
- Significantly reduced clearance rates and increased plasma levels in elders.
- Clearance increased by smoking.

Mechanism of action

- Complex dual action
  - √ Parent compound is a serotonin reuptake inhibitor (most potent among all the TCAs).
  - √ Metabolite demethylclomipramine (DMC) is a more potent NA reuptake inhibitor.
    - ▫ In some patients DMC may make up 70% of circulating drug concentration.
  - √ Down-regulation of beta, alpha-2, $5HT_2$ receptors.
  - √ Lowers seizure threshold.

Therapeutic actions by indication

Despite anticholinergic side effects and cardiac toxicity, may be well tolerated by some elderly patients and may be considered if other agents are ineffective.

- Case reports
  - √ Efficacy in persistent OCD in old age.
  - √ Clomipramine more effective than SSRIs in OCD in younger subjects.
  - √ Effectiveness in OCD with comorbid schizophrenia (general adult data).

Choosing a Drug

- Significant side-effect profile
  - √ Hypotension
  - √ Anticholinergicity
  - √ Weight gain
  - √ Sedation
  - √ Cardiotoxicity
- Clomipramine not recommended as first-line therapy for depression in elders.
  - √ May be a useful third-line agent.
- Similar limitations for OCD and off-label indications.

Dosing

- Daily dose regimen

  - √ Depression and OCD: tid dosing reduces peak plasma level effects.
  - √ May be given once daily with equal effectiveness if tolerated.
- Initiating therapy
  - √ In healthy elders, begin with once daily doses.
  - √ For frail elders, bid or tid schedules are often better tolerated.
    - ▫ Base decision on tolerance of side effects and general frailty; efficacy does not seem to be affected by schedule of administration.
- Initial dose 10–25 mg po hs

Increasing dose and reaching therapeutic levels

- Increase by 10–25 mg every 5–7 days (keep in mind the long time to steady state and increase dose slowly).
- Therapeutic target range is 50–75 mg (range 10–100 mg/day).
- Therapeutic dose for OCD and panic disorder not established for elders.
  - √ 75–150 mg probably the best range (case report data).
  - √ Higher end of range may be necessary for OCD.
- Chronic pain 25–150 mg/day (general adult data).
- Maintenance: See page 54 for general guidelines.

Side Effects

See also: general TCA side effects (pp. 101–106).

Table 1.47. Side Effects of Clomipramine

Side Effects	Most Common	Most Serious and Less Common
Autonomic system	• Dry mouth • Sweating	
Body as a whole	• Weight gain • Increased appetite • Fatigue	
Cardiovascular	• Postural hypotension √ May be exacerbated by once daily dose regimen • Cardiotoxic effects	
Central and peripheral nervous system	• Sedation/somnolence • Tremor • Myoclonus • Dizziness • Headache • Insomnia	• Seizures (dose related) • Serotonin syndrome • Tardive dyskinesia-like syndromes (usually associated with concurrent antipsychotic drugs)
Endocrine		• Agranulocytosis
Eye		• Increased intraocular pressure in glaucoma

(cont.)

Continued

Side Effects	Most Common	Most Serious and Less Common
Gastrointestinal	• Constipation • Nausea • Dyspepsia • Anorexia	
Liver and biliary		• Elevated liver enzymes
Metabolic and nutritional		• SIADH—rare
Reproductive	• Decreased libido • Ejaculation failure • Impotence	• Painful ejaculation

Special monitoring (see also p. 108)

- Plasma levels not well established—suggested range 160–400 ng/ml; levels > 500 ng/ml considered toxic (general adult data).
- BP
- Cardiac rhythm

Withdrawal effects

- Taper drug gradually.
- Syndrome includes dizziness, nausea, vomiting, headache, malaise, sleep disturbance, hyperthermia, irritability.

Drug Interactions

- Many interactions reported.
- Anticholinergics produce additive effects (see Table 1.14, pp. 71–72).
- Inhibits demethylation of some tertiary amine tricyclics under clinical conditions.
  √ Doubles imipramine half-life but no effect on desipramine.
- Enzyme-inducing agents may reduce plasma levels of the drug (e.g., carbamazepine). See Table 1.32, page 95.
- Enzyme-inhibiting agents (see Table 1.29, p. 92): Avoid combination with fluoxetine and fluvoxamine.
  √ Inhibit P450 enzymes and increase clomipramine plasma levels to toxic range.
- Avoid SSRIs—danger of serotonin syndrome.
- Avoid combinations of sedative agents—additive sedative effects.
- Drugs that may prolong QT interval
  √ Antiarrhythmics (amiodarone, bepridil, disopyramide, dofetilide, ibutilide, procainamide, quinidine, sotalol)
  √ Cisapride
  √ Antipsychotics
  √ Mefloquin
  √ Quinolones, especially sparfloxacin

- √ Beta-2 agonists (albuterol, bitolterol, formoterol, isoproterenol, levalbuterol, metaproterenol, pirbuterol, salmeterol, terbutaline)
- Antihypertensives: Clomipramine reduces or blocks antihypertensive effectiveness of guanethidine, bethanidine, clonidine, reserpine, and alpha-methyldopa.
- OTC/alternative medications
  - √ Cold preparations (antihistamines)
  - √ Calendula
  - √ Capsicum

Special Precautions and Contraindications

- Reduce dose with impaired liver or renal function.
- Contraindicated when
  - √ Predisposition to, or history of, seizure, CVS pathology (cardiac arrhythmias, AV block), stroke, hypotension
  - √ Acute recovery phase after MI, and during acute CHF

Overdose, Toxicity, Suicide

See pages 107–108.

Clinical Tips

- Some patients are rapid metabolizers (demethylators) of clomipramine.
  - √ This will diminish concentration of SRI parent compound (clomipramine) and increase action of NA reuptake inhibitor action of the metabolite (desmethyclomipramine).
  - √ Before concluding that patient is not responsive, check to see if patient is rapid metabolizer and extensive demethylator.
    - ▫ Use therapeutic drug monitoring (see p. 108).
      - ○ Patients genetically deficient in isoenzyme 2D6 will have clearance much higher than 1 ng/ml/mg.
      - ○ If so, switch to another SRI.
- Many side effects are dose related.
  - √ Important to titrate dose to achieve maximal therapeutic effect at the lowest dose.

DESIPRAMINE

Drug	Manufacturer	Chemical Class	Therapeutic Class
desipramine (Norpramin and others)	Aventis	dibenzazepine secondary amine	TCA AD

Indications: FDA/HPB

- Endogenous depressive illness

Indications: Off label

- Some efficacy for pain relief.
  - √ Said to equal amitriptyline in some studies (general adult data).

Pharmacology

See Table 1.34, page 98.

- Mechanism of action: Strong NA reuptake inhibition.
- Lipophilic
- Highly tissue and protein bound.
- Linear pharmacokinetics, in general.
  - √ Nonlinear pharmacokinetics in one-third of patients (general adult and geriatric data).
- Clearance
  - √ Reduced by acute alcohol intake.
  - √ Increased by smoking and chronic alcohol intake.
- Least anticholinergic of the TCAs and not as sedating as tertiary amines.
- OH metabolite excreted by kidney.
  - √ Unclear whether reduced kidney function leads to clinically significant increases in the plasma concentrations of the metabolite, but caution warranted.
  - √ Prudent to avoid desipramine in such patients if possible.

Choosing a Drug

- Little specific geriatric data available.
- Little sedation.
- More favorable anticholinergic profile (but only four times less potent than amitriptyline) makes it somewhat more tolerable than tertiary amines.
  - √ May still produce significant anticholinergic symptoms in elders.
- Hypotension—less than some other members of the class but still significant.
- May be stimulating and agitating.

Dosing

- Initiating therapy: Start with lowest available dose and increase slowly, especially in frail elders.
- Initial dose: Begin at 10–25 mg hs.

Increasing dose and reaching therapeutic levels

- Increase dose by 10–25 mg q 7 days (or longer interval in very sensitive patients).
- Therapeutic dose generally 50–150 mg (range 25–250 mg).
- Plasma levels are a key guide to dose increases and determining final therapeutic dose.
- Maintenance—see guidelines on page 54.

Side Effects

Milder compared to amitriptyline or imipramine.

- *Most common* are anticholinergic effects—activation/disinhibition/agitation, insomnia, tremor, and sweating (see also, pages 101–106).
- Isolated reports of testicular swelling.
- Cardiovascular: Significantly prolonged PR and QRS interval in about 40% of cases.

Monitoring

- Therapeutic plasma concentration level: 115–200 ng/ml

Drug Interactions

- Potentiation: Paroxetine increases desipramine plasma concentrations.
- See also, Tables 1.14 and 1.32 on pages 71–72, 95.

Overdose, Toxicity, Suicide

See pages 107–108.

Clinical Tips

- Watch for postural hypotension and, very occasionally, hypertension.
- If insomnia is a problem, consider prescribing desipramine in the morning.

DULOXETINE

Drug	Manufacturer	Chemical Class	Therapeutic Class
duloxetine (Cymbalta)	Lilly		SNRI AD

Indications

- Not yet approved by FDA/HPB.
- Treatment of depression.
- Efficacy demonstrated for treatment of urinary incontinence, and it is being investigated for this indication.

Mechanism of action: Serotonin and noradrenaline reuptake inhibitor.

Efficacy: Meta-analysis of premarketing studies (age $\geq$ 55 years) indicates effectiveness for major depression.

Dosage range 40–120 mg/day (general adult data); geriatric dose finding not established in premarketing trials to date.

Overall reported to be safe and well tolerated in meta-analysis of 7 geriatric (age $\geq$ 55 years) premarketing trials; no cardiac or weight effects noted to date, but clinical experience remains very preliminary; geriatric data still to come.

Main side effects include nausea, dry mouth, fatigue, dizziness, constipation, sleepiness, loss of appetite, and sweating.

Discontinuation syndrome: Dizziness, nausea, and anxiety if abruptly discontinued.

ESCITALOPRAM

See Appendix A for drug profile.

FLUOXETINE

Drug	Manufacturer	Chemical Class	Therapeutic Class
fluoxetine (Prozac)	Lilly	trifluoro propylamine	SSRI AD

Indications: FDA/HPB

- Depression, OCD, Bulimia nervosa
- Also marketed for premenstrual dysphoric syndrome (Sarafem).

Indications: Off label—Anxiety/panic

Pharmacology

- Nonlinear pharmacokinetics means increasing dose can disproportionately increase plasma concentrations.

- Is a substrate of CYP2D6 and can inhibit own metabolism, leading to higher than expected plasma levels during dose escalations.
- Pharmacokinetics not modified by age or renal impairment but half-life is prolonged by hepatic disease.
  - √ Requires dose reduction of 50% in hepatic disease.
- May take 2 months for the active drug to disappear from the body, especially in frail elders.

Mechanism of action

- Fluoxetine enhances serotonergic neurotransmission by selectively inhibiting reuptake of serotonin into the presynaptic terminals.
- Little affinity for histaminic, alpha-1 adrenergic, dopaminergic, and muscarinic receptors.

Therapeutic actions by indication

- Similar effectiveness profile to other antidepressants; improves
  - √ Dysthymia
  - √ Severe and mild forms of depression with associated behavioral and functional impairments, including the very old.
  - √ Comorbid anxiety associated with depression.
  - √ Bipolar II disorders and for relapse prevention.
    - ▫ Risk of manic switch rate not known for elders.
- Appears to be less effective than heterocyclics, venlafaxine, and mirtazapine in melancholic depression and atypical depression (general adult data).
- Case reports of efficacy in OCD in elders.
- Low remission rates of 21–35% in some intent to treat study samples.
- Fluoxetine improves depression associated with medical illness, including
  - √ Renal dialysis
  - √ Depression associated with comorbid dementia
  - √ Diabetes (general adult data)
  - √ Poststroke depression and emotionalism
    - ▫ Improvement in emotionalism as early as 3 days after treatment onset.
    - ▫ May enhance rehabilitation.
  - √ May counter postural hypotension (a common problem in Parkinson's disease) if used as adjunctive therapy.
    - ▫ Data should be viewed as preliminary, based on a pilot study.
  - √ Some effectiveness demonstrated in pain syndromes in samples that include geriatric patients (e.g., diabetic neuropathy), but overall effectiveness in geriatric pain syndromes not demonstrated.

Choosing a Drug

- In practice, generally as well-tolerated as other SSRIs and better than TCAs.
  - √ Fewer impairments in cognitive and psychomotor performance, no anticholinergic effects, and little cardiotoxicity.
- A second-line SSRI choice only because side effects may be prolonged after discontinuation due to long half-life.
  - √ Makes more problematic intolerant patients who have to be switched.
  - √ Longer washout also requires slowing therapeutic timetable.
- May be less effective and produce more side effects than sertraline in older patients.
- May induce agitation as do other SSRIs in early stages of therapy that can be interpreted by patient as panic symptoms and lead to discontinuation (general adult data).
  - √ Introduce slowly in lower doses to patients with panic symptoms to avoid premature discontinuation.
- Compliance may be marginally better than secondary TCAs (geriatric data scarce).

Quality of the data: Several open and controlled/blinded geriatric studies.

Dosing

Daily dose regimen

- Once daily, in morning with food.
- Fluoxetine weekly preparation—once a week (but no studies in elders).
- Some patients do better with every second- or third-day dosing schedule (taking advantage of long half-life).

Initial dose

- Fluoxetine
  - √ Geriatric dose not established by dose-finding studies.
  - √ Recommended starting dose, especially in frail elders, 5–10 mg.
  - √ Use liquid form for doses <10 mg or patients with pill-swallowing problems.
  - √ Many tolerate initial full 20 mg dose.
- Weekly preparation (Prozac Weekly)
  - √ 90 mg is only available dosage form. Not studied in elders, so effectiveness and safety unknown.
  - √ Not a recommended routine treatment.
    - ▫ However, may be useful in controlled individual circumstances for otherwise noncompliant patients.

Increasing dose and reaching therapeutic levels

- Increase dose based on side-effect tolerance q 1 week.
  - √ Some patients respond to low dose (5–10 mg), but many otherwise well elders require full adult therapeutic doses of 20–40 mg.
- If no indication of response to first plateau of 20 mg, in 2–3 weeks, consider increasing to 30 mg and then to 40 mg.
  - √ Note: General adult studies suggest that dose increases have limited effect in improving response rates, but this is still the first step in addressing nonresponse to initial dose.
- If patient is frail, has liver/kidney impairment, or side effects emerge at low doses, try reducing size and frequency of dose to q 2–3 days, titrating up slowly thereafter.
- If once daily dosing is not tolerated, try bid dose, morning and noon.
  - √ Note: When treating panic, start with a lower dose and increase more slowly, since initial doses may transiently increase symptoms; daily doses may not be necessary.

Maintenance dose (see also p. 54)

- Usually the same as the therapeutic dose.
- Dosing for off-label indications.
  - √ Poststroke emotionalism: Clinical reports indicate response at 20–40 mg.
  - √ Poststroke depression: Majority responsive to 20 mg.
  - √ OCD: Dosage range 40–60 mg (clinical case reports).
    - ▫ Required dose is generally higher than for depression, but side effects may limit tolerance.

Combination Therapy

- Augmentation strategies with fluoxetine not well established for elders.
- Combined therapies have higher potential for side effects in elders and should be used with caution.
- Desipramine–fluoxetine combination has shown effectiveness (general adult data).

Discontinuation and Withdrawal

Discontinuation

- Depression: See page 54.
- Poststroke emotionalism: Tendency to relapse if drug discontinued.
- Dysthymia: Risk of relapse is high after discontinuation.
  - √ Restarting medication often leads to improvement.

Withdrawal

- Long duration of action makes withdrawal syndromes less problematic than with short-acting SSRIs.
  - √ Has been used to "cover" withdrawal of shorter-acting SSRIs to prevent withdrawal syndrome.
- Long duration of action may require washout of 4–5 weeks or longer
  - √ Before switching to an MAOI, or
  - √ To avoid serotonergic side effects (or even serotonin syndrome in vulnerable patients) if switching to another SSRI, especially if using doses of 40 mg or more.
- After withdrawal, preexisting side effects may persist for days (or occasionally weeks, in very vulnerable patients).

Side Effects

- See also pages 70–90, 129.
- Specific geriatric data limited.

Most common side effects are headache, nervousness/anxiety, insomnia, fatigue, tremor, GI complaints, and sweating.

Table 1.48. Side Effects of Fluoxetine

Side Effects	Most Common*	Most Serious and Less Common
Body as a whole	• Fatigue • Asthenia • Mild initial weight loss, generally not of clinical concern √ Followed by weight gain in some patients	• Weight loss in medically ill may be significant • Rare systemic vasculitis (lung, kidney, liver) • Anaphylactoid reaction
Cardiovascular	• Little evidence of adverse cardiac effects √ Some reports of generally mild increased BP (age effect not reported)	• Bradycardia (unusual) Syncope (in one controlled study) • Case reports √ Atrial fibrillation √ Bradycardia √ Delirium (associated with high serum fluoxetine levels) √ Acute angle closure glaucoma √ Sudden death in patients with unstable respiratory disorders and/or unstable atrial arrhythmias
Central and peripheral nervous system	• Headache (31%) • Jittery nervousness • Insomnia (14%) • Tremor • Dizziness • Some patients complain of subjective experience of fogginess in thought and mild decline in attention	• Rare EPS (dystonia, choreiform movement, may involve masticatory/palatal muscles, Parkinsonism, akathisia) √ Onset rapid and may remit quickly when drug discontinued √ Symptoms sometimes persist √ Very rare tardive dyskinesia

(*cont.*)

Continued

Side Effects	Most Common*	Most Serious and Less Common
GI	• Nausea (18%) • Vomiting • Anorexia (12%) • Diarrhea (16%) • Dry mouth (7%)	
Endocrine		• Impaired glycemic control in diabetics—hypoglycemia √ May need to adjust insulin dose
Hematological		• Rare platelet dysfunction √ Hence prolonged bleeding times (associated with GI bleeding in elders) √ Remits with discontinuation or dose reduction
Metabolic and nutritional		• SIADH occurs infrequently √ 0.47%, with onset usually within 3–12 weeks √ Elevated serum levels of fluoxetine may be associated but hard to determine, since normal ranges of serum fluoxetine and norfluoxetine levels in geriatric patients not well established
Psychiatric	• Anxiety (12%) • Agitation	• Increased suicidal intensity (rarely) • Precipitation of manic/hypomanic state √ Unusual effect but may be more likely than with other drugs in class □ Reported higher potential to induce manic switch in bipolar patients than TCAs (0.98% vs. 0.39%)
Reproductive	• Women may experience loss of interest and sensation in sex • In men, erectile dysfunction, decreased libido, disturbed orgasm/ejaculation	
Skin and appendages	• Sweating	• Skin rash—may be severe and lead to discontinuation √ Associated with generalized allergic reactions (i.e., fever, arthralgia, leukocytosis, edema, respiratory distress, proteinuria, increased transaminase) √ Remits with discontinuation

* Percentages are general adult data.

Routine monitoring

- ECG
- Blood pressure

Special monitoring

- Maintain an index of suspicion for SIADH.
- Monitor serum sodium in susceptible patients with risk factors.
- Therapeutic effect not known to be related to serum concentrations, so blood level monitoring not useful.
  - √ Usual range of serum concentration of total fluoxetine in otherwise healthy elders is 90 ng/ml (range 40–140) and norfluoxetine 119 mg/ml (range 60–150).
- Monitor appetite and weight in frail elders.

Drug Interactions

- See also Table 1.26 on page 90.
- Key potentiating interactions of fluoxetine occur with drugs affected by fluoxetine-induced inhibition of CYP 2D6, 2C9, and 2C19, including:
  - √ TCAs
    - ▫ Especially imipramine and clomipramine.
    - ▫ Increases plasma levels of TCAs by up to 7-fold.
    - ▫ Combination of TCA and fluoxetine may induce toxic delirium.
    - ▫ Overall, few reported cases of significant problems, but there is also little age-specific data.
  - √ Citalopram
  - √ Paroxetine
  - √ Venlafaxine
    - ▫ Anticholinergic effects, including difficulty with urination, blurred vision, dry mouth, constipation.
  - √ Metabolites of nefazodone and trazodone
  - √ Barbiturates
  - √ Codeine
  - √ Dextromethorphan
  - √ Antipsychotics
    - ▫ Increased serum concentrations of haloperidol and clozapine
    - ▫ Type 1c antiarrhythmics
    - ▫ Beta-blockers
    - ▫ Verapamil
    - ▫ Phenytoin (toxicity and delirium)
- MAOI combination contraindicated.
  - √ High incidence of side effects, especially serotonin syndrome.

- √ Case report of serotonin syndrome with selegiline coadministration.
- Weakly inhibits isoenzyme 3A4, so weak potential for increased concentration of coadministered drugs metabolized by it, including:
  - √ Terfenadine (rarely, accumulation can induce *Torsades de Pointes*)
  - √ Astemizole
  - √ Carbamazepine
  - √ Quinidine
  - √ Lidocaine
- May increase or decrease lithium concentration.
  - √ Monitor levels more closely during coadministration, until stabilized.
- Tryptophan—agitation
- Tightly protein-bound drugs, including
  - √ Warfarin—Loss of anticoagulant control
  - √ Digoxin

Case reports of toxicity with fluoxetine combinations

- Fluoxetine–cimetidine
  - √ Parkinsonism (inhibitor of 2D6 and 3A isoenzymes, possibly increasing serum concentration of norfluoxetine).
- Fluoxetine–warfarin
- Fluoxetine–venlafaxine
- Fluoxetine–alprazolam
  - √ Increased alprazolam plasma levels

Overdose, Toxicity, Suicide

- Relative safety in overdose; similar to other SSRIs (see p. 129).
- Symptoms include
  - √ Nausea, vomiting
  - √ CNS excitation
  - √ Agitation
  - √ Restlessness
  - √ Seizures

Clinical Tips

- To get precise dosing of fluoxetine using liquid form, try a diabetes syringe.
- Some evidence (general adult data) that a response occurring earlier than 2 weeks may be placebo effect, although it may still be enduring.

- Sexual dysfunction may be masked in, or unreported by, elders.
  - √ Requires specific inquiry about pretreatment sexual patterns and interest and specific changes after drug therapy was started.
- Missed doses leading to rapid return of depressive symptoms are not as problematic as with shorter-acting SSRIs.
- Rare drug-induced dyskinesia may emerge rapidly after beginning drug and remit spontaneously and rapidly with discontinuation.
- Inhibition of 2D6 and its clinical effects on other drugs may last for weeks after discontinuing fluoxetine.
- Cognitive function is unimpaired after prolonged therapy (1 year).

Monitoring tips

- Although clinically significant weight loss secondary to drug effect is unlikely, it does occur.
  - √ Prudent to monitor weight in frail elders.
- Residual symptoms of depression are common and often significant even in responders.
  - √ Risk factor for relapse and an indication for ongoing clinical monitoring.
- Observe for increased agitation/akathisia and (rare) increase in suicidality.
- Observe for skin rash and discontinue drug if it occurs.
- Common side effects often spontaneously improve as patient accommodates to therapy in first few days after dosage increases.

MIRTAZAPINE

Drug	Manufacturer	Chemical Class	Therapeutic Class
mirtazapine (Remeron, Remeron sol tab)	Organon Inc.	tetracyclic piperazinoazepine	noradrenergic and specific serotonergic AD (NaSSA)

Indications: FDA/HPB

- Depression

Indications: Off label

- Anxiety associated with depression
- Panic disorder (preliminary data)
  - √ Case reports (unconfirmed by controlled data)
- Depression associated with Alzheimer's disease
  - √ Non-Alzheimer dementia (recent unpublished data)
- SSRI-induced sexual dysfunction when added to the treatment regimen (general adult data)

- Tremor (resting and essential) and levodopa-induced dyskinesias when added to other regimens (geriatric data)
- Night sweats and hot flushes (general adult data)

Pharmacology

Mechanism of action

- Receptor-blocking drug related to mianserin
- Minimum effect on monoamine reuptake
- Low affinity for muscarinic, cholinergic, and dopaminergic receptors
  - √ Primary site of action—noradrenergic neurons

Actions

- Increases release of NA by blocking inhibitory alpha-2 adrenergic presynaptic autoreceptors.
  - √ Occurs at two sites
    - ▫ Terminal region: Increases amount of NA released per nerve impulse.
    - ▫ Cell body region: Cell-firing and transmitter synthesis increased.
- Indirect increase of serotonergic transmission via the following mechanisms:
  - √ Increases noradrenaline release at the 5HT (serotonin) cell bodies in the raphe nuclei.
  - √ NA, in turn, acts at the excitatory alpha-1 adrenoreceptors on the 5HT dendrites and cell body to stimulate cell firing and release increased 5HT in the terminal regions.
  - √ Blockade of inhibitory alpha-2 adrenoreceptors on the 5HT terminals increases release of 5HT.
- Secondary 5HT receptor action
  - √ Antagonizes $5HT_2$ (reduces sexual side effects) and $5HT_3$ receptors (reduces GI side effects), channeling effect by stimulating $5HT_1$ receptor that is not blocked.
    - ▫ But $5HT_1$ stimulation remains somewhat controversial; not confirmed in some studies.
- Blockade of H_1 (histamine) receptors (strong antihistaminergic activity related to sedative quality of drug).

Therapeutic actions by indication

- Moderate and severe depression.
- Dysthymia (emerging general adult data).
- Medically compromised depressed patients.
- Sleep difficulties
  - √ Improves continuity and architecture in depressed (general adult) patients.

Table 1.49. Pharmacokinetics of Mirtazapine*

Bioavailability	Plasma Protein Binding	Volume of Distribution	Elimination Half-Life	T_{MAX}	Absorption	Excretion	Metabolism	Linearity
50%	85%, nonspecific	4.5 l/kg	20–40 hrs—longer in females (general adult data); clearance reduced by up to 40% in male elders; steady state in 3–5 days	2 hrs. after oral intake	Unaffected by food; higher plasma concentrations in elders but not clinically relevant	100% of dose within 4 days; urine 85%, feces 15%; clearance reduced by hepatic impairment (up to 30%) or renal impairment (up to 30–50%)†	Metabolized by 2D6 (demethylation), 3A4, and 1A2 (oxidation); metabolite demethylmirtazapine has weak pharmacological activity; no enzyme-inducing or-inhibiting effects (based on in vitro studies—no in vivo data)	Linear

* Generally derived from adult data.

† *Note:* Reduced dosage (30–50%) necessary in elders and with significant hepatic or renal impairment; elimination correlates with creatinine clearance.

- Comorbid anxiety/agitation and psychomotor retardation (general adult data with geriatric-aged patients included).
- PTSD—may be effective in some patients.
- Relapse prevention, long-term maintenance, and depression prophylaxis (general adult data).

Choosing a Drug

- Available data indicate drug is safe and tolerated in elders.
  - √ Drug of second choice for elders, since there is still very little specific data for this age group.
  - √ The few data available indicate effectiveness in elders.
    - ▫ Should be monitored cautiously for effectiveness and side effects.
    - ▫ Highly sedative and induces dizziness—may be more likely to lead to gait instability and falls in elders.
- Efficacy
  - √ Equal or superior effectiveness compared to standard TCAs, trazodone, some SSRIs (fluoxetine, citalopram), venlafaxine (general adult data), but conflicting data suggest less effective antidepressant action compared to imipramine (general adult data).
  - √ Evidence for earlier onset of action compared to paroxetine and possibly better tolerability in elders.
    - ▫ May be the result of primary antidepressant effect or anxiolytic and sedative action to which tolerance develops; the evidence is not robust.
- Similar mode of action to nefazodone, but mirtazapine produces greater sedation, decreased REM sleep time, and more weight gain than nefazodone; nefazodone has more potential for drug–drug interactions and increased REM sleep.
- Available in soluble tablet that dissolves on the tongue.

Dosing

- Initial and titration dosing schedules not well established for elders.
- Linear dose response makes dose titration necessary.
- Increased clinical response at higher levels.

Daily dose regimen

- Administer in the evening as single dose.
- Note: Drowsiness, sedation (antihistaminergic effects) predominate at lower doses; with increasing doses, noradrenergic neurotransmission increasingly counters the antihistaminergic effects;

if sedation is a problem at initial dose, may resolve spontaneously when dose is increased.
  - √ Because of this effect, manufacturer suggests that doses below 15 mg are not recommended.
  - √ However, because of prolonged half-life and higher plasma levels, elders (especially men), may be more sensitive to the drug, so it is prudent to start at the lower dose to begin.
  - √ If somnolence is significant but the drug is otherwise well tolerated, then increase to the next therapeutic level (general adult data).
- Guidelines are approximations derived from clinical experience, general adult, and limited geriatric data.

Initiating therapy

- Begin at 7.5–15 mg/day po hs.

Increasing dose and reaching therapeutic levels

- Increase by 7.5 mg at 7-day intervals or longer, as tolerated.
- Elders respond well at 15–30 mg/day (maximum 45 mg).

Maintenance dose

- Maintain a minimum effective therapeutic dose.

Combination Therapy

- Little augmentation data yet available.
- Case report of successful augmentation with lithium in previously refractory patient (age 64).

Discontinuation and Withdrawal

- Discontinue cautiously—SSRI-like withdrawal syndromes reported (general adult clinical case).
  - √ Dizziness, nausea, anxiety, insomnia, paresthesia

Side Effects

- Very few controlled geriatric studies or clinical case reports; side-effect data largely extrapolated from general adult samples.
- Side-effect vulnerability increases with coexisting brain disease such as dementia, even in mild forms (case reports).
- Few GI symptoms.
- Improves sleep parameters in depressed patients but at the expense of inducing daytime sedation or somnolence (general adult data).
- Little EPS reported (i.e., tremor).

- Little effect on CVS reported.
  - √ No quinidine-like effect on cardiac function.
- Minor effects on libido and sexual function.
  - √ Some evidence of improvement in sexual function in depressed subjects if mirtazapine is substituted for SSRI or other drug inducing sexual dysfunction (general adult data).
- Most common side effects include
  - √ Somnolence (> 50%)
  - √ Increased appetite (17%)
  - √ Weight gain (12%)
  - √ Dizziness (7%)

Table 1.50. Side Effects of Mirtazapine

Side Effects	Most Common*	Most Serious and Less Common
Body as a whole	• Weight gain (12%); (1–3 kg), mostly in first 4 weeks of therapy • Appetite increase (11–24%) • Malaise; flu-like symptoms • Sweating • Nausea, vomiting	
Cardiovascular†	• Orthostatic hypotension	
Central and peripheral nervous system	• Drowsiness may be a significant tolerance problem in some patients. √ Often transient over a few days of therapy. √ May be more pronounced at lower daily doses • Impaired cognition • Impaired motor performance • Dizziness (7%) • Headache • Confusion	• Tremor • Incoordination • Possible serotonin syndrome in combination with serotonergic compounds √ Fluoxetine (geriatric case report) • Delirium—unusual effect, based on current data. √ May occur at therapeutic doses in vulnerable patients (e.g., with coexisting dementia) • Sleep disturbance with vivid dreaming reported • Akathisia (case reports) • Theoretical risk of serotonin syndrome
Eye	• Blurred vision (23%)	
Gastrointestinal	• GI side effects more common in elders than younger individuals • Dry mouth (25%) • Constipation	• Abdominal pain √ May mimic acute abdomen
Hematological		• Agranulocytosis (mostly mild; very rarely, severe) • Neutropenia
Liver and biliary		• Increased liver enzymes √ Often transient with continued use, but significance not certain in elders

(*cont.*)

Continued

Side Effects	Most Common*	Most Serious and Less Common
Metabolic and nutritional	• Thirst	• Increased serum cholesterol
Musculoskeletal		• Arthralgia • Back pain
Psychiatric	• Anxiety • Agitation	• Single geriatric report of • hypomania following discontinuation of mirtazapine • Induction of mania (in right hemisphere poststroke depression)
Skin and appendages		• Photosensitivity • Rash

* Percentages are general adult data.

† *Note:* CVS symptoms may emerge, but relationship to drug is unclear; symptoms include hypertension, bradycardia, arrhythmias.

Monitoring

- Therapeutic drug monitoring not recommended.
- Monitor differential WBC—danger of neutropenia (and possible agranulocytosis).

Drug Interactions

Low propensity for interaction but geriatric data not available.

- Mirtazapine metabolism inhibited by drugs that inhibit 2D6, 3A4, 1A2 (see pp. 90–96)
- Warfarin—possible potentiation of anticoagulant effect.
  √ Extra monitoring advisable.
- Benzodiazepines—additive sedative and cognitive impairing effects.
- MAOI combinations contraindicated.
  √ 14–21-day washout switching from MAOI to mirtazapine.
  √ 7–14 days switching from mirtazapine to MAOI.
- Additive CNS depression with sedative hypnotics, barbiturates, antihistamines, opiates, and other agents with sedative properties (e.g., phenothiazines, tricyclics, trazodone, nefazodone).
- Serotonergic drugs—possible danger of serotonin syndrome (see pp. 79–82).
- Case report of levodopa-induced psychosis when combined in a Parkinson's disease patient.

Disability Interactions

- Reduce dose in patients with severe hepatic or renal impairment.

Effect on Laboratory Tests

- Uncommon: Transient increases in
  - √ ALT
  - √ Random cholesterol and triglycerides (may be related to weight gain)

Special Precautions and Contraindications

- History of, or vulnerability to, seizure disorder
- Hypotension
- Cerebrovascular disorder
- States of dehydration
- Additive effects with CNS depressants such as benzodiazepines and alcohol
- MAOIs

Overdose, Toxicity, Suicide

- Little reliable data available.
- Geriatric clinical reports suggest drug is safe in overdose.
- Commonest symptoms
  - √ Somnolence, lethargy, anxiety, confusion, tachycardia
  - √ Duration transient—spontaneous resolution with conservative treatment.
- No seizures reported.
- Serious symptoms generally related to concurrent overdose substances.
- Treatment for mirtazapine component of overdose.
  - √ Prudent to observe patient over period of half-life of drug (30–60 hrs.).
  - √ Provide general supportive measures (e.g., regarding airway and circulation).
  - √ Monitor ECG, vital signs (although changes are not usually serious).
  - √ Administer activated charcoal within first 24 hrs. in severe overdoses.
  - √ Induce emesis/gastric lavage in first hour or 2 after ingestion.
    - ▫ Not likely useful after that (peak serum concentration reached in 2 hours).
  - √ Run toxicology screen for other substances.
  - √ Take suicide precautions.

Caregiver Notes

- Because mirtazapine produces drowsiness, especially in the early stages of treatment, may be increased risk of falls.
  - √ Observe for instability of gait, especially when patient gets up at night.

Clinical Tips

- Sol tab: Use immediately after removing from blister pack; handle with dry hands; do not crush, chew, or cut tablet.
  - √ Slight price advantage over standard form of mirtazapine.
- Dry mouth, constipation, and dizziness are more likely in elders.
- Ask family and patient to report on sedation and gait steadiness.
- Monitor for signs of infection with low white blood cell counts.
  - √ Possible neutropenia, which can progress to agranulocytosis in rare cases.
  - √ Discontinue drug if this side effect emerges.

MOCLOBEMIDE

Drug	Manufacturer	Chemical Class	Therapeutic Class
moclobemide (Manerix)	Roche	benzamide	selective, reversible inhibitor of MAO-A (RIMA)

Indications: HPB

- Depression
- Not marketed in the United States, marketed in Canada.

Indications: Off label

- Panic disorder (general adult data)
- Case reports of successful treatment of depression in dementia, Parkinson's disease, and vascular dementia.

Pharmacology

- 50% increase in plasma concentrations with increased age.
- Clearance reduced by about 40%.
- Increase dose more slowly in elders.
  - √ Some may require reduced total dose.
  - √ Reduced dose necessary with hepatic but not renal impairment.

Mechanism of action

- Preferentially inhibits MAO-A (80%).
- 20–30% inhibition of MAO-B.
- MAOI action is reversible and of short duration (24 hrs.).

Choosing a Drug

- Equivalent efficacy, although some studies suggest not as effective as some other antidepressants.
  - √ Head-to-head studies in elders suggest equivalent efficacy to fluoxetine, fluvoxamine, nortriptyline.

- Does not affect sleep patterns.
- No negative cognitive effects and may improve cognition in some.
- In general, dietary restrictions are not necessary, with some exceptions.
  - √ Some evidence to support low-tyramine diet in patients susceptible to cardiac arrhythmias because of compromised myocardium.
  - √ MAO diet advisable during very high-dose therapy.

Dosing

Daily dose regimen

- Generally well tolerated by elders.
- Dosing bid or tid necessary.
- Always take after meals.

Initial dose

- Otherwise healthy elders often tolerate 300 mg/day.
  - √ 100–150 mg/day, especially for frail or otherwise sensitive patients.

Increasing dose and reaching therapeutic levels

- Optimal therapeutic dose for elders not established.
- Target dose is 300–450 mg/day in divided doses; range 300–600 mg/day.
- Increase by 100–150 mg increments usually no more often than q 7 days.
  - √ More rapid increases may produce undue plasma level increases because of metabolic nonlinearity.

Maintenance dose

- Minimum effective therapeutic dose

Combination Therapy

- Reports (general adult data) of depressed patients who were refractory to other therapy responding to high dose moclobemide (750–1500 mg) in combination with lithium and/or trazodone augmentation.
  - √ Not recommended routinely for elders, but high-dose therapy may be considered for treatment-resistant patients who are in settings where they can be carefully monitored.
- Safely used in combination with SSRIs (general adult data).
- Severe side effects may emerge with TCAs—combination contraindicated.
- No data with MAOIs.

Table 1.51. Pharmacokinetics of Moclobemide

Bioavailability	Plasma Protein Binding	Volume of Distribution	Elimination Half-Life	T_{MAX}	Absorption	Excretion	Metabolism	Linearity
55% after single dose (because of first-pass metabolism); 85–90% after multiple doses	50%	1.2 l/kg (general adult data)	1–2 hrs. (parent compound); becomes more prolonged at higher doses	45 min. (0.5–3.5 hours)	Peak plasma concentrations within 0.5–2 hrs. (general adult data); food reduces rate but not extent of absorption	95% in urine; clearance almost exclusively due to hepatic metabolism; < 1% excreted unchanged in urine	A substrate of CYP2C19 and 2D6; inhibits CYP2C19, 2D6, 1A2 (uncertain clinical significance); metabolites have little or no clinical activity	Linear up to doses of 200 mg, but nonlinear thereafter

Side Effects

- Commonest side effects include insomnia, headache, dizziness, and dry mouth.
- In general, an alerting/activating drug, reflected in side effects such as restlessness, sleep disturbance, and agitation.
  - √ Placebo-related incidence of these effects similar to moclobemide.
  - √ One study suggests elders may experience fewer side effects than general adults.
- Little weight gain and few cardiovascular or sexual effects.
- No negative cognitive effects and may improve cognition in some as result of improvement in depression and possibly because of activating effects.
- Well tolerated when used for depression associated with dementia.
- Similar tolerability to fluoxetine (general adult data).

Table 1.52. Side Effects of Moclobemide

Side Effects	Most Common*	Most Serious and Less Common
Cardiovascular	• Orthostatic hypotension	• Hypertension (case reports)
Case reports		• Intrahepatic cholestasis
Central and peripheral nervous system	• Sleep distrurbances √ Activating, with initial, terminal insomnia (3.6%) • Sedation/somnolence (1%) • Headache (4.6%) • Dizziness (2.9%) • Paresthesias • Restlessness	• Confusion • Agitation • Coma
Eye	• Visual disturbances	
Gastrointestinal	• Nausea (3.6%) • Dry mouth (3.9%) • Constipation (3.2%) • Diarrhea (1.7%) • Loss of appetite	
Metabolic and nutritional		• Raised liver enzymes without clinical sequelae • Serotonin syndrome—danger with all serotonergic drugs
Psychiatric	• Restlessness • Anxiety • Irritability	• Manic switch • Hypersexuality—case reports in patients with stroke and Parkinson's disease. • Exacerbation of psychosis in schizophrenia.
Skin and appendages	• Rash • Pruritis • Flushing	
Urinary		• Urinary retention

* Percentages are general adult data.

Drug Interactions

- Geriatric data limited, so caution appropriate.
- Inhibitors of 2D6 and 2C19 may reduce metabolic rate and increase plasma concentrations (see Table 1.32, p. 95).
- Overall, much less concern than with irreversible MAOIs about washout period when switching between moclobemide and other antidepressants (general adult data).

Switching and coadministration

- When switching *from* another serotonergic agent *to* moclobemide, wait 4–5 half-life periods of the original drug (e.g., 5 weeks with fluoxetine).
- From HCA to moclobemide, employ washout period.
- From moclobemide to HCA, conservative management employs 2-day washout.
- Combination of HCA and moclobemide not recommended.
  - √ May induce significant adverse effects, but data conflict.
    - ▫ Combination with desipramine has been used without problems.
- Sympathomimetics (norepinephrine and isoproterenol, and weight-reducing drugs) risk hypertension.
- Dextromethorphan (OTC decongestants, cold preparations)—reported severe CNS symptoms.
- Metoprolol increases serum concentration and hypotensive effect of the beta-blocker.
- Does not interfere with nifedipine or hydrochlorothiazide.
- Alcohol—no interaction in moderation (healthy elders).
- Cimetidine elevates moclobemide concentrations by prolonging its action.
  - √ Reduce dose to one-third to one-half.
- Clomipramine—danger of serotonin syndrome (case report).
- SSRIs—coadministration reasonably well tolerated.
  - √ Common side effects are headache, dizziness, nausea, dry mouth, myoclonic jerks (general adult data).
  - √ Caution advised because of potential for serotonin syndrome.
- Anesthesia—discontinue drug 2 days prior.
- Potentiates action of narcotics; avoid meperidine.

Effect on Laboratory Tests

Nonsignificant increase in liver enzymes.

Special Precautions and Contraindications

- Reduce dose one-third to one-half with hepatic impairment.

- Thyrotoxicosis or pheochromocytoma—theoretical potential to induce hypertensive reaction.
- Dietary restrictions as noted above; avoid large servings of tyramine-rich foods (see p. 118).
- Avoid if hypersensitive to the drug.

Overdose, Toxicity, Suicide

- No overdose fatalities reported to date with moclobemide alone.
  - √ Fatalities associated with combined AD overdoses that induce serotonergic syndrome.
- Symptoms include
  - √ Nausea; Vomiting
  - √ Drowsiness; Disorientation
  - √ Slurred speech
  - √ Hypertension
  - √ Seizures
  - √ Delirium (i.e., agitation, aggressiveness, behavioral change)

Management

- Provide supportive care.
- Administer gastric lavage, charcoal, emesis.

Clinical Tips

- Although useful for the treatment of anxiety associated with social phobia and depression, agitation as side effect can be mistaken for anxiety.
- No pressor effect with < 100 mg/day of tyramine.
  - √ But eat tyramine-containing food in moderation.
- Caution with
  - √ OTC drugs such as cimetidine or nasal decongestants.
  - √ Meperidine.
  - √ SSRIs and venlafaxine (may cause serotonin syndrome).

NEFAZODONE

Drug	Manufacturer	Chemical Class	Therapeutic Class
Nefazodone (Serzone, Dutonin, Nefadore, Nefirel, Rezeril)	Bristol-Myers Squibb	phenoxyethyltriazoline phenylpiperazine	AD

Indications: FDA

Note: Withdrawn from the market in Canada because of liver toxicity.

- Depression

Indications: Off label

- Pain
  - √ Improves diabetic neuropathy in some patients (open label, geriatric data).
  - √ Chronic daily headache (open label, nongeriatric data).
- PTSD (open label, general adult data)
  - √ Improvement in depression, intrusive recollection, avoidance, and hyperarousal.
- Generalized social phobia (general adult data)

Pharmacology

- Values in Table 1.53 are for healthy elders; no data for depressed, frail, or medically ill patients.
- Cmax increased in elders; initiate therapy at 1/3–1/2 the general adult dose.
- Nonlinear kinetics: Plasma level concentrations are greater than expected with higher doses, possibly secondary to inhibition of CYP3A4 (as well as being a substrate of that isoenzyme).
- Reduced dose (50%) necessary with hepatic but not renal impairment.
- Plasma concentrations 2-fold higher in elderly women.
  - √ May diminish with repeated doses.
  - √ Likely the result of decreased metabolic clearance combined with lower mean body weight.
- May be given without regard to timing of meals.
- Inhibitor of CYP3A4; weak inhibitor of CYP2D6.

Mechanism of action

- Thought to be due to a net effect of increased serotonin neurotransmission.
- Action more specific than most SSRIs (which produce a general increase in 5HT neurotransmission).
  - √ Potent antagonist of action of $5HT_2$ receptor sites, resulting in greater $5HT_{1A}$ serotonin binding, thereby enhancing neurotransmission mediated by that site.
    - ▫ Similar action to mirtazapine but via a different mechanism.
  - √ Down-regulation of $5HT_{2A}$ receptors.
  - √ $5HT_2$ stimulation induces anxiety, insomnia, and sexual dysfunction.
    - ▫ Nefazodone blockade of $5HT_2$ leads to fewer of these side effects.
- Limited, dose-dependent reuptake inhibition of serotonin and noradrenaline
  - √ Significantly weaker than venlafaxine.

Table 1.53. Pharmacokinetics of Nefazodone

Bioavailability	Plasma Protein Binding	Volume of Distribution	Elimination Half-Life (hrs.)	T_{max}	Absorption	Excretion	Metabolism	Linearity
20% (variable general adult data); increases with dosage because it inhibits its own first-pass metabolism	Extensive: 85–99% (parent; general adult data)	0.2–1.0 l/kg	7 (parent, HO-Nef); 18–33 (TAD); 4–8 (mCPP) steady state in 3–4 days (general adult data)	1–3 hrs.	Rapid after oral dose; food delays absorption by about 20% and increases oral bioavailability by 18%, but not usually clinically significant; peak plasma concentrations 2-fold higher in elders on single-dose administration, but only 10–20% higher after multiple dosing	Urine 55%; feces 30%	Metabolized by dealkylation and hydroxylation (CYP 3A4 and 2D6) to active metabolites hydroxynefazodone (HO-Nef), triazoledione (TAD), and m-chlorophenylpiperazine (mCPP)	Nonlinear increases in plasma concentrations (greater than expected with increased dose)

ANTIDEPRESSANTS

- Lacks affinity for alpha-2 adrenergic, muscarinic, cholinergic, histamine H_1, dopamine D_2, and gamma-aminobutyric acid sites.

Choosing a Drug

Note: Withdrawn from market in Canada and Europe because of liver toxicity.

- Efficacy similar to other antidepressants.
  - √ Sometimes effective when other agents have failed.
- Less disruptive to sleep patterns and sexual function.
  - √ Improves sleep in some patients during early treatment stages (general adult data).
- Generally safe in overdose.
- Used as second line to SSRIs at the present time.

Dosing

- Starting dose is about half general adult dose.
  - √ Special caution in women.
- Therapeutic window 300–500 mg/day in general adults.
  - √ Window not established for elders.
  - √ At lower or higher doses, therapeutic effect diminishes.

Daily dose regimen

- Dosing bid.
- Give hs when possible.

Initial dose

- Geriatric starting dose 50 mg once or twice daily.

Increasing dose and reaching therapeutic levels

- Increase dose q 7–10 days by 50 mg/day depending on patient's tolerance.
  - √ Patient may complain of sedation or mental clouding.
  - √ Observe for side effects during dose increases especially because of nonlinearity of plasma concentration increases.
- Optimal upper dose not well established for elders, but close to general adult levels.
- Therapeutic range 200–400 mg/day.
  - √ Therapeutic dose of 400 mg/day used in some studies.
- Clinically, wide variation in tolerance of nefazodone in individual cases.
  - √ Maximum dosage range may be as wide as 200–600/day.
    - ▫ Caution necessary at higher doses because of sedating side effects.

Maintenance dose

- Maintain as for other antidepressants (see p. 54).
- Long-term prophylactic effectiveness not established for elders.

Discontinuation and withdrawal by indication

- Effective in relapse prevention.

Side Effects

- Note "black box" warning from FDA and HPB of potential liver failure with nefazodone: 1/250–300,000 after 1 year of use.
- Most data are not age-specific.
- Few geriatric studies, but emergence of side effects similar in elders and general adult populations.
- Few anticholinergic effects reported.
- Induces less sexual dysfunction than SSRIs.
- Less disruptive of sleep patterns.
  √ Improves sleep efficiency.
  √ Does not suppress REM sleep (geriatric data not available).
- Some modest weight gain with long-term use, but less than SSRIs.
- Does not appear to adversely affect driving performance.
- Adaptation to many of the common side effects occurs over several weeks of therapy.

Table 1.54. Side Effects of Nefazodone

Side Effects	Most Common*	Most Serious and Less Common
Body as a whole	• Sweating • Asthenia (11%)	• Flu-like symptoms • Rash
Cardiovascular		• Sinus bradycardia (usually asymptomatic) • Hypotension • Orthostatic hypotension (probably due to alpha-1 adrenergic blockade); especially relevant to √ Patients with autonomic dysfunction related to Parkinson's disease, hypovolemia, and coadministered antihypertensive drugs or nitrates √ Cardiovascular or cerebrovascular disease that could be exacerbated by hypotension (e.g., MI angina, ischemic stroke) • Prolonged QT interval • AV block • Arrhythmias
Central and peripheral nervous system	• Sedation (19%) • Dizziness (12%) • Lightheadedness (10%) • Headache • Insomnia • Subjective mental confusion • Tremor	• Confusion • Visual Trailing √ Described by elders as double vision or even visual hallucinations • Mild psychomotor impairment • Abnormal dreaming • Memory impairment • Ataxia • Paresthesias (case report) • Seizures

(cont.)

Continued

Side Effects	Most Common*	Most Serious and Less Common
Gastrointestinal	• Nausea (21%) • Constipation (11%) • Dry mouth (19%) • Diarrhea • Anorexia	
Hematological		• Pancytopenia
Liver and biliary		• Rare reports of hepatitis and liver failure √ Onset for two-thirds of patients within 4 months (range from a few weeks to 1–2 years) of beginning treatment (general adult data) √ Usually improves with discontinuation of nefazodone √ Rarely fatal
Metabolic and nutritional		• Hypoglycemia in susceptible patients (e.g., diabetic) • Increased plasma prolactin levels • Serotonin syndrome
Musculoskeletal		• Myalgia • Arthralgia
Psychiatric	• Agitation/anxiety	• Activation of mania/hypomania
Reproductive	• Decreased libido	• Priapism √ Isolated cases √ Discontinue the drug immediately
Respiratory	• Rhinitis	
Sensory	• Blurred vision (6%)	• Abnormal taste
Skin and appendages		• Photosensitivity • Stevens–Johnson syndrome

* Percentages are general adult data.

Monitoring

- Liver function tests if premonitory signs of liver disease emerge.
  - √ Watch for anorexia, fatigue, asthenia, malaise, abdominal pain, nausea, discolored stools, dark urine, prolonged coagulation, confusion, asterixis, encephalopathy.
  - √ Laboratory indications of liver pathology include elevated levels of ALT, AST, alkaline phosphatase, gamma-glutamyl transpeptidase, bilirubin, and increased prothrombin times.

Drug Interactions

Nefazodone is a potent 3A4 inhibitor (see Table 1.28, p. 92).

- Alcohol—minimal potentiation of sedative hypnotic or psychomotor effects.
- Alprazolam—reduce dose by 50%.
- Calcium channel blockers.
- Carbamazepine—increased plasma concentrations of carbamazepine and decreased concentrations of nefazodone.
- Clarithromycin, erythromycin.

- Cyclosporine—plasma levels substantially increased (7-fold)
- Diazepam—not recommended.
  - √ Nefazodone increases plasma concentration of long-acting metabolite.
- Digoxin—increased digoxin levels; monitor levels closely.
- Fluoxetine (and likely other SSRIs)—serotonin syndrome (case report data).
- Haloperidol—may require reduced dose when coadministered with nefazodone.
- HMG-CoA reductase inhibitors—coadministration not recommended, especially simvastatin, lovastatin, atorvastatin, and cerivastatin.
  - √ Rarely associated with severe myopathy and rhabdomyolysis (pravastatin and fluvastatin are less problematic).
- Ketoconazole, itraconazole—coadministration relatively contraindicated.
- MAOIs—*do not use* in combination or within 3 weeks of discontinuing an MAOI.
  - √ Wait 1–2 weeks before introducing an MAOI after discontinuing nefazodone.
- Midazolam
- Propranolol—caution when coadministering.
  - √ Increased nefazodone metabolite mCPP levels possible.
- Terfenadine, astemizole, and cisapride contraindicated; may cause potentially fatal ventricular tachycardia (*Torsades de Pointes*).
- Triazolam—coadministration not recommended (data conflict).
  - √ Reduce dose by 75% when coadministered.
  - √ Nongeriatric data suggest nefazodone combination does not cause increased sedation, but caution in elders warranted.
- Vinblastin

Special Precautions and Contraindications

- Hypersensitivity to the drug or class is a contraindication.
- Coadministration with MAOIs, astemizole, cisapride, and terfenadine contraindicated.
- Caution in cirrhosis—reduce dose by 50%.
- Caution in conditions that may be worsened by CVS effects.
  - √ History of MI or stroke (hypotension), heart block, arrhythmias.
- 5–8-week washout period necessary when switching from fluoxetine (long half-life).
  - √ Higher than expected levels of active metabolite mCPP may result, producing transient but significant nausea, lightheadedness, and headache.
  - √ Start with lower dose of nefazodone.
- Discontinue medication immediately if liver complications arise.

Overdose, Toxicity, Suicide

- Relatively safe in overdose
- Symptoms of overdose:
  - √ Nausea, vomiting, somnolence, bradycardia, hypotension, respiratory depression, ECG changes (PVCs, prolonged QT interval), possibly seizures (in combination with alcohol).
  - √ Generally resolves in 8–24 hrs. (general adult data).
- Severe cases of very large overdoses may require intubation.
- Coma and death may result if taken in combination with other drugs.

Management

- Provide supportive interventions.
- Administer gastric lavage.
- Consider multiple drug involvement.

Clinical Tips

- Gender differences in metabolism, but clinical relevance not known.
  - √ Exercise additional caution when prescribing for elderly women.
    - ▫ Starting dose no more than half the adult dose (or less) and titrate slowly.
- May be better tolerated by patients who have developed akathisia on other SSRIs.
- Monitor BP in patients with coadministered antihypertensives.
  - √ Prudent to avoid nefazodone in such cases.

NORTRIPTYLINE

Drug	Manufacturer	Chemical Class	Therapeutic Class
nortriptyline (Pamelor, Aventyl, and others)	Eli Lilly (and others)	secondary amine	HCA AD

Indications: FDA/HPB

- Depression

Pharmacology

- Clearance markedly lower with concurrent medical illness.
- Highly protein bound
- Lipophilic
- Metabolite concentrations higher in elders (reduced renal clearance).

- Nortriptyline the only TCA that has therapeutic window (50–150 ng/ml).
  - √ I.e., therapeutic response increases with plasma level to a certain point and then begins to diminish.
  - √ Window is similar in all age groups.
- See table on page 98.
- Unclear whether age, per se, increases plasma concentrations over those found in younger patients.

Mechanism of action (see pp. 99–101)

- Inhibition of
  - √ NA reuptake
  - √ Some 5HT reuptake inhibition

Choosing a Drug

- Not a drug of first choice mainly because of potential cardiac toxicity as well as general TCA side-effect profile.
  - √ Long-term therapy not well studied but cardiac side effects limit its use in vulnerable populations over the long term.
- However, it remains a useful drug in selected patients, and among the TCAs, nortriptyline (with desipramine) is the drug of choice because
  - √ It has the most benign HCA side-effect profile
  - √ The relationship between the drug plasma level and clinical response has been established.
- Evidence that nortriptyline is more effective than SSRIs in very severe depressions, acute treatment of poststroke depression (studied against fluoxetine), and in depression in frail nursing home elders (studied against sertraline).
- Dropout rates in clinical studies are in the 12–19% range.

Prognostic indicators of response to treatment

- Poorer therapeutic response in presence of increased ventricular size (ventricle–brain ratio)—one study only.
- Drug effectiveness improved for all forms of depression when combined with IPT, possibly including bereavement-related major depression.
  - √ This may be true for other forms of psychotherapy as well (e.g., CBT or dynamic therapies), but no specific geriatric data yet available.

Dosing

Daily dose regimen

- Generally once daily hs dose.

- Some patients cannot tolerate a single daily dose and should be given a bid or tid dose.
  - √ Multiple-dose regimens decrease compliance.

Initial dose

- For frail elders use lowest available starting dose.
- Begin at 10–25 mg hs.

Increasing dose and reaching therapeutic levels

- Increase dose as quickly as tolerated—by 10–25 mg q 7 days, waiting longer between dose increases in sensitive patients.
  - √ Usual daily range is 50–100 mg but up to 150 mg in some patients who metabolize the drug well.
  - √ Some patients require full adult doses to reach therapeutic plasma levels.
  - √ Especially in the very old (>80 years), lower therapeutic doses of 30 mg have been shown to produce adequate blood levels in some patients.

Monitor

- Therapeutic response.
- Serial ECGs—cardiac toxicity is best indicator to follow and evaluate drug tolerance.
- Plasma levels of the drug—target therapeutic window of 40–150 ng/ml (most improve between 40–100 ng/ml) has been recommended (with a narrower window of 80–120 ng/ml suggested by others).
  - √ Maintain at lower range of therapeutic window, especially in frail elders, to see if antidepressant effect is achieved.
  - √ If not, increase dose to achieve higher therapeutic range (80–120 ng/ml), staying within the upper limit of the window.
  - √ Tolerability of higher general adult plasma levels may not be as good in elders.
  - √ Cognitively intact elders require plasma levels closer to younger patients, whereas cognitively impaired patients respond to lower levels.

Maintenance dose

- Maintain on minimum therapeutic dose.
- Reported relapse rates of 17% in first 4–8 months of continuation therapy.
- May require 8-week trial of therapy before deciding that patient is not responsive.

Combination Therapy

- Combination of nortriptyline and interpersonal psychotherapy appears to improve overall response rate and possibly long-term maintenance.

Side Effects

- See pages 101–106, and pages 70–88
- Overall, well-tolerated in acute treatment of young-old elders who are relatively free of medical contraindications such as heart disease.
  - √ Some evidence that initial side-effect burden declines during maintenance phase of therapy.
  - √ Somatic worry and complaints (i.e., physical tiredness, sleep disturbance, daytime sedation) not strongly endorsed by fully remitted patients on long-term maintenance therapy.
    - ▫ Those who complain of these effects often have residual symptoms of depression.
- Less sedating, hypotensive, and anticholinergic than tertiary amines, but still significant effects that need to be monitored (e.g., glaucoma, urinary retention).
- Not strongly associated with weight gain in long-term therapy.
- Significant interindividual variation in tolerability of significant side effects.
- Discontinuation rates compared to newer antidepressants appear to be higher, although there are few direct comparisons of new antidepressants with nortriptyline.

Table 1.55. Side Effects of Nortriptyline

Side Effects	Most Common	Most Serious and Less Common
Autonomic	• Anticholinergic effects	
Body as a whole	• Sweating • Asthenia	
Cardiovascular	• Orthostatic hypotension—not always associated with dizziness √ No worse in patients with preexisting hypertension • Tachycardia—increase in the range of 6–11 beats/min. √ May be mild or clinically significant	• Note: *Acts as a class 1 antiarrhythmic,* which increases risk of cardiac death after MI or in presence of ischemic heart disease • In therapeutic doses sometimes has similar potential to induce adverse cardiac effects (e.g., 2:1 AV block)
Central and peripheral nervous system	• Headache • Somnolence • Dizziness	• Lowers seizure threshold
Gastrointestinal	• Dry mouth—remains present throughout maintenance therapy √ Usually tolerable and a nuisance rather than a limiting effect of the drug • Constipation—may persist throughout treatment	

Routine monitoring

- Plasma levels in geriatric patients should be monitored routinely.
  - √ Therapeutic window is 50–150 ng/ml.
  - √ Do not exceed 150 ng/ml.
  - √ Hydroxymetabolites sometimes associated with cardiac toxicity even when nortriptyline levels are within the therapeutic window.
    - ▫ Especially relevant when 2D6 inhibitors are coadministered.
- Note: Plasma levels may not be useful indicators in presence of comorbid cognitive impairment, when side effects may emerge at lower levels.
- ECG weekly in patients at cardiac risk while dose is being increased; periodic monitoring thereafter for emergent cardiac side effects.
- BP monitoring during dose increases.
- BS, especially in diabetic or prediabetic patients.

Drug Interactions

- See pages 93–96.
- Lorazepam—some indication of improved antidepressant response when used in combination for anxiety associated with depression.
- Perphenazine—significant increase in plasma nortriptyline levels.
- Usual cautions to avoid alcohol, concurrent MAOIs, SSRIs (serotonin syndrome).
- Cimetidine—significantly increases anticholinergic action.
- Fluoxetine—increases plasma concentration of nortriptyline.
- Caution with sympathomimetics.
- Caution with inhibitors of CYP2D6.

Contraindications

- Ischemic heart disease—choose another drug class and/or monitor cardiac effects.
- Diabetes—some data to suggest a primary hyperglycemic effect of nortriptyline, but improvement in management of depression overall improves diabetes control, despite hyperglycemic effect of nortriptyline.
- Hyperthyroidism—increased risk of cardiac arrhythmias.
- Seizure vulnerability—reduce dose or choose another class of drug in presence of history of seizures or other significant vulnerabilities.

Overdose

See page 107.

Clinical Tips

- When monitoring blood levels, it is important to measure both nortriptyline and its active metabolites.
  - √ Metabolites are cardiotoxic, and can be unexpectedly high in elders.
- Anxiety relief is an important component of depression therapy.
  - √ Time-limited antianxiety medication may hasten or improve antidepressant action of the primary antidepressant agent.
- Long-term maintenance is effective in preventing relapse.
  - √ However, capacity to produce persistent tachycardia and dangers associated with ischemic heart disease (tachycardia associated with ischemic heart disease, associated with increased mortality) make less cardiotoxic drugs a better choice for long-term use, especially in frail or cardiovascularly compromised patients.
- Maintenance therapy has persistent effect on increasing sleep latency, decreasing REM sleep time, increasing REM sleep density, and reducing sleep apnea.
  - √ No effect on total sleep time or on improving sleep maintenance.
- Orthostatic hypotension not always a major problem with nortriptyline, per se, but the problem is exacerbated when other antihypertensives are used concurrently.
  - √ Dizziness not a good marker for hypotension, so supine and standing BP should be monitored regularly while increasing the drug dose, until a steady state has been established.
  - √ Patients with an orthostatic drop should be warned about the increased danger of falls, especially upon arising during the night.
  - √ Instructions include rising slowly from a sitting or lying position, sitting on the edge of the bed for 1–2 min. before standing, and routine use of support stockings in problematic cases.
- Monitor glycemic control in diabetic patients—may be a tendency to hyperglycemic dyscontrol.

PAROXETINE

Drug	Manufacturer	Chemical Class	Therapeutic Class
Paroxetine (Paxil), paroxetine CR, oral suspension	GlaxoSmithKline	phenylpiperidine	SSRI

Indications: FDA/HPB

- Depression
- Panic disorder
- OCD
- Social anxiety disorder
- GAD
- PTSD (recent FDA-approved indication)

Indications: Off label

- Chronic headache—no geriatric data; effectiveness in general adult populations but data still limited.
- Premature ejaculation (general adult data).

Pharmacology

See page 126.

- Maximum plasma concentrations are 3–4 times higher in elders and patients with severe hepatic and renal impairment (creatinine clearance < 30 ml/min.); half-life is longer.
  - √ Initiate treatment at lower doses and titrate up as necessary.

Mechanism of action

- Selective inhibition of neuronal uptake of serotonin.
- Somewhat more selective than fluoxetine in blocking serotonin reuptake.
- The most potent inhibitor of serotonin reuptake.
- Fairly potent noradrenergic reuptake inhibitor.
- Weak inhibitor of dopamine transporters.
- In vitro potent muscarinic antagonism, but in vivo effects more modest.
  - √ Greater affinity for muscarinic receptors than other SSRIs.
  - √ 20% of the anticholinergic potency of imipramine in vivo.
  - √ No apparent anticholinergic-related adverse effect on cognitive function.

Therapeutic actions by indication

- Effective in many forms of depression in elders, including minor depression (although not more effective than psychotherapy for this indication), depression comorbid with medical illness, dementia, and dysthymia.
  - √ Clear efficacy demonstrated in depression associated with MI—superior to nortriptyline.
  - √ No major advantage over other SSRIs for treatment of depressive symptoms.

- Panic disorder—reduces frequency of attacks (general adult data; no geriatric studies).
- Improves depressive symptoms of dementia.
  - √ Cognition may improve during therapy of depression associated with dementia, secondary to antidepressant effect.
    - ▫ No strong evidence for primary positive effect on cognitive performance.
- Effective in severe depression, including inpatients.
- Treats depression and concomitant anxiety symptoms.
- Efficacy demonstrated in PTSD (general adult data).
- Effective for relapse prevention (general adult data).
- Prevents development of depression with interferon-alpha for malignant melanoma.

Choosing a Drug

- A drug of first choice in depression, OCD, panic disorder, social anxiety, GAD, and PTSD.
- As effective as other antidepressants in elders.
  - √ Paroxetine equal in effectiveness to TCA antidepressants in head-to-head studies in elders.
  - √ Well-controlled study versus nortriptyline in moderately depressed young-old patients showed paroxetine to be equal in efficacy and superior in safety and tolerability.
- May impair sleep efficiency in some patients.
- Effective for continuation and maintenance therapy for relapse and recurrence prevention.
- The most potent CYP2D6 inhibitor among the antidepressants.
- Anticholinergic activity occasionally may limit utility in some patients.
- A severe discontinuation syndrome emerges frequently upon abrupt withdrawal from paroxetine.
  - √ Symptoms include agitation, anxiety, nausea, sweating, abnormal dreams, paresthesia, dizziness.
  - √ This drug requires a long taper to discontinue it, which is sometimes a disadvantage in those patients requiring a switch to alternative therapies.
    - ▫ Somewhat longer half-life in elders may attenuate discontinuation syndrome.
  - √ Cross-tapering strategies are not effective.
- Once daily dosing schedule is an advantage.
  - √ CR form now available (no geriatric data yet).
    - ▫ Flexible dosage forms available—12.5 mg, 25 mg, and 37.5 mg.
  - √ Liquid form available.

Quality of the data

- Several geriatric double-blind efficacy studies comparing paroxetine to other antidepressants (i.e., fluoxetine, clomipramine, amitriptyline, doxepin, mianserin).

Dosing

Daily dose regimen

- Administer once daily, in the evening if daytime somnolence is a problem, or in the morning, if insomnia occurs.
- Flexible dosing now possible using the liquid formulation (10 mg/5 cc).
  √ Employ for low dose initiation of therapy in sensitive patients.

Initial dose

- Base initial dosing decision on patient's overall clinical state, including frailty, hepatic and renal function.
- Initial dose 5–10 mg/day hs.
  √ Administer with food.

Increasing dose and reaching therapeutic levels

- No specific guidelines available for the timing of dose increases in elders.
  √ Clinical experience suggests dose increases of 5–10 mg q 2 weeks, based on tolerance and clinical response.
  √ May increase more quickly if tolerated.
- Usual therapeutic dose range is 10–20 mg.
- Maximum geriatric dose is 40 mg (very occasionally higher dose range for OCD and panic disorder may be necessary but not suggested as general rule).
- Maintenance dose and duration for bipolar disorder not established.
- In younger patients antipanic and OCD effect occurs at higher dose levels of 40 and 40–60 mg respectively.
  √ Dosing in elders not established for panic or OCD, but clinical experience indicates higher dose levels required, although doses greater than 40 mg are not suggested.
- Premature ejaculation helped by standard doses given on a chronic basis or an on-demand basis 3–4 hours before intercourse (oldest man in study 61 yrs.).

Maintenance dose

- Maintain at full therapeutic dose (see pp. 54–55 for guidelines on duration of antidepressant therapy).
- Continuation therapy in panic treatment prevented relapse over 6–9 months (general adult data).

Discontinuation and Withdrawal

- Discontinuation syndrome may be more common and intense with paroxetine than other SSRIs (because of short half-life and anticholinergic properties).
- When switching from paroxetine, taper very slowly over several weeks for sensitive patients.
- Substituting another SSRI to counter discontinuation effect may not be helpful and can aggravate potential for serotonin syndrome in patients who clear drugs slowly.

Side Effects

- See also page 129.
- Generally well tolerated.
- Side-effect profile similar in elders and general adult populations.
- Side-effect profile of CR form appears similar to IR form.
- Paroxetine side effects profile similar to other SSRIs.
  - √ Less activating and more sedative and anticholinergic than other SSRIs, which are troublesome to some elders.
  - √ Possesses about one-fifth the anticholinergic potential of nortriptyline.
- Side effects in elders generally less frequent than with some TCAs.
  - √ Paroxetine 61% vs. TCAs 74% (studied with active controls vs. amitriptyline, mianserin, doxepin, clomipramine).
  - √ Few head-to-head data for the generally better-tolerated secondary amines (i.e., nortriptyline and desipramine).
  - √ More GI side effects with paroxetine than with TCAs.
- Most common side effects include nausea, sexual dysfunction, asthenia, headache, constipation, dizziness, sweating, tremor, decreased appetite, sedation, dry mouth.

Table 1.56. Side Effects of Paroxetine

Side Effects	Most Common*	Most Serious and Less Common
Body as a whole	• Asthenia (12%) • Sweating (14%)	• Weight loss in elders who are frail can lead to weakness and impair ability to engage in rehabilitative activities, slowing recovery from illness or surgery • Weight gain
Cardiovascular	• Reduced heart rate in some patients. √ Not usually clinically significant	• Postural hypotension

(*cont.*)

Continued

Side Effects	Most Common*	Most Serious and Less Common
Central and peripheral nervous system	• Headache (19%) • Somnolence (12%) √ Daytime fatigue, especially in afternoon √ Can be especially hard for elders who mistake it for "old age" • Dizziness • Fine tremor • Sleep disturbance √ Insomnia √ Reduced REM sleep time. □ REM rebound after withdrawal √ Vivid dreaming	• Myoclonus • EPS • Serotonin syndrome • NMS
Endocrine		• Statistical association with increased risk of breast cancer (general adult data) √ Inhibition of CYP2D may be associated with increased cancer risk √ Avoid use in patients at high risk for breast cancer
Eye	• Blurred vision • May be especially troubling in the context of already compromised vision	• Acute angle closure glaucoma √ Caution in patients with history of angle closure glaucoma, age over 40 yrs., dilated pupils, history of eye pain or other ocular symptoms, and personal or family history of glaucoma √ Monitor intraocular pressure
Gastrointestinal	• Nausea (22%) √ Usually a transient problem accommodated to in the first week(s) of treatment • Dry mouth (14%) • Constipation (9%) √ Not usually a major problem with this drug • Diarrhea • Loss of appetite √ Especially relevant in demented elders with comorbid depression • Flatulence	
Hematological		• Bleeding—reduces platelet activation
Liver		• Elevated LFTs; isolated reports of hepatotoxicity √ Hepatitis with abnormal AST and ALT described sporadically √ Treat by discontinuing the drug; levels may remain abnormal for several weeks but usually remit spontaneously √ Occasionally, severe liver toxicity emerges

(*cont.*)

Continued

Side Effects	Most Common*	Most Serious and Less Common
Metabolic and nutritional		• SIADH in about 0.1–0.3% of patients; onset usually within 3 but up to 12 weeks √ Case report of □ Rapid onset SIADH within 48 hrs. □ Hyponatremia shortly after acute overdose
Musculoskeletal		• Myopathy—unusual
Psychiatric	• Nervousness/agitation/ anxiety	• Suicidal agitation—rare • Activation of mania
Reproductive	• Impaired sexual functioning √ Dose related—lower incidence at lower doses √ Higher incidence in treatment of panic and OCD because of use of higher doses √ May be relevant to some patients and not to others, depending on their level of sexual activity √ Do not assume that age alone makes this side effect irrelevant for elders • Men √ Delayed ejaculation (13%) √ Impotence √ Anorgasmia √ Erectile difficulties • Women √ Reduced sexual desire √ Inhibited orgasm	
Urinary		• Possible urinary retention

* Percentages are general adult data.

Management

- Dizziness
  - √ Monitor for gait instability because of increased danger of falls.
  - √ Rarely a reason to discontinue therapy, but precautions and instructions to families and patients are important.
- Appetite loss
  - √ Advise supplemental nutrients such as Ensure, or easy-to-eat foods such as milkshakes with egg added.
- Impaired sexual functioning.
- Inquire about partners and premorbid sexual performance to set a baseline to evaluate side effects.
- May require special sex counseling, emphasizing that this is a drug-related side effect that may continue for the duration of treatment, but not an age-related loss of capacity.

Monitoring

- If sudden decline in cognition or development of confusion, suspect SIADH or serotonin syndrome.
  - √ Monitor serum electrolytes, urine osmolarity, serum creatinine, BUN, and urine sodium.

Drug Interactions

- See pages 93–96 for other specific drug interaction cautions.

Monitor carefully or avoid

- Cimetidine (increased paroxetine levels)
- Codeine (reduced pain control—inhibition of conversion to morphine)
- Digoxin
- Flecainide (increased flecainide levels)
- Haloperidol (increased haloperidol levels)
- Lithium (increased risk of serotonin syndrome)
- Phenobarbital (reduced plasma concentration of paroxetine)
- Phenytoin (increased phenytoin levels, decreased paroxetine levels)
- Procyclidine
- TCAs (increased TCA levels)
- Theophylline (increased theophylline levels)
- Warfarin (increased risk of bleeding; monitor INR)

Paroxetine may inhibit metabolism and increase plasma concentrations of

- Flecainide
- Haloperidol
- Metoprolol
- Perphenazine
- Phenytoin
- Propafenone
- Risperidone
- TCAs
- Theophylline
- Thioridazine

Drugs that may increase risk of serotonin syndrome in combination with paroxetine include:

- $5HT_1$ agonists (sumatriptan, naratriptan, rizatriptan, zolmitriptan, almotriptan, frovatriptan)
- 5-hydroxytryptophan
- Buspirone
- Lithium

- MAOIs
  - √ Do not administer paroxetine for at least 14 days after an MAOI has been discontinued.
  - √ This is a general adult guideline that may be too short a time for elders who metabolize drugs more slowly.
- Meperidine
- Mirtazapine
- Moclobemide
- Nefazodone
- OTC cold remedies containing dextromethorphan, paracetamol, doxylamine, and pseudoephedrine
- Sibutramine
- SSRIs
- Tramadol
- Trazodone
- Venlafaxine

Drugs that may decrease paroxetine levels and antagonize therapeutic action include

- Barbiturates
- Phenytoin

Drugs that may increase paroxetine levels include

- Bupropion
- Cimetidine
- Clozapine
- Flecainide
- Quinidine

Disability Interactions and Contraindications

- Dementia—paroxetine does not exacerbate cognitive deficits.
- Severe renal or hepatic dysfunction—caution.
  - √ Severe renal impairment (creatinine clearance < 1.8 l/hr.) leads to increased plasma drug concentrations.
  - √ Reduce dose of drug.
- Hypersensitivity to the drug.
  - √ History of serotonergic syndrome and SIADH.

Effect on Laboratory Tests

No clinically significant effects on laboratory parameters.

Overdose, Toxicity, Suicide

Symptoms include

- Nausea
- Vomiting

- Tremor
- Involuntary muscle movements
- Dilated pupils
- Dry mouth
- Irritability, agitation
- Fever
- Headache
- Tachycardia
- ECG changes
- Occasionally coma
- Fatalities if in combination with other drugs such as alcohol

Management

- No specific treatment.
- General intervention and supportive care, as with any overdose.
  - √ Observe carefully.
  - √ Run toxic screen for concurrent drugs.
  - √ Induce emesis or administer gastric lavage.
  - √ Consider activated charcoal 20–30 mg q 4–6 hrs. within first 24 hrs. after ingestion.
  - √ Monitor vital signs and ECG.
  - √ Monitor airway.
  - √ Provide fluids.
  - √ Dialysis, forced diuresis, hemoperfusion, and exchange transfusion are not helpful.

Clinical Tips

- Generally not considered sedating, but some patients report feeling fatigued.
- Long-term therapy (1 year) shows no detrimental effect on cognitive function; cognition improves with effective treatment of depression.
- CR form—do not cut or crush.
- If a sudden change in clinical state after beginning therapy or increasing the dose, monitor serum electrolytes for hyponatremia.

PHENELZINE

Drug	Manufacturer	Chemical Class	Therapeutic Class
phenelzine (Nardil)	Pfizer	hydrazine	MAOI AD

Indications: FDA/HPB

- Depression—most effective for "atypical, nonendogenous or neurotic depression with mixed anxiety, hypochondriacal and phobic features."

Pharmacology

- Plasma levels higher in elders.

Choosing a Drug

- Usually a drug of final resort.
  - √ Used only after other drug regimens have failed.
  - √ Patients unresponsive to other medications may respond to MAOI (general adult data).
  - √ The safest of the MAOIs for elders.
- Carefully chosen geriatric patients tolerate this drug surprisingly well.
  - √ Not suitable for cognitively impaired patients, unless caregiver is fully responsible for all medications.
  - √ Patients should be able to be monitored regularly and frequently.
- Onset of action may be delayed up to 4 weeks.
- Some sedative effect.

Dosing

- Dosing schedule is tid.
- Initial dose 7.5 mg/day orally.
- Increasing dose and reaching therapeutic levels
  - √ Increase by 7.5 mg/day every 4–7 days.
  - √ Usual target dose 30–45 mg/day (range 22.5–60 mg/day) in divided doses.
- Maintenance dose
  - √ In early months of treatment monitor weekly for delayed onset BP changes (orthostatic hypotension)

Discontinuation and Withdrawal

- Taper drug slowly to discontinue.
- Abrupt withdrawal syndrome.
  - √ Onset within 1–3 days.
  - √ Symptoms include
    - ▫ Agitation
    - ▫ Nightmares
    - ▫ Sleep disturbance
    - ▫ Very occasionally, psychosis and seizures
- Manage by reintroducing drug and tapering slowly.

Side Effects

- See pages 116–121.
- Greater number of side effects overall than tranylcypromine.
- Side effects similar in type and severity to nortriptyline.

Table 1.57. Side Effects of Phenelzine

Side Effects	Most Common	Most Serious and Less Common
Cardiovascular	• Postural hypotension • Edema—pedal or sometimes more generalized	
Case reports		• Paradoxical transient Parkinsonian syndrome • Visual hallucinations in conjunction with macular degeneration
Central and peripheral nervous system	• Insomnia • Sedation/drowsiness afternoon sleepiness, ("nardil nod") • Myoclonus • Headache • Dizziness • Fatigue	• Tremor
Eye		• Blurred vision
Gastrointestinal	• Constipation • Dry mouth	
Hematological		• Leukopenia
Liver and biliary		• Elevated AST/ALT
Metabolic and nutritional	• Weight gain	• Hypertensive crisis • Serotonin syndrome • Temperature dyscontrol
Psychiatric	• Hypomania/mania switch	• Anxiety • Exacerbation of psychosis
Reproductive	• Impaired orgasm/ejaculation	
Respiratory	• Nasal congestion	
Skin and appendages	• Rash, pruritis	
Urinary	• Hesitancy	

SERTRALINE

Drug	Manufacturer	Chemical Class	Therapeutic Class
sertraline (Zoloft), oral concentrate	Pfizer	nanphthalenamine	SSRI AD

Indications: FDA/HPB

- Depression
- Panic disorder
- PTSD
- OCD
- Nongeriatric: premenstrual dysphoric disorder

Indications: Off label

- Emotional lability after stroke
- Unexplained pain of noncardiac origin

Pharmacology

- Pharmacokinetics (see p. 126) in the elderly are similar to younger adults: 3-fold elevation of generally inactive metabolite n-desmethylsertraline.
  - √ Clinical significance not known.
- Inhibits CYP2D6.
  - √ Not a strong effect but occasionally clinically significant.
  - √ Overall, minimal inhibitory effect on the P450 system.
    - ▫ Hence few major pharmacokinetic drug interactions.
- Renal and hepatic impairment reduce elimination and increase half-life.

Mechanism of action

- Selectively inhibits the neuronal reuptake of serotonin.
- Little affinity for other binding sites and weak effects on NA and dopamine neuronal reuptake.

Therapeutic actions by indication

- Depression
  - √ Improves
    - ▫ Cognition
    - ▫ Energy
    - ▫ Anxiety
    - ▫ Sleep
    - ▫ Quality of life and satisfaction with physical, psychological, and social health.
  - √ Patients with late-stage Alzheimer's disease do not show robust antidepressant effects.
    - ▫ Some require dose in the 100 mg range
  - √ Minor depression in nursing home patients responsive to treatment.
  - √ Effective for depression in the medically ill.
    - ▫ Demonstrated safety in depression associated with vascular disease—hypertension, cardiovascular disease, and poststroke lability of mood.
    - ▫ May have special effectiveness for tearfulness in poststroke lability of mood.
- Noncardiac chest pain
  - √ This form of pain often associated with anxiety and panic symptoms.

- √ Sertraline reduces the frequency and intensity of the daily pain experience.
- Panic
  - √ Reduces panic, including situational, phobic avoidance, unexpected, and limited symptom attacks.
  - √ Reduces time spent worrying (general adult data).
- PTSD
  - √ Reduces avoidance and arousal (general adult data).

Choosing a Drug

- In general, effectiveness equal to other SSRIs.
- May not be as effective as nortriptyline in frail elders in nursing home settings.
  - √ Studies difficult to interpret (e.g., nortriptyline samples often exclude patients with cardiac pathology, limiting the overall utility of that drug, compared to populations who may be included for sertraline treatment).
- Recent MI: Effective and safe, with no apparent effect on key cardiac measures.

Prognostic indicators of response to treatment

- Nursing home residents: favorable response of minor depression.
- Somewhat less effective than secondary amine antidepressants in medically ill or demented elders.
- Poststroke mood lability: Onset of remission achieved earlier than in depression—at 4 weeks.

Dosing

Daily dose regimen

- Once daily administration.
- Morning often best to reduce effects on sleep.
- Patients who experience daytime somnolence respond better to an hs regimen.
- Administer with food.

Initiating therapy for depression

- Begin at low dose.
- Increase within tolerance of side effects.
- Full adult doses often required for elders.

Initial dose

- Usual starting dose 25–50 mg orally in the morning.
- Start at lowest available dose for very frail elders.

Increasing dose and reaching therapeutic levels

- Increase dose weekly by 25 mg based on tolerance and clinical response (steady state achieved 1 week after each dose increase).
- Usual therapeutic dose 50–100 mg/day (range 25–200 mg).
  √ Many respond at 50 mg.
- Onset of early therapeutic action may be as early as first 2 weeks.
- Full clinical trial in elders is 8 weeks.
  √ Likelihood of response diminishes considerably if there has been no response at all after 4 weeks.

Maintenance dose for depression

- Similar to other antidepressants (see p. 54 for detailed discussion of maintenance therapy).

Dosing for other indications

- PTSD-50–200 mg range (general adult data).
- Poststroke lability of mood responsive at 50 mg.
  √ Continue the drug; often there is a rapid return of symptoms if drug is discontinued.
- Non-cardiac chest pain-50–200 mg.
- Panic/anxiety may respond better to higher doses of 100–200 mg.

Side Effects

- Similar to other SSRIs.
- Most common side effects are GI upset (diarrhea, nausea, dyspepsia), anorexia, headache, insomnia, somnolence, tremor, sweating, dry mouth, dizziness, male sexual dysfunction, agitation, and fatigue.

Table 1.58. Side Effects of Sertraline

Side Effects	Most Common*	Most Serious and Less Common
Body as a whole	• Sweating • Hot flushes	
Cardiovascular		• Tachycardia
Central and peripheral nervous system	• Headache (most common side effect reported in some studies) • Insomnia (13%) • Somnolence (13%) • Tremor • Impaired concentration	• Agitation • Twitching • EPS • Serotonin syndrome

(cont.)

Continued

Side Effects	Most Common*	Most Serious and Less Common
Eye	• Visual disturbances	
Gastrointestinal	• Nausea (15%) • Diarrhea/loose stools (22%) √ Greater incidence than other SSRIs • Anorexia (10%) • Dyspepsia • Dry mouth • Constipation • Vomiting	
Hematological		• Purpura/bleeding (impaired platelet aggregation)
Metabolic and nutritional		• SIADH
Musculoskeletal		• Arthralgia
Psychiatric	• Anxiety (15%) • Nervousness/agitation	• Activation of mania
Reproductive	• Males: ejaculatory delay, loss of libido • Females: loss of libido, delayed or impaired orgasm	
Skin and appendages		• Stevens–Johnson syndrome (case report data)

* Percentages are general adult data.

Monitoring

- Sertraline plasma levels do not correlate with clinical effect.
- Special monitoring
  - √ Serum sodium in hospitalized elders
  - √ Blood levels of concurrent phenytoin

Drug Interactions

See also, Tables 1.28 through 1.32, pages 92–96.

- Drugs that may potentiate sertraline effect.
  - √ Cimetidine—decreases clearance.
  - √ Grapefruit juice inhibits metabolism.
    - ▫ Clinical significance uncertain.
  - √ Drugs that may increase risk of serotonin syndrome in combination with sertraline include.
    - ▫ $5HT_1$ agonists (sumatriptan, naratriptan, rizatriptan, zolmitriptan, almotriptan, frovatriptan).

- Other SSRIs
- 5-hydroxytryptophan
- Buspirone
- Lithium
- MAOIs (do not administer sertraline for at least 14 days after an MAOI has been discontinued; this is a general adult guideline that may be too short a time for elders who metabolize drugs more slowly).
- Meperidine
- Mirtazapine
- Moclobemide
- Nefazodone
- OTC cold remedies containing dextromethorphan, paracetamol, doxylamine, and pseudoephedrine.
- SAMe
- Sibutramine
- St. John's Wort
- Tramadol
- Trazodone
- Venlafaxine

- Sertraline may inhibit metabolism and increase plasma concentrations of:
  - √ Coadministered nortriptyline (and other TCAs); usually small increase but occasionally may be clinically significant in some elders.
  - √ Phenytoin: Increases plasma concentration because of CYP2C9 inhibition (geriatric clinical case data).
  - √ Haloperidol: May increase plasma concentration to a small but possibly clinically significant degree, especially in patients of Asian heritage.
    - Related to CYP2D6 inhibition by sertraline and larger numbers of slow metabolizers among this population.
  - √ Tolbutamide
  - √ Antiarrhythmics (e.g., propafenone, flecainide)
  - √ Warfarin
    - Monitor prothrombin times.
  - √ Diazepam
  - √ Lithium
  - √ Clozapine
  - √ Galantamine
- Sertraline may inhibit metabolism and impair the effect of codeine.
  - √ Reduces analgesic effect (blocks conversion to morphine).

Disability Interactions

- Safe and effective in depression after MI.
- Seems to be well tolerated in frail nursing home population (open uncontrolled study).
- Caution (reduce dose) in renal and hepatic impairment.

Special Precautions and Contraindications

- Taper drug to discontinue to avoid discontinuation syndrome (see pp. 132–134).
- Hypersensitivity to drug or class a contraindication.

Overdose: Toxicity and Suicide

- Generally safe in overdose.
  √ Deaths in combination with other drugs.
- Symptoms include
  √ Somnolence
  √ Nausea/vomiting
  √ Tachycardia
  √ ECG changes
  √ Anxiety
  √ Dilated pupils
- Management
  √ Provide general support (i.e., airway, fluids).
  √ Monitor vital signs and cardiac function.
  √ Activated charcoal with sorbitol quite effective.
  √ Administer gastric lavage or induce emesis.
  √ Careful history and toxicology screen for concurrent drugs essential.
  √ Forced diuresis, hemoperfusion, exchange transfusion, or dialysis is not effective.

Clinical Tips

- PTSD best treated with combination of psychological and pharmacological interventions.
  √ Underdiagnosis common in primary care settings.
- Monitor plasma levels of coadministered nortriptyline, which may increase significantly in a few patients.
- First signs of therapeutic response may be intermittent periods of relief of depression or increased energy without subjective relief of depression.
- Improvement may continue for 3 months or longer before reaching a plateau of effect.

  - √ 75% of improvement occurs over 8 weeks but remaining 25% of improvement occurs only after 8 weeks of therapy.
- Note that in comparison to nortriptyline
  - √ Side-effect profile similar except for anticholinergic affects of nortriptyline (i.e., increased dry mouth and constipation and mild adverse effects on cognition).
  - √ Efficacy similar regardless of severity of depression.
  - √ Time to onset of clinical effect similar.
  - √ Sertraline may be better tolerated in > 70-yr.-olds.
- While clinical impact of grapefruit juice remains unknown, best to restrict its use during treatment with sertraline.
- Rapid dose escalation does not speed onset of therapeutic effect but may induce diarrhea.

ST. JOHN'S WORT

- No licenced indications
  - √ An OTC drug
- Extracts of *Hypericum perforatum.*
- A widely used antidepressant especially in Germany.
- Experience in elders still limited to clinical lore.
- Review of placebo-controlled trials shows efficacy for mild–moderate depression in general adult populations.
  - √ Compared to standard antidepressants recent trials are less favorable to St. John's Wort than earlier studies.
- Unproved claims for other psychiatric actions include
  - √ Antianxiety
  - √ Dysthymia
  - √ Insomnia
  - √ OCD
- Pharmacokinetics
  - √ Inducer of CYP3A4: Reduces plasma concentration of drugs metabolized by this enzyme (see p. 95).
- Dose
  - √ Geriatric doses for depression not determined; all data for general adults and should be modified for elders based on tolerance.
  - √ Increase dose slowly.
    - ▫ Hypericin standardized extract 0.3% oral doses—300 mg tid or 1200 mg/day or 300–600 mg po daily.
    - ▫ Hypericin standardized extract 0.2% 250 mg bid.
    - ▫ Hyperiform 3% standardized extract 300 mg tid.
    - ▫ Also may be prepared as tea: 2–4 g of dried tea leaves.

Table 1.59. Side Effects of St. John's Wort*

Side Effects	Most Common	Most Serious and Less Common
Body as a whole	• Fatigue	
Case reports	• Intracranial hemorrhage (subarachnoid and subdural)	
Central and peripheral nervous system	• Dizziness • Headache • Insomnia	• Paresthesias
Gastrointestinal	• Dry mouth • GI discomfort	
Metabolic and nutritional	• Serotonin syndrome	
Psychiatric	• Agitation • Anxiety • Restlessness • Irritability	• Hypomanic switch
Skin and appendages	• Skin rash • Photosensitivity	

* Reliable controlled data not available for this agent, especially for elders.

Drug Interactions

- Risk of serotonin syndrome in combination with
  - √ Antidepressants, including MAOIs, SSRIs, mirtazapine, venlafaxine, and nefazodone.
  - √ $5HT_1$ agonists—triptans such as sumatriptan, naratriptan, and rizatriptanal.
- Reduces plasma levels of several drugs (induces p-glycoprotein metabolism in gut or CYP3A4 hepatic enzyme): carbamazepine, cyclosporine, digoxin, diltiazem, fentanyl, TCAs, verapamil, theophylline, and coumadin.
- May intensify or prolong the effects of narcotics, anesthetics.

Withdrawal

- Withdraw slowly to avoid reaction to abrupt discontinuance.

TRAZODONE

Drug	Manufacturer	Chemical Class	Therapeutic Class
trazodone (Desyrel)	Bristol (many generics)	triazolopyridine	AD

Indications: FDA/HPB

- Depression

Indications: Off label

- Hypnotic
  - √ hs sedation
  - √ Also used to treat insomnia associated with antidepressant therapy.
- Behavioral control
  - √ For "agitation" in patients with dementia-related behavioral disturbances.
  - √ May be best for repetitive, verbally aggressive and oppositional behaviors.
- May be useful in improving
  - √ Painful diabetic neuropathy.
  - √ Negative symptoms of late-onset schizophrenia as adjunct to neuroleptic medication.
  - √ Symptoms of delirium unresponsive to neuroleptics (case series).

Pharmacology

Note:

- Plasma levels of mCPP may be higher than trazodone.
  - √ mCPP is anxiogenic.
- Substantial interindividual variability in trazodone metabolism.
- Reduced doses necessary in elders.
- Food delays and enhances absorption.

Mechanism of action

- Mixed serotonin agonist
  - √ Parent compound antagonizes $5HT_{2A/2C}$ receptors.
  - √ Metabolite mCPP is $5HT_{1c}$ agonist and alpha-2 antagonist but probably not responsible for mediation of trazodone's antidepressant action.
- Significant blockade of alpha-1 and histaminic receptors.
- Little anticholinergic effect.

Therapeutic actions by indication

- Hypnotic
  - √ Improves subjective quality of sleep.
    - ▫ Reduces arousals but not sleep latency or duration.
  - √ Evidence of rebound insomnia if treatment withdrawn.
- Dementia-related psychosis, agitation, and aggression.
  - √ Trazodone often improves this constellation of symptoms, especially verbally aggressive and oppositional behaviors.
  - √ Doses of 100–250 mg/day.

Table 1.60. Pharmacokinetics of Trazodone

Bioavailibility	Plasma Protein Binding	Volume of Distribution	Elimination Half-Life	T MAX	Absorption	Clearance	Excretion	Metabolism
70–90 %	89–95% (general adult data)	Higher in elders (1.15 vs. 0.89 l/kg) (Trazodone is lipophilic and there is higher fat to lean body mass ratio in elders)	11.6–13.6 hrs.	1–2 hrs.	Food may delay absorption but increase extent of absorption (by up to 20%)	6.3 l/hr.	60–70% renal clearance; rest in feces; < 1% excreted unchanged	Hydroxylation, oxidation, N-oxidation, cleavage of pyridine ring; active metabolite mchlorophenylpiperazine (mCPP) is metabolized by CYP2D6; trazodone does not affect metabolizing enzymes

- √ Improvement may occur within a week, with some continuing to improve over 1 month.
- √ BPSD-recent study of effectiveness: Compared to haloperidol and placebo, showed little benefit.
  - ▫ Most RCTs show positive results for this indication.

Choosing a Drug

- Not suggested as an antidepressant for elders.
- More useful as adjunct for hs sedation.
- Avoid use after recent MI.
- Antidepressant effect
  - √ Equal efficacy to amitriptyline, imipramine, and fluoxetine when used in full therapeutic doses.
  - √ Because lower doses often used with elders, efficacy in this age group is not equal to better tolerated drugs.
- Since introduction of new-generation antidepressants, not used routinely as antidepressant for elders, since sedative and orthostatic hypotensive side effects are not well tolerated in antidepressant doses.
  - √ But has been shown to be effective antidepressant in earlier studies, with beneficial anxiolytic properties early in treatment.
  - √ Less likely than amitriptyline to produce impairment in skills performance.

Dosing

Daily dose regimen

- Dosing tid the norm when using the drug as an antidepressant but not for sedation.
- For optimal speed of absorption, do not administer with food.

Initiating therapy

- Sedative dose often reached before antidepressant dose.
- If used as an antidepressant, side effects such as sedation and orthostatic hypotension may be reduced by giving more of the daily dose at night.

Initial dose

- Starting dose for depression is 25–50 mg/day.
  - √ May give as single dose hs.

Increasing dose and reaching therapeutic levels

- Antidepressant regimen
  - √ Antidepressant dose is 150–300 (maximum of 400 mg).
  - √ Increase dose in 25–50 mg increments every 3–4 days.

Hypnotic regimen

- Begin at 12.5–25 mg/day.
  - √ Increase in 12.5–25 mg increments of 3–4 days to target level of 25–200 mg hs.

Dementia behavioral control regimen

- Optimal dosing not established.
- 25–100 mg bid or tid.
  - √ RCTs (pilots) suggest average dose of 100–250 mg/day.
  - √ Doses as high as 500 mg/day have been used effectively in elders (e.g., for behaviors associated with DLB).

Painful diabetic neuropathy

- 50–100 mg hs

Delirium

- 50–100 (up to 200) mg

Maintenance dose

- Depression: Same as therapeutic dose.
- Sedation: Use should be time-limited in most cases.
  - √ In some instances may be used chronically for intractable insomnia.
    - ▫ Dose should be titrated down to lowest effective dose.

Side Effects

- Few anticholinergic and cardiovascular side effects.
- Most troublesome side effect is sedation.

Table 1.61. Side Effects of Trazodone

Side Effects	Most Common	Most Serious and Less Common
Body as a whole	• Weight gain • Edema	
Cardiovascular	• Orthostatic hypotension (may occur at lower doses of 50–175 mg) • Dizziness	• Cardiac arrhythmias—PVCs, possible ventricular tachycardia, especially with preexisting ventricular disorders

(cont.)

Continued

Side Effects	Most Common	Most Serious and Less Common
Case reports		• Movement disorders • Nightmares • Serotonergic syndrome
Central and peripheral nervous system	• *Drowsiness/sedation/somnolence* • Gait instability • Morning grogginess when used for sedation • Headache • Mild cognitive interference (e.g., impairment of memory and alertness, especially in vulnerable elders)	• Seizures (dose related)
GI disorders	• Nausea/vomiting • Dry mouth	
Hematological		• Decreased WBC count • Agranulocytosis
Musculoskeletal	• Myalgia	
Psychiatric		• Switch to mania • Anxiety associated with coadministration with 2D6 inhibitors √ Leads to increased concentrations of anxiogenic metabolite mCPP
Reproductive	• Sexual impairment	• Prolonged erections • Priapism in men • Clitoral priapism √ Not an emergency, as it is in males

Drug Interactions

Drugs that potentiate effects of trazodone include

- Alcohol, sedatives, other CNS depressants.
  √ Produces excessive drowsiness.
- MAOIs—serotonin syndrome (see pp. 79–82).
- Neuroleptics—hypotension with low-potency drugs.
- Antihypertensives—additive hypotension.
- Serotonergic drugs—serotonin syndrome with SSRIs, SNRIs, and others (see Table 1.19, p. 81).
- Fluoxetine—may slow trazodone metabolism.
- Inhibitors of CYP2D6—may lead to accumulation of active metabolite mCPP, predisposing to agitation and anxiety (see Table 1.31, p. 95).

Trazodone may reduce the effect of

- Warfarin
- Methyldopa
- Clonidine

Trazodone increases plasma levels of

- Digoxin
- Phenytoin

Trazodone potentiates antihypertensive effects of prazosin.

Special Precautions

- Caution in patients with preexisting cardiac disease—risk of arrhythmias.
- Caution as with other sedative medications—danger of falls, especially at night, caution driving or operating other machinery.

Overdose, Toxicity, Suicide

- Relatively safe in overdose (mixed age data).
- Generally, fatalities occur when taken in combination with other agents.

Symptoms include

- Drowsiness
- Hypotension
- Respiratory arrest
- Seizures
- Priapism

Routine management including

- Administering gastric lavage.
- Administering activated charcoal.
- Forced diuresis may be useful.
- Monitor vital signs and institute supportive measures, as required.

Clinical Tips

- Use of this drug for sedation carries risks (albeit rare or uncommon) such as priapism, orthostatic hypotension, or serotonin syndrome not associated with other classes of hypnotics such as benzodiazepines; use with cautions in mind.
- Some elders may not tolerate even low doses.
- Side effects can be limited by giving larger part of the daily dose hs.
- Advise all male patients of danger of priapism.
  - √ Incidence between 1/1,000–10,000 (general adult data).
- Ask patients to report erections lasting longer than 2 hrs.
  - √ Requires urgent intervention to prevent morbidity (urinary retention, fibrosis of the cavernosa, impotence, gangrene).
    - ▫ Occurs at doses of 50–400 mg.
    - ▫ Onset usually within first month (range 2 days–18 months).

Management of priapism

- Treat as urological emergency.
- Urgent treatment required within 4–6 hrs.
- Surgical correction in > 30% of reported cases.
- Permanent impotence may occur in 40–50% after surgical correction of priapism.

Caution in withdrawal from trazodone, as with all SRI medications (see withdrawal syndrome, p. 132).

VENLAFAXINE

Drug	Manufacturer	Chemical Class	Therapeutic Class
venlafaxine (Effexor, Effexor XR)	Wyeth-Ayerst	bicyclic phenylethylamine	AD

Indications: FDA/HPB

- Symptomatic treatment of depressive symptoms, including poststroke depression in the acute poststroke period.
- Generalized anxiety disorder (XR form).

Indications: Off label

- Pain
  - √ May be effective in painful diabetic neuropathy in younger and older patients; headache and fibromyalgia in younger patients.
  - √ Data should be seen as predominantly anecdotal, clinical, and uncontrolled.
- Control of hot flashes in androgen ablation therapy for prostate cancer.

Pharmacology

- Novel structure unrelated to TCAs or other antidepressants.
- Reduce dosage in liver and renal impairment.
  - √ By 25% in renal impairment, 50% in dialysis patients, and 50% in hepatic impairment.
- Pharmacokinetics not known to be affected by age (although ODV clearance reduced 15% in > 60-yr.-olds).

Mechanism of action

- Similar to TCAs.
- At lower doses, most potent effect is blockade of neuronal reuptake of serotonin.

Table 1.62. Pharmacokinetics of Venlafaxine

Bioavailability	Plasma Protein Binding	Volume of Distribution	Elimination Half-Life	Clearence	T_{MAX}	Absorption	Excretion	Metabolism	Linearity
Unclear—probably > 45% (general adult data)	Low: < 30% (general adult data)	Parent 2–23 l/kg ODV 9–13 l/kg	5 hrs. 10 hrs. for active metabolite (ODV); XR form 15 hrs. (non geriatric subjects)	Parent- 49 +/− 27 ml/h/kg; ODV 94 +/− 56 ml/h/kg; no difference in elders; ODV steady-state clearance 15% lower in > 60-yr.-olds	2–4hrs. peak levels not as high with XR and are achieved later (6+ hrs.)	Well absorbed (90%); food does not impair absorption; steady state in 3 days for adults; may be longer in elders	Primarily renal (87%); 5% excreted unchanged; decreased clearance of ODV in elders	Extensive first pass metabolism by CYP2D6 to active metabolite ODV and other minor metabolites; n-desmethylvenlafaxine is metabolized by CYP3A3/4; induces mild inhibition of 2D6	Linear kinetics over normal dosage range

- At higher dosage levels (> 300 mg), inhibition of neuronal uptake of noradrenaline predominates and is probably responsible for the anticholinergic-like effects, such as dry mouth.
- Some inhibition of dopamine reuptake also occurs.
- Lacks affinity for muscarinic, cholinergic, histaminergic, and alpha-1 adrenergic receptors.

Therapeutic actions by indication

- Diabetic neuropathy: Improves sharp or burning pain peripherally.
- Anxiety: Improves anxiety/somatization in depressed patients (general adult data).
- Poststroke depression: Improves mood and may also improve neurological symptoms and rehabilitation scores.
- Hot flashes: Reduces (but generally does not eliminate) number of episodes/day.

Choosing a Drug

- IR generally requires bid dosing.
  - √ A disadvantage to compliance with some elderly patients.
  - √ Some indication that once daily dosing is as effective and may be tried if compliance is a factor and XR preparation unavailable.
- XR once daily form preferable.
  - √ May have slightly superior side-effect and efficacy profile.
- Overall, effectiveness and tolerance in elderly comparable to general adult populations.
- Appears to be effective in prophylaxis of recurrence of depression in elderly subjects.
- Growing evidence (general adult) for efficacy in refractory depression (i.e., unresponsiveness to adequate or maximal doses of other antidepressants).
  - √ Meta-analytic data show better efficacy for venlafaxine over SSRIs but not tricyclics (general adult data).
- Efficacy reported in psychotic depression (general adult data).
- XR effective for generalized anxiety disorder (geriatric and general adult data).
- Efficacy in longstanding dysthymic disorders in younger patients (open label).
- Bipolar disorders not specifically studied, but viewed by some as useful after SSRIs and bupropion (general adult data).

Prognostic indicators of response to treatment

- Shown effective in hospitalized patients with severe depression.
- Comorbid anxiety or other psychiatric illness may decrease responsiveness.

Quality of the data

- Efficacy data
  - √ Limited double-blind studies
  - √ Clinical data (open label) indicate efficacy in elderly.
- Depression
  - √ Some studies included elderly patients and a few focused specifically on geriatric patients, such as in the poststroke data.
- Diabetic neuropathy
  - √ Clinical uncontrolled data
- Anxiety
  - √ No specific data for elderly treated for anxiety disorder.

Dosing

Note: Curvilinear dose-response curve; hence increased response at higher doses.

Daily dose regimen

- Geriatric doses not well established.
- Geriatric patients often respond at 75–150 mg range.
- In younger patients best results occur at higher dosage ranges (225 mg) using XR preparation.
  - √ Hence it is important to titrate this drug to maximum tolerated therapeutic dose to get full effect.

Initiating therapy

- No age effect on pharmacokinetics and studies in elderly do not strongly support need for reduced dosages, but clinical experience suggests prudence.
- Start with lowest available dose (12.5/18.75 mg–25/37.5 mg (U.S./ Canada available IR dosage forms).
  - √ Lowest dose of XR form is 37.5 mg (hard capsule).
- Initial antidepressant response may be evident as early as the first week of therapy.
  - √ Early response may be placebo effect rather than true antidepressant effect.
    - ▫ Placebo effect associated with increased risk of relapse.
  - √ Similar response pattern for GAD.

Initial dose

- Administer IR preparation bid (or tid, if side effects warrant) with food.
- Administer XR preparation once a day with food.

Increasing dose and reaching therapeutic levels

- Increase slowly based on clinical response and tolerance over next few weeks.
  - √ IR form: 12.5/18.75–37.5/50 mg/day q 5–7 days.
  - √ XR form: Start 37.5 and increase to 75 mg after 1 week, and increase by 37.5 mg weekly thereafter, based on tolerance.
- Geriatric dose (especially XR form) generally does not exceed 225 mg (in contrast to reported general adult doses up to 600 mg).
  - √ Wide range of effective doses reported in the elderly: 37.5–375 mg/day.
- Although steady-state drug levels generally achieved much more slowly in elders, level not established for this drug and speed of dose increases and target dose should be individualized, based on clinical response and tolerance of side effects.

Maintenance dose

- See general guidelines, page 54.
- If patient relapses while on lower-dose therapy, often will improve if dose is increased.

Off label dosing

- Pain: Clinical reports suggest effectiveness at 37.5 mg bid (general adult data).
- In poststroke study, good results obtained with doses of 75–150 mg/day (IR form).
- Hot flashes: Low dose effective—25 mg/day (12.5 mg bid).

Combination Therapy

- Augmentation with methylphenidate.
  - √ May enhance response in refractory or partially improved patients.
- Lithium
  - √ Added sequentially to adequate trial of venlafaxine produced further improvement in some patients (well tolerated in a generally younger, pharmacologically uncomplicated patient group, with some geriatric patients included).
  - √ Lithium level of 0.7 recommended target.
  - √ Use caution with lithium combination in the elderly (see also p. 516).
- Bupropion
  - √ Augmentation may enhance antidepressant effect.
    - ▫ Increased theoretical danger of hypertension with this combination secondary to 2D6 inhibition by bupropion and increased plasma concentrations of parent compound venlafaxine.

Discontinuation and Withdrawal

Discontinuation syndrome

- Withdrawal syndromes reported within hours of abrupt discontinuation.
- Taper slowly to avoid emergence of
  - √ Anxiety
  - √ Nervousness/agitation
  - √ Insomnia
  - √ Nausea
  - √ Diarrhea
  - √ Dry mouth
  - √ Dizziness
  - √ Headache
  - √ Paresthesias
  - √ Malaise
  - √ Sweating
  - √ Autonomic instability (blood pressure and heart rate swings; occasionally severe)
  - √ Confusion
  - √ Visual hallucinations
  - √ Hypomania
- May be prolonged over several days or weeks.

Side Effects

- Generally well tolerated.
- Believed to have little effect on muscarinic, histaminic, and adrenergic receptors.
  - √ Although there are low general rates of anticholinergic, sedative, and hypotensive effects in therapeutic doses, these effects in elders may be clinically significant and should be watched for.
- Side effects tend to be dose dependent.
- Commonest side effects (e.g., nausea and dizziness) remit with continued administration over a few weeks.
  - √ Sometimes may persist longer before remitting spontaneously.
- Drug-related discontinuation rates are dose dependent in the 17–30% range (general adult data).
- Commonest adverse effects are
  - √ Nausea/vomiting
  - √ Dizziness
  - √ Insomnia
  - √ Somnolence
  - √ Asthenia
  - √ Sweating
  - √ Constipation

√ Anorexia
√ Dry mouth
√ Anxiety/nervousness
√ Tremor
√ Blurred vision
√ Sexual dysfunction—abnormal ejaculation

Table 1.63. Side Effects of Venlafaxine

Side Effects	Most Common*	Most Serious and Less Common
Autonomic system	• Sweating	• Anticholinergic symptoms in combination with fluoxetine
Body as a whole	• Asthenia • Slight weight loss • May experience short-lived waves of nausea and subjective temperature changes • Case reports of dose-dependent sweating (nocturnal and daytime)	
Cardiovascular	• Tachycardia • Palpitations • Postural hypotension	• Older patients at somewhat greater risk for BP increases that may occur during treatment √ Increases are usually small (2–5 mm Hg), but sustained hypertension may occur in up to 13% of patients at higher doses √ Effect is dose dependent □ Less evident at lower dosage ranges; may be greater at high doses (≥225 mg) √ Appears not to persist with continued use √ Preexisting hypertension not adversely affected and so far seems safe in patients with cardiovascular disease □ Systematic data still limited √ Caution in patients with angina and transient ischemic attacks
Case reports	• Bruxism (case reports in younger patients treated successfully with buspirone)	
Central and peripheral nervous system	• Insomnia—reduced REM, increased wake time (general adult data) √ May be persistent • Headache • Dizziness • Nervousness • Somnolence • Psychomotor impairment	• Possible dystonic reactions • Isolated reports of confusion, convulsions • Seizure risk (small)

(*cont.*)

Continued

Side Effects	Most Common*	Most Serious and Less Common
Eye		• Mydriasis • Increased intraocular pressure in patients with narrow angle glaucoma
Gastrointestinal	• Nausea √ Most common (31%) side effect from pooled data, especially in first week of therapy √ Spontaneous accommodation in about 1 week with continued administration • Dry mouth • Constipation • Anorexia • Weight loss	
Hematological		• Bleeding
Liver and biliary		• Drug-induced hepatitis
Metabolic and nutritional		• Hyponatremia • SIADH (see pp. 82–83)
Psychiatric		• Drug-induced manic switch √ Short-term therapy risks appear small √ (Data from younger populations suggest greater risk in women with bipolar I or II diagnosis)
Reproductive	• Sexual dysfunction	
Skin and appendages	• Pruritis reported with XR form √ May emerge after several weeks of treatment	
Urinary	• Hesitancy	• Urinary retention (isolated report)

* Percentages are general adult data.

Monitoring

- Routine
  - √ ECG (baseline)
  - √ Blood pressure (initially over 1–2 weeks and at points of dose escalation)
- Special monitoring
  - √ Liver function
  - √ Serum sodium

Drug Interactions

- Venlafaxine exerts little effect on cytochrome P450 enzyme system.

- Use cautiously in combination with other psychotropics that do have P450 or anticholinergic action.
  - √ Significant exacerbation or emergence of anticholinergic side effects reported (nonsystematic, individual case reports) with coadministration of clomipramine, fluoxetine, nortriptyline, haloperidol, and desipramine.
- Cimetidine and fluoxetine increase serum levels of venlafaxine.
- Case report of severe anticholinergic side effects with venlafaxine–fluoxetine combination.
- *Do not use with MAOIs*—risk of serotonin syndrome.
  - √ If switching *to* MAOI, washout period is 2–5 weeks.
  - √ If switching *from* MAOI, wait 2 weeks (longer in frail patients with compromised liver/kidney function).
- Alcohol—no major interactions but prudent to avoid.
- Caution with all serotonergic drugs—danger of serotonin syndrome (see Table 1.19, pp. 79–82).
- May inhibit metabolism of imipramine, desipramine, and risperidone.
  - √ Clinical relevance uncertain and no geriatric-specific data.
  - √ Exercise usual caution when coadministering these drugs or others metabolized by the CYP2D6 enzyme (see Table 1.31, p. 95).
- Tramadol—increased risk of CNS depression, serotonin syndrome, and psychomotor impairment.

Note: In case reports venlafaxine has been administered concurrently with ECT with few adverse effects (but controlled data not available).

Effect on Laboratory Tests

- QTc prolonged occasionally.
- Elevated serum cholesterol.

Disability Interactions

- Not suggested as first-line agent for geriatric patients with hypertension.
  - √ If used, monitor BP carefully.
- Reduce dosage by 50% in hepatic cirrhosis.
- Reduce dosage by 25% in renal impairment and 50% in dialysis patients.
  - √ Administer 4 hrs. after dialysis is completed.

Special Precautions

- Reduce dosage if creatinine clearance declines to below 30 ml/min.

- Several weeks washout period needed when switching from fluoxetine (long half-life), since higher than expected blood levels may occur.

Contraindications

- Recent or concurrent MAOI.
- History of hypersensitivity to the drug.
- For maximum caution, relative contraindications include
  - √ During acute postmyocardial infarction period.
  - √ Acute cerebrovascular events.
    - ▫ Reasons may be related to small increases in systolic blood pressure and heart rate.
    - ▫ Some data also suggest increased platelet activity with venlafaxine.

Overdose, Toxicity, Suicide

- No good geriatric data available.
- Commonest effects include
  - √ Drowsiness
  - √ Lethargy
  - √ Seizures
  - √ Paresthesias
  - √ QTc prolonged
  - √ Sinus tachycardia
  - √ Reports of increased hepatic enzymes LDH, SGOT/AST, SGPT/ALT in overdose (younger patient).
  - √ Report of tonic/clonic contractions in overdose (younger patient).
- Management
  - √ Provide general support of airway, oxygenation, fluids, and electrolytes.
  - √ Monitor vital signs.
  - √ Monitor cardiac function/ECG.
  - √ Run toxicology screen for concurrent drugs.
  - √ Administer gastric lavage.
  - √ Administer activated charcoal.
  - √ Forced diuresis, hemoperfusion, dialysis, or exchange transfusion not helpful.

Clinical Tips

- Caution when transitioning from MAOI to venlafaxine.
  - √ May need longer-than-usual washout.
- At lower doses the pharmacological profile of venlafaxine is identical to that of SSRIs.

  - √ Dose increases produce a larger antidepressant effect in general adults.
    - ▫ May be due to additional NA reuptake inhibition at higher doses (i.e., inhibition of neuronal uptake pump for noradrenaline).
- Severe sweating may be controlled in some patients with benztropine, if switching to another antidepressant is not possible, but caution necessary regarding anticholinergic side effects.
- Demonstrated prophylaxis of generalized anxiety disorder in younger patients.
  - √ Hence responsive patients should remain on active treatment.
- Improvements in activities, social and occupational functioning may not emerge for up to 8 months (general adult data).
- Assess blood pressure and heart rate initially.
  - √ Extra caution needed in patients with hypertension, tachyarrhythmias, or other CVS disorders.
- Caution when administering ECT concurrently with venlafaxine.
  - √ Case report of bradycardia in younger patient.
- Although venlafaxine has dual action, it can act like an SSRI in terms of drug interactions, toxicity, and side effects (e.g., serotonin syndrome).
- When monitoring mental status, once drug has been instituted, keep in mind hyponatremia as a rare contributor to new-onset confusion or cognitive changes.
  - √ Monitor serum sodium concentration as necessary.
- If SIADH noted with another antidepressant, observe carefully for emergence of similar problem when switching to venlafaxine.
  - √ One of several drugs associated with SIADH.
- Monitor mood—switch to bipolar mania reported.
- Monitor intraocular pressure in patients with narrow angle glaucoma.

2. Antipsychotic Agents

OVERVIEW

Antipsychotics are used for a wide array of symptoms and diagnoses, including primary psychoses, behavioral disturbances associated with dementia, delirium, severe agitation, and psychosis associated with depression and bipolar disorder.

They are divided into two broad classes: typical and atypical. Most of the typicals are no longer routinely used for elders, having been replaced by the better-tolerated atypical agents. The main exception is haloperidol; mid-potency loxapine and perphenazine are also used for some patients; depot preparations are useful for chronic psychotic states in noncompliant elders.

Members of the class

Table 2.1. Antipsychotic Agents

Generic Name	Usual Starting Dose (mg/day)	Usual Therapeutic Range (mg/day) (Maximum Dose)
	TYPICAL NEUROLEPTICS	
aliphatic phenothiazines		
chlorpromazine (Thorazine, Largactil)	5–10 (IM is 4 times the potency of oral dose)	10–200
	PIPERIDINE PHENOTHIAZINES	
thioridazine (Mellaril)	10–25	10–200
mesoridazine (Serentil)	10	10–200
	PIPERAZINE PHENOTHIAZINES	
perphenazine (Trilafon)	2–4	2–24 (32)
trifluoperazine (Stelazine)	1–2	2–15
fluphenazine (Prolixin),	0.25–0.5	0.25–4.0
• injectable depot forms	6.25 mg every 14–21 days, depending on preparation	12.5 mg q 2–4 weeks (100)
fluphenazine decanoate (Modecate)		12.5 mg (25 mg) every 3 weeks or more

(cont.)

Continued

Generic Name	Usual Starting Dose (mg/day)	Usual Therapeutic Range (mg/day) (Maximum Dose)
fluphenazine enanthate (Moditen)	begin with test dose of 2.5 mg	12.5 mg (25) every 2–3 weeks or more
	BUTYROPHENONES	
haloperidol (Haldol)	0.25–0.5	0.25–4.0
haloperidol decanoate, • injectable depot form		Use low doses 20–40 (100) mg (about 10 times the daily oral dose as a single injection every 4 weeks); lasts about 30 days
	THIOXANTHINES	
thiothixene (Navane)	1	1–15
	DIBENZOXAZEPINES	
loxapine (Loxitane)	5–10	10–40 (80)
	DIHYDROINDOLONES	
molindone (Moban)	5–10	5–20 (100)
	DIPHENYLBUTYLPIPERIDINE	
pimozide (Orap)	0.25	2–3
	ATYPICAL NEUROLEPTICS	
aripiprazole (Abilify)	2	10
clozapine (Clozaril)	6.25–12.5	25–200
olanzapine (Zyprexa)	1.25–2.5	2.5–10
quetiapine (Seroquel)	25–50	25–200 (400)
risperidone (Risperidal)	0.25–0.5	0.5–3
ziprasidone (Geodon)	10–20, IM form 2–5	40–80 (160)

Wide scope of use of this class of drugs in elders.

- 40% of antipsychotic drug prescriptions in the U.S. are for elders.
- Where the patient is located influences treatment with drugs.
  - √ In the acute medical hospital setting, antipsychotics are used in 10% of patients, with increased length of stay in those who receive it.
  - √ Nursing homes: 32–65% receive antipsychotics, often for various symptoms associated with dementia.
- Rates of psychosis
  - √ Community: 1–5%
  - √ Nursing homes: 10%
  - √ Alzheimer's patients: up to 63%

Indications for prescribing antipsychotic agents in elders include

- Psychosis and severe behavioral disturbances associated with
  - √ Schizophrenia and related disorders
  - √ Mood disorders
  - √ Delirium
  - √ Dementias (BPSD)
  - √ Neurological disorders

ATYPICAL ANTIPSYCHOTICS

- Atypical refers to
  - √ The dual dopamine-serotonin antagonism of this class of drugs.
    - ▫ Atypicality requires $5HT_2$ affinity to be greater than D_2 affinity.
- Significantly reduce both negative and positive symptoms of schizophrenia.
  - √ Some negative symptoms develop secondary to treatment-induced EPS; improvement with atypicals compared to typicals may be due to apparent advantage because they produce fewer EPS.
- Growing body of data suggests that atypicals exert therapeutic effects on depression and hostility as well as psychosis.
- Decreased propensity to produce EPS.
- Reduced propensity to produce elevations in prolactin concentrations (not all atypicals–e.g., risperidone- are less prolactin sparing).
  - √ Potency in enhancing prolaction release: risperidone > haloperidol, > olanzapine > clozapine.

Limitations of atypicals

- Paucity of randomized controlled studies in elders.
  - √ Publication bias in favor of positive findings may artificially enhance effectiveness findings.
- Few nonindustry-sponsored trials.
- Side effects.
- Uncertainty about dosing with some agents (e.g., quetiapine) in some patient populations.
- High cost with subsequent limitations on access.

Effectiveness

- Majority of atypical drug prescriptions now are for nonschizophrenia indications.
  - √ Bipolar disorder (general adult data) and "geriatric agitation."
- Still too early to be sure that all drugs in the class have equal effectiveness and tolerability in general adults.
  - √ Data for elders is thin but promising.
- Clinical evidence suggests that members of this class of drugs have different efficacy profiles.
  - √ Hence worth trying another member of the class if there is no or inadequate response to one drug.
- Overall, they have replaced typical antipsychotics as drugs of first choice for geriatric psychosis and especially for management of BPSD.
  - √ Some evidence that low-dose atypicals are more effective in dementia-related psychosis and agitation than in nondemented schizophrenia.

- √ Generally appear to have broader and superior efficacy, especially for treatment of negative symptoms of schizophrenia (e.g., decreased verbal fluency and apathy).
- Some evidence that patients who had been chronically refractory to typical antipsychotics may be responsive to atypical antipsychotics—but evidence inconclusive on this indication.
  - √ Except for clozapine, for which data are more convincing.
- Response time of symptoms.
  - √ Sleep, agitation, and aggression respond most rapidly.
  - √ Positive symptoms respond in 3–6 weeks.
  - √ Negative symptoms respond in 6–12 weeks.
- Cognitive function
  - √ Atypicals have an inconsistent beneficial effect on improving core cognitive impairments of schizophrenia.
    - ▫ Verbal fluency, attention, working memory, and executive function.
- Cost effectiveness (all general adult data)
  - √ Clozapine is the most cost effective.
  - √ Risperidone and olanzapine are cost neutral.
  - √ No data for quetiapine, ziprasidone, aripiprazole.

TYPICAL ANTIPSYCHOTICS

- Unfavorable side-effect profile in elders.
- May be grouped into high-, intermediate-, and low-potency agents.
  - √ Dosing ranges for low-potency agents are much wider than high-potency agents because of wide individual variations in bioavailability of low-potency drugs.

Pharmacology

- All highly lipophilic.
- Well absorbed from GI tract but undergo extensive first-pass hepatic metabolism and hence have low bioavailability (variable levels of about 40–60%).
- T_{max} in 2–3 hours.
- High interindividual variability in pharmacokinetics.
- Pharmacokinetics all generally linear.
- All share common action.
  - √ Blockade of dopamine, especially D_2, receptor sites.
    - ▫ Motor symptoms caused by blockade in the nigrostriatal system.
- Effective for positive symptoms of schizophrenia but not negative symptoms.
- Serum levels generally not useful for routine clinical practice, with some exceptions.

Table 2.2. Pharmacokinetics of Atypical and Typical Antipsychotics

TYPICAL ANTIPSYCHOTICS						
Drug	**Bioavailability (%)**	**Plasma Protein Binding (%)**	**Elimination Half-Life (hours) (range)**	**Excretion***	**Metabolism**	**Linearity**
Aripiprazole†						
Olanzapine		High > 90%, especially to albumin and alpha-1 glycoprotein	48 (41–55) (geriatric)	Clearance 26 l/hr (12–47) (general adult data); excretion 2/3 renal, 1/3 feces; clearance 30% lower in women and 40% higher in smokers	Primarily by CYP1A2 and 3A4 (to minor degree by 2D6 and 2C19) and by flavine mono-oxygenase system	Linear (general/ adult data)
Risperidone	66% in extensive metabolizers; 82% in slow metabolizers (general adult data)	90%	25 for risperidone plus active metabolite	Predominantly renal excretion of metabolite	By CYP2D6; active metabolite 9-OH-risperidone (equipotent to parent compound; may cause emergence of EPS)	Linear
Quetiapine	Low—9%	83%	6.2–6.8; clearance is 30–50% lower in elders		Mainly CYP3A4 and to much lesser extent 2D6; many metabolites including dihydrosertindole and norsertindole; not clinically relevant	Linear
Ziprasidone (general adult data)	60% if taken with food	99% (to albumin and alpha-1 acid glycoprotein)	4–10 (oral form); 3 (IV form)	Urine and feces	Mainly CYP3A4 and aldehyde oxidase; 1A2 may be involved. Methyldihydro-ziprasidone the only active metabolite.	Linear
Clozapine	50–60%	97% protein bound	4–16 (acute dose); 66 hours (chronic dosing) (general adult data)	Urine—50% of metabolites; feces—30% of metabolites	Completely metabolized before excretion by CYP1A2, 2D6, 3A4; metabolite nor-clozapine may be active.	

(cont.)

* In general, clearance of atypicals may be faster in men than women.

† For data see Appendix A: Newly Approved drugs.

Continued

Drug	Bioavailability (%)	Plasma Protein Binding (%)	Elimination Half-Life (hours) (range)	Excretion	Metabolism
TYPICAL ANTIPSYCHOTICS					
Chlorpromazine (oral, rectal, liquid, and IM forms)	10–33 variable due to first pass metabolism	> 90 (to albumin)	17.7 (7–119)	< 1% excreted unchanged	CYP2D6 and 3A4; complex metabolism both hepatic and prehepatic produce pharmacologically active metabolites 7-OH-chlorpromazine sulfoxide and several others.
Thioridazine	25–33	99	Biphasic: 7.5 (4–10); 21 (11–37)		2D6 (and 2C19, 1A2); active metabolites mesoridazine, sulphoridazine, and cardio-toxic metabolite thioridazine 5-sulfoxide
Perphenazine	25	92	20–40	Urine and bile	2D6; main metabolites n-dealkyl-perphenazine and 7-OH-perphenazine; 1A4, 2C19, and 3A4 likely responsible for dealkylation metabolic step; metabolite perphenazine sulfoxide inactive.
Fluphenazine (injectable depot forms; in sesame oil)	50	90–95	33 (oral)		2D6 substrate and inhibitor; unconjugated metabolites sulfoxide and 7-OH-fluphenazine are active; conjugated metabolites are inactive
Fluphenazine decanoate			7–10 days after single injection, and 14+ days after multiple injections (general adult data)		
Fluphenazine enanthate			3.5–4 days		
Haloperidol (oral form; general adult data)	60–70	92	21 (12–36)		CYP3A4, 2D6, 1A2 involved in metabolism; metabolites are reduced hydroxy-haloperidol which oxidizes back to haloperidol.
Haloperidol decanoate (injectable depot form; in sesame oil)	100		3 weeks		
Thiothixene	50	90–95	34		Sulfoxidation, dealkylation, glucuronic acid conjugation
loxapine			Biphasic: 5/12–19 (1–19) oral (general adult data); IM 8–23 hours	Urine and feces	n-demethylation and hydroxylation to active metabolite amoxapine followed by glucuronidation.
molindone		76 (general adult data)	Rapid elimination 2–4	Urine and feces	2D6 substrate

Table 2.3. Potency of Typical Antipsychotics

High Potency	Intermediate Potency	Low Potency
haloperidol (and decanoate form) thiothixene chlorprothixene fluphenazine (and decanoate and enanthate forms) pimozide	loxapine molindone perphenazine trifluoperazine	chlorpromazine thioridazine mesoridazine

Depot antipsychotics

- Depot forms are indicated for noncompliant patients but not usually for routine use for elders because of less predictable absorption, danger of increased side effects, and prolonged duration of side effects, if they occur.
  - √ Despite these problems, for selected noncompliant patients with chronic primary psychosis, depot forms may be necessary and very helpful.
  - √ Studies are poorly constructed to show clear advantages.

Pharmacokinetic properties of depot antipsychotics (general adult data)

- Depot forms are dissolved in oil (sesame, coconut, or Viscoleo).
- Diffusion and availability of the drug released from the oily depot site is the initial rate-limiting kinetic step.
  - √ Therefore, the apparent rate of elimination is controlled by the rate of absorption and release from the injection site rather than by hepatic metabolism.
- Bypasses first-pass metabolism.
- Time to peak concentration varies considerably from one preparation to another.

Plasma levels of typicals

- Plasma concentrations in elders vary widely from levels in younger patients.
  - √ General adult data not reliable for elders.
- Currently, plasma level measurement is useful to determine decreased bioavailability or noncompliance.
- A nondetectable level in the presence of confirmed compliance indicates decreased bioavailability and the need for increased dose, switch to depot form, or discontinuation of a competing drug that induces hepatic enzymes (e.g., carbamazepine).
  - √ IM forms bypass first-pass hepatic metabolism and increase bioavailability.

- Optimal therapeutic levels have been suggested for
  - √ Thioridazine (0.8–2.4 ng/ml-general adult data) above which EPS is more common with no therapeutic gain.
  - √ Fluphenazine 0.2–2.0 ng/ml (general adult data).
- Large interindividual variations in relationship between dose and plasma concentrations.
- Phenothiazines detectable in plasma up to several months after drug discontinuation.

CLINICAL CONDITIONS TREATED WITH ANTIPSYCHOTIC AGENTS

Behavioral and Psychological Symptoms of Dementia (BPSD)

BPSD is not a formal diagnostic term but

- An umbrella term that describes a constellation of symptoms and behaviors commonly associated with various dementias.
- These behaviors constitute the most common forms of behavioral disturbance in nursing homes
- Markedly increases caregiver burden.
- Epidemiology
  - √ Sixty-six percent of dementia patients demonstrate BPSD at some time during the illness course.
    - ▫ May be more common in frontotemporal dementias and DLB.
  - √ Most common in nursing homes (80–90%) but occurs in 33–45% of community-dwelling elders.
- BPSD is comprised of
  - √ Discrete disorders
    - ▫ Psychosis or depression
  - √ Nonspecific behaviors
    - ▫ Psychomotor agitation, apathy, wandering, aggression
- Wherever possible, a specific diagnosis should be sought and diagnosis-specific interventions and management used.

Agitation and psychosis associated with dementia have a different psychobiology and course than phenomenologically similar behaviors associated with other disorders (e.g., schizophrenia) or age groups. For example, psychosis in Alzheimer's disease, in contrast to schizophrenia, is associated with

- Dopaminergic deficits (i.e., reduced dopamine neurotransmission, reduced D_2 receptor density and numbers of uptake sites).

- Greater prevalence of EPS.
- More rapid rate of decline.
- Greater impairment of frontal lobe function.
- Increased risk of aggressive behavior, wandering, agitation, disruptive behavior, family problems, lack of self-care.

Nondopaminergic mechanisms seem to play a major role in psychosis associated with dementia, perhaps accounting for the modest effect of antipsychotic agents.

- Emergence of psychosis may be related to decline in cholinergic activity in Alzheimer's disease.
  - √ Theory is supported by the antipsychotic effect of cholinergic agents such as physostigmine and the AChEIs.
- Behavioral disturbances (i.e., agitation) reflect preserved dopaminergic function and may account for effectiveness of antipsychotic agents in controlling this aspect of BPSD.
- Aggression/anger emerges in 50% of patients with BPSD.
  - √ Associated with deficiencies of inhibitory neurotransmitters.
    - Serotonin and 5HIAA: In Alzheimer's disease there are reduced levels of 5HT metabolites in cerebrospinal fluid, cell loss in raphe nucleus, and loss of $5HT_1$ and $5HT_2$ receptors; serotonergic drugs are sometimes effective in controlling aggression.
    - GABA: benzodiazepines and possibly valproic acid are GABAergic.

Frontotemporal dementia behavioral symptoms are associated with dopamine depletion, leading to symptoms of hyperexploration, failure to inhibit response strategies, and perseveration. Antipsychotic (dopamine blocking) agents should be used with caution or not at all in these conditions. These differences in pathophysiology may require treatment strategies substantially different from those extrapolated from studies of other types of psychosis, such as schizophrenia (e.g., nicotine patches or dopaminergic agents such as bromocriptine may be effective in agitation and dementia-related psychosis, respectively).

Clinical Presentation of BPSD

- Characterized by inappropriate vocal, motor, affective, or verbal behavior.
- Usually most evident during the moderate and moderately severe stages of dementia.
  - √ Some symptoms (agitation, apathy, aberrant motor behaviors) continue to increase throughout the illness.

- Behavior fluctuates in intensity and form during the day.
  - √ BPSD (angry, agitated, resistive) exacerbated in unfamiliar environments (e.g., admission to a hospital) and by tasks beyond patient's cognitive capacities, as well as by pain, physical illnesses, or drug effects.

Table 2.4. Symptoms of BPSD*

Withdrawal, passivity
Global agitation
Disturbance of diet and appetite
Impaired ideation
Anxiety
Perceptual disturbance—hallucinations
Sleep disturbance
Aggression—verbal
Perceptual disturbance—misperception
Affective/mood disturbance
Agitation—wandering
Aggression—physical
Aggression—resistive/uncooperative

* In rank order of frequency of expression; from Tariot et al., 1997.

Psychotic Symptoms Associated with Dementia

- Mostly new onset, but sometimes longstanding chronic psychosis is complicated by the emergence of coincidental dementia. New psychotic symptoms emerge in 40–80% of patients with dementia by the seventh year of their illness.
- Usually occur in middle stages of the dementing disease, but the apparent decline in later stages may be due only to patients' inability to articulate psychotic symptoms.
- Delusions develop in 10–73% (median 34%) of demented patients.
  - √ 21% develop persecutory beliefs.
  - √ Characteristics of delusions
    - ▫ Variable, evanescent, relapsing.
    - ▫ Sometimes chronic.
    - ▫ Often concrete and simple (e.g., theft of misplaced articles, abandonment, delusional misidentification, unfaithfulness of partner), but may be more complex.
  - √ May be associated with rapid clinical deterioration.
- Hallucinations develop in 21–49% (median 28%) of demented patients; illusory misperceptions of environment are also common (upto 49%).
  - √ Hallucinations may involve any of the following sensory modalities:
    - ▫ Visual (range from unformed shadows to well-formed people, animals, sometimes bizarre forms such as tiny figures,

clowns; not always frightening but often so, and become the source of delusional distortions).
    - Auditory (sounds, voices, music).
    - Touch (tactile hallucinosis such as parasitosis).
    - Olfactory (noxious odors leading to delusional misinterpretation, e.g., fear of being poisoned).
    - Gustatory (not common, but changes in taste sensation may cause patient to develop delusional ideas about food being bad or poisoned).
  - √ May be more troubling and difficult to manage than the effects of the cognitive impairment per se.
  - √ Psychotic symptoms may be more prominent in presence of concurrent sensory impairments (e.g., visual hallucinations are commonly associated with visual disturbances, auditory with hearing impairment).

BPSD-Related Aggression

- Prevalence not well documented: Reported in up to 65% of demented elders in the community.
- Delusions are predictors of aggression.
- Aggression is often the most troubling symptom to caregivers.
- Physically aggressive behavior characterized by
  - √ Hitting, biting, kicking, pushing, scratching, spitting, clutching.
- Physically nonaggressive behavior (in 26–45%) characterized by
  - √ Pacing, wandering, disinhibition, inappropriate disrobing/dressing, repetitive mannerisms.
    - Wandering and restlessness are the most common forms of nonaggressive agitation.
  - √ Sexually inappropriate behavior.
- Verbally aggressive behavior characterized by
  - √ Inappropriate complaining, intrusive requests for attention, resistance, negativism, insults (e.g., racial), obscenities (sometimes out of character, based on past personality) and screaming.
- Physically nonaggressive behavior often calmed by
  - √ Familiar caregivers/family
  - √ Predictable and familiar surroundings.
  - √ Distracting input (visual, tactile, or auditory).

BPSD-Related Affective States

- Occurs in 19% and include
  - √ Apathy
  - √ Emotional lability
  - √ Depression
  - √ Anxiety

Management of BPSD

- Principles of management
  - √ Appropriate and limited use of medication
  - √ Flexibility
  - √ Patience (change takes time)
  - √ Divide the components of behavior.
    - ▫ Intervene with specific interventions rather than trying to modify everything at once.
  - √ Attend to sensory input, environment, and daily behavior.

Table 2.5. Initial Management of BPSD

Clinical Intervention	Comment
Initial workup • Fully describe behaviors based on direct observation. • Establish specific etiology, when possible: √ Neurological (e.g., recent stroke, occult head trauma) √ Psychiatric (e.g., mood, anxiety, or psychotic disorder) √ Medical conditions (e.g., pain, delirium) √ Medication effects (e.g., adverse effects of dopaminergic or anticholinergic drugs) √ Sleep impairment √ Sensory impairment √ Social issues (e.g., losses, support structure)	
Optimize treatment of all medical conditions and pain syndromes, including sensory impairments.	
Optimize medications.	
Attend to safety issues of patient, co-patients, and staff.	• Especially address aggressive, wandering, or intrusive behaviors that provoke retaliation.
Define and document the BPSD target symptoms.	• Shotgun therapy not advisable (and may contravene OBRA guidelines and regulations); determine precipitants and avoid provocative events (e.g., overly intrusive personal care).
Define behaviors unlikely to respond to pharmacological interventions.	• Behaviors unlikely to respond include √ Wandering, pacing, exit seeking √ Screaming, inappropriate verbalizing √ Resistance to toileting √ Inappropriate voiding or spitting √ Hoarding √ Withdrawal (although apathy may respond to stimulating drugs such as methylphenidate) √ Some sexual behaviors (although SSRIs or estrogen can be useful)

(cont.)

Continued

Clinical Intervention	Comment
Define behaviors likely to respond to pharmacological interventions.	• Likely behaviors include √ Coexisting Axis 1 disorder √ Sleep-cycle disturbance √ Assaultiveness √ Hyperexcitability √ Hallucinations √ Delusions √ Suspiciousness √ Hostility
Define psychosocial factors.	• Psychosocial factors include √ Losses √ Family conflict √ Cultural/language barriers √ Personality-based issues
Utilize nonpharmacological interventions initially, as appropriate.	

Table 2.6. Non-Pharmacological Interventions for BPSD

Intervention	Comment
Optimize environment	• Reduce noise levels (e.g., loud TV, institutional procedures like floor cleaning, staff shouting, or hilarity). • Attend to conflicts with roommates. • Provide background music—nonpercussive and familiar, from patient's youth and culture. • Create simplified predictable environment, calm solid colors; visual (labels, signs, pictures), auditory, and tactile cues. • Create safe "wandering environment" (e.g., wandering garden, closed units). • Consider white noise and pet therapy.
Social and stimulation therapy	• Use calm low-volume interventions by staff. • Make simple statements. • Provide repetition, as necessary. • Use supportive but not patronizing tone. • Validate, encourage, and support reminiscences. • Help maintain personal identity. • Redirect repetitive behaviors to familiar, formal tasks (e.g., wiping counters, folding clothes).
Individualize/optimize daily routines	• Increase daily activity (e.g., exercise, group games). • Evaluate need for daytime naps—try to prevent reversal of sleep cycle.
Behavior modification	Example: A-B-C method • Determine *A*ntecedents (i.e., precipitants) of behavior. • Identify *B*ehaviors. • Initiate appropriate behavior-modifying *C*onsequences.
Bright light therapy	Advances sleep-phase syndromes.
Education	Benefits patient, caregivers, and family.

Medication Management of BPSD

No medications have been specifically approved for BPSD.

- Some suggest that antipsychotic use in elders for nonpsychotic conditions is controversial.
  - √ But, on balance, antipsychotic agents remain the best pharmacological therapeutic agents available to date.
- Studies on improvement with antipsychotics commonly employ rating scales (e.g., the Brief Psychiatric Rating Scale (BPRS)).
  - √ Improvement rating requires at least 20% improvement in the BPRS score—modest at best; helps to put expectations for improvement based on outcome studies into perspective.
  - √ Improvement of BPSD is only modest with typical agents, but a more favorable response to atypical agents likely, especially for agitation.

Medications are used for

- Urgent control of medication-responsive symptoms: acute behaviors, hyperactivity, depressive symptoms, psychotic symptoms.
  - √ To a lesser extent: physical or verbal agitation, especially the more severe aggressive/uncooperative subtypes that may be unresponsive to behavioral, social, or environmental interventions.
  - √ Note: the term *agitation* is not favored under OBRA legislation but sometimes is unavoidable, as the basic causes of behavior may not be definable/diagnosable.
  - √ A long-term medication strategy required in some cases.

Table 2.7. General Principles of Drug Management of BPSD

1. Drug choice: There is no definitive drug treatment; each patient is a mini-clinical trial; adequate trial is about 12 weeks.
2. Medications are used with specific goals in mind, such as axis 1 disorders.
3. Clusters of symptoms may guide treatment, even if atypical from accepted nosological diagnoses (e.g., the association of depressive symptoms with agitation, irritability, dysphoria, and anxiety may indicate antidepressant as first intervention).
4. Employ regular scheduled therapy; PRN or standing orders may lead to inadvertent, inappropriate use of medication.
5. Avoid polypharmacy; for complex refractory cases, polypharmacy is sometimes essential, but only under close supervision.
6. Monitor for adverse effects.
7. Conduct periodic trials of medication withdrawal; many symptoms are self-limiting over time (required under OBRA legislation).

Both antipsychotic and non-antipsychotic treatments are used for BPSD.

- Antipsychotic medications
  - √ Class of choice for psychosis and severe agitation.
  - √ Nonpsychotic symptoms for which antipsychotics are most likely to be effective include suspiciousness, sleeplessness, excitement, hostility, emotional lability, restlessness, aggression, irritability, uncooperativeness.
  - √ Atypical antipsychotics are the drugs of first choice.

Table 2.8. Antipsychotic Agents in BPSD

Drug	Dosing for BPSD	Side Effects	Comments
	ATYPICAL ANTIPSYCHOTICS		
Aripiprazole	Starting dose used in one trial is 2 mg with average daily therapeutic dose of 10 mg		No other geriatric data
risperidone	Start at 0.125–0.25 mg bid and increase to 1–2 mg/day in divided doses, as needed	Orthostasis and sedation; low incidence of significant EPS at this dose range, but this side effect occurs even at low doses and should be monitored	Best tolerated at the 1 mg dose (range 0.5–1.25 mg/day; higher doses for functional psychosis 0.5–3 mg/day); direct, abrupt switch to risperidone from haloperidol improves response and is well tolerated
olanzapine	Begin at 2.5 mg/day and increase as necessary	Initial sedation, some anticholinergic effects, but not prominent at this dose level	Best response appears to be at the 5–10 mg/day dose (with range up to 20 mg); higher ranges may be best for psychotic symptoms; some data suggest it is superior to risperidone and haloperidol
quetiapine	25–200 mg/day	Commonly sedation, dizziness, agitation, postural hypotension	Wide range of effective doses
clozapine	6.25–200 mg/day	Significant anticholinergic effects, orthostatic hypotension, fatigue, hypersalivation, and nausea; many side effects are dose dependent and diminsh with reduced dose; significant risk of agranulocytosis—requires careful monitoring	Caution in raising dose; elders more sensitive to serious side effects; useful in refractory cases of psychosis (especially if associated with Parkinson's and Lewy body dementia) unresponsive to other atypicals or when EPS side effects emerge with them

(*cont.*)

Continued

Drug	Dosing for BPSD	Side Effects	Comments
Ziprasidone	Not well established; mean dose 100 mg/d.	Commonly sedation that responds to 20 mg dose reduction; occasional EPS.	Few drug interactions reported. Utility still in early phases of investigation
	TYPICAL ANTIPSYCHOTICS		
		High-potency drugs associated with EPS and TD in this population, which is especially vulnerable to Parkinsonian side effects (rates of 5–90%), typicals often worsen already-compromised cognition; best choice is often a mid-potency agent	About 1/3 of patients with BPSD symptoms of agitation and/or psychosis respond to typical antipsychotics, although studies are often flawed; no longer recommended as first-line therapy in dementia; effectiveness is only modest and side-effect rates are high; apathy, withdrawal, and general deterioration are unresponsive to typical antipsychotics
loxapine	10–50 mg/day		Considered by some as a drug of first choice for BPSD, including aggression
haloperidol	2 mg/day	Significant risk of side effects with higher doses over 2 mg/day	Still commonly prescribed; low doses in the 0.5 mg/day range are ineffective in many cases; overall, agitation does not respond to this drug, but aggression may be moderated
thiothixene	1–10 mg/day	EPS risks increase with dose, including TD	Little data for elders, but effective for short-term treatment of acute agitation
thioridazine	10–50 mg/day	*Prolonged QTc;* other key side effects include sedation, anticholinergic effects, orthostasis	lower doses of this useful drug required in light of documented prolonged QTc
Other typical agents are rarely used now and are not commonly used for routine management	• Chlorpromazine 10–100 mg/day • Trifluoperazine 1–10 mg/day • Perphenazine 2–16 mg/day		

√ Base choice of specific drug on side-effect profile.
√ Doses usually substantially lower than those in nondemented psychotic patients.

- Nonneuroleptic medications for BPSD
  √ Serotonergic agents, SRI-type antidepressants (see p. 123).

Table 2.9. SRI Drugs for BPSD

Drug	Dose	Comments
citalopram	20–30 mg/day	May outperform other SSRIs in depression associated with AD (data still preliminary); advantage over placebo, and on some measures over perphenazine, in control of psychosis and behavioral disturbance
sertraline	25–100 mg/day	
paroxetine	5–20 mg/day	
fluoxetine	5–20 mg/day	
trazodone	75–400 mg/day (mean about 75–150 mg)	Useful for agitation (has been successfully augmented with 2.5 g/day of L-tryptophan); sedative side effects are one limiting factor; rare risk of priapism

Table 2.10. Other Drugs for BPSD

Drug	Dose	Side Effects	Comments
		BENZODIAZEPINES	
			Useful for short-term management of event-stimulated agitation; use shorter- and intermediate-acting agents (e.g., oxazepam, lorazepam), not long-acting; avoid ultrashort-acting agents (e.g., triazolam)
oxazepam lorazepam clonazepam zolpidem	10 mg 0.25–0.5 mg 0.5–1.5 mg 2.5–5 mg	Paradoxical disinhibition (particularly problematic in demented or otherwise brain-damaged patients), oversedation, risk of falls, dependence, interdose withdrawal (especially with PRNs), discontinuation syndromes, cognitive and psychomotor side effects	Single dose as necessary 30–45 min. before a known agitating event, such as bathing; useful for intermittent agitation associated with anxiety, tension, and sleep problems (but not irritability); efficacy diminishes over time; use for short term
buspirone	initial dose 5 mg tid, titrating up to 15–20 mg tid as necessary (clinical data only)		Onset of action 1–8 weeks; moderately useful for aggression; latency to antiaggression effects of 4–6 weeks

(*cont.*)

Continued

Drug	Dose	Side Effects	Comments
		MOOD STABILIZERS	
valproate (mood stabilizer of choice)	250–1500 mg/day (range up to 2500) in 2–3 divided doses	Observe for hepatic and hematological toxicity (platelet counts for thrombocytopenia), sedation, ataxia, dizziness, weight gain	GABA-enhancing agent; may counteract GABA deficits in Alzheimer's patient; effectiveness similar to antipsychotics; sometimes improved response if used in combination with antipsychotic; reduced verbal/physical aggression by about 50% in one study, but results more modest in other studies; target plasma levels 30–90 μg/ml, but levels not clearly associated with effect
carbamazepine	300 mg/day (range 100–600 mg/day, maximum of 1000 mg/day used by some)	Not suggested; serum concentrations above 9 μg/ml associated with increased rates of adverse events; blood dyscrasias; strong propensity for drug–drug interactions, which limit its utility; skin reactions, sedation, ataxia, electrolyte disturbance; monitor for infection; regular CBC	Inhibits limbic kindling; effective for agitation, hostility, uncooperativeness; ineffective for anergia, anxiety/depression, thought disturbance; plasma levels of 5μg/ml (range 4–9)
gabapentin	300 mg/bid		Reported useful
		BETA-BLOCKERS	
		Caution re side effects of beta-blockers; contraindicated in CHF and COPD, diabetes, angina, severe peripheral vascular disease, hyperthyroidism; may induce bradycardia and hypotension	Evidence not clear, response variable; a useful third- or fourth-line option to antipsychotics; latency of several weeks before antipsychotic–antiaggression effects emerge; maintain on maximum dose for 8 weeks to determine efficacy
propranalol	10–800 mg/day	Begin at 20 mg test dose; increase by 20 mg/day every 3 days; some patients tolerate faster dose increases of 60 mg every 3 days	Dosage ranges are very wide for frail elders; some have increased dose to 12 mg/Kg, up to maximum of 800 mg/day (however, doses in this range are uncommon in practice, and not suggested routinely); avoid sudden discontinuation, especially in presence of hypertension; taper by 60 mg/day to daily dose of 60 mg, then by 20 mg/day until stopped

(*cont.*)

Continued

Drug	Dose	Side Effects	Comments
pindolol	40–60 mg/day, in bid divided doses		Data limited; may offer some therapeutic advantage due to sympathomimetic properties (in contrast to propranolol), which may make it less likely to induce bradycardia or hypotension
		OTHER AGENTS	
cholinesterase inhibitors			Sometimes useful (see p. 551)
physostigmine	6 mg/day administered in divided doses every 2 hours		Has been used in investigational units for treatment of psychosis associated with Alzheimer's disease; duration of action about 3–4 hours
estrogen or medroxyprogesterone			For disruptive sexual behavior
melatonin	3 mg each evening		Used to control "agitation"; improvement may occur over a period of days to weeks (data preliminary)

For all medications

- Monitor side effects.
- Maintain therapy trial for 6–12 weeks; lack of response is an indication to switch to another medication.
- Attempt periodic withdrawal of medications once patient is stabilized.
  - √ Often necessary to maintain therapy for prolonged periods for some syndromes (e.g., aggression, depression, or psychosis; other symptoms [e.g., agitation] tend to be more transient).
- When withdrawing medication, do it gradually to avoid withdrawal syndromes.
- About 50% of patients experience recurrence of symptoms within 3–6 months after withdrawal (relapse rate is 90% in the first year for adult schizophrenia).

Psychosis Associated with Parkinson's Disease and Parkinsonism

Causes of parkinsonism (in addition to idiopathic Parkinson's disease) include various drugs (see Table 2.20, pp. 268–271) and neurological disorders such as PSP, DLB, SDAT, and multiple systems atrophy.

- Parkinson's disease (PD) prevalence in nursing homes (> 75 years) up to 35%.
- Psychosis and parkinsonism usually associated with dopaminergic medication, but may also correlate with presence of lewy bodies.
- Risk of psychosis in PD
  - √ Increases with age.
  - √ With levodopa, 20% incidence of psychosis; increases to > 30% with adjunctive dopamine agonists.

Pathophysiology

- Psychosis may be associated with hypersensitivity of postsynaptic monoaminergic receptors in pathways that loop through the striatum and frontal cortex.
  - √ Chronic stimulation with dopamine agonists (e.g., levodopa, amantadine, MAO-B inhibitors, catechol-O-methyltransferase inhibitors) may kindle psychotic symptoms.
  - √ Postsynaptic serotonergic receptor hypersensitivity may be implicated in hallucinations and delusions induced by dopamine agonist.

Clinical presentation

- Premonitory signs of psychosis
  - √ Progressive cognitive impairment
  - √ Generalized sleep disturbance—daytime somnolence, insomnia, nocturnal myoclonus
  - √ Personality change
  - √ Confusion or hallucinations with retained insight
- Symptoms
  - √ Visual hallucinations in 20% of patients taking dopaminergic agents, especially levodopa.
    - ▫ Onset after prolonged therapy of 2 years or more with levodopa.
    - ▫ Risk increases at higher doses.
    - ▫ Hallucinations often well formed and convincing to the patient (e.g., Lilliputian), often emerge at night, are sometimes frightening; auditory and tactile hallucinations, especially early in course of dopamine agonist therapy, suggest DLB or SDAT.
  - √ Delusions less common than hallucinations (3–17%), but delusional interpretation of hallucinations occurs; case reports of delusional misidentification.

Management

- Challenging, often requires compromise between optimal control of psychosis and side effects.

- Treat other contributing medical conditions and sleep disturbance.
- Atypical neuroleptics are the drugs of choice.
  - √ Typical antipsychotics no longer used in most cases.
    - If they must be used, a low-potency drug (molindone or thioridazine) in low doses is sometimes very cautiously tried.
- Caution with all antipsychotics because DLB may mimic drug-induced psychosis of Parkinson's disease.
  - √ Antipsychotic medication generally should be avoided in DLB.
- Typical neuroleptics (i.e., dopamine blocking agents) should be avoided.
  - √ Worsen parkinsonian symptoms, especially mobility and tremor.
- ECT is sometimes effective for both the psychosis and the movement component of Parkinson's disease.
  - √ Effect is transient and treatment generally requires continuation ECT therapy.
- Reducing levodopa or other dopaminergic therapeutic agents is not the best option.
  - √ May improve symptoms of psychosis but worsen PD symptoms and induce postural instability, hypotension, and falls.
- Anticholinergic drugs may increase hallucinosis and delirium.

Table 2.11. Medication Summary for Psychosis with Parkinsonism

Drug	Comments
quetiapine	Drug of first choice; well tolerated, effective; a better initial option than reducing dopaminergic drugs.
risperidone	Drug of choice but caution re induction of parkinsonian symptoms.
olanzapine	Second-line option because may induce parkinsonian symptoms even in low doses.
clozapine	Doses much lower than those for schizophrenia (1–10% of usual dose) produce good therapeutic results, but is difficult to use safely in the older segment of this population because of serious side effects and blood monitoring requirements (see p. 318); onset of action within a few days of treatment initiation; may be effective for control of otherwise refractory mixed tremor; D_1 blocking action of clozapine responsible for effect in suppressing dyskinesias in PD patients.

Diffuse Lewy Body (DLB) Disease

- Accounts for 15–25% of dementia cases in elders; DLB found in 50% of patients with dementia and persistent psychosis.
- Identified genetic relationship to Parkinson's and Alzheimer's disease.

Pathophysiology

- Named for the rounded eosinophilic inclusion bodies in brainstem nuclei of all patients with Parkinson's disease and in the cortex of about 10–25% of patients with dementia (at autopsy).
  - √ Alpha synuclein a characteristic immunochemical feature, similar to Parkinson's disease and multiple systems atrophy.
- Pathology probably related to D_2 receptor blockade in the striatum.
  - √ Reduced choline acetyltransferase in temporal and parietal cortices

Clinical presentation

- A special case of dementia because cognitive, parkinsonian, and psychiatric features coexist, and symptoms of agitation or psychosis respond unfavorably to neuroleptic treatment.
- Rapidly progressive cognitive decline.
  - √ Cognitive impairment may fluctuate widely.
- Psychiatric symptoms that emerge at onset of the disorder are a better diagnostic indictor of DLB dementia than the occurrence of psychosis later in the course of dementia.
- Symptoms include one or more of the following
  - √ Hallucinations—vivid, well-formed visual or auditory
  - √ Delusions—paranoid, persecutory
  - √ Mild spontaneous EPS
  - √ Frontal release reflexes—glabellar, snout, sucking, palmomental
  - √ Neuroleptic sensitivity syndrome—marked adverse reactions to standard doses of neuroleptics
  - √ Repeated unexplained falls
  - √ Syncope
  - √ Transient clouding of consciousness or difficulty with arousal (may resemble narcolepsy)
  - √ Fluctuating confusion
  - √ Depression
  - √ Disturbed sleep common, including REM sleep behavior disorder
    - ▫ Yelling, striking out, grabbing, twitching, teeth grinding.
    - ▫ Appears to be attempting dream enactment.
    - ▫ May lead to injury of self or sleep partner.
  - √ Aggression
  - √ CT-nonspecific atrophy
  - √ Parkinsonism evident in about 9% of DLB
    - ▫ Responds to antiparkinsonian agents early in the course of DLB, but less so later on.

- Treat with l-dopa.
- L-dopa response is variable and unpredictable.
- Theoretical danger of increasing psychosis but clinically does not generally happen.

Management of Psychiatric and Behavioral Features of DLB

DLB patients are very sensitive to neuroleptic effects.

- 80% have adverse reactions, including increased mortality.
- Use extreme caution with all antipsychotics, including atypicals; some atypicals (e.g., clozapine, quetiapine) not as dangerous with regard to neuroleptic sensitivity syndrome, but none is risk free.
- 25–80% of patients with DLB treated with typical antipsychotics develop neuroleptic sensitivity syndrome.
  - √ Severe parkinsonism—tremor, bradykinesia, rigidity, gait disturbance, masked facies
  - √ Autonomic dysfunction
  - √ Delirium/clouding of consciousness
  - √ Catatonic states
  - √ Irreversible cognitive decline (perhaps caused by acceleration of neuronal loss)
  - √ Decline in functional ability
  - √ Many falls
  - √ Reactions may be fatal in rare cases

Pharmacological management

- Try AChEIs and nonpharmacological interventions before resorting to antipsychotics.
- AChEIs have shown promise in controlling DLB-associated.
  - √ Hallucinations
    - Auditory and visual especially marked in mild cognitive impairment.
  - √ Delusions and delusional misidentification
  - √ Confusion
  - √ Agitation
  - √ Depression
  - √ Attentional deficits
  - √ Hypersomnolence
  - √ Apathy
- If antipsychotics are to be initiated in DLB, consider initiating therapy in inpatient unit.
  - √ Quetiapine, olanzapine, and clozapine are tolerated, but be very cautious with these too and observe for toxicity.

Delirium

Delirium is a transient organic mental syndrome caused by any endogenous or exogenous disturbance that affects central brain function and produces a syndrome characterized by global impairment of cognition and attention, reduced level of consciousness, abnormal psychomotor activity, and disturbed sleep–wake cycle. The following table summarizes the causes of delirium.

Table 2.12. Causes of Delirium

Cause	Specific Agents/Conditions
Intoxication	• Medication—antiparkinsonian agents; anticholinergic agents, including antihistaminics (e.g., diphenhydramine); psychotropics (especially lithium, TCAs, benzodiazepines), antispasmodics, eye drops, narcotics, analgesics, steroids, psychostimulants, analgesics, anti-inflammatory agents, alcohol, antineoplastic agents, anticonvulsants, antiarrhythmic agents (especially digoxin). • Substance intoxication • Poisons
Withdrawal syndromes	• Alcohol, sedative hypnotics
Anesthesia and postoperative states	• Postoperative delirium often results from hypoxemia or use of opiates and benzodiazepines.
Infections	• Systemic sepsis, urinary tract infection, pneumonia, and upper respiratory infections with dehydration.
Metabolic disturbance	• Glycemic dyscontrol; electrolyte (Na, K, Ca, Mg), fluid (dehydration), and acid/base imbalance; hypoxia, hypercapnia, temperature dyscontrol, nutritional deficiencies (especially thiamine deficiency and vitamin B_{12} deficiency), liver/renal failure, anemia.
Cardiopulmonary disturbances	• CHF, arrhythmia, MI, malignant hypertension, shock, pulmonary embolus.
Neurological disturbances	• Tumor, subdural hemorrhage, infections (meningitis, encephalitis, brain abscess), cerebrovascular diseases, seizure syndromes, head/brain trauma.
Endocrine disturbance	• Thyroid, parathyroid
Other	• Sleep disorders—apnea, sleep deprivation, sensory deprivation, bedsores.
Contributing factors include	• Use of restraints, polypharmacy, malnutrition.

Epidemiology

- Occurs in 10–31% of all hospital admissions
  - √ Wide variations, depending on the population (e.g., much higher in postsurgical patients).
- High-risk patients include those with drug dependence, cognitive impairment, multiple medical illnesses, and patients on intensive care units (especially burn and open heart surgery patients).
- Delirium is a marker for increased risk of death and institutionalization.

- Predisposing factors
  - √ Advanced age
    - ▫ Elders may *not* be at increased risk of agitation in ICU settings, solely because of age.
  - √ Comorbid medical illness
  - √ Preexisting cognitive impairment, neurological disorder
  - √ Multiple concurrent drug use
    - ▫ Especially anticholinergics, antihistamines, digoxin, anticonvulsants, steroids.
  - √ History of delirium
  - √ General physical frailty
- Diagnosis
  - √ Up to 70% of delirium cases are not diagnosed by clinical staff physicians.
  - √ Acute confusional states are caused by acute onset of new medical illness or exacerbation of preexisting chronic illness.
  - √ Toxic confusional states are caused by drug toxicity due to age-related sensitivity, overdose, or drug interactions (especially anticholinergic additive effects, which produces CNS anticholinergic syndrome), infections, or fever.

Symptom picture of delirium

- Onset: develops acutely over hours or days.
- Incipient delirium
  - √ Characterized by personality change, irritability, distractibility, loosening of associations, disinhibition.
- Key diagnostic features.
  - √ Fluctuating symptoms.
  - √ Clouded consciousness.
    - ▫ Impaired focusing, sustaining concentration.
  - √ Attention deficit.
    - ▫ Inability to maintain shift and focus attention.
  - √ Disorganized thinking, indicated by rambling, irrelevant, or incoherent speech.
    - ▫ Inaccurate word usage.
    - ▫ Slurred articulation.
    - ▫ Repetitive, disjointed context.
    - ▫ Impaired volume, rate, rhythm—pressured or halting speech
  - √ Disorientation.
    - ▫ Time of day and place; person, in extreme cases.
    - ▫ Marked confusion.
  - √ Memory impairment (especially recent but also remote).
  - √ Misidentification of familiar places and persons.
  - √ Perceptual disturbances.
    - ▫ Psychosis (visual, tactile, auditory hallucinations, paranoid ideation).

    - Not often volunteered; symptoms need to be actively sought.
    - Often nocturnal delusions are not as systematized or fixed across time as in other forms of psychosis.
  - √ Sleep–wake cycle disturbance.
    - Excessive daytime sleeping.
    - Nocturnal agitation and hyperalertness.
    - Nightmares.
  - √ Behavioral/psychomotor disturbance.
    - Often fluctuating.
    - Agitation, extreme restlessness, combativeness, screaming.
    - May alternate with hypoactivity.
    - Slowed speech, passivity, lethargy, apathy.
  - √ Affective disturbance.
    - Fear.
    - Lability of mood.
    - Irritability.
  - √ Autonomic nervous system signs.
    - May include flushing, pupillary dilatation, sweating, hypertension.

Management

- Identify and correct underlying cause of delirium.
  - √ Complete history and chart review.
  - √ Laboratory/special investigations, including CBC, RBC, B_{12} folate, electrolytes, FBS, CO_2, thyroid screen, AST/ALT, CK, creatinine, BUN, urinalysis, chest X-ray, ECG, EEG, O_2 saturation on all patients; obtain medication levels, toxic screens, blood cultures, neuroimaging, and LP as indicated.
  - √ Identify any medical pathology, including sleep pathology such as apnea.
  - √ Observation of vital signs.
  - √ Conduct careful clinical mental status examination.
  - √ Rule out other diagnoses (e.g., dementia, psychotic illnesses such as schizophrenia, mania/hypomania, depression).
  - √ Identify and correct sources of toxicity.
    - Optimize drug dosages, treat infections.
- O_2 may be sufficient therapy in low O_2 saturation delirium.
  - √ Provide supportive measures: fluid/electrolyte balance (especially important because dehydration and electrolyte imbalance implicated in delirium), nutrition, and vitamin replacement.
- Optimize environment.
  - √ Provide appropriate levels of stimulation.
    - Orientation cues (e.g., clock, calendar, familiar photos, personal items).
    - Reduced noise levels.

- Light, but avoid constant bright light because it impairs diurnal cycles.
  - √ Provide calming, reassuring interactions.
  - √ Limit casual visiting and unnecessary examinations (especially an issue in teaching facilities).
  - √ Educate, reassure, support family.
  - √ Encourage close, familiar family members to stay with patient within limits of their tolerance.
  - √ Bedside nursing, observation and support (often sufficient in mild cases).
  - √ Restraints rarely necessary.
    - Exceptions: temporary use for severe, uncontrollable aggression or agitation that interferes with essential medical management.
    - Avoid, whenever possible, because of side effects (injury or even death).
    - Consider nursing alternatives (e.g., private-duty nursing/ companions).
- Target specific symptoms
  - √ Psychosis.
  - √ Severe agitation, aggression.

Initiate medications for more severe states

- Use least anticholinergic agents (to avoid exacerbating delirium).
- Avoid hypnotics.
- Psychotropics contraindicated in elders who are drowsy and hard to rouse.

Agent of choice is low-dose antipsychotic in oral, IM or IV formats. Haloperidol recommended for short-term management.

- Begin with 0.25–0.5 mg/day orally or half that in IM form and increase to 0.5–1.5 mg daily in three divided doses.
  - √ IV form has rapid onset of action and is useful for severe agitation.
    - Dose 0.5–2 mg repeated q 30 min. until patient is calm.
  - √ IV not an approved indication but often effective for emergency sedation.
    - Danger of widening QTc interval and acute emergence of EPS.
  - √ Maintain on a daily dose one-half to one-third the 24-hr. dose required to calm the patient.
- Repeat oral or IM dose q 30–60 min. for severe cases.
- Taper dose over 3–5 days once delirium begins to remit.
- Risperidone (1–1.5 mg/day, available in liquid form) and olanzapine (5–10 mg/day) orally reported effective in 2 open studies and individual case reports.

- √ Use of IM and sublingual forms not yet well studied in elders but show promise in management of acute agitation.
- Physostigmine 1–2 mg IM/IV to counter anticholinergic delirium.
  - √ Caution in heart disease, asthma, diabetes, peptic ulcer, bladder/bowel obstruction.
- Short-acting benzodiazepines should be avoided for general management of delirium; occasionally may be useful if used judiciously for insomnia or withdrawal syndromes (e.g., delirium tremens, benzodiazepine withdrawal).

Delusional Disorder

- Definition: nonbizarre delusions without hallucinations or organic dysfunction and without schizophrenia or mood disorder
- Classified according to predominant delusional theme
  - √ Erotomanic
  - √ Grandiose
  - √ Jealous
  - √ Persecutory
  - √ Somatic
  - √ Poverty
- Onset
  - √ Usually in mid or late life.
  - √ Women later than men (ages 60–69 vs. 40–49).
- Risk factors: sensory impairment (hearing loss), personality disorders, immigration status, early life trauma, low socioeconomic status.
- Clinical picture
  - √ Paranoid subtypes often predominate.
    - ▫ Shared delusions (folie à deux) between couples sometimes emerges.
    - ▫ Paranoid misidentification.
    - ▫ Capgras syndrome—delusion of doubles.
  - √ Associated with agitated and disruptive behaviors.
  - √ Often but not invariably associated with organic features; increased rate of cerebral infarctions (compared to late-onset schizophrenia/paraphrenia).

Management

- Not well studied in elders.
- Patients often have little insight and are resistant to treatment.
- Pharmacological treatment described in clinical cases and uncontrolled studies.
  - √ Atypical antipsychotics
    - ▫ Drugs of first choice based on side-effect profile.

    - Not well studied for delusional disorder in elders, but no reason to think they would not be effective in usual antipsychotic doses.
  - √ Typical antipsychotics
    - Pimozide is the most commonly used drug for this purpose, with sporadic reports of other agents (e.g., depot preparations such as fluphenazine enanthate).
    - Pimozide oral dose of 1–4 mg/day, with best results achieved at 2–3 mg/day; EPS a significant side-effect problem.
    - Fluphenazine enanthate dose 5 mg q 2 weeks; depot route may more effective because of better compliance.

Visual Hallucinations without Accompanying Psychopathology

Visual hallucinations occur commonly in elders and are usually associated with other pathology such as dementia, but also occur less commonly in clear sensorium, without accompanying or preexisting psychopathology.

Charles Bonnet Syndrome

Charles Bonnet syndrome (CBS) originates from ophthalmological pathology, such as macular degeneration in association with sensory deprivation, aloneness, and neuronal stimulation secondary to retinal distortion. Symptoms include

- Sudden onset of persistent, stereotyped, complex visual hallucinations of figures.
  - √ Especially faces, animals, humans, miniature people, flowers, inanimate objects, complex patterns.
- Themes may be rich or simple, usually colorful, and often pleasant, curious, or humorous to patient; rarely frightening.
- May be continuous, periodic, or episodic.
- Normal sensorium involved.
- Full or partial insight available.
- Absent delusions or hallucinations in other modalities.
- No dementia or neurological disorders present.
- Preserved function in other spheres.

Treatment

- Treat underlying visual pathology where possible.
- Carbamazepine (clinical case reports only).
- Valproate (clinical case reports only).
- Typical neuroleptics not often effective but atypicals may be better.

Occipital Vascular Lesions

- Complex images sometimes emerge, but more often are unformed.
- Balint's syndrome
  - √ Hallucinations and past-pointing when reaching for or fixating on parts of objects.

Retinal Stimulation

- Usually results in unformed visual images (e.g., blobs or zigzag lines).

Stroke and Tumors

- Forms of visual hallucinations vary, depending on site of the lesion.
- Arise on the side opposite the stroke.
- Visual hallucinations more likely to occur with lesions of the right hemisphere.

Schizophrenia

- Incidence: 1% of those over age 65; 85% reside in the community.
- Cognitive impairment intrinsic to schizophrenia:
  - √ Memory
    - ▫ Episodic and semantic memory disproportionately impaired.
  - √ Executive functioning
    - ▫ Poor social, problem solving, community functioning, and skill acquisition.
- Two forms accepted, although not part of DSM-IV: early (EOS) and late (LOS) onset schizophrenia.

Table 2.13. Common Features of EOS and LOS

- Positive symptoms, chronicity of course, and family history.
- Negative (deficit) symptoms; may be more pronounced in elders with EOS.
  - √ Do not develop as much in LOS form.
- Cognitive impairment less severe in LOS, although similar in general form to EOS.
  - √ Even the most cognitively intact patients show some impaired executive function.
- Similar MRI findings: increased white matter hyperintensities.
- Paranoid subtypes often predominate in both.

Early onset schizophrenia

- Onset before age 45.
- Paranoid symptoms often predominate.
- Sometimes more florid symptoms (i.e., positive symptoms) diminish in old age, but not invariably.
  - √ Negative symptoms tend to persist.
  - √ Hallucinations are less frequent and less disturbing.

- √ Delusions may be less frightening.
- √ Incidence of severe agitation decreases.
- Vulnerable to increased stress, which exacerbates preexisting psychosis.
- Depression levels high.
  - √ About 40% have comorbid clinical depression.
  - √ Often responds to neuroleptic therapy and remits along with psychotic symptoms.
- Some develop superimposed age-related disorders, such as dementia or Parkinson's disease, which makes their management much more complex and difficult.
  - √ Prominent cognitive impairment often found in chronic schizophrenia, but does not seem to progress in late life in the same way as the dementias.
  - √ But cognitive impairment in late-life schizophrenia is common and significantly impairs function.
  - √ No evidence of typical neurodegenerative brain pathology.
- Symptoms generally remain stable or improve (in 80%) with increasing age; 20% decline.
- Social disability tends to remain in late life, but there is some improvement in coping skills.

Late onset schizophrenia (LOS)

- Onset after age 45.
- 15% of schizophrenia is late onset.
- LOS not formally distinguished by age of onset in DSM but has some distinctive features.
  - √ 2–5 times more common in women.
  - √ Larger ventricles and thalami on MRI neuroimaging.
  - √ Usually require lower doses of antipsychotics.
    - Exquisitely sensitive to development of TD and drug-induced EPS.

A profile of LOS is provided in the following table.

Table 2.14. Profile of Late-Onset Schizophrenia

- Bizarre persecutory delusions
- Auditory (occasionally visual) hallucinations
- Fewer negative symptoms than EOS
- Inappropriate affect, loosening of associations (uncommon)
- MRI evidence
  - √ Larger thalamic size in LOS
  - √ White matter hyperintensities
- Often responsive to low-dose antipsychotics (one-third the dose of early onset form)
- Increased risk of tardive dyskinesia
- Dementia and affective disturbance not present

Management

Data on treatment of schizophrenia in elders is sparse, especially detailed studies of response to pharmacotherapy, long-term tolerance of treatment, compliance, and outcome. Full range of therapies is required, as with younger patients. The following two tables summarize management issues involved in treating elders with schizophrenia.

Table 2.15. Management of Schizophrenia in Elders

Management Factors	Comment
Attend to general factors affecting pharmacological therapy in elders.	• Factors complicating management include sensory deficits, multiple-drug regimens, cognitive impairment, and impaired compliance.
Full physical workup is even more important in this population, which often has had poor medical care, contributing to increased severity of disorders.	• Elders of minority races may be a greater risk in this regard. • 58% of elders with schizophrenia has at least one significant comorbid medical illness.
Choice of antipsychotic	• Response rate to antipsychotics in the 60–75% range. • Select agent with least EPS potential, demonstrated clinical efficacy for target symptoms (including negative symptoms), and that is well tolerated by elders.
Drugs of choice—atypical antipsychotics for nonacute therapy	• Favorable side-effect profile. • More effective for negative symptoms in elders.
Drugs of choice for acute/emergency situations when speed of action is necessary	• Typical antipsychotic (e.g., haloperidol), followed by atypical agent once acute symptoms are controlled. √ Parenteral atypical agents (ziprasidone) or rapidly absorbed forms (zydis form of olanzapine) may make atypicals more practical in urgent care situations. √ Otherwise well elders may tolerate combination of typical and atypical agents concurrently during acute management situations.
Negative symptoms	• Often respond best to non-antipsychotic medication or other interventions. √ Example: Dysphoria responds best to antidepressants and psychotherapies; psychosocial dysfunction to social–environmental intervention and psychotherapies.
Dosing	• Geriatric dosing not well studied. • Some indication that elders improve on lower doses of haloperidol (2–3 mg/day) than younger people with schizophrenia. • Low-dose perphenazine (< 15 mg per day) is relatively ineffective in elders without dementia in first 10 days of therapy; response rates may improve with extensions to 3 weeks. • EPS rate during acute therapy is very low if low-dose antipsychotic therapy is used, regardless of the drug.

Table 2.16. Relapse Prevention and Maintenance Treatment

- Long-term maintenance therapy has positive effect on symptoms and prevents relapse in the majority of patients.
  - √ Relapse remains a substantial risk, even on maintenance therapy.
- High relapse rate of > 50% if antipsychotic drugs are discontinued.
- EPS sometimes more limiting to long-term outcome than primary symptoms of schizophrenia.
  - √ Indicates need for trial of dose reduction by gradual tapering or switching to an atypical drug.
- Continuous maintenance regimes more effective than targeted medication regimens (i.e., giving medication intermittently in response to onset of early prodromal symptoms of relapse).
- Prophylaxis and prevention of relapse often difficult because of
  - √ Poor compliance (in about 50% of patients).
  - √ Problems with follow-up.
  - √ Side effects of long-term therapy (e.g., TD).
- Relapse prevention may be improved by weekly follow-up visits; however, this schedule is often burdensome and unacceptable to patients, so negotiation is necessary.

Psychosis and Behavioral Disturbances in Mood Disorders

- Psychotic depression (see p. 35).
  - √ Agitated behavior may emerge in psychotically depressed patients in old age.
  - √ Hoarding behavior often associated with schizophrenia and dementia.
    - ▫ Often responsive to antipsychotic treatment.
  - √ Psychotic features of depression occur in 28–45% of patients with depressive episode.
  - √ Important to distinguish depressive agitation from anxiety states (see following table).

Table 2.17. Depressive Agitation versus Anxiety

Depressive Agitation	Anxiety
Primarily physical and behavioral activation	Inner apprehension/dread
Often correlates with cognitive decline	Cognition less affected
Independent of past history of anxiety	History of anxiety
Treat with antidepressants and/or antipsychotics (possibly ECT)	Treat with psychotherapy, SRIs, benzodiazepines
Worse in early evening—"sundowning"—and at night	Often worse in early A.M. but sometimes at night
Rage and irritability commonly associated	Anger not prominent

- Bipolar disorder (see p. 37)
- Release hallucinations associated with sensory impairment (i.e., visual or auditory loss)
  - √ Response to medication variable.
    - ▫ Low-dose atypical antipsychotics may be useful.

- Huntington's disease
  - √ Psychiatric symptoms occur early in the disease (i.e., depression, apathy, irritability, mania, psychosis, dementia).
  - √ Atypical antipsychotics appear effective (e.g., risperidone 3 mg/day; clinical case reports).
- Multiple sclerosis
  - √ A disease of young adults that may graduate into old age.
  - √ Only case reports of atypical antipsychotics being effective for psychosis in these patients.
- Psychosis secondary to general medical conditions
  - √ Examples: metabolic encephalopathies, toxic/drug/alcohol encephalopathies
  - √ Treat/stabilize primary condition.
  - √ Use low-dose atypical antipsychotic.

Table 2.18. Differential Diagnosis of Medical Conditions That May Predispose to Psychosis*

Illness Type	Disorders
Toxic/drug induced	Benzodiazepines, anticholinergic agents, antiparkinsonian agents, alcohol and other substances of abuse, cortisone
Cerebrovascular disease	Stroke, intracranial hemorrhage, lupus cerebritis, hypertensive encephalopathy
Infectious diseases	Common infections including UTI, pneumonia, STDs, prion diseases (e.g., Creutzfelt–Jacob)
Traumatic brain injuries	Subdural/arachnoid hemorrhage, direct brain trauma (frontal)
Neurological disorders (including degenerative)	Alzheimer's disease and related disorders, Parkinson's disease, seizure disorders
Neoplastic brain disease	Primary/metastatic
Endocrine/metabolic	Hypo/hyperthyroidism, hypo/hyperglycemia, hypo/hypercalcemia, sodium/potassium imbalance, endocrinopathies (e.g., Cushing's disease)
Nutritional deficiencies	Vitamins (thiamine, folate, B_{12}, niacin)

* Transient and/or long-lasting.

PRINCIPLES OF TREATMENT WITH ANTIPSYCHOTICS

- Neuroleptics should be prescribed for target diagnoses or symptoms.
- Use of antipsychotic agents with this population is governed by general principles of clinical pharmacology of elders.
  - √ Lower doses are required.
  - √ Select agent previously helpful to patient.
  - √ Use less sedating agents unless specific reason to sedate patient.

- √ Rapid tranquillization has not been studied in elders and is not suggested.
- Many patients (up to 75%), especially those with dementia-related symptoms, can have antipsychotics reduced or discontinued with no adverse effects.
  - √ Psychosis without dementia does not respond well to dose reduction—symptoms reemerge.
- Antipsychotics with anticholinergic side effects are often more difficult to taper because of anticholinergic rebound syndrome.

OBRA

- U.S. Omnibus Budget Reconciliation Act (OBRA–87 legislation) defined guidelines for standards of practice (Psychotropic Utilization Protocol–PUP), including
  - √ Dosages of specific psychotropic drugs.
  - √ Required dose-reduction trials and monitoring of side effects.
  - √ Rationale required for exceeding recommended doses, using non-recommended agents, or diverging from recommended utilization protocol.

Regulations predated atypicals but the guidelines have been updated.

- Specific approved diagnostic indications include
  - √ One of the DSM psychoses (i.e., schizophrenia, schizoaffective disorder, delusional disorder, acute psychotic episodes, brief reactive psychosis, schizophreniform disorder, atypical psychosis, psychosis in an organic disorder [i.e., delirium or dementia], Tourette's disorder, or Huntington's disease).
  - √ The specific diagnosis must be documented on the record.
  - √ Psychosis in an organic condition
    - ▫ Documentation must be both objective and quantitative.
    - ▫ Not due to a preventable cause.
    - ▫ Causing danger to self or others.
    - ▫ Continuous crying, yelling, screaming in functionally impaired patient.
  - √ Emergency situations or when patient cannot be managed by any other means.
- OBRA specifically *prohibits* antipsychotic use in
  - √ Nonspecific agitation (wandering, poor self-care, unsociability, restlessness, fidgeting, nervousness, uncooperativeness, or other agitation not a danger to self or others).
  - √ Memory impairment.
  - √ Depression without psychosis.
  - √ Insomnia

  - √ Apathy
  - √ Anxiety
- OBRA specifically requires
  - √ Regular reassessment and documentation of need for continuing the medication.
  - √ Regular assessment and documentation of side effects.
  - √ Avoidence of PRN medication, wherever possible.
  - √ Periodic attempts to reduce or discontinue the medication.

Table 2.19. Pharmacological Characteristics of Antipsychotics

Pharmacology	Comment
Generally well absorbed	Gastric emptying time and passage through gut may be delayed by: • Age-related decline in gut motility. • Commonly used drugs. • Anticholinergic effects of antipsychotics themselves. • Antiparkinsonian drugs. • Antacids
Generally highly protein bound	• Affinity for alpha-1-acid glycoprotein (AGP) and albumin.
Lipid soluble	Stored for prolonged periods in lipid compartment, leading to: • Prolongation of clinical and toxic effects. • Prolonged persistence of active drug in the body after discontinuation of treatment (for months, in some cases).
Increased sensitivity of elders to effects	• Secondary to age-related decreases in central dopamine and ACh, especially in presence of structural brain pathology.
Metabolized by phase 1 (oxidation) and 2 (glucuronidation) liver metabolism, followed by renal excretion	• Metabolism of atypical antipsychotics less age-dependent and doses more similar to younger patients than for typical antipsychotics. • Drugs (e.g., clozapine) metabolized by CYP1A2 and 3A4 may be cleared less efficiently with aging, since these enzymes decline in elders.

Neuroleptic Pretreatment Evaluation

- Establish a working diagnosis and appropriate indication for drug therapy.
- Conduct comprehensive psychiatric history and examination, including:
  - √ Past/current medication use/side-effect history.
    - ▫ History of prior EPS reaction increases likelihood of repeat occurrences.
    - ▫ Prior use and response to neuroleptics.
    - ▫ Polypharmacy
  - √ History of symptom development.
- Examine cognitive functions.
- Assess ADL/IADL.
- Conduct family history.

- √ Naturally occurring parkinsonism in blood relatives increases potential for EPS side effects.
- Conduct psychosocial/support history.
  - √ A crucial component to successful therapy.
    - ▫ Reducing psychosis alone does not necessarily translate into improved quality of life in the absence of addressing nonsupportive psychosocial factors.
  - √ Evaluate
    - ▫ Family structure
    - ▫ Conflicts
    - ▫ Support available
    - ▫ Access to social assistance
- Conduct medical history.
  - √ Assess for medical problems, depending on presentation, especially
    - ▫ Reversible medical conditions that may produce/mimic behavioral disturbances.
    - ▫ Sensory deficits.
- Conduct physical and neurological examination.
  - √ Include instrumental assessment for parkinsonian EPS.
    - ▫ Positive signs are predictive of EPS side effects during neuroleptic treatment; common in Alzheimer's patients, especially bradykinesia and rigidity.
    - ▫ Special care should be taken to rule out DLB because of marked sensitivity to neuroleptic drugs, which are relatively contraindicated in this condition.
  - √ Assess for
    - ▫ Potential intolerance of neuroleptic side effects.
    - ▫ Potential for exacerbation of physical illnesses.
- Screen for substance abuse.
- Order baseline laboratory screening.
  - √ CBC
    - ▫ Especially baseline WBC in patients being treated for the first time with a neuroleptic, especially phenothiazines.
  - √ TSH (S)
  - √ Chemistry screen
    - ▫ Including liver functions (i.e., AST, ALT, alkaline phosphatase, serum bilirubin).
    - ▫ Electrolytes
  - √ Urinalysis
  - √ Fasting blood sugar, serum triglycerides (especially with olanzapine and clozapine).
  - √ Medication levels
  - √ ECG, serum B12, and folate, as indicated.
- Consider neuroimaging.

NEUROPHARMACOLOGY OF NEUROLEPTICS

Dopamine Receptors

- D_2 or D_4 antagonism is essential for antipsychotic effect.
  - √ Therapeutic response requires 60–70% D_2 occupancy.
    - ▫ EPS caused by > 80% D_2 occupancy, but akathisia is produced by lower occupancies of 55–65%.
- Conventional neuroleptics are
  - √ Nonselective antagonists of D_2 and D_3 receptors.
  - √ Significantly active at H_1 receptors, alpha-1 adrenergic receptors, and M_1 muscarinic receptors.

Serotonin System

- $5HT_2$ receptor antagonists (e.g., one of the actions of atypical antipsychotics) may inhibit serotonin system and disinhibit dopamine system, thereby ameliorating EPS.

Glutamate and Aspartate Systems

- Glutamate and aspartate transmitter roles are now under investigation.
  - √ As excitatory neurotransmitters, they are implicated in schizophrenia.
  - √ Glutamatergic and dopaminergic systems are interactive, modulating one another.
- Clinical relevance
  - √ Clozapine differs from typical antipsychotics in its glutamatergic effects.
  - √ Elders may be at increased risk of glutamate-mediated neurotoxicity.

CHOOSING AN ANTIPSYCHOTIC DRUG

- Overall, atypicals have displaced typical antipsychotics for routine use.
- All agents are about equally effective for positive symptoms.
  - √ Distinguished only by side effects.
  - √ Select drug based on side-effect profile, ease of administration, dosage forms available, speed of onset of action, patient's history of response.
    - ▫ Atypicals may have slower onset of action in acutely psychotic patients

- Atypicals show superior efficacy for negative symptoms and overall safer side-effect profile.
- Some atypicals, especially clozapine, may be more effective than typicals in treatment-resistant psychosis and for both positive and negative symptoms of schizophrenia.
- For acute psychotic agitation, administer
  - √ Typical antipsychotic, especially haloperidol in IV or IM form; may be the best initial treatment to control urgent situations.
  - √ Switch to atypical agent once acute symptoms controlled.
- Some otherwise robust elders may tolerate concurrent administration of typical and atypical agents, but not suggested for routine use.
- Low-potency typicals (e.g., thioridazine, chlorpromazine) differ in side-effect profile from high-potency ones, largely because of high affinity for muscarinic receptors.
- However, both high- and low-potency drugs, have significant disadvantages.
- Middle-potency typicals (e.g., perphenazine, loxapine) are sometimes preferred for routine typical antipsychotic use because of compromise on intensity of side effects.
- 5–10 % of patients are poor metabolizers of antipsychotics, due to 2D6 metabolism (e.g., haloperidol, perphenazine, risperidone, and thioridazine.
  - √ This and other age-related factors promote highly variable tolerance of antipsychotics.
  - √ This variability is especially important when considering the impact of inhibitors of 2D6 metabolism on the efficacy and side-effect profile of drugs metabolized by this enzyme (see p. 95).
  - √ *Note:* Poor CYP2D6 metabolizers are at threefold risk of parkinsonian side effects.
- Although atypical neuroleptics are now the drugs of choice in most situations requiring antipsychotic treatment, haloperidol and thioridazine are still commonly prescribed.
  - √ Typicals are necessary for patients who are unresponsive to atypicals.
  - √ Typicals are sometimes needed in combination with atypicals.
  - √ Thioridazine is no longer generally indicated, since FDA black-box warnings in 2000, requiring labeling about prolonged QTc and dangers of Torsades de Pointes.
- Response to antipsychotics in elders is best predicted by presence of positive symptoms (e.g., delusions or hallucinations).
  - √ Negative symptoms (social withdrawal, motivational impairments) respond poorly to neuroleptics.

Table 2.20. Comparative Side Effects of Antipsychotic Agents

Generic Name	Sedation	Hypotension	EPS	Anticholinergic Symptoms	Other Side Effects	With Medical Conditions	As Drug Choice
chlorpromazine	+++	+++	++	+++	Jaundice, skin disorders, agranulocytosis, temperature dysregulation, seizures		Aliphatic side chain; low potency; not suggested in elders; pharmacokinetics make it less predictable and possibly more toxic in elders
clozapine	+++	++/+++	0/+	+++	Agranulocytosis may be higher in elders; respiratory distress (including arrest) with doses >100 mg/day; impaired glycemic control	Avoid in diabetes I and II, closed angle untreated glaucoma, prostatic hypertrophy, and seizure disorders (unless concomitant anticonvulsant used)	Often effective for cases of treatment resistant schizophrenia, other forms of psychosis, and agitation where other drugs have not been effective; Parkinson's disease or cases of severe TD; usually used in inpatient settings where close monitoring is possible; use very low doses initially and monitor WBC weekly, and BP and mental status
fluphenazine enanthate	+	+	+++	+			

injectable depot fluphenazine enanthate							Depot not suggested for dementia; reserve for psychosis
injectable depot fluphenazine decanoate							Decanoate form may release significant proportion of drug within hours of injection increasing risk of EPS; overall, similar doses used in elders and younger patients
haloperidol	+	+	+++	+	EPS is common	Usually well tolerated after recent MI and in CHF	Useful for a range of psychotic, excited, and agitated states; psychosis requires 2–3 mg range despite danger of EPS
injectable depot haloperidol decanoate					Long-lasting severe EPS a danger with depot form; steady state in about 3 + months (general adult data)	Usually safe after MI and with CHF	IV Injectable form useful for emergency sedation but danger of acute EPS and prolonged QTc
loxapine	++	++	++	++			Useful in elders; similar indication as perphenazine
mesoridazine	+++	+++	+	+++			Side effects similar to thioridazine; little data for elders
molindone	++	+/++	+/++	++	*No* weight gain;		Not commonly used in elders

(*cont.*)

Continued

Generic Name	Sedation	Hypotension	EPS	Anticholinergic Symptoms	Other Side Effects	With Medical Conditions	As Drug Choice
olanzapine	+	+	+	+	Anticholinergic properties sometimes problematic for elders; impaired glycemic control	Avoid in diabetes I and II	May lose effect in doses > 10 mg/day
perphenazine	++	++	++	++			Useful for excitation, aggression, agitation; for psychosis/agitation of dementia, 6 mg range found effective; higher ranges necessary for nondementia-related psychoses
pimozide	+	+	+++	+		Avoid with arrhythmias and QTc prolongation on ECG	Not suggested in elders
quetiapine	++	+	0	+			
risperidone	++	++	+	0			Low doses (0.25 mg/day) often effective for BPSD-like symptoms; higher dose ranges (4–6 mg/day) may be necessary for schizophrenia; parkinsonism emerges at high ranges

thioridazine	+++	+++	+/++	++/+++	Danger of QTc prolongation and Torsades de Pointes; T-wave changes; pigmentary retinopathy	Avoid in presence of arrhythmias and when QTc is prolonged on ECG	Piperidine side-chain; low potency; most frequently used drug for elders in the past; great precaution and possible contraindication in elders because of cardio-toxicity; may be useful to counter agitation
thiothixene	++	++	++/+++	+/+++			Not widely used for elders; clinical reports of utility with acute confusional states, agitation, sundowning, and aggression with dementia, psychosis, restlessness, excitement; reduce EPS by using lower doses
trifluoperazine	++	++	++/+++	+/++			Not widely used in elders
ziprasidone	+	+	+	+			

+ = mild; ++ = moderate; +++ = marked

Note: Although low-potency antipsychotics are less likely to produce EPS, they still induce a high incidence of these symptoms in elders (about half the rate of high-potency agents). Different formulations offer advantages and sometimes significant variations in side effects and potency when used for elders.

- IV (fastest acting)
  - ✓ Sometimes exacerbates hypotensive side effects.
  - ✓ Haloperidol most effective IV drug for acute emergencies.
  - ✓ Injectable forms of olanzapine and ziprasidone are being developed; geriatric data not available.
- IM and oral liquid forms act at about the same speed.
  - ✓ May produce high peak plasma levels with acute side effects (e.g., hypotension).
  - ✓ IM haloperidol effective in subacute situations.
- Long-acting depot forms
  - ✓ Advantages
    - ▫ Improved compliance, ease of administration.
    - ▫ Especially useful for chronically psychotic elders who are noncompliant, resistant toward oral medication or live in the community and are not in frequent contact with physicians.
    - ▫ Consider longer-acting depot preparations (haloperidol, fluphenazine, clopenthixol) if compliance is compromised by
      - ◦ Unwillingness to take medications.
      - ◦ Resistance to taking oral medications.
      - ◦ Swallowing difficulties.
      - ◦ Family or caregiver ambivalence to medications.
      - ◦ Practical compliance considerations, such as incapacity to travel to appointments or to acquire drugs.
  - ✓ Disadvantages
    - ▫ Not well studied in elders.
    - ▫ Dosage cannot be readily and flexibly adjusted if side effects emerge.
    - ▫ Painful at injection site, especially in thin frail elders with reduced muscle mass.
    - ▫ Absorption may be erratic.
    - ▫ In long-term use, patient must attend a medication clinic or get office injections.
    - ▫ Rapid release of fluphenazine decanoate may predispose to EPS.
    - ▫ Depot formulations sometimes have different pharmacokinetics (e.g., increased bioavailability, less interindividual variations in plasma concentrations) than oral (see specific drug sections).
  - ✓ Dosing

- Use 10 times the stable oral dose IM every 4 weeks, adjusting based on clinical response and side effects.
- Variations for specific drugs.
  - Fluphenazine decanoate: Stabilize on oral form first if possible; taper oral and D/C; begin depot with test dose; base depot dose on oral dose. When danger of clinical decline during oral taper; consider concurrent IM (6.25 mg); repeat IM in 2–4 weeks (6.25 mg) and then continue oral taper; dosing intervals vary from 2 weeks to 2 months. Some geriatric patients can be maintained on q4 month regimens. Absorption and release of depot may be variable in elders with reduced muscle mass.

ADMINISTRATION AND DOSING

Recent studies of dopamine receptor site occupancy reveal that low doses of antipsychotics are often adequate for therapeutic response—that is, to produce D_2 occupancy of 60–70%. This is especially true in elders with compromised brain function or altered metabolic capacity.

- Discuss risk–benefit ratio of therapy with patients or/and caregivers.
- Starting dose one-fifth to one-quarter of general adult dose, especially in frail elders.
- Begin with divided doses to reduce intolerance of single-dose high peak plasma levels.
  - √ May initiate trial of once daily regimens of high-potency typical antipsychotics after tolerance to drug is determined and patient is clinically stable.
    - Most atypicals and low-potency typicals are given bid
    - Although olanzapine can be given once daily after the desired daily dose has been achieved.
  - √ Special caution with drugs with higher potential for hypotension and sedation.
- Nocturnal agitation: Administer drug 1–2 hours before usual time of behavior onset to maximize effect of sedation when useful and appropriate.
- Sedative effect of some antipsychotic drugs, such as nonsedating atypicals, can be augmented by trazodone.
  - √ Benzodiazepines and antihistamines have undesirable side effects and should be avoided as routine sedating agents in elders, although they are sometimes unavoidable.
- OBRA guidelines specify drug doses and require clear rationales for exceeding them.

Regularity of drug administration

- Psychosis therapy usually requires regular rather than PRN dosing.
- Intermittent unpredictable behavior (e.g., BPSD) may be managed with closely monitored PRN dosing.
  - √ Frequent use of PRNs should be converted to regular daily dose.
- PRNs also useful when added to regular dose to control unexpected upsurge in agitated psychotic behavior.

Increase/decrease dose according to tolerance and clinical effect. Consider medical comorbidities and concurrent drug use, metabolic factors, and substance use such as smoking, alcohol, and drugs.

- Some elders require larger doses comparable to younger adults, especially for treatment of psychosis not associated with dementia.
- IM forms are more potent (e.g., fluphenazine injectable is 5 times more potent than oral form).
  - √ Use IM when oral is not possible or practical.
    - ▫ Empirical data on IM use lacking for elders, although widely used.
    - ▫ IM may be necessary in emergency situations (e.g., aggression, self-harm dangers, severe agitated delirium).
  - √ Liquid forms may be useful in presence of swallowing difficulties.

Monitoring

- Precautions in patients with
  - √ Impaired liver and kidney function
  - √ Hypotension
  - √ Cardiovascular disease
  - √ Respiratory disturbances
  - √ Glaucoma especially if untreated
  - √ Prostatic hypertrophy
  - √ Seizure disorder
  - √ Photosensitivity
  - √ Retinopathy
  - √ Anesthesia

Patient's physical condition may decline over time. Pharmacodynamics/kinetics, and hence dosage requirements, may change with aging, over the long course of treating chronic conditions.

- Routine daily monitoring during dose increases includes
  - √ BP
  - √ Temperature
  - √ Other vital signs
  - √ Observation for EPS

- At baseline and 6-month intervals, establish
  - √ Fasting plasma glucose levels
  - √ Fasting cholesterol levels
  - √ Triglyceride levels
  - √ Blood-sugar levels

Maintenance Phase

- Duration of therapy varies depending on target symptoms.
  - √ Acute agitation of BPSD is usually time limited and antipsychotic may be discontinued after few days or used as PRN for upsurge in behavioral disturbance.
  - √ Psychotic depression (see pp. 35–36)
  - √ Chronic psychosis requires long-term therapy.
    - ▫ Increasing age alters pharmacokinetics and dynamics of the drugs used and may require dose or medication alterations through the course of treatment.
  - √ Aging may reduce intensity of positive symptoms and therefore decrease need for antipsychotic medication.
    - ▫ Trial of discontinuation in some chronic, stable patients with schizophrenia may be considered with careful observation and caution.
- Find lowest effective dose for control of symptoms by very slowly tapering dose from acute levels.
- Observe carefully and increase dose at earliest sign of symptom return.
- Reassess need for medications periodically to ensure use of lowest effective dose.

Regular monitoring includes

- Ascertaining compliance (see p. 47).
  - √ Compliance may be improved with depot preparations, but safety concerns (high risk of EPS with prolonged treatment) should be taken into account.
- Periodic blood screens.
  - √ Especially WBC, with differential within first 2 months and every 6 months thereafter.
- Weight
  - √ Introduce weight-reduction program immediately if undue and undesireable weight gain emerges
- Gait, rigidity, abnormal movements (e.g., use AIMS) every 3–6 months.
- LFTs 2–3 times per year
- Renal function
- FBS q 6 months and serum triglycerides annually especially with clozapine and olanzapine.

- √ If hyperglycemia emerges, measure fasting plasma glucose level.
- √ Glucose tolerance test, as indicated.
- √ Reassess risk/benefit of drug.
  - ▫ Consider quetiapine or ziprasidone as substitutes for clozapine, olanzapine, or risperidone.

Discontinuation of a Drug

- If there is a need to discontinue a drug, risk of relapse is reduced by
  - √ Gradual tapering and withdrawal (weeks or months), but risk of relapse is still very high (> 50% in first year).
  - √ Adding new drug and tapering first agent.
    - ▫ Monitor for additive side effects, such as cardiac conduction.
- Taper high-potency typical antipsychotics over at least 2 weeks.
- Taper highly anticholinergic agents (e.g., clozapine, thioridazine) over at least 4 weeks.
  - √ Often takes 3–6 months.
  - √ Anticholinergic rebound symptoms may emerge, especially with low-potency and highly anticholinergic agents, even if dopaminergic agents are substituted (such as high-potency antipsychotics or atypicals).
    - ▫ Key symptoms include insomnia, rebound anxiety, restlessness, nausea/vomiting, and emergent EPS.
    - ▫ Symptoms may look like components of psychotic relapse.
  - √ Withdrawal symptoms may discourage patients from complying with withdrawal schedule.

Switching from a conventional to an atypical antipsychotic drug is far from an exact science.

When switching because of ineffectiveness of the typical antipsychotic, maintain the conventional drug until target dose of the atypical is reached and then taper typical slowly.

When switching because of side effects, taper typical antipsychotic while increasing atypical.

- This cross taper can take a long time—several weeks or months, depending on patient's tolerance and side effects.
- Tapering schedule is about 10% per week.

In either case, frail elders should be watched with more care; sometimes they are not tolerant of having 2 drugs on board at the same time. If so, reduce one before beginning the other, recognizing that there is increased risk of relapse. Of course, in urgent situations (e.g., NMS), the offending drug must be discontinued abruptly and the new drug introduced gradually, if appropriate at all.

Treatment Resistance

- Maximize dose within tolerance of side effects.
- If refractory to typical agent, switch to atypical.
  - √ Usually best to avoid initiating clozapine in an ambulatory setting unless patient can be carefully monitored.
  - √ Inpatients may be switched to clozapine, with cautions, after failure of 1 typical and 2 atypical agents.
- Drug response time varies, depending on the symptom target.
  - √ If there is partial response, continue trial for 6–12 weeks.

Augmenting strategies

- Consider adding a typical antipsychotic to an atypical in nonresponsive patients.
- Consider adding mood stabilizer.
- Use a concurrent antidepressant if significant depressive symptoms.
- Short-acting benzodiazepine sometimes helpful for short-term management of agitation.
  - √ Avoid in combination with clozapine.
- Other augmenting strategies not well investigated in elders include the use of lithium (with caution because of high risk of neurological side effects), trazodone, psychostimulants, beta-blockers, and calcium channel blockers.

Compliance issues (see also p. 47)

- High degree of noncompliance among patients taking antipsychotics (general adult data); clues of noncompliance include
  - √ Worsening of symptoms.
  - √ Absence of expected side effects.
- Elders generally err by taking too few pills, but sometimes confusion may cause accidental overdoses.
- Patient may hoard pills with suicidal intent.
- Observation and monitoring may be necessary.
  - √ Watch patient while taking medication, but be sensitive to patient's sense of being policed.
  - √ Count pills at office checkups.
  - √ Discuss prescription management with pharmacist.
  - √ Review therapeutic working alliance for tension, including family resistance and collusion with patient's noncompliance.
  - √ Take plasma drug levels 12 hours after oral dose.

Refusal of all antipsychotic medication by a patient who clearly will benefit or has benefited in the past is a special case in point.

- Resistant patients are sometimes given medications in disguised forms in food or juice.
- This practice should be carefully considered, since it poses ethical/legal dilemmas for caregivers and institutions; nevertheless it is often done, even though not widely discussed.
- Consider and address the many clinical, ethical, and legal issues.
  - √ Obtain family cooperation and approval.
  - √ Patient is declared legally incompetent.
  - √ Obtain external second opinion on clinical necessity of covert medication.
  - √ Discuss fully with team of caregivers to get common agreement.
  - √ Policy and rationale is documented clearly in patient's record.
  - √ Monitor patient carefully for response and side effects.
  - √ Be aware of OBRA psychotropic utilization protocol.

Table 2.21. Symptom-Specific Interventions

Target Symptoms	Intervention	Comments
Positive psychotic symptoms	• Antipsychotic	• Increase or decease dose according to patient's response and tolerance; change drug, as necessary, based on response
Negative symptoms with active psychosis	• Antipsychotic	• Atypical is best choice
Negative symptoms with akinesia secondary to antipsychotics	• Reduce antipsychotic, add anticholinergic	• Observe for anticholinergic side effects
Negative symptoms with affective disorder or anxiety	• Add antidepressant and/or anxiolytic, reduce antipsychotic, consider adjunctive psychotherapy	• Psychotic depression requires antipsychotic and antidepressant combination, but ECT is most effective; depression in schizophrenia may not respond to antidepressant, and some general adult evidence that tricyclics retard response to antipsychotic therapy
Negative symptoms unresponsive to antipsychotic	• D/C antipsychotic and substitute social, environmental, and psychotherapeutic interventions	
Acute agitation with dementia	• Single dose oral or IM typical antipsychotic (e.g., haloperidol) best for single dose use; interpersonal support and environmental change; supportive psychotherapy	• Reevaluate with trial of reduction or discontinuation of drug therapy periodically; these agitated states are often self-limiting; examine for other causes of agitation, including masked depression and physical illness

SIDE EFFECTS OF ANTIPSYCHOTICS

- Most frequently overlooked side effects include tardive dyskinesia (TD), subtle movement disorders, mild cognitive impairment, falls, akathisia, drug-induced dysphagia, and fecal impaction.
- Preexisting neurological conditions (e.g., DLB, Parkinson's disease) negatively influence tolerance of antipsychotic treatment.
- Dystonias have been reported in patients with dementia when treated with atypical antipsychotics.
- Neuroleptic-induced parkinsonism may be caused by very low-dose typical neuroleptic, either low or high potency.
- EEG changes include slow wave activity, increased alpha rhythm (not clinically relevant).

Side Effects of Atypicals

- Lower (but still significant) incidence of EPS compared to typicals, especially in elders.
  - √ Rank order of EPS potential: clozapine < quetiapine < olanzapine = ziprasidone
  - √ Risperidone hard to classify
    - ▫ At low doses, risk is low.
    - ▫ At higher doses, it is the atypical drug most likely to induce EPS.
- Elders are more susceptible to EPS with these drugs, and it is important to monitor patients for emergence of EPS, especially in the presence of comorbid Parkinson's disease.
- Conversely, atypicals have an antidyskinetic effect when given in the presence of preexisting dyskinesia, especially buccolinguomasticatory symptoms.
- Less perturbation of prolactin levels (but some, e.g., risperidone, have clinically relevant effects).
- Many side effects are related to periods of dose escalation, especially with clozapine.
  - √ In long-term care settings, dose can be titrated more slowly, but in acute-care hospitals there is pressure to discharge quickly, and dose escalation is often more rapid; these patients are at greater risk of dose-related emergence of side effects.
- As a class
  - √ Members share common characteristics but vary considerably in pharmacology and side-effect profile.
    - ▫ Side effects mainly due to muscarinic and histaminic receptor blockade.
    - ▫ Side effect profile includes
      - ◦ Hypotension and orthostatic hypotension

- Sedation
- Weight gain
- Especially with clozapine and olanzapine and exacerbated by concurrent lithium or valproate (general adult data), geriatric data on amounts of weight gain not available.
- Anticholinergic side effects
- Significant impairment of glycemic control in some patients (emergent diabetes mellitus and possible ketoacidosis).
- Most common with clozapine and olanzapine; quetiapine also implicated (general adult data); risperidone is less likely to produce diabetes in those over age 40; geriatric data less clear. Clozapine seems less likely to produce diabetes in elders based on a recent study but overall it's best to be cautious and monitor blood sugars.
- Reports of diabetic ketoacidosis shortly after initiating treatment with these drugs (usually within first 6 months).

√ Abnormal lipid levels—hypertriglyceridemia with clozapine and olanzapine, but not risperidone and ziprasidone which may lower levels.

- Receptor affinities are not fully determined and there are inconsistencies in the data.
  - √ Clozapine and olanzapine block histaminic and muscarinic receptors more strongly than risperidone and therefore cause more anticholinergic side effects; however, clinical effect on cognitive function is probably low.
  - √ Clozapine blocks D_4 accounting for some of its antipsychotic action.
  - √ Alpha-2 blockade is associated with priapism and inhibits clinical effects of some antihypertensive agents.
    - Atypicals, especially clozapine, may have significant activity at glutamatergic receptor sites accounting for some of their antipsychotic effectiveness through secondary inhibition of subcortical dopamine.
- Some atypicals (e.g., risperidone share features of both typical [at higher doses] and atypical agents [at lower doses]).
- Discontinuation rates are generally on the low side.
- Onset of action of atypicals may not be as fast as typicals in acute psychosis but they work quite rapidly for agitation and secondary psychosis.
- Atypicals are less affected by age-related clearance factors than typical agents.
- Atypicals may be more rapidly metabolized by men than by women.
- Cost-benefit analyses—the jury is not back on elders but indications are that atypicals reduce the number and extent of

hospitalizations with improved compliance and fewer severe side effects (general adult data).

SIDE EFFECTS OF ANTIPSYCHOTIC DRUG CLASS

Sedation

- Common; may be useful property of the drug in controlling agitation and inducing sleep.
- May impair mental functioning and produce confusion/disorientation.
  - √ When this is a problem, consider high-potency neuroleptics or risperidone weighing the potential for EPS.
- Oversedation common even with drugs that have mild sedative side-effect profiles and in combination with other sedative agents or narcotics.
- Many patients accommodate to sedative side effects in 1–3 weeks of treatment.
  - √ Effect can be chronically problematic for some.

Management

- Wait for effect to diminish with time.
- Try lower dose.
- Switch to less sedating neuroleptic.
- Prescribe full-dose HS if tolerated and appropriate for the drug.

Cardiovascular Side Effects

- Tachycardia over 90 beats per minute.
  - √ Anticholinergic vagal inhibition effect or reflex tachycardia secondary to vasodilatation and alpha-1 adrenergic blockade.
  - √ Manage with
    - ▫ Lower drug dose
    - ▫ Change antipsychotic.
    - ▫ Beta-blocker or antiarrhythmic.
  - √ Other arrhythmias include ventricular tachycardia, bigeminy, ventricular fibrillation.
- ECG changes
  - √ Nonspecific T-wave changes and QT interval prolongation (especially with thioridazine or high-dose antipsychotics).
- Prolonged QT interval associated with secondary (i.e., noncongenital form) Torsades de Pointes.
  - √ Presyncope, syncope, or sudden death.
  - √ Polymorphic ventricular tachycardia.
  - √ Generally unresponsive to antiarrhythmic drugs.
- *Sudden cardiac death:* 2-fold increased risk with moderate/

large doses of neuroleptic, especially in those with severe cardiovascular disease

Drugs that prolong QT interval

- √ Alcohol (hypomagnesemia)
- √ Antiarrhythmics (class Ia and III)
  - ▫ Amiodarone
  - ▫ Bepridil
  - ▫ Disopyramide
  - ▫ Dofetilide
  - ▫ Ibutilide
  - ▫ Procainamide
  - ▫ Quinidine
  - ▫ Sotalol
- √ Astemizole
- √ Beta-blockers
- √ Budesonide
- √ Digoxin (bradycardic effects)
- √ Diuretics (hypokalemia)
- √ Moxifloxacin
- √ Pimozide
- √ Potassium channel blockers
- √ Propoxyphene
- √ Sparfloxacin
- √ TCAs
- √ Thioridazine

Conditions increasing risk of Torsades de Pointes include

- Metabolic abnormalities.
- Electrolyte disturbances.
  - √ Hypokalemia, hypomagnesemia.
- CVS disease
- CNS disease
- Congenital long QT interval.

Thioridazine

- In doses higher than 100 mg/day, associated with greater cardiac side effects and dangers.
- Dose–response relationship to higher risk of cardiac arrest and ventricular arrhythmias.
- Highest risk of Torsades de Pointes.
  - √ Avoid in QT prolongation with persistent QTc > 500 msec. recent MI, CHF, cardiar arrhythmia.

Other drugs causing torsades de pointes include

- Quinidine, antimalarials (quinine, halofantrine), terfenadine,

astimozole (no longer marketed) in combination with CYP3A4 inhibitors.
  - √ Antifungals (azoles and sparofloxin, grepafloxen) or
  - √ Macrolide antibiotics such as erythromycin and gastric motility enhancer cisapride.
- Avoid concurrent use with antipsychotics
  - √ Especially thioridazine
  - √ Haloperidol is usually safe post MI and in CHF.
    - Haloperidol in both oral and IV routes rarely causes Torsades de Pointes.
  - √ Pimozide may cause prolongation of the QT interval and flattened/inverted T-waves and U waves; monitor ECG during dose adjustment.
- Avoid concurrent use of drugs that lengthen QT interval (see p. 282).

Atypical antipsychotics show little, if any, cardiac advantage over typicals.

- Clozapine associated with myocarditis.
  - √ Myocarditis associated with eosinophilic/lymphocytic infiltrate.
- Ziprasidone
  - √ Inceased QTc at higher doses.

High-risk patients with preexisting cardiovascular disease require careful evaluation before treatment. Risk factors include

- Heart failure, history of arrhythmias, MI.
- Electrolyte disturbances and autonomic dysfunction.
- Use caution in using neuroleptics (especially low-potency in high doses) in vulnerable patients.

Postural (Orthostatic) Hypotension

- More common in elders.
- Caused by effect of drug on CNS vasoregulatory centers.
  - √ Blockade of alpha-1 adrenergic receptors.
- Increased risk in patients with low cardiac output and concurrent use of other alpha-1 adrenergic receptor blockers.
- Symptoms
  - √ Dizziness
  - √ Fainting/syncope on standing up.
- Avoid low-potency agents, atypical antipsychotics.
- Generally occurs early in course of treatment and at peak blood levels.
- Special risk with IM medications.
- Hypotension associated with increased risk of falls (especially at night), MI, or stroke.

Management

- Reduce dose of neuroleptic.
- Switch to less hypotensive neuroleptic.
- Educate patient/family about risk, especially nocturnal risks.
  - √ Rise slowly from sitting or lying position (15–60 secs).
  - √ Use elastic stockings for external support (use both day and night).
- Avoid ephedrine and amphetamine, which aggravate psychosis and agitation, and epinephrine and isoproteronol which lower BP secondary to beta-adrenergic agonist action.
- Maintain fluid/electrolyte balance.
  - √ Increased risk with low salt intake, dehydration, antihypertensive agents, hypothyroidism, stimulant withdrawal.
  - √ Consider sequential trials of increasing blood volume (salt and water loading), but beware of cardiovascular overload.
- Use alpha-agonists (e.g., metaraminol, phenylephrine, norepinephrine) or fludrocortisone acetate cautiously (0.1 mg daily); try to avoid antihypertensive medication.

Anticholinergic-Induced Reactions

See also anticholinergic side effects, pages 71–75.

- Potentially serious and occasionally life-threatening for elders.
- Risks increased by
  - √ Age-related reductions in general cholinergic functions.
  - √ Concurrent anticholinergic medications (e.g., antiparkinsonian agents, TCAs, meperidine.
- Thioridazine among the most anticholinergic agents; avoid use with other anticholinergics.
- Caution with clozapine.
- Avoid anticholinergic agents in delirium.
  - √ Use haloperidol and observe for fecal impaction (easily missed).
- Long-term anticholinergic therapy can cause reversible bilateral diffuse glucose hypometabolism.

Management

- Reduce dose of drug, switching to quetiapine, risperidone, ziprasidone, or higher-potency antipsychotic.
- For blurred vision consider
  - √ Pilocarpine 1% eye drops
  - √ Bethanechol 5–10 mg po repeated q 60–90 minutes up to maximum of 50 mg/day
    - ▫ Caution re. occasional hypotensive reaction and reflex tachycardia
  - √ Eye glasses

- For dry eyes
  - √ Caution with contact lenses.
  - √ Use artificial tears.

Sexual Effects

- Breast enlargement and rarely galactorrhea
- Diminished libido
- Impaired orgasmic response and quality
- Painful retrograde ejaculation
- Priapism associated with alpha-adrenergic antipsychotics.

Management

- May require dose reduction or switch to non-alpha-adrenergic agent.
  - √ Severe priapism constitutes an emergency (see pp. 216–217).

Movement Disorders

Acute (Early) Onset EPS—Akathisia

- Common side effect in elders and may be very distressing.
- Objective symptoms
  - √ Semipurposeful leg and foot movements
  - √ Shifting weight while sitting or standing
  - √ Muscle tension
  - √ Nervousness and agitation especially characterized by leg movements
    - ▫ Crossing/uncrossing legs, stamping feet; rocking, swaying, pacing
- Subjective symptoms:
  - √ Muscle stiffness, jitteriness, a restless desire to move associated with inner tension
  - √ Inner restlessness may be present without observable movement and agitation.
- Movement component may be further masked by presence of coexisting hypokinesia, which may inhibit restless movements.
- May be increased suicidal agitation associated with extreme dysphoria.
- Variant—pseudoakathisia
  - √ Objective movement but no subjective component.
  - √ If persists longer than 6 months, called "chronic akathisia."
- Onset: rapid—may occur within hours of first dose.
  - √ Most occur within first week of treatment and up to 2 weeks.
  - √ Associated with maximal plasma concentrations of the drug.

Severity of EPS correlates with potency of the drug: less with low-potency and atypical antipsychotics, more with higher-potency typicals.

May be caused by D_2 dopaminergic blockade and serotonergic mechanisms, but the pathophysiology is not yet clearly defined.

Emerges in medically ill patients (e.g., terminally ill), for whom morphine, sodium valproate and sodium bicarbonate are reported to increase risk.

Management

- Distinguish akathisia from anxiety and agitation of other origins (e.g., dementia, pain, psychosis).
- Evaluate and respond to suicidal ideation/agitation.
- Lower dose of drug.
  - √ If agitation increases, consider another cause and manage accordingly.
- Add propranolol (20–80 mg/day).
  - √ *Note caution:* If antipsychotic causes alpha-1 blockade, addition of beta-blocker can produce hypotension and cardiac decompensation.
- Switch to atypical agent.
- Add benzodiazepine (e.g., lorazepam, clonazepam) with appropriate cautions.
- Biperiden (anticholinergic agent) IM or IV offers rapid but short-term (4 hours) relief in severe cases, or when diagnosis not clear.
  - √ In general, anticholinergic agents are less helpful.

Acute (Early) Onset EPS—Parkinsonian Symptoms

- Rates of up to 75% of typical neuroleptic-treated elders.
  - √ Peak incidence in 70–80-year-olds.
- May unmask idiopathic Parkinson's disease in about 11% of patients.

Parkinsonian symptoms are indistinguishable from idiopathic Parkinson's except by drug history. Predominant symptoms are:

- Bradykinesia
  - √ Mask-like facies, decreased arm swing when walking, shuffling gait, weak voice, difficulty initiating movement, stooped posture.
- Rigidity (with cogwheeling)

Additional symptoms include

- Perioral tremor (rabbit syndrome)
  - √ Rare in drug-induced parkinsonism.
  - √ No tongue involvement.
  - √ Continues in sleep.
  - √ Responds to anticholinergics and discontinuing antipsychotics.

- Resting tremor
  - √ Not as common in drug-induced states, but can be the primary symptom.
  - √ Onset usually in the upper extremities.
    - ▫ Pill rolling tremor is unusual.
- Loss of postural reflexes (impaired righting reflex).
- Hypersalivation secondary to decreased rate of swallowing, with drooling.
- Autonomic instability.
- Micrographia

Symptoms usually symmetrical but may be asymmetrical.

- Onset may be detectable within 48 hours of beginning therapy in susceptible patients.
  - √ More typically within 10–14 days.

Drug-induced parkinsonism is less likely to be unilateral than idiopathic Parkinson's. Parkinsonism probably associated with increased risk of falls; may be associated with increased negative symptoms of schizophrenia. Factors that increase risk of neuroleptic-induced parkinsonism include

- Older age
- Female gender
- Higher baseline EPS
- Family history of essential tremor
- Severity of dementia or other comorbid brain damage (EPS may occur at low doses of neuroleptic)
- Use of IM neuroleptic

EPS reaction is a marker for increased mortality in the year after beginning neuroleptic treatment. EPS is associated with

- Increased expression of TD
- Secondary negative symptoms
- Dysphoria and poor compliance and cognitive dysfunction

Other drugs associated with drug-induced parkinsonism include

- Benzamides (metoclopramide, sulpiride, clebopride)
- Reserpine
- Tetrabenzine
- Methyldopa
- Calcium channel blockers (flunarizine, cinnarizine, nimodipine, nifedipine, verapamil, diltiazem)

Management

Monitor weekly, especially early in treatment to detect initial changes, and then periodically thereafter. Early EPS (e.g., rigidity or micrographia), often evident within 4 days of treatment onset, correlates with later severity of EPS.

- Distinguish akinesia from depression.
- Reduce dose of drug.
- Switch to lower risk/agent (e.g., atypical neuroleptic).
- Add anticholinergic agents (e.g., benztropine, procyclidine, biperiden, or diphenhydramine) with caution (anticholinergic CNS syndrome).
- Consider dopaminergic agent (amantadine, levodopa) or benzodiazepine.

Dopamine agonists carry increased risks in the presence of:

- Cognitive dysfunction
- Orthostatic hypotension
- History of psychosis

With treatment, most symptoms resolve in 7 weeks (range 1–36 weeks).

Acute Dystonic Reaction

- Overall, uncommon in elders.
- Rates of 1.5–2% (compared to 30% in younger patients).

Clinical picture

- Slow, sustained muscular contraction or spasm.
  - √ May be painful.
- Muscle spasms of the neck (torticollis or retrocollis), face, jaw (forced opening leading to dislocation or trismus), tongue (protrusion or twisting), extraocular muscles (oculogyric crisis), and back.
  - √ Can cause dysphagia, dysarthria, difficulty breathing.
- Pisa syndrome may occur early in treatment.
  - √ Onset 48–96 hours after beginning neuroleptic or increasing dose.

High-potency typical neuroleptics pose greatest risk of acute dystonic reaction but may occur with any neuroleptic (e.g., risperidone).

- Cause may be imbalance between acetylcholine and dopamine in basal ganglia.
  - √ Anticholinergics restore balance.
- Most commonly seen in afternoon and evening.
  - √ Rarely at night or morning.
- Recurrent acute dystonia may be a sign of noncompliance with medication.

Management

- Rapidly responsive to anticholinergic agent.
  - √ Benztropine 0.5–1 mg or diphenhydramine 25 mg.
- Discontinue typical antipsychotic immediately.
  - √ If not possible to discontinue, lower dose of drug.
- Switch to atypical.
- Use anticholinergics for the minimum time required to bring symptoms under control.
- For extreme cases unresponsive to other interventions, consider botulinum toxin.
- Pisa syndrome may be unresponsive to these interventions.
  - √ Amantadine may be effective.
- *Try to avoid prophylactic anticholinergics in elders.*

Dysphagia

- Occurs both in Parkinson's disease and as a drug side effect.
- Inquire actively about dysphagia.
- Observe swallowing during meals.
  - √ Watch for evidence of gagging, coughing, or choking.
- Examine gag reflex in patients on antipsychotics.

Management

- Reduce or discontinue antipsychotic.
- Avoid anticholinergics, which may exacerbate the condition.
- Instruct re. dietary modification (e.g., chopped or pureed food).
- Instruct competent patients on eating habits (i.e., small mouthfuls, active attention to swallowing).

Tardive Dyskinesia (TD)—Late Onset Movement Disorder

TD is a hyperkinetic movement disorder that persists after the drug has been discontinued.

- Onset later in course of treatment (usually after at least 4 weeks).
- Prevalence: increases with age and duration of therapy.
  - √ Up to 60% of patients on typical antipsychotics after 3 years, 23% of which are severe.
    - ▫ Much lower rates with atypical antipsychotics (e.g., 2.6% on risperidone after 1 year).
  - √ Longer-term follow-up rates not available for elders.
  - √ Six-fold increase in elders over general adult populations.
  - √ African Americans at increased risk.

Symptoms:

- Orofacial muscles most often involved, especially chewing movements; other movements include writhing tongue movement

and/or thrusting, vermicular movements, puffing of cheeks, pursing/pouting/puckering of lips, lip smacking, blowing, vigorous eye blinking.
  - √ Orofacial tardive dystonia has been described as emerging only during eating.
  - √ Distinguish orofacial movements from other symptoms
    - ▫ Associated with ill-fitting dentures.
- Writhing, jerking limb movements (choreoathetoid).
  - √ Rhythmic low-frequency movements that may resemble tremor.
    - ▫ 3 cycles per second, in contrast to finer tremor of Parkinson's at 7 cycles per second.
- Hand movements include writhing finger movements, repetitive flexion extension of thumbs, repetitive hand clasping.
  - √ Finger movements impair writing and other fine motor activity.
- Toe movements, foot tapping, squirming.
- Severe forms involve rolling neck movements, rocking of trunk.
- Respiratory dyskinesias involving the diaphragm and respiratory muscles can be life-threatening, though rarely.
  - √ Aerophagia, belching, or grunting
- Movements disappear during sleep or exacerbate under stress.

Especially in early stages, patient is often unaware of movements but also may become embarrassed by them.

Course

- Variable—but may remain stable over many years.
- Spontaneous partial remission occurs, but less likely in elders.
- If drug dose is decreased or discontinued, symptoms either may improve over next months to 2 years or may persist.
  - √ May worsen especially initially after drug is reduced or discontinued.

Risk

- Relatively high, even in elders on relatively low-dose typicals (e.g., haloperidol < 2 mg/day or thioridazine < 75 mg/day) and for short periods of time (1–12 months).
- Associated and risk factors include
  - √ More advanced age
  - √ History of cumulative neuroleptic exposure
  - √ Alcohol abuse
  - √ Early EPS
  - √ Cognitive impairment
  - √ Female gender
  - √ African American descent

- √ Diabetes mellitus
- √ Possibly concurrent mood disorder, concurrent anticholinergic medication
- Reduce risk by using minimal effective doses of any antipsychotic. Use atypical antipsychotics preferentially. If typical antipsychotic is necessary, opt for intermediate-potency drug. Discontinue unnecessary treatment.

Monitor for early EPS; more than one movement disorder (Parkinson's or TD plus tardive dystonia) may occur in the same patient.

Management

- Advisable to monitor, using a standard involuntary movement scale (e.g., AIMS) to assess patients on antipsychotics at baseline.
- Workup
  - √ Physical/neurological workup.
  - √ History of exposure to antipsychotics (including total duration and dose), l-dopa, lithium, estrogens, amphetamine and other stimulants, toxins, and metals.
    - ▫ Rheumatic fever and neurological disorders in early life (e.g., Sydenham's chorea).
    - ▫ Family history of movement disorders.
    - ▫ Medical history of thyroid disease, polycythemia, SLE.
  - √ Laboratory/imaging.
    - ▫ Routine blood work/chemistry
    - ▫ TSH(s)
    - ▫ Urine screen
    - ▫ Testing for stimulants and transitional metals, if suspected and warranted by history.
    - ▫ Consider EEG and CT scan.
- Differentiate from Parkinson's Disease which is often comorbid with TD.
  - √ Note that some anti-parkinsonian drugs (i.e., anticholinergics) often worsen TD.
- Initial management
  - √ Best strategy is to substitute atypical for typical antipsychotic after discontinuing typical antipsychotic.
    - ▫ For choreic TD, risperidone appears to be the most powerful suppressant, but avoid in other forms of TD.
    - ▫ Clozapine has demonstrated some efficacy in younger patients but fully controlled empirical data lacking and side effects are a concern.
    - ▫ If discontinuation is impossible use lowest possible dose of antipsychotic and add
      - ◦ Benzodiazepine

    - Vit E 400–1600 IU/day (but expect modest response in severe/longstanding cases).
    - Also consider: beta-blocker (e.g., high dose propranolol—increased risks in elders; adult dose 500–800 mg/d), clonidine (0.2–0.9 mg/day), alpha-methyldopa (750–1500 mg/day) (all general adult doses).
  - ECT may be effective in severe cases especially with depression.
- √ Alternative management strategies
  - Discontinue offending drug (half of patients improve over next 2 years; general adult data)
  - Reduce the dose to lowest effective.
  - Both discontinuation and dose reduction are risky although either alternative is sometimes possible
    - > 50% risk of relapse of psychosis in first 9 months or worsening of symptoms of TD in the short term
  - Increased neuroleptic dose may suppress movements (sometimes temporarily).
  - Younger patients on low-dose antipsychotic with TD are more likely to remit spontaneously, but elders less likely.
- √ Systematic trial of other interventions
  - Acetazolamide 1.5–2.0 g daily (TID dose). Coadminister thiamine 0.5 g TID.
  - Ondansetron, dose 4–8 mg daily.
  - Benzodiazepines may be effective (especially clonazepam) but empirical data remain few in number and quality.
  - Also consider bromocriptine, buspirone, choline, cyproheptadine, deanol aceglumate, lecithin, lithium, nifedipine, tryptophan, verapamil
    - All reported useful, but overall evidence for treatments of TD is inconsistent and sparse.
  - GABA agonists (e.g., baclofen, sodium valproate, progabide) probably not effective.
  - Botulinum toxin injected locally every few months can relieve regional syndromes such as torticollis or retrocollis.
  - Educate patients about symptoms and how to tell others about them and avoid embarrasment.
    - Provide tips: Avoid buttons (use Velcro); advise re. balance, footwear, shower and bath precautions (e.g., no-slip mats, grab bars, shower chair, long-handled bathing aids).
  - Recommend gait training to prevent falls.

Dystonia, Akathisia, Myoclonus, and Tourette's

Tardive dystonia (sustained twisting, involuntary muscle contraction) is unusual in elders—rates of 1.5–2%. Usually develops insidiously, increases with duration of exposure to drug, and may be associated with changes in drug therapy (switching agents, reducing doses).

- Usually presents with focal dystonia (e.g., torticollis, blepharospasm, gait disturbance, dysphagia).
- Progressive from one part of body to another
  - √ Usually in ascending pattern; general adult data.
- Pisa syndrome (flexion of trunk to one side; slight axial rotation)
  - √ Risk factors include old age and organic brain disorder.
  - √ Onset 48–96 hours after beginning neuroleptic or increasing dose.
- Akathisia may occur after drug is withdrawn (tardive form).
- Rabbit syndrome: Perioral involuntary EPS, manifested as quickly alternating vertical movements, resembling movement of a rabbit's mouth.
  - √ May be accompanied by "popping sound" as mouth opens.
  - √ Tongue not involved.
  - √ Slower, writhing movement of TD not evident.

Management

- Withdraw offending agent, if possible.
- Akathisia not usually responsive to anticholinergics.
  - √ More responsive to beta blockers (e.g., propranolol 40–80 mg/day), clozapine, or possibly reserpine.
- For other tardive disorders, consider tetrabenzine, benztropine, or botulinum toxin injection.
- Rabbit syndrome responds to antiparkinsonian medication (in contrast to TD).

Catatonia

- Uncommon; associated with high-potency neuroleptics.
- Onset within a few weeks of beginning therapy.
- Catatonic symptoms include immobility, waxy flexibility, cogwheeling, withdrawal, refusal, to eat, negativism, mutism, verbigeration, echolalia, echopraxia, drooling, urinary incontinence.
- Lethal catatonia resembles NMS and is often indistinguishable.

Management

- Stop neuroleptic.
- Provide supportive measures and trial of IM lorazepam 1–2 mg, increasing to maximum tolerated doses over 2–3 days.
- Continue lorazepam orally thereafter if necessary.
- If symptoms do not resolve, institute ECT.
- Other possible drugs include clonazepam, amantadine, and sometimes anticholinergics.

Neuroleptic Malignant Syndrome (NMS)

NMS is an acute, life-threatening disorder, with mortality rates (general adult data) of 11–25%. It is especially lethal in conjunction with organic brain pathology, alcohol/opiate abuse, and depot antipsychotics.

- Uncommon; rate of 0.2–2% at any time during course of treatment.
- May increase in frequency in elders and possibly with depot medications.
- Increased risk at time of dose changes.
- Prior episode a significant risk factor.
- Etiology unknown. Theories include
  - √ Thermodysregulation secondary to dopamine blockade which releases serotonin action.
  - √ Skeletal muscle defects increasing Ca release.

Diagnosis and symptoms

- Neuroleptic treatment started within 7 days of symptom onset, (and usually within 24–72 hours)

Exclude other causes of symptoms. Diagnostic criteria vary. One set requires two major symptoms—hyperthermia and muscle rigidity (lead-pipe)—plus at least five other symptoms, which include

- Severe parkinsonism (especially coarse tremor) other symptoms include dystonia, dyskinesia, akinesia, flexor-extensor posturing, festinating gait
- Autonomic dysfunction (fever 101–107 degrees F; diaphoresis)
- Fluctuating consciousness especially mutism, agitation, confusion, coma
- Autonomic dysfunction
  - √ Tachycardia
  - √ Rapid respirations
  - √ Hyper/hypotensive BP fluctuation
  - √ Urinary incontinence
  - √ Increased salivation
  - √ Sweating
  - √ Dysphagia
  - √ Pallor
- Changes in blood chemistry
  - √ Increased creatinine phosphokinase (CPK), sometimes with very high levels (CPK 350–4300 u/mL)
  - √ Metabolic acidosis
  - √ Myoglobulinemia
- Often severe leukocytosis—15,000–30,000/mm^3 (often with left shift)
- Abnormal LFTs
- Low serum iron levels
- Rhabdomyolysis may lead to acute renal failure.

- √ Raises mortality rate to 50%.
- Dysphagia may lead to pulmonary insufficiency secondary to aspiration.
- Nonlethal but permanent sequelae include residual myoclonus, dysarthria, dysphagia.
- Occasional cases of atypical NMS
  - √ Absent muscle rigidity or fever.

DSM-IV criteria require hyperthermia and muscle rigidity plus *two* of the following: tremor, mutism, agitation/coma, tachycardia, BP fluctuation, sweating, dysphagia, elevated CK and WBCs.

Neuroleptics implicated in NMS are strong D_2 dopamine receptor antagonists, most commonly haloperidol (although haloperidol appears less likely to lead to fatal outcome than other causal agents).

- Low potency agents have lower risk. Atypicals reported to induce NMS (quetiapine and olanzapine)
- Sudden change in neuroleptic dose (up or down) can precipitate NMS independent of dose and duration. Other dopaminergic blocking agents such as amoxapine have been implicated.
- Rarely, withdrawal from dopamine agonists may induce NMS-like state, as may withdrawal from SSRIs or lithium.

Predisposing factors include

- Dehydration
- Highly agitated state
- History of ECT
- Organic brain pathology (especially retardation and substance abuse)
- Use of high therapeutic and loading doses of neuroleptic
- Use of long-acting neuroleptics and high potency agents
- Simultaneous use of more than one neuroleptic
- Stress
- Concomitant use of lithium or antidepressants
- Possibly low serum iron levels
  - √ Reported with haloperidol/clozapine/venlafaxine combination.
- High ambient temperature.

Management

Differentiate from other conditions with hyperthermia: Anticholinergic syndrome, drug-induced hyperthermia (meperidine, NSAIDs, amphetamine), hyperthyroidism, acute lethal catatonia, CNS infection, heavy metal poisoning (lead, arsenic), lithium toxicity, sepsis, serotonin syndrome, thyrotoxicosis, drug withdrawal (alcohol, benzodiazepine).

Educate patients and caregivers re risks and early detection.

NMS considered an emergency. When it occurs

- Discontinue neuroleptics and anticholinergics immediately.
- Provide aggressive, supportive medical care.
  - √ Fluid replacement
  - √ Correct electrolyte imbalance.
  - √ IV fluids
  - √ Control malignant hyperthermia via cooling and antipyretic agents.

Pharmacological interventions may or may not be necessary, are not well studied in elders, and are somewhat controversial. If no improvement on supportive measures within 2–4 days pharmacological alternatives include

- Dantrolene used most often.
  - √ 0.25–2 mg/kg body weight qid IV until stabilized.
  - √ Then switch to oral or IM routes.
  - √ May be increased to 1–2 mg/kg qid (4–8 mg/kg/day either orally or IM).
  - √ Watch for hepatic toxicity at high cumulative doses above 10 mg/kg/24 hrs.
- Bromocriptine 5 mg tid PO or by NG tube and increased to 10 mg tid as necessary.
  - √ Observe for hypotension.
- Amantadine 100 mg PO/ or via NG tube; may titrate to 200 mg bid.
- Slowly metabolized decanoate forms may require plasmaphoresis.

Recent data suggest managing NMS as aggressively as malignant catatonia to reduce mortality.

Some recommend vigorously using

- IV lorazepam 3–4 mg/day, increasing to high doses (up to 16 mg/day; general adult data) over 3–4 days.
- Followed by ECT (the definitive treatment for presumptive malignant catatonia, often indistinguishable from NMS).
- If there is no response in 7–14 days, ICU admission for severe "malignant" cases.
  - √ Consider plasmapheresis in extreme cases.

If continuing psychosis cannot be managed any other way, use an antipsychotic with a different mode of action, preferably an atypical agent if that has not been tried.

- Rechallenge with the same neuroleptic leads to NMS recurrence in 80% of cases.
- Avoid haloperidol, trifluoperazine, thiothixene and fluphenazine.

- Inform patient, caregivers, and family about risks, obtaining informed consent to proceed.
- Use atypicals (low potency agents or atypical drug; may be safer but data unclear).
  - √ Increase dose slowly
- Hospitalize patient during dose titration phases.
- Monitor
  - √ Vital signs and temperature carefully
  - √ WBC, CPK

Grand Mal Seizures

EEG changes may herald seizures comprised of slow dysrhythmic waves, sharp waves, or spike and slow wave responses. Risk factors include

- History of seizures or epilepsy
- ECT
- Rapid increase/decrease in dose
- Comorbid organic CNS disorders
- Polypharmacy with other drugs that reduce seizure threshold

Management

- Avoid rapid increases in blood levels of neuroleptics.
- Raise dose slowly to reduce seizure risk.
  - √ Clozapine risk relatively low at low doses but risk higher during dose titration phase or at high maintenance doses. Monitor for high plasma levels (450 μg/ml) in patients at high risk.
- If seizure occurs
  - √ Reduce antipsychotic dose by at least 50%
  - √ EEG
  - √ Anticonvulsant
  - √ Neurology consult

Ophthalmologic Syndromes

- Pigmentary retinopathy
  - √ Caused by high-dose thioridazine (> 800 mg), mesoridazine.
- Skin-eye syndrome
  - √ Sometimes encountered in elders who have been treated chronically for years with phenothiazines.
  - √ Characterized by progressive pigmentation of skin areas and conjunctiva and sclera, with irregular stellate opacities of cornea and lens.
- Blurred vision
  - √ Anticholinergic effect

Management

- High doses of thioridazine contraindicated.
- Order complete eye examinations periodically.
  - √ As much as every 6 months in vulnerable patients.
- Lenticular changes persist after drug discontinuation.
- Corneal changes may resolve slowly over years.

Jaundice

- Phenothiazines may induce obstructive (cholestatic) jaundice, though rarely.
- Phenothiazines contraindicated in patients with history of obstructive jaundice or liver disease.
- Discontinue medication; generally reversible.

Hematological Effects—Agranulocytosis

- Induced by clozapine in about 1% of cases.
  - √ Onset sometimes abrupt, within hours of treatment or within first month–12 weeks but very occasionally will occur after prolonged use of > 1 year.
  - √ More common in women and elders.
- Rare effect with chlorpromazine (0.7%) and occasionally other phenothiazines (< 0.02%).
- Spike in WBC of > 15% predicts onset of agranulocytosis within 75 days.
- Signs include acute sore throat, high fever, mouth sores or ulcers, weakness, lethargy.
  - √ High mortality if drug is not discontinued.
- WBC < 3500/mm^3—do not begin low potency antipsychotic.
- Management
  - √ Hematopoietic growth factors and granulocyte-macrophage colony stimulating factor.

Weight Gain

- Weight gain is a side effect of most antipsychotics in all subclasses. Little geriatric-specific data are available.
- Among atypicals, clozapine (4–5 kg) and olanzapine have the greatest potential for weight gain, with ziprasidone the least (0.5–1 kg).
- Among typicals, haloperidol and molindone are least likely to induce weight gain; perphenazine and chlorpromazine induce the greatest amount (4–6 kg; general adult data) over about 10-week period, with greater weight gain likely over longer periods.

- Cause of weight gain unknown
  - √ May be related to the increased insulin and leptin levels associated with clozapine and olanzapine.
- Monitor weight of obese patients, especially with comorbid physical disorders such as COPD, emphysema, sleep apnea, diabetes, hypertension, risk of stroke, gall bladder disease.
- Chronic schizophrenics may be at greater risk of drug-induced obesity as they age; may lead to poor compliance in some patients.

Management

- Changing medication often possible but not always very helpful.
  - √ Discontinuation, although sometimes recommended, is problematic because of the high likelihood of psychotic relapse in some patients.
- Weight control programs (calorie-restricted balanced diets) for institutionalized elders likely to be effective.
- Educate patient in advance about weight gain potential and strategies for prevention.
  - √ Diet counseling and education.
- Caution patients about discontinuing medication.
- Orlistat 120 mg tid is effective (general adult data) and does not interact with neuroleptics.

Endocrinological Disorders—Increased Prolactin Levels

Prolactin is normally inhibited by dopamine (neurons projecting from the hypothalamus); TRH or serotonin also may be involved. Inhibition of dopamine by antipsychotic D_2 receptor blockade releases increased prolactin.

Clozapine and quetiapine unlikely to produce this side effect. Clinical manifestations include

- Breast tenderness or enlargement
- Gynecomastia
- Very rarely, galactorrhea
- Increased breast tumor growth
- Osteoporosis

Management

- Very rarely requires changing medications (e.g., to quetiapine).
- Prolactin inhibited by
  - √ Bromocriptine—starting dose 1.25–2.5 mg/day, increasing by 1.25–2.5 mg/week to optimal dose 5–7.5 mg/day. (range 2.5–15 mg/day) (all general adult data) or
  - √ Amantadine 50–100 mg bid—start low, go slow.

Skin Disorders

- After prolonged high dose therapy
  - √ Most serious effects rarely seen with modern therapeutic approaches, especially low-dose therapies and atypicals.
- Photosensitivity a potential side effect with most typicals.
- Allergic reaction
  - √ Maculopapular, itchy, whole-body rash
  - √ Purple skin pigmentation
    - ▫ Predominantly chlorpromazine; very rarely other phenothiazines

Management

- Warn patients about the danger of sun exposure
  - √ Burning may occur despite the presence of a tan.
- Prevent sunburn with generous use of high SPF sun blockers, especially on highly vulnerable body parts such as the face.
  - √ Caution against sun bathing or prolonged sun exposure (including winter sun on ski slopes or hazy/foggy days).
  - √ Wear sun-protective clothing even in the shade (e.g., wide-brimmed hats, dark T-shirts).
  - √ Advise UVA/UVB screening sunglasses.
- Control rash by changing to another type of neuroleptic.
  - √ Avoid skin pigmentation by using low to moderate doses.
  - √ Pigmentation is reversible over months or years after discontinuing neuroleptic.
  - √ For seborrhea use topical skin lotions, soaps, and discontinue drug.

Cognitive Impairment

- Likely caused by anticholinergic properties of some antipsychotics.
- Short-term verbal memory impaired.
- May lead to frank delirium in susceptible patients.
- Usually associated with higher dose ranges.
- Symptoms of anticholinergic toxicity include
  - √ Dilated pupils
  - √ Hot dry skin
  - √ Dry mucous membranes
  - √ Tachycardia
  - √ Absent bowel sounds

Management

- Avoid concomitant anticholinergic agents; in cases of confusion, discontinue offending drug.
- Anticholinergic delirium (see pp. 76 and 252).

SIADH

SIADH is especially evident in the physically frail. Even modestly low sodium levels can cause confusion/disorientation in vulnerable elders. (See also pp. 82–83).

Distinguish SIADH from water intoxication occasionally seen in patients on neuroleptic medication.

- In SIADH, urine osmolarity is high.
- In water intoxication, urine osmolarity very low.

Impaired Glycemic Control

- Emergence of de novo diabetes mellitus, usually type II (noninsulin dependent).
- Hyperglycemia
- Exacerbation of type I and II diabetes mellitus.
- Ketoacidosis (can be fatal)

Onset within 3 months (10 days–18 months; general adult data).

Not dose-dependent and seems independent of weight gain associated with antipsychotics.

- Mechanism of action may be decreased insulin action, induction of hypertriglyceridemia.
- Risk factors for type II diabetes include
  - √ Increased age
  - √ Diagnosis of early-onset schizophrenia independent of medication effects.
  - √ Overweight prior to treatment
  - √ Weight increase > 10% during treatment.
  - √ Pretreatment history of glucose dysregulation and/or hypertension.
  - √ Family history of diabetes.
  - √ Female gender
  - √ Ethnicity (Hispanic, African and Native American, Asian Indian, Polynesian, Australian aborigines)

Antipsychotic treatment markedly increases the incidence of diabetes in schizophrenia. Impaired glycemic control probably (but not conclusively) occurs

- Especially with clozapine and olanzepine.
  - √ Very occasionally, risperidone and quetiapine.
- With typical agents, especially thioridazine, loxapine and chlorpromazine.
  - √ Reported with other agents.

ANTIPSYCHOTIC AGENTS

Management

Discuss risk with patients based on presence or absence of various additive risk factors; tailor drug choice to risk level.

- High-risk patients avoid clozapine and olanzapine, if possible, or monitor more cautiously.
- Establish baseline and 6-month fasting plasma glucose levels, fasting cholesterol levels, triglycerides levels.
- Monitor blood sugar levels along with other routine monitoring during therapy with neuroleptics.
- Drug discontinuation usually reverses the glycemic impairment, with reappearance if drug is reintroduced.

Liver Impairment

- Elevated liver enzymes (AST, ALT, GLD).
- Usually benign and elevations are slight (about 50 U/L, especially ALT).
- Very rarely associated with jaundice or significant hepatocellular damage.

Management

- Continue therapy and monitor LFTs.
- If levels increase, reduce dosage.
- Consider changing drugs if allergic form of obstructive jaundice is suspected (diagnosed with increased bilirubin and urobilinogen).
  - √ If levels exceed 2–3 times normal, reevaluate therapy and switch to less liver-toxic medication (i.e., atypical antipsychotic other than clozapine).

Temperature Dyscontrol

- Occasional hypothermia
  - √ Less commonly, hyperthermia (unassociated with NMS)
  - √ Temperatures in excess of 104° may occur.
- Onset within few hours of administering drug.
- May be aggravated by decreased sweating (anticholinergic effect).
- Hypothermia
  - √ Occurs especially with phenothiazines haloperidol and olanzapine.
  - √ Also associated with hypoproteinemia, cachexia, digitalis toxicity, and hypothyroidism.

- √ Severe hyperthermia associated with subcortical disorders of the hypothalamus or hypothalamic pituitary axis (case report data).
- Commonest cause of hypothermia is sepsis.
  - √ Associated with high mortality rates.

Management

- Warn patients of dangers of hypo/hyperthermia and ensure appropriate ambient temperature.
- Hyperthermia: Cooling (e.g., body ice packs) and antipyretic agents may be necessary, in addition to discontinuing the drug.
- Hypothermia: In addition to addressing suspected drug side effect, treat as suspected infection until proved otherwise.
  - √ Discontinue antipsychotic drug.
  - √ Administer warmed IV fluids, heating lamps, and warm blankets.

Sudden Death

Cause of antipsychotic-associated sudden deaths not well defined.

- May have cardiac origin.
- Most commonly associated with thioridazine.

Edema

Edema usually occurs in lower extremities.

Cause unknown. May be due to dopamine–aldosterone or prolactin interaction.

ANTIPARKINSONIAN AGENTS

- Often used to control some forms of EPS.
  - √ Acute dystonic reactions
  - √ Parkinsonism
  - √ Rabbit syndrome
- Anticholinergics and dopaminergics are most common agents.
  - √ Drugs of first choice are benztropine or procyclidine; amantadine is drug of second choice.
- Because of side effects and potential dangers of combining these drugs with other psychotropics, use only for emergent symptoms (not prophylaxis) and for time-limited periods.
  - √ For acute EPS (akinesia, dystonia) use acute dose and follow with maintenance doses only as necessary.

- √ Not useful for akathisia.
- √ In most cases may be discontinued after several weeks to 1–6 months.
- √ Caution with SSRIs—delirium reported.

- Administer with meals.
- Caution patients about impaired reflexes, use of machinery, and driving.
- Other anticholinergic–related precautions and interventions (see pp. 71–75).

Side Effects

Management of side effects

See page 75.

Withdrawal

- Taper slowly over 1 week to avoid withdrawal effects.
  - √ GI—nausea, vomiting, diarrhea, hypersalivation.
  - √ CNS—headache, insomnia, nightmares
  - √ Other—rhinorrhea, dizziness, tremor.
- Effects may persist for 2 weeks.

Drug Interactions

- Caution with coadministration of
  - √ Drugs with anticholinergic properties
  - √ CNS depressants
  - √ Antihypotensives
  - √ Epinephrine (hypotension)
  - √ Drugs that lower seizure threshold
- For all antipsychotics
  - √ Antiparkinsonian therapeutic action of levodopa and other antiparkinsonian medications may be reduced by dopamine receptor blockade of antipsychotics.
  - √ Absorption is impaired by antacids, metamucil.
  - √ Additive CNS depression with
    - ▫ Alcohol
    - ▫ Barbiturates, other CNS depressants.
- For low-potency neuroleptics
  - √ Anticholinergic effects exacerbated by additive effects of anticholinergic drugs (see Table 1.14, p. 71).

Table 2.22. Profile of Antiparkinsonian Agents

	Amantadine	Benztropine	Biperiden	Procyclidine	Trihexyphenidyl
Brand	Symmetrel	Cogentin	Akineton	Kemadrin	Artane
Chemical group	Dopaminergic	Anticholinergic	Anticholinergic	Anticholinergic	Anticholinergic
Dose	50–100 mg bid	0.5–2 mg daily Acute dystonia: use IM injection followed by daily oral drug for 1–2 weeks with trial of discontinuation.	1–2 mg IM/IV; repeat every ½–1 hour until acute symptoms have resolved; maximum 4 injections per 24 hours; use lower range for frail elders.	2.5 mg/day, increasing by 2.5 mg/day until effective (range 5–10 mg, with greater caution in demented or otherwise frail elders).	Begin with 1 mg/day, increasing as necessary (range 5–10 mg/day).
Indications	• Dystonia • Parkinsonism • Rabbit syndrome	• Acute dystonic reactions • Parkinsonism • Rabbit syndrome	• Acute dystonic reactions • Parkinsonism • Rabbit syndrome	• Acute dystonic reactions • Parkinsonism • Rabbit syndrome	• Acute dystonic reactions • Parkinsonism • Rabbit syndrome
Contraindications	*Urinary* Retention Prostatic hypertrophy *GI* Paralytic ileus Bowel obstruction Megacolon *Metabolic* Heat stroke Hyperthermia *CVS* Heart failure Peripheral edema *Eyes* Narrow angle glaucoma	*Urinary* Retention Prostatic hypertrophy *GI* Paralytic ileus Bowel obstruction Megacolon *Metabolic* Heat stroke Hyperthermia *CVS* Tachycardia CHF Angina Peripheral edema *Eyes* Narrow angle glaucoma *CNS* Dementia	Same as for benztropine	Same as for benztropine	Hypertension plus those for benztropine
Precautions	• Withdrawal √ Observe for emergent NMS. • Monitor WBC for leucopenia.	• Withdrawal (see p. 304)	• Withdrawal (see p. 304)	• Withdrawal (see p. 304)	• Withdrawal (see p. 304)

Table 2.23. Side Effects of Anticholinergic Drugs and Amantadine

Side Effect	Most Common	Most Serious and Less Common
Body as a whole		• Fever
Cardiovascular	• Palpitations • Tachycardia • Dizziness	
Central and peripheral nervous system	• Confusion • Reduced concentration • Restlessness • Tremor • Ataxia • Weakness • Lethargy • Slurred speech • Insomnia	• Delirium • Disorientation • Short-term memory impairment, fatigue, inertia, confusion √ Especially with benztropine as compared to amantadine
Endocrine		• Galactorrhea (amantadine)
Eye	• Blurred vision • Photophobia • Dry eyes	• Narrow angle glaucoma
GI disorders	• Dry mouth • Nausea/vomiting • Constipation • Dry throat	• Paralytic ileus • Acute intestinal pseudo-obstruction
Psychiatric	• Depression • Anxious excitement (especially with trihexyphenidyl)	• Psychosis (especially with amantadine)
Respiratory	• Nasal congestion	• May aggravate respiratory ailments
Skin and appendages	• Dry skin/reduced sweating • Flushing	• Skin rash
Urinary	• Hesitancy • Retention	

DRUG–DRUG INTERACTIONS

Table 2.24. Drug–Drug Interactions*

Antipsychotic	Metabolizing CYP Enzymes	CYP Inhibitors**	CYP Inducers***
Haloperidol	Probably 2D6 but metabolic pathway unclear; possible 1A2 or 3A involvement	*Inhibitors of 3A:* amiodarone, cimetidine, SSRIs (fluoxetine, fluvoxamine) clarithromycin, erythromycin, troleandomycin, metronidazole, norfloxacin, fluconazole, ketoconazole, itraconazole, nefazodone, grapefruit juice, quinidine, indinavir, nelfinavir, saquinavir, ritonavir	*Inducers of 1A2:* polycyclic aromatic compounds (smoking), phenytoin, omeprazole, rifampin, carbamazepine *Inducers of 3A:* barbiturates, dexamethasone, rifampin, ritonavir, phenytoin, carbamazepine, oxybutynin, St. John's Wort

(*cont.*)

Continued

Antipsychotic	Metabolizing CYP Enzymes	CYP Inhibitors**	CYP Inducers***
Clozapine	1A2 (primary pathway); 2D6 (secondary pathway)	*Inhibitors of 1A2*: cimetidine, fluvoxamine, grapefruit juice, ketoconazole *Potent inhibitors of 2D6:* fluoxetine paroxetine, quinidine, possibly bupropion *Other inhibitors of 2D6:* amiodarone, chlorpheniramine, cimetidine, clomipramine, sertraline, citalopram (weak inhibitor), haloperidol, methadone, perphenazine, propafenone, ritonavir, indinavir, terbinafine, propranolol, valproate	*Inducers of 1A2:* (see haloperidol)
Olanzapine	1A2, 2D6	*Inhibitors of 1A2* (see clozapine) *Potent inhibitors of 2D6* (see clozapine) *Other inhibitors of 2D6* (see clozapine)	*Inducers of 1A2* (see haloperidol)
Perphenazine	2D6	*Potent inhibitors of 2D6* (see clozapine)	Not inducible
Thioridazine	2D6	*Inhibitors of 2D6* (see clozapine)	Not inducible
Risperidone	2D6	*Inhibitors of 2D6* (see clozapine)	Not inducible
Chlorpromazine	2D6, 3A	*Inhibitors of 2D6* (see clozapine) *Inhibitors of 3A* (see haloperidol)	*Inducers of 3A* (see haloperidol)
Desipramine	2D6	*Inhibitors of 2D6* (see clozapine)	Not inducible
Pimozide	3A4	*Inhibitors of 3A* (see haloperidol)	*Inducers of 3A* (see haloperidol)
Quetiapine	3A4	*Inhibitors of 3A* (see haloperidol)	*Inducers of 3A* (see haloperidol)

* Predominantly general adult data.
** May increase plasma concentrations.
*** May reduce plasma concentrations.

OVERDOSE WITH TYPICAL ANTIPSYCHOTICS

Symptoms

- CNS effects
  - √ Restlessness
  - √ Confusion/delirium
  - √ Coma
  - √ Severe EPS
  - √ Sedation
- Hypotension
- Cardiac effects
  - √ Tachycardia
  - √ Arrhythmias

- Vasomotor/respiratory collapse
- Miosis: Hyperthermia, Death

Management

- Gastric lavage, emesis (in a conscious patient)
- One dose of activated charcoal with saline cathartic
- Supportive measures
  - √ Airway, oxygenation, fluids
  - √ In coma-endotracheal tube, tracheostomy in prolonged coma, respirator
- Electrolyte balance
- Monitor: Cardiac function, BP
- Hypotension
  - √ Place patient in Trendelenburg position
  - √ Administer: IV fluids, Concentrated albumin, Dopamine or norepinephrine
  - √ Note: *Avoid epinephrine.*
- Seizures
  - √ Benzodiazepine (lorazepam IV) or phenytoin, if necessary
- EPS
  - √ Benztropine (maintain for 48 hours)
- Hemodialysis not useful

OVERDOSE WITH ATYPICAL ANTIPSYCHOTICS

- As a class show wider variation in symptoms than typicals
  - √ See individual drugs for detailed discussions.

INDIVIDUAL ANTIPSYCHOTIC DRUG PROFILES

ARIPIPRAZOLE

See Appendix A for drug profile.

CLOZAPINE

Drug	Manufacturer	Chemical Class	Therapeutic Class
clozapine (Clozaril)	Novartis	dibenzodiazepine	antipsychotic

Indications: FDA/HPB

- Treatment-resistant schizophrenia

Indications: Off label

- Most effective atypical (general adult and sporadic geriatric clinical data) for treatment of

- √ Resistant psychosis
  - √ Bipolar disorders (including rapid cycling and treatment-refractory mania with or without psychosis)
  - √ Schizoaffective (manic phase) disorder
- Refractory BPSD
- Clinical reports indicate utility in behavioral disruption, aggression, agitation, and depression associated with dementia.
- Controls aggression associated with schizophrenia.
- Effective for levodopa- and dopamine-agonist-induced psychosis associated with treatment of Parkinson's disease.
  - √ Permits increased doses of antiparkinsonian medication while controlling psychotic side effects and improving parkinsonian symptoms.
    - ▫ Slow initiation and dose titration leads to improved tolerance and reduced side effects.
    - ▫ Efficacy in managing emergent paraphilias in Parkinson's disease (clinical case).
- Nonpsychiatric uses
  - √ Control of tremor in Parkinson's disease (based on more prominent D_1 receptor blocking action).
  - √ Control of levodopa-induced dyskinesia in Parkinson's disease.
  - √ Effective antitremor agent (equal to benztropine) but not a first-line treatment because of side-effect profile.
  - √ Other movement disorders
    - ▫ Huntington's disease (variable effectiveness on movement disorder).

Pharmacology

See Table 2.2 on page 233.

Blood levels

- Correlate with dose.
- Reduced by smoking (especially in men).
- Lower in men compared to women.
- Increased with age.

Mechanism of action

- $5HT_{2a}$ receptor affinity ($5HT_2$ antagonism) much greater than D_2 affinity ($5HT_{2a}/D_2$ ratio > 2).
  - √ Affinity for $5HT_{2c}/_{3c},_{1a}/_{b}/_{c}$ receptors; $5HT_6$ and $_7$ receptors recently identified with high affinity for clozapine.
  - √ $5HT_3$ blockade possibly associated with anti-emetic effects and inhibition of dopamine release.

- D_4 receptor blockade equal to or greater than D_2, with blockade evident at the $D_1/_3/_5$ receptors.
  - √ Relatively low D_2 occupancy in basal ganglia may account for lower incidence of EPS.
  - √ More selective for mesolimbic (A10 region) and mesocortical dopamine pathways.
  - √ Does not appear to block midbrain substantia nigra dopamine neurons.
- M_1 anticholinergic (tachycardia, constipation, diaphoresis, delirium, urinary dysfunction), alpha-1/2, beta-antiadrenergic (orthostatic hypotension, sexual dysfunction, sedation), and H_1-antihistaminic (sedation) effects.
- Possible glutamate and GABA affinities.

Therapeutic Actions by Indication

- Suppresses levodopa-induced dyskinesia in Parkinson's disease patients.
- Antipsychotic response in Parkinsonian patients often evident after a few days.
- Positive symptoms and aggression may improve the most in schizophrenia and other forms of psychosis.
- Modest improvement in negative symptoms (apathy, abulia, anhedonia, social withdrawal).

Choosing a Drug

- Very few controlled studies on efficacy in elders.
- Available data show positive but modest effect in older patients with severe schizophrenia.
- Most data based on open or uncontrolled clinical trials.
- Often not suitable for general use in elders, because of
  - √ Orthostatic hypotension
  - √ Need for monitoring for agranulocytosis
  - √ Confusion/delirium
  - √ Cardiac effects
  - √ Sedation/lethargy
  - √ Anticholinergic effects
- Despite side-effect profile, tolerated by many demented elderly in low doses.
- Equipotent with chlorpromazine.
- Other atypicals with more favorable side-effect profiles (e.g., risperidone) may be equally effective, although some general adult studies suggest greater efficacy of clozapine over risperidone in severe chronic schizophrenia.

- √ Some guidelines suggest it be used after failure of 263 other antipsychotics (including a typical agent).
  - ▫ This may be too cautious, in light of its efficacy and that it is often well tolerated, for some hospitalized severely psychotic elders with long histories of psychosis.
  - ▫ In hospitalized patients with severe psychosis who can be monitored, it is very effective and useful (clinical data).
  - ▫ Efficacy in unselected psychotic, naturalistic, inpatient populations suggests that elders may be somewhat less responsive to drug than younger cohorts, although still responsive overall.
- May have prolonged latency to response of 2–4 months.
- Less likely to induce TD and often improves preexisting TD symptoms.
- Agranulocytosis may be more common in elders (data only suggestive).
- Do not initiate in patients with
  - √ WBC count < 3500/mm3
  - √ History of myeloproliferative disorder
  - √ History of clozapine-induced agranulocytosis or granulocytopenia

Race/ethnicity

- Agranulocytosis may be more common in patients of Ashkenaz Jewish background.

Dosing

- Plasma level monitoring: therapeutic level for schizophrenia about 200–350 ng/ml (general adult data).
- Use divided doses at every dose range.

Initial dose

- Day 1: Begin 6.25 mg/day (or even every second day).
- Day 7: Increase in 6.25 mg increments every week.

Increasing dose and reaching therapeutic levels

- Very wide effective dose range in elders: 12.5–450 mg, depending on target symptoms.
  - √ As with all neuroleptics, higher doses generally required for primary psychotic disorders such as schizophrenia: 200–450 mg/day; a common dose is about 200 mg.
  - √ Bipolar: 25–112.5 mg/day (clinical case data).
  - √ 12.5–125 mg/day suffice for secondary psychosis (e.g., dementia or Parkinson's disease-related).
    - ▫ Psychosis associated with Parkinson's disease often responds to 25–50 mg (range 6.25–150 mg/day).

  - √ Levodopa-induced dyskinesia may respond to the 50–100 mg/day dose range (data on young-old elders), but dosing empirically determined, case by case, especially in physically frail elders who often require lower doses.
- Timetable for increasing dose in elders not well established but advisable to go very slowly over weeks to months.
  - √ Rapid dose increases lead to intolerance of the drug and frequent rejection of further trials.
  - √ Wide variation in recommended dose-increase schedules for elders, but in general, slow increase of 6.25–12.5 mg/day increments every 7 days.
- Once maintenance dosage achieved, may use once or twice daily dosing schedule.

Off-label indications dosing

- BPSD: wide range, 12.5–125 mg/day.
- Suppression of dyskinesias in Parkinson's disease.
  - √ Dose for older patients not well established, but try one-fifth to one-third of adult dose (100–200 mg).
    - ▫ Clinical data suggest tremor in Parkinson's disease responds to 12.5 mg daily in elders.
  - √ Because response may be delayed, especially for negative symptoms, therapeutic benefit may continue to accrue for a year.

Combination or Substitution Therapy

- Olanzapine: Case reports (general adult data) of successful augmentation.
- Switching from clozapine to another agent (e.g., see quetiapine, p. 345).
  - √ Strategies and protocols for elders not well established.
  - √ Consider adding new agent (e.g., risperidone, olanzapine, or quetiapine) to clozapine first in small doses, gradually increasing dose while cross-tapering clozapine.
    - ▫ Added side-effect burden always potentially problematic in elders with this strategy.
    - ▫ Suggested protocol for olanzapine: Add 5 mg olanzapine for a week, then begin to taper clozapine at 12.5–25 mg/day weekly.

Discontinuation and Withdrawal

- High discontinuation rates (40 + %), but similar to rates in younger adults.
- Discontinuation after effective therapy of chronic psychosis often induces exacerbation (rebound?) of psychosis and agitation.

- √ In non-urgent situations, discontinue gradually over 4–6 weeks, or longer.
  - ▫ Symptoms include dramatic increase in psychotic symptoms, diaphoresis, confusion, nausea, vomiting, headache, diarrhea, agitation, EPS, and restlessness.

Side Effects

Percentages given are usually from general adult data.

- Anticholinergic side effects are significant.
  - √ Similar to low-potency antipsychotics.
- Orthostatic hypotension, fatigue, hypersalivation, and nausea are common.
- Side effects are more significant in elders who have pre-existing parkinsonism, postural instability, and osteoporosis.
- Low incidence of EPS.
- Agranulocytosis is a serious risk; requires careful monitoring.
  - √ 0.8% at 1 year, 0.91% at 1.5 years (general adult data).
  - √ Risk seems to be higher in elders.
- Significant side effects (e.g., confusion) may emerge even at low doses of 12.5 mg/day.
- Common side effects often emerge during dose titration phase.
- Many side effect are dose dependent and diminish with reduced dose of drug.
- Side effects are a limiting factor when using higher doses in primary psychosis.

Autonomic Side Effects

- Hypersalivation (31%)
  - √ Surprising side effect in light of anticholinergic profile of drug.
  - √ May be profuse, especially during sleep, and limit tolerance of therapy.
  - √ May be very distressing to elders, producing drooling, especially at night when swallowing rate diminishes.
  - √ Benztropine or amitriptyline have been used but not generally recommended for elders because of toxicity risk; consider clonidine, an alpha-2 agonist.
- Sweating (6%)

Body as a Whole Side Effects

- Fever, especially during initiation of therapy, but may occur at any time.
  - √ Usually benign, transient, and self-limiting, but occasionally requires discontinuation of therapy, reinstituting cautiously when temperature returns to normal.

        - Most patients can tolerate reinstitution of therapy at lower dose and slow dose escalation.
    - √ Benign form sometimes associated with elevated white count.
    - √ Do complete CBC and differential to rule out agranulocytosis.
- Weight gain—may be substantial.
    - √ Sometimes problematic in elders, especially if prone to diabetes or cardiovascular disorders.
    - √ Consider nutritional counseling and exercise.
        - Sometimes more useful theoretically than practically, since many elders taking clozapine are unable to cooperate with these regimens.
    - √ Usually most evident in first 12 weeks of therapy (general adult data) but may continue for up to 4 years.
- Sleep disturbance

Most serious and less common

- NMS
    - √ Many symptoms of NMS are also associated with clozapine alone (i.e., tachycardia, diaphoresis, fever, leukocytosis, and delirium).
        - Muscular rigidity is an important differentiating symptom present in NMS.
- Rare: Sudden death in combination with benzodiazepines.

Cardiovascular Side Effects

- Tachycardia (25%)
    - √ Dose related.
    - √ May persist throughout treatment.
    - √ May respond to beta-blocker (e.g., atenolol).
    - √ Probably due to both anticholinergic and noradrenergic effects.
- Postural hypotension (9%)
    - √ Caused by anti-adrenergic effects.
    - √ Generally emerges during initial dose titration.
    - √ Reduce by lengthening intervals between drug dose increases and increasing by smaller dose increments.
    - √ Do not use epinephrine to treat hypotension.
- Hypertension

Most serious and less common

- Deep vein thrombosis (incidence 1/3,000; general adult data) and venous thromboembolism reported.
    - √ Risk of pulmonary embolism.
    - √ Unclear if related to all antipsychotic therapies or whether clozapine poses a specific risk.

- Syncope and rare respiratory arrest.
  - √ Associated with hypotension and possibly with concurrent benzodiazepine medication.
- Falls
- Possible bradycardia
- ECG
  - √ T–wave changes, depression of ST segment (and may prolong QTc, but not clinically significant).
- Eosinophilic cardiomyopathy (general adult data).
- Myocarditis—rare (0.06%; general adult data; no geriatric patients reported to date) but potentially lethal (in 0.02%; general adult data).
  - √ Occurs especially in first month of therapy and during titration phase.
  - √ Associated with flu-like symptoms, fever, sinus tachycardia, hypotension, chest discomfort, and heart failure.
- Occasional reports of pericarditis, pericardial effusion, and cardiomyopathy.

Case Reports of Side Effects

- Nocturnal combativeness
- Acute interstitial nephritis
  - √ Presents with sudden rise in serum urea and creatinine and sometimes fever.
- Various arrhythmias, CHF

Central and Peripheral Nervous System Side Effects

- Sedation (39%)
  - √ Some patients feel "washed out" and lethargic.
  - √ Give bulk of dose hs to reduce daytime sedation.
- Dizziness (19%)
- Delirium/confusion
- Headache
- Tremor (6%)
  - √ Fine fast tremor
- Akathisia
- D_1 frontal blockade may impair some aspects of cognitive performance.
- Restlessness

Most serious and less common

- Myoclonic jerks.
- Seizures and EEG changes—dose dependent.
- Increase dose slowly to minimize risk.
- EEG patterns change in 53–74%.
  - √ Most commonly, general slowing (general adult data).

- Seizures probably dose-related.
  - √ Occur during dose titration phase with lower doses and in maintenance phase at high doses.
  - √ Rates (general adult data)
    - ▫ 1–2% < 300 mg/day
    - ▫ 3–4% 300–600 mg/day
    - ▫ 5% 600–900 mg/day
- Increased caution in elders with increased vulnerability to seizures.
  - √ History of seizures, dementia, or other CNS disorder, concurrent medications that reduce seizure threshold.
    - ▫ Valproate is anticonvulsant of choice.
- Confusional state
  - √ Elders more predisposed.
  - √ May occur at low doses (< 25 mg).
  - √ May progress to delirium.
- TD possible but rare.

Endocrine Side Effects

- Emergence (or exacerbation) of diabetes mellitus or impaired glycemic control in a substantial subset of patients (general adult data).
  - √ Onset 1–5 weeks after beginning therapy.
  - √ May emerge at relatively low doses (e.g., 50 mg).
  - √ Severe hyperglycemia occasionally emerges.
  - √ May worsen pre-existing diabetes, requiring increased insulin dosage.
    - ▫ Management of emergent diabetes mellitus: Most patients require oral hypoglycemic; 5% require insulin or discontinuation of drug.
- May lower plasma cortisol.

Visual Side Effects

- Visual disturbances.
- May precipitate narrow angle glaucoma.

Gastrointestinal Side Effects

- Constipation
  - √ High fiber diet and attention to fluid intake helps.
  - √ Laxatives PRN
- Nausea/vomiting
  - √ Manage with dose reduction, antacids, or ranitidine (not cimetidine).
  - √ Dry mouth (6%)

Most serious and less common

- Ileus
- Eosinophilic colitis syndrome (clinical report not yet confirmed in studies; general adult data).

Hematological Side Effects

- Agranulocytosis (< 1% in general adult population; geriatric data not clear but probably 5 times or more higher in elders).
  - √ A toxic rather than allergic response.
  - √ May be more common in women, elders, and medically/physically frail.
  - √ Gradual development, hence can be controlled by careful monitoring of blood counts.
  - √ Dose and duration of therapy not clearly correlated with emergence of this potentially fatal side effect.
    - ▫ Onset usually within first 3 months of treatment, but occasionally emerges after longer periods of > 1 year.
    - ▫ Usually a benign course if found early and drug discontinued.
- Eosinophilia (i.e. $> 4 \times 10^9$)
  - √ Rates not clear—0.2–13% reported (general adult data).
  - √ Onset within 3–5 weeks
- Other blood dyscrasias
  - √ Leucopenia
  - √ Leukocytosis
  - √ Neutrophilia

Liver and Biliary Side Effects

- Increased serum liver enzymes and CPK levels.
  - √ Usually transient.
  - √ Occasionally substantial and leads to hepatitis.
  - √ Lower dose or suspend treatment.
- Pancreatitis

Metabolic and Nutritional Side Effects

- Increased serum triglycerides levels.

Musculoskeletal Side Effects

- Myopathic features, muscle weakness.

Psychiatric Side Effects

- Occasional paradoxical emergence of psychotic symptoms after initiation of clozapine in Parkinson's disease (case report data).
- Anxiety disorder

- √ Unmasking or precipitation of OCD-like picture and social phobia (general adult data).

Reproductive Side Effects

- Erectile and ejaculatory dysfunction in males.
- Orgasmic impairment in females.

Respiratory Side Effects

- Rare pulmonary embolism associated with deep vein thrombosis.
  - √ Causal relationship to clozapine not well established.
- Respiratory depression

Urinary Side Effects

- Urinary retention.
- Incontinence
  - √ Ephedrine has been used but only with caution in elders.

Monitoring

Routine

- Use caution when giving this drug to elders and monitor for all side effects, not just blood dyscrasias.
- When monitoring WBC, include differential counts routinely in light of range of blood dyscrasias occasionally found.
- Agranulocytosis—absolute neutrophil count (ANC) < 500/mm^3.
  - √ May be fatal, but monitoring reduces risks very substantially.
  - √ Baseline pretreatment WBC count required.
  - √ At least weekly WBC counts necessary for first 6 months.
    - ▫ Do not initiate treatment if WBC is < 3500/mm^3.
  - √ Reduce frequency of WBC counts to q 2 weeks thereafter, if WBC count has remained above 3000/mm^3 (ANC > 1500/mm^3).
  - √ Continue WBC monitoring for at least 4 weeks after discontinuation of the drug (general adult data—may be longer washout in elders).
  - √ If clozapine is discontinued for 1 month, or longer, and then reinstituted, the clock restarts and monitoring is required weekly for another 6 months before reducing to q 2 weeks.
  - √ Discontinue treatment if
    - ▫ WBC falls below 3000/mm3.
    - ▫ ANC falls below 1500/mm3.
    - ▫ May reinstate therapy if
      - ◦ No signs of infection emerge, and
      - ◦ WBC and ANC counts return to above-threshold levels.
  - √ Consider bone marrow aspiration to determine granulopoietic status if WBC drops below 2000/mm^3 or ANC < 1000/mm^3.

- √ *Note:*
  - ▫ Patients cannot be restarted on clozapine if WBC has fallen below 2000/mm3 or ANC below 1000/mm3.
  - ▫ WBC spike of > 15% may be marker of incipient agranulocytosis, with onset within 75 days; heightened vigilance recommended.
- Eosinophil count necessary weekly, especially in first 2 months and then monthly.
  - √ Discontinue drug if count is > 3×10^9.
    - ▫ Do not rechallenge until level returns below 1×10^9.
  - √ Levels below 1.5×10^9 usually self-limiting (general adult data), but observe carefully.
  - √ Eosinophilia may be precursor to neutropenia.
- Serum triglycerides necessary annually.
- Monitor weight on regular basis.
- Monitor LFTs.

Special monitoring

- Plasma levels of 350 ng/ml–450 ng/ml (clozapine plus norclozapine) a possible target level (general adult data), but clear relationship between plasma levels and clinical effect not yet determined.
- Plasma levels above 1000 ng/ml may be associated with seizures (general adult data); geriatric data unavailable.

Drug Interactions

- Avoid benzodiazepines during dose titration phase—potentially fatal cardiorespiratory depression.
- Avoid combining with other anticholinergic agents (see Table 1.14, p. 71).
- Fluvoxamine and, to a lesser but often clinically significant degree, sertraline and fluoxetine, increase plasma concentrations of drug and metabolites.
  - √ Especially important to monitor side effects when using high-dose clozapine in combination with SSRIs.
- Caution in combination with antihypertensive medication.
- Caution with cimetidine, enoxacin, chloroquine, warfarin and digoxin—increased plasma concentrations.
- Caffeine—as seizure augmenter in ECT, associated with supraventricular tachycardia (case report).
- Case report of perphenazine combination increasing clozapine plasma concentrations to toxic levels.

Clozapine action antagonized by

- Smoking—induces CYP1A2 and may reduce plasma concentrations of drug.

Disability Interactions and Contraindications

- Parkinson's disease
  - √ High incidence of side effects such as delirium.
  - √ Low-dose therapy reduces side effects.
- Diabetes
  - √ May induce new-onset type II diabetes.
  - √ May induce impaired glucose tolerance.
  - √ May worsen previously controlled diabetes.
- Monitor patients with hypertension and cardiac arrhythmias more closely because of danger of these side effects.
- Caution advised in patients with preexisting seizure disorders.
  - √ May be advisable to use concurrent anticonvulsant therapy, with appropriate cautions for age-related issues.
- Prior emergence of hematological impairment on clozapine—agranulocytosis—contraindication.
- Contraindicated in patients with preexisting severe heart disease.
- Special caution
  - √ In patients with seizure disorders.
  - √ In patients with diabetes or family history of vulnerability.
  - √ In women—may be more sensitive to side effects.

Overdose, Toxicity, Suicide

Contents of this section reflect general adult data.

Presents with

- Altered states of consciousness
  - √ Sedation
  - √ Delirium
  - √ Coma
- Tachycardia, hypotension
- Respiratory depression/failure
- Hypersalivation
- Occasional seizures
- *Note:* Emergence of toxic effects may be delayed.
  - √ Observe for several days.

Management

- General support—establish and maintain airway, oxygenation, fluids, and electrolytes.
- Administer activated charcoal/induce emesis.
- Monitor cardiac and vital signs.
- *Note:* Avoid epinephrine (for hypotension) and quinidine or procainamide for cardiac arrhythmias.
- Dialysis not indicated.

Caregiver Notes

- Caregivers should be alerted to side effects
  - √ Sore throat, fever, lethargy, weakness, or other signs of infection.
  - √ Excessive thirst, increased frequency of urination, weakness—may be a sign of emergent diabetes.
  - √ Difficulty with urination, cyc pain, severe constipation.
  - √ Persistent tachycardia (rapid heart rate), chest pain, shortness of breath, hypotension (low blood pressure with dizziness), or flu-like symptoms.
- Advise patients not to stop and restart drug on their own.
  - √ If medication discontinued for more than 2 days, it is dangerous to restart the drug at the same dose. *Contact physician for instructions.*
- Advise not to take OTC medications.

Clinical Tips

- "Start low and go slow" rule especially important for clozapine to control orthostatic hypotension.
  - √ Greater caution advised in acute care settings where there is pressure to escalate doses faster in order to discharge patients more efficiently.
    - ▫ Observe for dose-related side effects.
    - ▫ Rapid dose escalation is false economy, since induction of side effects lengthens ALOS.
- Reduce or discontinue benzodiazepines during initiation phase of treatment to reduce risk of orthostatic hypotension.
- Improves treatment of Parkinson's disease by controlling psychosis (often drug-induced) and allowing optimization of antiparkinsonian therapy.
  - √ Hematological monitoring may be a limiting factor in using this drug in some patients, but other side effect risks are reduced by responsiveness to relatively low doses.
- Occasional intense hypersensitivity with initial doses.
  - √ Syncope/hypotension, bradycardia, EPS at initial low dose (25 mg).
  - √ Begin therapy at 6.25–12.5 mg.
  - √ As dose increases, observe for emergence of anticholinergic side effects.
- Although often effective for psychosis symptoms in dementia, side effects are common and prominent in frail elders with dementia, even at doses in the 25–75 mg range.
- Special caution
  - √ In patients with seizure disorders.

- √ In patients with diabetes or family history of vulnerability.
- √ In women—may be more sensitive to side effects.
- Antipsychotic effects sometimes wear off in second year of therapy.
  - √ Sometimes increased doses help, but side effects may be a limiting factor.
- Fever management (over 100° F)
  - √ Routine workup
    - ▫ Physical examination
    - ▫ Urinalysis
    - ▫ WBC/differential
    - ▫ Chest X-ray
    - ▫ Blood cultures, if indicated
    - ▫ CPK level
  - √ Discontinue clozapine if NMS suspected.
  - √ If no other cause found, consider diagnosis of clozapine-induced fever and continue treatment cautiously, if fever does not increase.
- Unexplained fever, flu-like symptoms, tachycardia, or symptoms of heart failure should alert physician to possibility of myocarditis or cardiomyopathy.
- ECT—generally safe when coadministered, but case reports of spontaneous seizures following ECT and occasional elevation of BP and tachycardia (all general adult data).

FLUPHENAZINE

Drug	Manufacturer	Chemical Class	Therapeutic Class
fluphenazine (Prolixin) enanthate (Moditen), decanoate (Modecate)	Geneva	piperazine phenothiazine	antipsychotic

Indications: FDA/HPB

- Psychosis

Indications: Off label

See pages 236–262.

Pharmacology

See Table 2.2 on pages 233–234.

Note: Following points reflect general adult data.

- 5–40-fold interindividual variations in steady-state blood levels, half-life, etc.
- Metabolic profiles of oral and depot forms differ.
  - √ Oral: Levels of metabolites higher than parent compound.
  - √ Depot: Levels of metabolites lower than parent compound.
  - √ Decanoate form has better bioavailability and more predictable plasma levels.
- Steady state achieved at about 3 months, but longer in elders.

Choosing a Drug

- Not recommended for general use in elders.
- Most potent of the phenothiazines.
- Produces marked EPS.

Dosing

- Enanthate form may require higher dose to achieve same therapeutic effect.
  - √ Plasma levels of fluphenazine enanthate lower than fluphenazine decanoate.
- Duration of action of enanthate is shorter (1–3 weeks) than decanoate (4–6 weeks, or longer) (general adult data).
- Absorption rate altered by reduced muscle mass in elders.
- IM forms about 5 times more potent than oral.

Daily dose regimen

- May use once daily dosing.

Initial dose

- Oral—0.25–1 mg/day.

Increasing dose and reaching therapeutic levels

- Increase by 0.25–1 mg once or twice a week.
- IM (hydrochloride, *not* depot forms): use one-third to one-half the oral dose; start with 0.25 mg.
- Depot form: Schedule of dosing not established for elders.
  - √ Try to reduce initial effective dose by about 25% after about 4–6 weeks of efficacy following the first dose.
  - √ Overlap with oral form not considered necessary unless patient relapses.
    - ▫ In that case, add oral medication temporarily.

Maintenance dose

- Target oral therapeutic dose 0.5–4 mg/day.
- Target decanoate dose level.
  - √ Psychosis
    - ▫ Range of 3.75–12.5 mg q 2–4 weeks.
    - ▫ Recommended ranges closer to 3.75 mg, especially at the beginning, before tolerance has been determined.
  - √ Dementia
    - ▫ 3.75 mg q 14 days.
    - ▫ Depot for dementia not recommended; reserve it for unusual circumstances in chronic psychosis.
  - √ Some geriatric patients can be maintained on much more infrequent dosing schedules (e.g., 3–6 months apart).

Side Effects

See pages 279–303, especially anticholinergic cardiovascular, neurological, and hematological effects.

- Compared to other phenothiazines, has weaker anticholinergic, sedative, and hypotensive effects.
  - √ But *strong EPS effects.*
- Depot forms
  - √ Side effects may persist for months after discontinuation.
  - √ Induce higher rates of NMS but lower rates of EPS than oral.
- Lens and corneal opacities after long-term use (17% after 5 years; general adult data) with decanoate form; enanthate and oral forms not reported.

Routine monitoring

- Therapeutic plasma levels not available for elders and generally not reliable indicators of therapeutic effect.
- Purported therapeutic steady-state levels are 1.2–1.4 (range 0.2–2.8) ng/ml.

Contraindications and Special Precautions

- Contraindicated in suspected subcortical brain damage.
  - √ Danger of hyperthermic reaction (onset sometimes delayed by 14–16 hours).
- Watch LFTs.
- May cause agranulocytosis in 4–10 weeks of therapy.

Drug Interactions

See pages 306–307.

- $2D_6$ substrate and inhibitor.
- Metoclopramide increases EPS.
- Metrimazide increases risk of seizures.

Overdose

See pages 307–308.

Clinical Tips

- Depot forms may produce long-lasting and sometimes severe toxicity.
  - √ Generally not recommended for routine use in elders.
  - √ If used (e.g., because of significant noncompliance in chronic psychosis), monitor closely and be very cautious.
- With liquid form avoid caffeine, tea, and apple juice.
- Sedative effect begins quickly, after about 1 hour, with either oral or IM forms.

HALOPERIDOL

Drug	Manufacturer	Chemical Class	Therapeutic Class
haloperidol (Haldol)	Ortho-McNeil	butyrophenone	antipsychotic

Indications: FDA/HPB

- Psychotic disorders
- Tourette's disorder

Indications: Off label

- BPSD: Management of severe agitation, confusion, aggression, and extreme hyperactivity.
  - √ Whenever possible, a specific diagnosis should be made.
- Delirium

Pharmacology

See also page 234.

- Binds with high affinity to a number of CNS sites.
  - √ CNS tissue concentrations can be much higher than plasma concentration.
- Little data on pharmacokinetics in elders.
  - √ Plasma levels may be much higher in elders: haloperidol by factor of 2 or more, and reduced haloperidol by a factor of 5.

- √ Probable age-related decline in hepatic metabolism (but data not definitive).
- √ In some elders plasma levels may be lower than expected despite full-dose therapy (occasionally undetectable in some patients).
  - ▫ Therapeutic implications not known.
  - ▫ Because of high tissue binding in the CNS, plasma levels may not mirror clinical effect.

- Reduced (hydroxy) haloperidol.
  - √ Accumulates during chronic administration and may prolong action of drug during dose reductions.
  - √ Clinically important because it reconverts to haloperidol.
- Decanoate form is more fat soluble, has a duration of activity measured in weeks (as opposed to days for the oral form), has a prolonged time to peak plasma concentration of 6–8 days, terminal phase half-life of about 21 days, and a time to steady state of 3–4 months (compared to 3–4 days; all general adult data).
- Grapefruit juice: Plasma levels unaffected.

Mechanism of action

- Dopamine, especially D_2 receptor, blockade.
- Increases rate of dopamine turnover.

Choosing a Drug

- No longer advisable for first-line long-term routine use—atypicals much preferred.
- Drug of choice for short-term rapid control of psychosis and agitation.
  - √ IM and IV forms facilitate this indication.
  - √ Patients with dementia are very sensitive to EPS side effects with this drug.
    - ▫ Almost all develop some symptoms with doses > 2 mg when used beyond the acute control period.
  - √ Studies of overall effectiveness in BPSD show very modest improvement beyond placebo, so clinical effect is weighed against side effects.
- Delirium and acute agitation—remains drug of choice.
  - √ Although effective for symptom control, side effects are often a significant limitation if used in doses above 5 mg/day or for a prolonged period of time.
- Most common agent associated with inducing NMS.
- Recognizing side-effect potential, depot form remains useful for managing noncompliant patients who require long-term therapy.
  - √ May reduce relapse rates.

- Although overall response of BPSD to antipsychotics is modest, haloperidol offers a better response rate when used in effective doses (2–3 mg for psychotic symptoms).
- Case reports of efficacy in monosymptomatic delusions of infestation.
- Flexible dosage forms and routes of administration an important advantage.

Race/Ethnicity

- Asian men appear to metabolize the drug more slowly than Asian women and Caucasians.
  - √ May require lower doses (general adult data), especially if higher dose ranges are used.

Dosing

Daily dose regimen

- Psychosis/agitation in Alzheimer's disease: Standard dosing (2–3 mg/day) more effective than low dose (0.5–0.75 mg).
  - √ Side effects are a trade-off.

Initiating therapy

- Oral
  - √ Begin with divided doses bid.
- Depot form
  - √ Available dose forms are too high for many elders, hence decanoate form may not be appropriate for routine use in elders because of risk of overmedication and side effects.
  - √ About 10 times the potency of oral form.
  - √ Initiating depot should be approached with caution.
    - ▫ Behavior of the decanoate form of haloperidol not well characterized in elders (e.g., half-life or dose response).
    - ▫ Danger of acute EPS with depot form.
    - ▫ Absorption may be erratic (e.g., because of muscle mass differences in young and old).
    - ▫ Elimination very slow, probably in the range of several months.
  - √ Depot dose should be 10–15 times the oral, with supplemental oral doses as necessary.
  - √ During conversion from oral to depot form, plasma concentrations can drop significantly with increased risk of relapse (general adult data).
    - ▫ Weeks 1–2: Taper oral haloperidol by 50%, then add depot.
    - ▫ Weeks 3–4: Further reduce oral by 50% and repeat depot dose.

  - Month 2: Taper remaining oral and decrease depot dose at this injection by 25% from month 1 total dose level.
  - Months 3–4: Steady state has been reached—reduce depot by a further 25% and titrate dose based on clinical response.
- √ Another technique: Use a full loading depot dose without supplemental oral doses.
  - Technique not well studied in elders.
  - Therapeutic advantage of this technique not well demonstrated.
  - May be an increased risk of EPS or akathesia.
  - Loading doses in elders riskier and not usually indicated, except in chronic psychosis that has been difficult to manage and subject to significant relapse if medication levels fall.
  - *Note:* After 2 or 3 doses, the plasma levels increase considerably compared to levels after the first dose; hence the need for reduced doses.

Initial dose

- Oral: In frail/demented elders begin with low daily dose of 0.25–1 mg in bid divided doses, when appropriate, and increase gradually based on clinical response and emergent side effects.
- Depot: 12.5 mg (approximate—doses vary widely in a given individual)
  - √ Administer monthly once steady-state achieved.

Increasing dose and reaching therapeutic levels

- Oral: Target dose is in narrow range of 1.5–3 mg for patients with Alzheimer's disease.
- Depot: Titrate dose based on clinical response.
  - √ Wide target depot range of 12.5–100 mg/month.
    - Higher end of dose range reserved for chronic schizophrenia and not used for dementia with associated psychosis.

Maintenance dose

- Oral: Once stabilized
  - √ A single nighttime dose of haloperidol is often appropriate and well tolerated.
  - √ Dose may be adjusted downward to lowest effective dose.
- Depot: Once efficacy has been established, maintain at effective dose indefinitely for treatment of chronic psychosis.

Discontinuation and Withdrawal

- Short-term tolerance usually good in dementia patients, but EPS emerges over longer term of weeks to months.

√ Attempt trial of discontinuation after symptoms stabilize and intermittently thereafter.
√ Maintain on lowest effective dose.

Side Effects

- Most common: EPS and other CNS effects.
- At low doses well tolerated.
- See pages 279–303, for detailed discussion of key side effects and their management
  √ Especially EPS, NMS, and TD.

Table 2.25. Side Effects of Haloperidol

Side Effects	Most Common	Most Serious and Less Common
Body as a whole		• Some weight gain but less than clozapine
Cardiovascular		• Postural hypotension (unusual) • Prolonged QTc and associated *Torsades de Pointes* (multiform ventricular tachycardia with IV bolus treatments)—*sometimes fatal*
Case reports		• Acute intestinal pseudo-obstruction in combination with benztropine
Central and peripheral nervous system	• Sedation • EPS √ Increased risk in elders with doses > 2–3 mg/day □ Risk—and effectiveness—reduced with doses lower than 1 mg/day. □ Lower but significant rates of EPS emerge even on low dose √ Akathesia √ Parkinsonism √ TD—higher rate than with atypicals • Risk of falls	• Catatonia
Endocrine		• Gynecomastia
Eye	• Blurred vision	
Gastrointestinal	• Dry mouth • Constipation	
Liver and biliary	• Increased LFTs—usually benign	
Metabolic and nutritional		• NMS • Hypothermia

(*cont.*)

Continued

Side Effects	Most Common	Most Serious and Less Common
Respiratory		• Laryngeal spasm • Respiratory spasms occur early in treatment, in contrast to TD √ Grunting, puffing, disturbed rate of respiration √ Responds to dose reduction or antiparkinsonian medication
Skin and appendages	• Decanoate form: inflammation at injection site	
Urinary		• Retention/obstruction with prostatic hypertrophy

Routine monitoring

- Clinically relevant plasma range not yet determined for elders, and routine plasma level monitoring not recommended.
  - √ Overall, ranges in elders are slightly lower than in general adults.
  - √ Older schizophrenic range is up to 10 ng/ml (15 ng/ml general adult data).
  - √ Ranges sufficient to produce about a 70% occupancy of D_2 receptor sites
    - ▫ Therapeutic improvement found in dementia cases at 0.3–1.4 ng/ml.
  - √ Very high interindividual dose/plasma level variability.
    - ▫ Plasma levels may be less variable and more reliable in previously neuroleptic-naïve patients with dementia treated with this drug.
  - √ Patients on long-term therapy with very high plasma levels sometimes benefit from dose reductions to bring levels into a "window" of up to 10 ng/ml.
    - ▫ Also reduces EPS side effects.

Special monitoring

- High-dose haloperidol rarely associated with prolonged QTc and *Torsades de Pointes*.
  - √ Monitor vulnerable patients with serial ECGs and discontinue promptly, if indicated.

Drug Interactions

See pages 306–307.

Action potentiated by

- Fluvoxamine—robustly elevates plasma concentrations.
- Indomethacin—may induce confusion and severe drowsiness.
- Methyldopa

Action antagonized by

- Carbamazepine—induces hepatic enzymes and reduces plasma concentration by as much as 60%.
  - √ Despite lower plasma levels, cardiotoxicity (prolonged QTc and heart failure) associated with concurrent use.
- Barbiturates—induce hepatic enzymes.
- Plasma concentration of haloperidol reduced by
  - √ Trihexyphenidyl
  - √ Phenytoin
  - √ Smoking (secondary to induction of isoenzyme 1A2)

Contraindications

- Thyrotoxicosis: Associated with neurotoxic reaction when haloperidol is used.
- DLB
- Parkinson's: relatively contraindicated for associated psychoses or agitation.
- Caution with concurrent lithium administration.
  - √ Encephalopathy, with weakness, lethargy, confusion, tremor, fever, EPS, and elevated WBC, BUN, FBS, and serum enzymes reported although not confirmed in controlled trials.

Overdose, Toxicity, Suicide

See also pages 307–308.

Symptoms

- Severe EPS
- Hypotension
- Sedation
- Respiratory depression
- Shock-like state
- Cardiac arrhythmias (including Torsades de Pointes)

Clincal Tips

Haloperidol used to be a gold standard for efficacy; it has been replaced by atypicals but is still widely used and may be preferable in patients who are very sensitive to the orthostatic hypotension or anticholinergic effects often induced by some atypicals.

IV form not recommended for elders as a general rule, but in special situations, especially in the ICU, may be very helpful (e.g., management of delirium).

- Danger of acute EPS is low but may be further lessened with concurrent benzodiazepine.

- √ Lorazepam (IM or IV) in a dose ratio of 4 haloperidol: 1 benzodiazepine (e.g., 4 mg haloperidol: 1 mg lorazepam).
- Very wide dosage ranges for IV use, but often in the 10–40 mg/day range.
- Sometimes much higher doses used.
  - √ Apparent resistance to drug treatment sometimes due to drug-induced akathisia masking target symptoms, leading to escalating dose of drug.
- Duration 1–5 days.
- Overall, serious side effects less evident with parenteral route.
- Has the advantage of being safe in presence of cardiac pathology.
  - √ *Note:* High-dose therapy (oral or IV) produces occasional prolonged QTc, which may be life-threatening.
  - √ Danger may be reduced by using continuous IV infusion, rather than IV bolus, but not well studied in elders.
- Substitute oral for IV form as soon as possible.
- Important to define target symptoms and evaluate response frequently.
- For patients on long-term therapy for agitation (usually in nursing homes), drug holidays of 2 nonsequential days a week may be used without increase in agitation.
- Relatively rapid onset of therapeutic action 30–60 minutes after IM, faster with IV.
- Absorption of depot form may be prolonged, requiring longer periods between doses.
- Specific danger from haloperidol/lithium interaction, previously suspected, not borne out in controlled trails.
  - √ However, lithium toxicity, in general, is higher in elders.

Rise in LFTs can be nerve wracking.

- Usually associated with higher-dose therapy not usually used in elders.
- Acute increase in first few days usually dose-dependent and responds to reducing dose.
- Otherwise, modest rises are frequent but benign unless they exceed 2–3 times normal.
  - √ Reevaluate the therapy unless they recede spontaneously, as they do in > 50%.

Monitor EPS especially for doses > 2 mg/day.

LOXAPINE

Drug	Manufacturer	Chemical Class	Therapeutic Class
loxapine (Loxitane)	Watson	dibenzoxapine tricyclic	antipsychotic

Indications: FDA/HPB

- Schizophrenia

Indications: Off label

See pages 236–262.

Pharmacology

Note: The antidepressant amoxapine is a metabolite of loxapine.

Mechanism of action

- High D_2 affinity.
- High affinity for binding to $5HT_2$ and dopamine D_4 receptors.
- Because in vivo D_2 affinity remains higher than $5HT_2$ occupancy, this drug is not an atypical antipsychotic (in contrast to in vitro action where $5HT_2$ affinity is greater than D_2).
  √ Recent PET data suggest equal occupancy.

Choosing a Drug

- Chemically distinct from other antipsychotics, but similar action and side-effect profile to perphenazine.
- Serotonin-blocking properties.
- Equipotent to other antipsychotics.
- Low propensity for antihistaminic and anticholinergic actions.
- Effective for aggression in dementia.
- May be more acutely sedating than IM haldoperidol.

Dosing

Daily dose regimen

- Divided doses bid–qid.

Initial dose 5–10 mg/day.

Increasing dose and reaching therapeutic levels.

- Increase dose by 5–10 mg once or twice a week.
- 60–80% D_2 occupancy produced by low doses of 15–30 mg/day, suggesting efficacy at lower than standard dosing.
- Useful dose 10–15 mg/day.
  √ Dose range used 10–100 mg/day.

Side Effects

Mostly general adult data; little geriatric-specific data available.

See table, pages 279–303.

- EPS
  √ Not as pronounced as with high-potency agents.

Table 2.26. Side Effects of Loxapine

Side Effects	Most Common	Most Serious and Less Common
Body as a whole	• Fatigue • Weight gain (chronic use)	
Cardiovascular	• Hypotension (orthostatic)	• Tachycardia • Dysrhythmias • ECG changes • Syncope • Dizziness
Eye	• Blurred vision	• Retinal pigmentation • Ocular pigmentation
Central and peripheral nervous system	• Sedation √ Especially evident with IM forms • TD	• NMS • Seizures
Gastrointestinal	• Dry mouth • Constipation	
Hematological		• Agranulocytosis • Leukopenia
Liver and biliary		• Hepatotoxicity • Allergic cholestatic jaundice
Urinary		• Urinary retention

For drug interactions, see pages 306–307.

For overdose, see pages 307–308.

OLANZAPINE

Drug	Manufacturer	Chemical Class	Therapeutic Class
olanzapine (Zyprexa)	Lilly	thienobenzodiazepine	atypical antipsychotic

Indications: FDA/HPB

- Short term treatment of Schizophrenia and bipolar disorder.

Indications: Off label

See also pages 236–262 for indications.

- BPSD, including psychosis, aggression, agitation, affective symptoms.
- OCD
- Delirium
- May be useful in managing depression associated with schizophrenia.
- Monosymptomatic psychosis (case report).
- DLB—reduces psychosis without increase in parkinsonism (preliminary data analysis).

Cost effectiveness

- More costly than risperidone, although effectiveness is similar for patient groups.
- In individual patients, the key issue is effectiveness and some patients will respond to and tolerate one agent and not another.

Pharmacology

See also page 233.

- Males and smokers have higher clearance (by 25%).
  - √ Women may have higher plasma levels than men.
  - √ Consider reducing dosage in frail women who are nonsmokers.
- Interindividual clearance varies by factor of 4 (general adult data).
- Low incidence of persistent hyperprolactinemia compared to haloperidol.
  - √ No difference with placebo after 6 weeks.

Mechanism of action

- Multiple receptor site affinities (in vitro) include $5HT_{2A}/_{2C}/_{3}/_{6}$ serotonin and $D_4/D_1/D_2$ dopamine antagonism, histamine H_1, alpha-1 adrenergic and antimuscarinic M_1/M_5; possibly a glutaminergic mechanism as well.
- D_2 occupancy similar to clozapine but may be lower than haloperidol.
- Blockade of serotonin receptors greater than that of D_2.

Choosing a Drug

- A drug of first choice in elders.
- Generally well tolerated in elders, even chronically psychiatrically impaired and institutionalized.
- Effective in acutely psychotic and otherwise agitated elders, including BPSD-related psychosis.
  - √ 75% of patients in a nursing home study showed substantial improvement in psychotic and agitation symptoms.
  - √ Not all placebo-controlled studies in elders show efficacy.
- Psychotic depression
  - √ Positive outcomes in preliminary trials of combinations with SSRI (i.e., citalopram, paroxetine; general adult data).
  - √ May be some antidepressant properties, better choice for patients with concurrent depressive symptomatology.
- Use in bipolar disorder inferred from double-blind, placebo-controlled general adult data.
  - √ More effective than placebo (48% vs. 24%) in treating acute mania.

  - √ Geriatric outcome/efficacy data for bipolar indications very limited.
- Once-a-day dosing an advantage.
- Zydis preparation dissolves readily in the mouth without liquid.
- Delayed onset of action: latency of 6 weeks to several months.
- Oral form not effective for prn use in acute situations (delayed peak plasma levels 5–6 hours).
  - √ Trials of IM form suggest positive effect in agitation associated with dementia.
- Probably fewer EPS than risperidone at comparable doses
  - √ but more than clozapine or quetiapine.
  - √ Aggravates parkinsonism and increases "off" time in treatment of hallucinations in Parkinson's disease, although it may reduce dyskinesias.
    - ▫ Psychosis does not respond robustly, especially when associated with dementia.

Dosing

- Optimal dosing not yet established for elders.
  - √ Data suggests efficacy is best at doses < 15 mg.
- Side effects have emerged even at relatively low doses, so caution is advisable when initiating therapy for the first time in a geriatric patient, especially if frail or debilitated.

Initiating therapy

- Start at lower dose range and increase slowly, watching for emergent side effects.
  - √ Especially EPS, sedation, and postural hypotension.

Initial dose

- For frail elders and those with dementia or preexisting EPS such as Parkinson's disease, begin at 1.25–2.5 mg/day.
- Otherwise uncomplicated psychosis, begin at 2.5–5 mg/hs.
- Begin with bid dosing when starting at 5 mg and switch to single hs dose once the daily dose has been determined and side effects are under control.
- IM form 2.5–5 mg
  - √ Onset of action in 30–60 minutes.
- DLB dose 5–10 mg
  - √ Dosing not well established.
  - √ Caution recommended, since this agent not well tested in this population.

Increasing dose and reaching therapeutic levels

- Increase dose 2.5 mg/day q 5–7 days.
- Patients with psychosis but without dementia respond at around 10 mg (range 2.5–10 mg/day).
- Patients with dementia and psychosis respond best to 5 mg/day (with ranges on either side: 2.5–10 mg/day).

Maintenance dose

- Not well defined—general rule of thumb is 5–10 mg for psychosis.

Side Effects

See also table on pages 279–303 for side effects, especially anticholinergic, cardiovascular, weight, impaired glycemic control.

- Generally well tolerated, based on limited geriatric data.
- Not associated with agranulocytosis or seizures.
- Low potential for EPS.
- Somnolence with risk of falls may be a significant problem.
- Commonest side effects include
  - √ Dizziness
  - √ Constipation
  - √ Increased ALT
  - √ Akathesia
  - √ Postural hypotension

Table 2.27. Side Effects of Olanzapine

Side Effects	Most Common*	Most Serious and Less Common
Anticholinergic effects	• Especially at higher doses; little anticholinergic action at 5 and 10 mg/day; some anticholinergic effects emerge at 15 mg/day • Constipation • Dry mouth	
Body as a whole	• Increased appetite • Weight gain √ May be significant √ May plateau at around 30 weeks but data scarce	
Cardiovascular	• Tachycardia	• Orthostatic hypotension uncommon but may be severe √ Sometimes self-limiting or managed by dose reductions √ Syncope, rare

(*cont.*)

Continued

Side Effects	Most Common*	Most Serious and Less Common
Central and peripheral nervous system	• Somnolence, lethargy √ Dose dependent √ Associated with abnormal gait √ Give dose hs to reduce daytime sedation • Delirium more frequent in chronically, often institutionalized, psychiatrically ill elders √ Increased rate in DLB √ Rates in community-dwelling elders not known √ Generally associated with concurrent medications • EPS √ Generally emerges at higher doses but may occur at lower doses, so caution warranted √ Parkinsonism (rate about one-third of haloperidol; sometimes severe) □ Akinetic symptoms—may worsen rigidity and bradykinesia □ Gait impairment ○ Stooped posture ○ Unsteadiness ○ Leaning ○ Ambulation dysfunction □ Speech impairment □ Patients with Parkinson's more susceptible to worsening of motor symptoms (tremor), even at low doses • Dizziness • Insomnia • Akathisia • Agitation/overactivation • Anxiety • Asthenia • Nervousness • Effects on cognition √ Impaired performance in elders probably marker of sedation □ Slowed reaction times, diminished alertness √ Accommodation to effects may occur over time	• Akathisia • Tardive dyskinesia (risk 1.5%/year, general adult data) • EEG abnormality
Endocrine	• Loss of glycemic control	• Impaired glycemic control (general adult case reports) fairly common (18% in one study) √ Often improves with discontinuation of the drug √ Induction of diabetes mellitus, especially in predisposed, in the first 3 months of treatment √ Treatment emergent hyperglycemia may be severe √ Diabetic ketoacidosis

(cont.)

Continued

Side Effects	Most Common*	Most Serious and Less Common
Gastrointestinal	• Dyspepsia	
Hematological		• Bruising
Liver and biliary		• Elevated liver enzymes
Metabolic and nutritional	• Elevation of serum triglyceride levels	• NMS cited in several case studies (general adult and geriatric data) • Elevated liver enzymes (ALT) √ Hypothermia (case reports) √ Fever
Musculoskeletal	• Myalgia • Back pain	
Psychiatric		• May induce mania/hypomania (general adult data)
Reproductive		• Priapism reported
Respiratory	• Rhinitis	

* Percentages are general adult data.

Monitoring

- BP in the initial titration phases until stabilized.
- Therapeutic plasma levels are > 9 ng/ml.
  - √ These levels not well established and not reliable for routine clinical use.
- Blood sugars, as needed.
- Annual liver enzyme monitoring.

Drug Interactions

See Table 2.24 on pages 306–307 for CYP enzyme-related drug interactions.

- Low overall risk of drug interactions.
- 1A2 inhibition significantly increases plasma concentrations of olanzapine and decreases clearance.
- Inhibition of 2D6 does not have major effect on metabolism of olanzapine in general adults, but may have more clinical relevance in vulnerable elders.
- Benzodiazepines and alcohol may increase heart rate, hypotensive effects, and sedation.
- Haloperidol—case report of increased parkinsonism with concurrent therapy.
- Epinephrine—hypotensive effect.

- General caution with
  - √ CNS depressants
    - Antihistamines
    - Barbiturates
    - Benzodiazepines/sedative hypnotics
    - Certizine
    - Clonidine
    - Cyclobenzaprine
    - Methyldopa
    - Opiates
    - Propoxyphene
    - Tramadol
  - √ Anticholinergic drugs (see Table 1.14, p. 71)

Effect on Laboratory Tests

- Transient increases in ALT.
- May increase prolactin levels, but less so than haloperidol (general adult data).

Disability Interactions

- Renal impairment: Dosage adjustment not required on this basis alone.
- Hepatic impairment: Caution advised until patient's response is clear.
- Anticholinergic cautions.
- Caution in patients with cardiovascular disease, cerebrovascular disease, and risk of seizures.
- Hypersensitivity to the drug a contraindication.
- Caution in chronic lung disease; respiratory depression may be secondary to sedative effects.

Overdose, Toxicity, Suicide

Dangers (general adult data)

- Symptoms include
  - √ Drowsiness
  - √ Slurred speech
  - √ Anticholinergic effects (i.e., agitation, altered mental state, hyperthermia, decreased bowel sounds, tachycardia without arrhythmia).
  - √ Antihistaminic symptoms (sedation, drowsiness).
  - √ Alpha-1/alpha-2 adrenergic antagonism (i.e., agitation, miotic pupils, orthostatic hypotension, reflex tachycardia).

- Combinations with other agents, including alcohol, associated with coma and death.

Management

- Absorption decreased by activated charcoal in conjunction with a laxative.
  - √ May be useful in treating early stages of olanzapine overdose.
- Hemodialysis not effective in overdose (large volume of distribution and high protein binding).
- Provide general supportive measures.
- Avoid agents with beta-agonist properties (e.g., epinephrine, dopamine).
  - √ May increase hypotension.

Clinical Tips

- History includes inquiry into tobacco smoking patterns.
  - √ Smoking induces CYP1A2 enzymes and reduces concentration of plasma olanzapine.
- Has been shown effective in reducing emergence of psychotic symptoms in nursing home patients, but prophylactic use not advised.
- If instituted with a concurrent typical antipsychotic drug, taper typical antipsychotic over period of 1–2 weeks.
- Not necessary to monitor serial WBC (as with clozapine).
  - √ Has been used safely in a few patients with clozapine-induced blood dyscrasias (general adult data) without impairing recovery.
- If side effects emerge, many can be managed by reducing the dose and then titrating it up again more slowly.
- Most effective dose range in institutionalized elders with dementia is 5 mg, although 10 mg/day is necessary for some.
  - √ Higher doses in this group are not usually effective and brings a higher rate of side effects.
- Delirium may emerge in vulnerable patients at relatively low doses of 2.5–5 mg.
- Management of delirium
  - √ Discontinue drug.
  - √ Evaluate for other contributing factors.
  - √ Reintroduce drug at lower dose.
  - √ Increase dose slowly.
  - √ Monitor serum glucose levels, especially in patients with risk factors for diabetes.
  - √ Monitor patients with history of NMS.

PERPHENAZINE

Drug	Manufacturer	Chemical Class	Therapeutic Class
perphenazine (Trilafon)	Schering	piperazine phenothiazine	antipsychotic

Indications: FDA/HPB

- Schizophrenia
- Severe nausea and vomiting

Indications: Off label

- Agitated, hyperexcited, aggressive patients

Pharmacology

See Table 2.2 on pages 233–234.

Mechanism of action

- Blockade of dopamine, adrenergic, and cholinergic receptor sites.
- Significant affinity for $5HT_{2A}$ receptors but less than for D_2.

Choosing a Drug

- Replaced as a drug of choice in elders by atypicals, although perphenazine has some characteristics of atypicals in that it has low incidence of EPS at lower plasma levels (< 1.2 ng/ml).
- Until recently, a drug of choice for BPSD.
- Response time may be longer in elders with psychosis without dementia (3 weeks) compared to younger subjects (within 10 days).

Dosing

Daily dose regimen

- For psychosis without dementia, low-dose therapy not very effective.
- Available in liquid and IM injectable forms.

Initial dose 2 mg daily (hs).

Increasing dose and reaching therapeutic levels

- Increase by 2–4 mg once or twice a week.
- Therapeutic levels for dementia-related symptoms is 2–8 mg.
- Higher range (up to 32 mg/day) for other forms of psychosis.

Side Effects

See also pages 279–303.

Table 2.28.

Side Effects	Most Common	Most Serious and Less Common
Anticholinergic	• Dry mouth • Constipation • Urinary retention • Blurred vision	
Cardiovascular	• ECG changes • Hypotension (orthostatic) • Tachycardia • Dysrhythmias	
Central and peripheral nervous system	• EPS • Restlessness • Anxiety	• TD • Seizures
Eye		• Retinal pigmentation
Hematological		• Agranulocytosis • Leukopenia
Liver and biliary		• Cholestatic jaundice
Metabolic and nutritional		• NMS
Skin and appendages		• Hyperpigmentation • Rash

Monitoring

- Few geriatric data.
- Optimal pre-dose blood level 0.8–2.5 nmol/l (range 0.8–6).
  - √ Higher ranges may be necessary for severe psychosis (general adult data).

Drug Interactions

See also Table 2.24 on pages 306–307.

- Potentiates
  - √ CNS depressants
  - √ Anticholinergics
- Antagonizes action of some antihypertensives.
- Action may be potentiated by fluvoxamine.
- Because of potent $2D_6$ antagonism, will inhibit metabolism of other drugs metabolized by this enzyme.

Disability Interactions and Contraindications

- Subcortical brain disease occasionally associated with severe hyperthermic reactions within first day of administration.

- Known hypersensitivity to perphenazine.
- Severely reduced levels of consciousness.
- Concurrent high dose CNS depressants (e.g., barbiturates, alcohol, narcotics, analgesics, antihistamines).
- Presence of significant bone marrow depression, blood dyscrasias, liver damage.

Overdose, Toxicity, Suicide

- Initiate emergency treatment immediately.
- Hospitalize.
- Signs and symptoms
  - √ EPS
  - √ Autonomic effects
  - √ CVS effects (e.g., hypotension, cardiac arrhythmia, cardiac arrest)
  - √ Stupor, coma

Management

- Induce vomiting (ipecac) even if spontaneous vomiting has already occurred, except if consciousness is impaired.
  - √ Give 8–12 oz. of water with ipecac.
  - √ Repeat dose if no vomiting in 15 minutes.
  - √ *Note:* Ipecac acts centrally as well as through local gastric irritation.
    - ▫ Perphenazine may inhibit action of ipecac through its central antiemetic action.
- Administer activated charcoal.
- Administer gastric lavage, if necessary.
- Manage shock.
  - √ Provide oxygen, airway, IV fluids, corticosteroids.
- Control temperature dysregulation.
  - √ Hypothermia and hyperthermia
- CVS management.
  - √ Cardiac monitoring for 5 days or more.
  - √ Arrhythmia: Administer neostigmine, pyridostigmine, or propranolol.
  - √ Cardiac failure: digitalis.
  - √ Hypotension: *avoid epinephrine.*
    - ▫ Use norepinephrine.
- Some effects may be delayed for hours or days.
- Acute EPS: benztropine mesylate or diphenhydramine.
- Dialysis of no value.

QUETIAPINE

Drug	Manufacturer	Chemical Class	Therapeutic Class
quetiapine (Seroquel)	AstraZeneca	dibenzothiazepine	atypical antipsychotic

Indications: FDA/HPB

- Short-term treatment of schizophrenia

Indications: Off label

See also pages 236–262.

Quetiapine studies include

- Psychosis in medical conditions
- Bipolar disorder
- Effective for psychosis associated with DLB (open small *n* study with no placebo control)

Pharmacology

See also page 233.

- 30–50% lower clearance in elders.
- Requires proportionally lower doses.
- Hepatic impairment: Reduce dose and use slow dose escalations.
  - √ Renal impairment does not require dose adjustment.
- Little propensity to produce sustained increases in plasma prolactin levels.

Mechanism of action

Antipsychotic action thought to be mediated through combined activity at D_2 and $5HT_2$ receptors.

- $5HT_{2A}$ receptor inhibition is greater than binding at D_2 receptors.
- Most potent action is histamine H_1 inhibition.
- Affinity for
  - √ D_1 receptor
  - √ $5\text{-}HT_{1A}$
  - √ Low affinity for D_2 receptors
    - ▫ Hence, little drug-induced parkinsonism.
- Modest alpha-1 inhibition.
  - √ Hence, less postural hypotension.
- Little cholinergic, muscarinic, or benzodiazepine receptor affinity.
  - √ Hence, insignificant anticholinergic effects.
- Little effect on prolactin levels.
- Mesolimbic selectivity after chronic administration.

Choosing a Drug

- A drug of choice for the elderly.
- Low potential for EPS even at higher dose ranges.
- Little anticholinergic or prolactin-elevating actions.
- May be the most rapidly absorbed of the atypicals.
  - √ Absorption enhanced with food.
- Appears to be better tolerated than other antipsychotic agents by patients with DLB.
- Improves positive and negative symptoms of schizophrenia.
- Effective in release musical hallucinations (case report).
- Improves psychosis associated with Parkinson's disease and, in general, does not worsen motor symptoms.
- Improves aggression and hostility in Alzheimer disease.

Dosing

Daily dose regimen

- Wide range of effective dosing but geriatric dosing is not well defined.
- Common mean about 120–150 mg/day in demented patients.
  - √ Recent study suggests dose < 120 mg is ineffective.
- Higher ranges necessary for nondemented patients with primary psychoses (schizophrenia) or bipolar disorder.
- Use bid-tid dosing regimens.
  - √ May be a disadvantage to compliance in some patients, unless in a controlled environment.

Initiating therapy

- Initial dose 25 mg/day po.

Increasing dose and reaching therapeutic levels

- Increase dose every 2–4 days by 25–50 mg, as required and tolerated.
  - √ Increase dose more slowly in frail elders.
  - √ Slower dose increases improve likelihood of completing course of treatment.
    - ▫ Consider giving larger dose in evening to reduce daytime sedation.
  - √ Consider tid dosing for patients less tolerant of side effects (e.g., hypotension).
  - √ Target ranges
    - ▫ Lower dose range 120–150 mg/day more usual for treating agitation and dementia-related psychosis.

- Target dose in Parkinson's disease may be even lower—50–75 mg/day (range 25–150 mg/day)—but not well established.
- Higher dose range 300–800 mg/day may be necessary in some elders with schizophrenia and other psychoses, who are otherwise well and can tolerate high-dose therapy.

Side Effects

- Overall tolerance in elders is good, based on limited data.
- Main common side effects are somnolence, dizziness, agitation, and postural hypotension.

Table 2.29. Side Effects of Quetiapine

Side Effects	Most Common*	Most Serious and Less Common
Body as a whole	• Weight change √ Gain or loss √ Significant gain in long-term general adult trials (5–6 kg)	• Flu-like symptoms • Sweating
Cardiovascular	• Postural hypotension 15% (but only 3% develop clinically significant orthostatic hypotension) √ Onset especially as dose is being increased, usually early in course of treatment (first 2 weeks) √ Mostly mild or moderate in degree √ Tachycardia √ Occasional syncope √ Caution in patients with preexisting conditions that predispose to hypotension √ Manage by starting with low doses and titrating slowly √ Observe for incoordination and gait disturbance □ Risk of accidental injury in 12%	
Central and peripheral nervous system	• Low incidence of EPS: 6–13% √ Tremor √ Dyskinesia √ Gait impairment √ Other movement disorders √ Few require antiparkinsonian medication √ Pre-existing TD often remits during treatment • Somnolence: 30% √ Occurs early in treatment and at relatively low doses (50 mg) √ Related to H1 inhibition • Relatively low incidence of insomnia • Dizziness: 12–17% • Headache	• Seizures √ May be more prevalent in presence of preexisting brain disorders (e.g., Alzheimer's disease) • Acute dystonia

(cont.)

Continued

Side Effects	Most Common*	Most Serious and Less Common
Endocrine		• T4 reduced infrequently in some patients √ TSH rarely increased √ Appears fully reversible when drug is discontinued • Sporadic reports of emergent diabetes
Eye		• Theoretical possibility of cataract induction
Gastrointestinal	• 8% affected • Constipation • Dry mouth • Anorexia/dyspepsia	
Hematological		• Leukopenia/neutropenia • Thrombocytopenia • Bleeding gums, bruising
Liver and biliary		• Transient increased hepatic enzymes (ALT/AST) early in treatment
Metabolic and nutritional		• Occasional increased serum cholesterol; usually resolves spontaneously • Weight gain • NMS
Psychiatric	• Agitation (16%) √ Usually transient (often 1 day), but may be severe	
Reproductive		• Priapism
Skin and appendages		• Rash

* Percentages are general adult data.

Routine monitoring

- Track blood pressure in patients who develop dizziness or faintness.
- Consider regular slit-lamp eye exams for cataracts at initiation of treatment and every 6 months.
  √ However, clinical experience since marketing of the drug shows very little danger of cataract induction.
- Obtain baseline thyroid indices.

Drug Interactions

See also Table 2.24 on pages 306–307.

- *Caution* in coadministration of drugs that inhibit CYP3A4 (e.g., ketoconazole, itraconazole, erythromycin, fluconazole) or are substrates for the enzyme.

Action potentiated by

- Ketoconazole, itraconazole, fluconazole, nefazodone, erythromycin.
- Alcohol.
  - √ Potentiates cognitive/motor effects of drug.
- Antihypertensives.
  - √ Effect may be potentiated by drug.
- Cimetidine reduces clearance.
  - √ Clinical relevance not described for elders.
- Lorazepam: quetiapine reduces its oral clearance.

Action antagonized by

- Phenytoin, carbamazepine, barbiturates, rifampin, glucocorticoids.
  - √ Phenytoin increases clearance 5-fold.
  - √ May need increased dose of quetiapine as long as phenytoin is administered, but reduce dose of quetiapine if phenytoin is discontinued.
- Increased clearance rate with thioridazine.
- Caution with CNS depressants, including OTC drugs.
- Increased dose of quetiapine may be required if these drugs are used concurrently.

Effect on Laboratory Tests

- Increased serum triglycerides (small, nonsignificant).
- Increased LFTs—otherwise asymptomatic (general adult data; no geriatric reports).
- T4 reduced.
  - √ Levels restored with discontinuation of the drug.

Special Precautions

- Usual precautions in using machinery or driving until patient's reaction to the drug is determined and a steady state has been reached.

Overdose, Toxicity, Suicide

- Little experience in elders.
- Expect hypotension, sedation/somnolence, tachycardia, possible seizures, dystonias, arrhythmias.
- Provide supportive measures, including airway support, ventilation.
- Administer gastric lavage.
- Institute cardiac monitoring.

- Caution in using disopyramide, procainamide, or quinidine—may prolong QT interval.
- Alpha-adrenergic blockers (e.g., bretylium) may aggravate hypotension.
- Administer antiparkinsonian medication for severe EPS.
- Support BP with IV fluids, sympathomimetic agents.

Clinical Tips

- Avoid rapid dose escalations.
  - √ Increases likelihood of intolerance of medication side effects and treatment noncompliance/discontinuance.
- If switching to quetiapine from clozapine, better success achieved if there is a slow titration of quetiapine while slowly decreasing clozapine.
  - √ Long overlap period best.
  - √ Increase quetiapine by 12.5 mg/day each week while decreasing clozapine by 6.25 mg each week for 2 weeks, 12.5 mg per week for next 2 weeks, and 25 mg per week thereafter, until discontinued.
- Clinical relevance of increased plasma levels of triglycerides and total cholesterol not known.
- Expect significant (> 20%) improvement in psychotic symptoms in about 50% of cases.

RISPERIDONE

Drug	Manufacturer	Chemical Class	Therapeutic Class
risperidone (Risperidal)	Janssen-Ortho	benzisoxazole derivative	atypical antipsychotic

Indications: FDA/HPB

- Psychotic disorders
- Specific forms of psychosis relevant to elders, in which risperidone has been reported as effective include
  - √ Schizophrenia (EOS, LOS)
  - √ Acute catatonia
  - √ Delusional parasitosis (case report)
  - √ Visual hallucinations (Charles Bonnet syndrome)
  - √ Psychosis (hallucinations) associated with parkinsonism
  - √ DLB—neuroleptic sensitivity reactions occur with risperidone
  - √ Levodopa-induced psychosis
  - √ Psychotic mood disorders
  - √ Psychosis with comorbid medical illness
- BPSD listed in Canada but not in U.S.

Indications: Off label

Effectiveness based on wide variety of investigations, most of which are general adult data, some geriatric. A few controlled trials have been conducted, but most are uncontrolled clinical data.

- BPSD: Effective for aggression and agitation.
- Bipolar disorder: General adult data are promising, but little controlled data to date, and none in elders.
  - √ Double-blind general adult data show equal efficacy to haloperidol for rapid control of manic symptoms.
- Movement disorders.
- Delirium

Cost Effectiveness

- High cost of drug relative to typical antipsychotics is not offset by reduction in readmission rates.
  - √ However, improved side-effect profile makes it a better choice for elders than typicals.

Pharmacology

- Elimination half-life increased in elders.
- Reduce risperidone dose in elders and all patients with renal impairment.
  - √ Recent study suggested no need for age-related dose reduction but caution is warranted.
  - √ Increased half-life in patients with renal insufficiency.
    - ▫ Reduced rate of clearance of active metabolite by 30%—reduce dose.
  - √ Decreased clearance with renal impairment.
    - ▫ May lead to increased plasma levels of 9-hydroxy metabolite.
    - ▫ Equipotent to parent compound in D_2 blocking action.
- Marked and sustained plasma prolactin levels.

Mechanism of action

- Highly potent $5HT_{2a/c}$ serotonin antagonism and substantial but less potent dopamine (D_2) antagonism.
  - √ $5HT_2$ receptor occupancy is 80% (greater than clozapine) at a dose of 3 mg/day (general adult data).
  - √ D_2 receptor occupancy in the striatum is 72% at a dose of 3 mg/day (general adult data).
    - ▫ D_2 affinity greater than other atypicals at higher doses (> 4 mg).

  - D_2 antagonism associated with elevations of plasma prolactin levels.
- Antagonizes alpha-1 and alpha-2 adrenergic receptors (associated with hypotension) and histamine H_2 and (with lower affinity) $5HT_{1c/a/d}$ receptors.
- Overall, acts as an atypical agent at lower doses and as a more typical agent at higher doses.
- Enhances prolactin release.

Therapeutic Actions by Indication

Dementia

- May be more effective than typical antipsychotics for aggression/agitation in dementia because of affinity for serotonin receptors.
- Improves nighttime sleep.
- May improve anxiety symptoms.
- May improve depressed mood, but generally dysphoria and apathy less responsive than other BPSD symptoms.
- Case report data of improvement in persistent vocalizations in severe dementia.
- Especially effective in control of aggression in patients with dementia.
  - √ Aggression may respond in about 3 weeks and agitation in 5–7 weeks.

Schizophrenia

- Improves positive and possibly negative symptoms of schizophrenia (general adult data).
  - √ Symptom improvement continues over 12 months in chronic non-dementia–related psychosis in elders.
- May indirectly improve cognitive performance.
  - √ Improved score on MMSE.

Parkinson's disease

- Improves psychotic symptoms and agitation in Parkinson's disease, but may increase EPS.
  - √ Should be used with caution in this population, even in lower dosage range of 1–1.5 mg/day.
  - √ In Parkinson's disease, higher doses are less benign and are avoided.

Safety profile

- A drug of choice for elders.
- More selective agent than clozapine.
- Does not have the risk of agranulocytosis associated with clozapine.

- Low incidence of persistent TD in demented elders (dose approximately 1 mg).
- No need for leukocyte monitoring.
- May have slight advantage in speed of onset of action over other atypicals (anecdotal evidence).
- Improves depressive symptoms associated with schizophrenia (general adult data).
- Recent warning posted
  - √ Increased risk of stroke or cerebrovascular-related events in demented patients.

Efficacy

- > 75% of patients significantly improved in a range of psychotic and agitation symptoms in nursing home sample.
- Comparable efficacy with clozapine in head-to-head trial, with somewhat more favorable side effect profile (general adult data).
- Onset of effective action within a few days.
- More effective than typical antipsychotics for negative symptoms and possibly also positive symptoms of schizophrenia (general adult data).

Race/Ethnicity

- Some evidence for slower metabolism in some Chinese patients.

Dosing

- Doses for BPSD are generally lower than for schizophrenia or other major psychotic disorders.
- Employ basic dosing strategy.
  - √ Cautious titration.
  - √ Many elders require about one-third the adult dose.
- Liquid form (1 mg/ml) useful for titrating dose or for patients unable or unwilling to swallow pill.
- Injectable and depot forms under investigation.
- Maximum doses may be lower in patients with DLB.

Daily dose regimen

- To avoid side effects from peak plasma levels, administer bid; if patient tolerates the drug well, administer once daily for convenience and to improve compliance.
- Dosing for specific disorders—guidelines only (geriatric dose-finding studies are not available yet).
  - √ Psychosis with Parkinson's disease: 0.25–1.25 mg/day.
  - √ BPSD: 0.25–1 mg/day.
  - √ DLB: 0.25–1 mg/day.

- √ Charles Bonnet syndrome: 1–2 mg/day (single case report).
- √ Schizophrenia/schizophreniform disorders: 2–4 mg/day.

Initiating therapy

- Begin at low dose and increase slowly to reduce emergence of side effects.
- Generally effective in once daily dosing regimen.
- Reduce to half recommended dose for first trials in Chinese patients, until capacity to metabolize the drug is established.

Initial dose

- Conservative: 0.125–0.5 mg/qhs.
- When starting at 0.5 mg in frail elders, use 0.25 mg bid for 2–3 days until stabilized, before considering a once daily dose.
- For DLB or Parkinson's disease, use even lower starting dose of 0.125 mg/day.
- Titrate slowly based on patient's tolerance.
- Oral solution (in BPSD–associated agitation)—begin at 0.25 mg/day.

Increasing dose and reaching therapeutic levels

- Over 1.5 mg, increase dose by 0.25–0.5 mg/day q 7 days, as tolerated (lower dose for patients with Parkinson's disease).
- Some patients tolerate more rapid increase (q 2–4 days in lower dose range, up to 1.5 mg).
  - √ Increased risk of emergence of side effects.
- Oral solution (in BPSD–associated agitation)—increase dose 0.25 mg/week.

Maintenance dose

- Effective doses range from 0.5–6 mg (in divided doses bid); 6 mg dose not usually needed and not well tolerated by many elders.
- Target range
  - √ Most elders respond to lower end of the dose range (1 mg/day), especially demented, frail, or medically ill elders and those with BPSD.
    - ▫ Common ceiling is 2–3 mg.
  - √ Some elders (including those who are extensive metabolizers) require larger doses, averaging about 3–4 mg.
    - ▫ Generally, patients with schizophrenia, drug-resistant agitation or bizarre behavior.

Combination therapy

- SSRIs: Clinical data suggest may augment antidepressant effect in refractory cases.

Discontinuation and Withdrawal

- Trial of discontinuation (gradual tapering):
  - √ Aggression: after 2–8 months.
  - √ Mild agitation: after 1–6 months (or earlier, if patient has responded quickly and fully).
  - √ Monitor long-term use and justify continuation therapies.

Side Effects

- Generally well tolerated.
- Adverse events occur in 30–40% of elders.
- Reduced by using low doses (side effect rates at doses < 1 mg/day equal to placebo).
- EPS side effects emerge at higher dose ranges (> 2 mg).
  - √ May be due to higher D_2 receptor site occupancy and loss of relative $5HT_2$-mediated protection from EPS.
- Warning signs of intolerance include
  - √ Excess sedation
  - √ Confusion
  - √ Dizziness
  - √ Bradykinesia

Table 2.30. Side Effects of Risperidone

Side Effects	Most Common*	Most Serious and Less Common
Autonomic	• Dry mouth • Blurred vision • Hypersalivation	
Body as a whole	• Fatigue	• NMS
Cardiovascular	• Orthostatic hypotension (10%) √ Dose-related; often improves if dose is reduced. √ Predisposing factors include preexisting cardiac pathology, hypertension, and use of antihypertensive medication. √ Monitor sitting and standing pressures during dose adjustments until tolerance established. • Nonorthostatic hypotension (29%) may be significant, especially in preexisting cardiac disease. √ Monitor BP, including orthostatic, until safe maintenance dose established. • Tachycardia/palpitations • Peripheral edema 16%	• Prolonged QT interval

(*cont.*)

Continued

Side Effects	Most Common*	Most Serious and Less Common
Case reports	• Breast enlargement/nipple sensitivity in males • Catatonia • Delirium in association with other medications and ECT • Severe allergic reaction √ Onset may be weeks into treatment √ Edema, disseminated maculopapular eruption, stridor √ Management includes discontinuation of risperidone, antihistamine. • SIADH • Induction of mania—direct relationship to risperidone therapy not entirely established (general adult data). • Leukopenia/neutropenia • Lithium combination—acute dystonia	• Sudden death
Central and peripheral nervous system	• Emergence of symptoms increases with √ Increasing frailty √ Presence of comorbid dementia or other neurodegenerative disorders √ Increased dose • Insomnia 16% • Dizziness 5–22% • Gait disturbance—weakness and difficulty walking • Sedation 4–15% • Confusion 2% • Agitation 1–15% • New-onset EPS 11% √ Especially tremor, as well as rigidity/bradykinesia, akathesia, drooling √ Factors predictive of EPS include □ Higher dose: > 1 mg, although may emerge (less commonly) with doses in the 0.5 mg/day range. ○ Doses under 1.5 mg/day: EPS rate after 1 year in the 2–3% range ○ Higher scores on pretreatment EPS severity measures □ Renal impairment □ Older age □ DLB □ Possibly concurrent use of SSRIs, valproate, levothyroxine □ Subcortical dementia √ Risk for new-onset TD about 20% that of haloperidol	• TD may emerge (uncommon); rate not well determined. √ One study in the 2% range during year 1 of treatment. √ Single case report of emergence after brief low-dose therapy. • Emergence of akathisia after withdrawal of risperidone. • EEG abnormalities: seizure (case report data) • Burning paresthesias • Stroke and TIAs associated in demented patients.

(cont.)

Continued

Side Effects	Most Common*	Most Serious and Less Common
Endocrine		• New-onset diabetes (case reports)
Gastrointestinal	• Constipation • Abdominal cramps • Nausea	
Liver and biliary		• Elevation of liver enzymes usually after several weeks. √ Case report of rapid onset after two doses.
Metabolic and nutritional		• SIADH
Reproductive		• Ejaculatory delay • Priapism (rare)
Skin and appendages		• Photosensitivity • Rare severe skin rash (Stevens–Johnson)
Urinary		• Urinary retention

* Percentages are general adult data.

Monitoring

- Routine
  - √ BP (including orthostatic) should be monitored until stable maintenance dose established.
- Special monitoring
  - √ Blood sugars
  - √ Serum sodium

Drug Interactions

See Table 2.24 on pages 306–307 for enzyme inhibition/induction.

- Caution when coadministered with drugs that may prolong QT interval (quinidine-like effect).
- Caution with some SSRIs and valproate.
  - √ May increase serum concentrations.
- Carbamazepine may decrease risperidone levels (case report).
  - √ Theoretical implication of induction of CYP3A isoenzyme, although 2D6 is main pathway of metabolism for risperidone.
- Diuretics, ACE inhibitors, other vasodilators, calcium channel blockers, and adrenergic antagonists increase hypotension.
- Case reports (cause and effect not well established) of
  - √ Donepezil—EPS
  - √ Lithium—delirium

Disability Interactions and Contraindications

- *Caution* in demented patients with history of stoke.
  - √ Risk of stroke or TIA doubles (4% risperidone vs. 2% placebo)
    - ▫ Mechanism unknown.
- DLB relative contraindication for use of neuroleptics, including risperidone.
  - √ Has been used successfully (clinical case reports).
  - √ If used, use very low doses of 0.25–1 mg/day.
- Parkinson's: Useful for levodopa-induced psychosis but may aggravate rigidity in sensitive patients or at higher dose levels.
  - √ Occasionally improves EPS and TD.
- *Caution* in cardiac patients, especially with concurrent medications that prolong QT interval.
- Vulnerability to hypotensive effects increases with preexisting cardiac condition, volume depletion, dehydration.
- Renal insufficiency: Reduce dose to half recommended daily dose.
- Hepatic insufficiency associated with decreased plasma proteins and hence reduced protein binding of drug, causing potential increased free fraction.
  - √ Consider divided doses.
- Diabetic vulnerability—may induce new-onset diabetes.
- Caution in seizure disorders.

Overdose, Toxicity, Suicide

- Little data of any kind available.
- Case reports (general adult data) suggest little danger in overdose.
- Symptoms an exaggeration of known pharmacological effects, including
  - √ Drowsiness
  - √ Tachycardia
  - √ Hypotension
  - √ EPS
- Manage with supportive measures, as indicated
  - √ Gastric lavage plus activated charcoal.
  - √ Monitor cardiac function during first few hours after ingestion.

Clinical Tips

- Reduce cardiovascular drugs and CNS depressants to a minimum.
- Preexisting EPS may improve with risperidone.

- Some evidence for antidepressant effects.
- For hallucinations and delusions, expect somewhat delayed onset of action over about 6 weeks.
  - √ May be useful to start treatment with a typical antipsychotic, which may have a more rapid onset of action.
    - ▫ May be given alone until patient's condition stabilizes.
    - ▫ When tolerated in some patients concurrently with risperidone, reducing the typical drug dose while increasing risperidone.
    - ▫ Latter strategy more problematic in frail elders.
- Caution in Parkinson's psychosis after 3–4 months of maintenance, when parkinsonian symptoms may worsen secondary to drug effect.
- Onset of action may be within a few days up to 2–4 weeks.

THIORIDAZINE

Drug	Manufacturer	Chemical Class	Therapeutic Class
thioridazine (Mellaril)	generic	piperidine phenothiazine	antipsychotic

Indications: FDA/HPB

- Management of psychotic disorders.
- Treatment of multiple symptoms in geriatric patients.
  - √ Anxiety/fear
  - √ Agitation
  - √ Depressed mood
  - √ Tension
  - √ Sleep disturbances
- Short-term treatment of moderate to severe depression with variable degrees of anxiety in adults.
- *Note:* one of the very few medications with age-specific geriatric indications.

Pharmacology

See Table 2.2 on pages 233–234.

- Plasma concentrations may be much higher in elders by a factor of 1.5–2.
  - √ Not invariably demonstrated.
- Higher level of cholinergic receptor binding than chlorpromazine.

Mechanism of action

- Nonselective dopamine receptor antagonist.
- Alpha-adrenoreceptor antagonist.
- Binds to serotonin and histamine receptors.

Choosing a Drug

- Not suggested for routine use in dementia, despite longstanding FDA approval for this indication.
- *Note:* FDA (U.S.A.) and HPB (Canada) require special labeling for QTc prolongation (blockade of the potassium rectifier channel [I_{kr}] that may induce Torsades de Pointes).
  - √ Previously the drug of choice, widely used, and generally effective for BPSD-like symptoms and psychosis in elders.
  - √ Recommended now only as a tertiary line drug in light of cardiac dangers.
  - √ Largely replaced by atypical antipsychotics.
- Controlled data for any indication in elders sparse.
  - √ Contrary to prior practice, no empirical controlled evidence for specific advantage in dementia, aside from positive effect on anxiety.
- Advantage is low incidence of EPS.
- Disadvantage is side-effect profile of low-potency agents
  - √ Induces hypotension, sedation, quinidine-like effects.

Dosing

Initial dose

- 10–25 mg/day po, single or divided doses.

Increasing dose and reaching therapeutic levels

- Target dose 10–75 mg/day range (upper range of 200).
- doses over 75 mg associated with sedation and cognitive impairment
  - √ Not recommended for frail impaired elders.

Side Effects

See also pages 279–303 regarding anticholinergic, sedative, and cardiovascular side effects.

- Despite a wide array of low-potency side effects, generally well tolerated by elders in low doses of 25–200 mg.

Table 2.31. Side Effects of Thioridazine

Side Effects	Most Common	Most Serious and Less Common	Comments
Anticholinergic			• See page 75
Cardiovascular	• Postural hypotension	• ECG changes √ Abnormal T and U waves • Prolongation of QTc interval √ Danger of Torsades de Pointes • PVCs, ventricular arrhythmia, syncope, seizure and death (rarely)	• Torsades de Pointes can occur in otherwise normal hearts √ Associated with prolonged QT interval > 450 msec √ Generally reverts to sinus rhythm spontaneously but not always √ May progress to ventricular tachycardia, fibrillation, and arrest
Central and peripheral nervous system	• EPS, generally of low level • Dizziness √ May collapse, black out • Delirium • Cognitive impairment • Sedation (mild) • Falls		• EPS emerges with significant frequency as dose increases to the 50–75 mg range √ Increases "sway" in elders, possibly increasing predisposition to fall
Eye			• Pigmentary retinopathy in high-dose therapy not employed for elders
Gastrointestinal			• See pages 279–303
Metabolic and nutritional	• Hypothermia		

Monitoring

- Routine
  - √ ECG pretreatment monitoring.
  - √ Pretreatment eye exam.
  - √ Therapeutic plasma concentration 2–5.2 ng/ml.
- Special Monitoring
  - √ Consider ongoing ECG monitoring in light of cardiac toxicity.
  - √ Consider repeat eye exams routinely thereafter, in the very rare circumstance that thioridazine is used in high dose for long-term therapy.

Drug Interactions

- Thioridazine increases concentration of phenylpropanolamine and quinidine.
- Caution with drugs that inhibit CYP2D6 (see pp. 306–307).
- Fluvoxamine inhibits metabolism by 2C19 and 1A2.
  - √ Increases plasma concentrations significantly.
- Drugs that prolong QTc
  - √ Alcohol (hypomagnesemia)
  - √ Antiarrhythmics (class 1a and III)
    - ▫ Amiodarone
    - ▫ Bepridil
    - ▫ Disopyramide
    - ▫ Dofetilide
    - ▫ Ibutilide
    - ▫ Procainamide
    - ▫ Quinidine
    - ▫ Sotalol
  - √ Astemizole
  - √ Beta-blockers
  - √ Budesonide
  - √ Digoxin (bradycardic effects)
  - √ Diuretics (hypokalemia)
  - √ Hydrochlorothiazide diuretic
    - ▫ Hypokalemia increases risk of arrhythmias.
  - √ Moxifloxacin
  - √ Pimozide
  - √ Potassium channel blockers
  - √ Propoxyphene
  - √ Sparfloxacin
  - √ TCAs
- Antacids may decrease effectiveness of the drug—administer at least 1 hour apart.
- General cautions with
  - √ CNS depressants
    - ▫ Antihistamines
    - ▫ Barbiturates
    - ▫ Benzodiazepines/sedative hypnotics
    - ▫ Certizine
    - ▫ Clonidine
    - ▫ Cyclobenzaprine
    - ▫ Methyldopa
    - ▫ Opiates
    - ▫ Propoxyphene
    - ▫ Tramadol
  - √ Anticholinergic drugs (see Table 1.14, p. 71).

Disability Interactions and Contraindications

These are general cautions; in the small doses usually used for elders, some of these interactions are less important.

- CVS disease
  - √ Arrhythmia
  - √ Hypotension
  - √ Prolonged QT interval
  - √ Severe hypertension
- Parkinson's disease
- Seizure disorder/vulnerability
- Prostatism
- Impaired liver function
- Glaucoma
- Hypersensitivity to the drug

Overdose, Toxicity, Suicide

See pages 307–308.

THIOTHIXENE

Drug	Manufacturer	Chemical Class	Therapeutic Class
thiothixene (Navane)	Pfizer	thioxanthene	antipsychotic

Indications: FDA/HPB

- Schizophrenia and other psychotic disorders

Indications: Off label

- Agitation
- Psychosis
- Excitement and restlessness.

Pharmacology

See Table 2.2 on pages 233–234.

Choosing a Drug

- High-potency antipsychotic with low hypotensive, sedative, and anticholinergic potential.
- High EPS potential.
- Use similarly to haloperidol.

- Not recommended for long-term use because of high risk of EPS.
  - √ Useful for acute symptom control before switching to atypical agent or discontinuing the drug.

Dosing

Initial dose

- Begin with 1 mg and increase by 1 mg increments.
- Use once-a-day schedule for low doses.
- If higher doses used, administer bid or tid.

Increasing dose and reaching therapeutic levels

- Target therapeutic dose 2–10 mg/day.

Side Effects

See pages 279–303.

- Commonest side effects are drowsiness, restlessness, agitation, and insomnia.

Table 2.32. Side Effects of Thiothixene

Side Effects	Most Common	Most Serious and Less Common
Anticholinergic	• Infrequent when used in low doses	
Body as a whole	• Weakness • Fatigue	• Peripheral edema • hyperpyrexia
Cardiovascular	• Tachycardia	• Hypotension with syncope (infrequent) • Nonspecific ECG changes
Central and peripheral nervous system	• EPS, especially akathesia • Excitement • Headache	• Delirium (rarely) • TD—generally with long-term therapy on higher doses
Eye		• Lenticular pigmentation after prolonged use (unlikely in elders on short-term therapy)
Gastrointestinal		• Nausea/vomiting
Hematological		• Transient leucopenia or leukocytosis occasionally
Liver and biliary		• Asymptomatic increase in liver enzymes
Psychiatric	• Depression	• Activation of psychosis (reduce the dose)
Skin and appendages		• Rash • Pruritis • Photosensitivity

Drug Interactions

- Caution with
  - √ CNS depressants
  - √ Anticholinergic drugs

Contraindications and Special Precautions

- Contraindicated if hypersensitive to the drug.
- General cautions in
  - √ CNS depression.
  - √ Seizure disorder or significant vulnerability.
    - ▫ Withdrawal states (e.g., benzodiazepines, alcohol).
  - √ Concurrent anticholinergic drugs.

Overdose, Toxicity, Suicide

Symptoms include

- Muscular twitching
- Drowsiness
- Dizziness

Severe overdose induces

- CNS depression
- Rigidity
- Weakness
- Torticollis
- Tremor
- Salivation
- Hypotension
- Coma

Management

- Administer gastric lavage, activated charcoal.
- Induce emesis.
- Provide supportive measures (e.g., airway, oxygenation, fluids).
  - √ Monitor airway, since EPS can induce dysphagia and respiratory difficulty.
- Restore electrolyte balance.
- For hypotension
  - √ Position patient (Trendelenburg)
  - √ Administer
    - ▫ IV fluids
    - ▫ Dopamine or norepinephrine

Note: Avoid epinephrine and other pressor agents.

- Seizures: benzodiazepine (lorazepam IV).
- EPS: benztropine (maintain for 48 hours).
- Hemodialysis not useful.

ZIPRASIDONE

Drug	Manufacturer	Chemical Class	Therapeutic Class
ziprasidone (Geodon)	Pfizer	benzisothiazolyl piperazine derivative	antipsychotic

Indications: Available in United States only.

- Schizophrenia, schizophrenic acute agitation

Pharmacology

- Plasma concentrations about 20% higher in elders.
- Increased plasma concentrations with cirrhosis.
- Renal impairment does not increase plasma concentrations.

Mechanism of action

- High affinity for $5HT_{1A}$ (agonist) and D_2 (less than for $5HT_2$).
- High affinity for $5HT_{2A/2C/1B/1D}$—antagonist.
  - √ Affinity for $5HT_{2A}$ 8–11 times D_2 affinity.
  - √ Highest serotonin/dopamine ratio among atypicals.
- Moderate affinity for D_1 and alpha-1 adrenergic receptors.
- Little alpha-2, beta-adrenergic, $5HT_{3/4}$, H_1, or M_1 receptor affinities.
- Increases prolactin levels.
- Appears to inhibit neuronal reuptake of serotonin and norepinephrine comparable to antidepressants.

Choosing a Drug

- Resembles risperidone, possibly with less risk of EPS.
- IM form available, with apparent efficacy for acute agitation (general adult data) with a 10–20 mg dose.
  - √ Geriatric data not available, but dose needs downward adjustment in elders, until shown otherwise.
- Safety and effectiveness in elders not established.
  - √ Data are promising for use in agitation in dementia and case reports in agitated dementia and delirium with mood disorders associated.

General adult data re the following factors

- Little or no weight gain (in contrast to other atypicals).
- Low risk of EPS (about equal to olanzapine).
- Reduced risk of elevated plasma glucose levels.
- Increased risk of prolonged QTc interval—may be significant.
- Effective for affective and anxiety symptoms at lower doses.
- Equivalent (but not superior) efficacy for schizophrenia to conventional antipsychotics, with possibly more favorable side-effect profile and better effect on negative symptoms.
- Appears to be useful for relapse prevention in schizophrenia.
- Acute mania: Similar to risperidone, clozapine and olanzapine in outcome of treatment.
- Effective for psychotic and affective schizoaffective disorders.
  - √ Dose-dependent response.
  - √ Comparisons with other agents not yet available.

Quality of the data: Trials are all relatively short term (up to 6 months) and very little geriatric data.

Efficacy data

- No geriatric data yet.
- Several double-blind, comparative, and open label marketing studies.
- Longest study about 6 months.

Dosing

No geriatric data available yet.

Initial dose

- Schizophrenia, schizoaffective disorder 4–10 mg bid.
  - √ Estimated dose for elders; each patient is trial and error.
- Dementia (BPSD) 10 mg po (25% recommended general adult dose) daily and increase or decrease as necessary.
- Administer with food.
- IM form effective and well tolerated in adult study for control of acute symptoms.
  - √ Limited general adult data but no data or reports on elders.
    - ▫ General adult IM dose in the 10 mg range for acute psychotic agitation.
    - ▫ For elders, reduce dose to 2–5 mg as a trial intervention—but *it is trial-and-error method at this point.*

Increasing dose and reaching therapeutic levels

- General adult therapeutic dose range 120–160 mg/day.

- Age, per se, does not appear to alter pharmacokinetics such as clearance.
  - √ Pharmacodynamic factors not yet determined for elders.
  - √ Suggest 20–50% rule of thumb approach at this stage (i.e., 25–80 mg/day in divided bid doses, increasing as necessary).

Switching to ziprasidone

- Abrupt discontinuation of the first drug and immediate switch to ziprasidone without cross-taper is well tolerated in general adult populations; no geriatric data.

Side Effects

Note: Side-effect profile based on general adult data; geriatric data not available.

- IM form causes pain at injection site.
- Higher incidence of nausea and vomiting than haloperidol.
- Early studies suggest somnolence is transient.

Table 2.33. Side Effects of Ziprasidone

Side Effects	Most Common*	Most Serious and Less Common
Body as a whole	• Asthenia	
Cardiovascular		• QTc interval prolongation by 6–10 msec √ Theoretical danger of Torsades de Pointes • Orthostatic hypotension √ Unusual with oral form, may be more marked with parenteral form
Central and peripheral nervous system	• Somnolence/sedation (14%) • Dizziness • Headache	• EPS • NMS
Endocrine		• Transient hyperprolactinemia
Gastrointestinal	• Nausea/vomiting (especially with parenteral form)	
Metabolic and nutritional		• Elevation of prolactin levels √ Often temporary
Respiratory disorders	• Transient rhinitis (7–8%)	
Skin and appendages	• Pain at injection site	• Rash (usually possible to continue treatment due to spontaneous resolution)

* Percentages are general adult data.

Routine monitoring

- Routine baseline and regular ECG (especially observing QTc interval) especially during dose modifications.

Drug Interactions

- Avoid use with drugs that prolong QTc interval.
  - √ Alcohol (hypomagnesemia)
  - √ Antiarrhythmics (class Ia and III)
    - Amiodarone
    - Bepridil
    - Disopyramide
    - Dofetilide
    - Ibutilide
    - Procainamide
    - Quinidine
    - Sotalol
  - √ Astemizole
  - √ Beta-blockers
  - √ Budesonide
  - √ Digoxin (bradycardic effects)
  - √ Diuretics (hypokalemia)
  - √ Hydrochlorothiazide diuretic
    - Hypokalemia increases risk of arrhythmias.
  - √ Moxifloxacin
  - √ Pimozide
  - √ Potassium channel blockers
  - √ Propoxyphene
  - √ Sparfloxacin
  - √ TCAs
  - √ Thioridazine
- Drugs that inhibit CYP3A4.
  - √ Although not clinically significant in general adults, possibly problematic in elders.
  - √ See also, pp. 306–307
- Cimetidine induces 3A4 isoenzyme and reduces plasma concentrations by 36%.
- Ketoconazole increases plasma concentrations by 39%.
- Antihypertensive agents.
- May antagonize dopamine agonists.
- Does not inhibit CYP2D6.

Disability Interactions and Contraindications

- Metabolism not affected by mild to moderate hepatic or renal impairment.

- √ Dose adjustment in elders, based on liver and kidney functional decline with aging, may be unnecessary.
- √ Other factors may require lower doses in elders.
- *Caution* in presence of risk factors for Torsades de Pointes.
  - √ QTc interval longer than 450 msec.
  - √ History of syncopal episodes.
  - √ Concurrent drugs that inhibit metabolism of the QTc prolonging drug.
  - √ Female gender.

Overdose, Toxicity, Suicide

- No geriatric data available.
- Provide general supportive measures.
- Induce emesis in conscious patient.
  - √ Caution re. risk of aspiration.
- Consider activated charcoal with laxative.
- Monitor for cardiac arrhythmias.
- Avoid epinephrine, dopamine, and bretylium.
- Dialysis not effective.

Clinical Tips

- Administer with food.
- Prudent to monitor ECG for 6–12 months in light of uncertainty about potentially serious effects.
  - √ Torsades de Pointes.

3. Antianxiety Drugs and Sedative/Hypnotics

OVERVIEW

Anxiety and sleep disorders are treated with six classes of agents:

- Benzodiazepines (most commonly used)
- Nonbenzodiazepine sedative/hypnotics
- Buspirone
- Antidepressants (see Chapter 1)
- Beta-blockers
- Antihistamines

This chapter covers benzodiazepines, nonbenzodiazepine sedative/hypnotics, and buspirone.

- Propranolol and other relevant drugs are addressed.
- Kava and valerian are herbal compounds briefly discussed.

Barbiturates, chlordiazepoxide, and meprobamate were commonly used in the past but are no longer used or advised for elders.

- Barbiturates, because of their serious side effects, significant drug interactions, abuse potential, danger in overdose, and strong withdrawal syndromes (nightmares, anxiety, rebound insomnia, and in higher doses or abrupt withdrawal, seizure potential).
- Meprobamate has similar significant side-effect problems, including abuse potential.
- Chlordiazepoxide is generally inappropriate for these indications.
- Chloral hydrate is occasionally used but not recommended.
  - √ Side effects include withdrawal syndrome, occasionally severe, (e.g., inducing delirium) and gastric irritation.
  - √ Has a narrow therapeutic index and induces hepatic enzymes leading to drug interactions.

- Antihistamines are not recommended for elders.
  - √ They induce sleep but are anticholinergic, interact with other drugs, and rapidly become ineffective for sleep induction.

Sleep disorders and alcohol misuse are discussed in detail. Other agents used for anxiety or sleep are addressed in other chapters. Antidepressants are often more effective antianxiety agents for some conditions (e.g., panic disorder, some phobias, OCD, PTSD) than some benzodiazepines.

- Trazodone, SSRIs, and mirtazapine are covered in Chapter 1.
- Gabapentin, occasionally used for sleep (but no controlled studies), covered in Chapter 4.
- Buspirone (non-benzodiazepine anxiolytic) is discussed in this chapter.

BENZODIAZEPINES

Chemical classification

- 2-keto compounds
  - √ Inactive compounds (prodrugs) that depend on metabolism to produce active compounds.
  - √ Slow metabolism in liver by oxidation.
  - √ Long half-lives.
- 3-hydroxy compounds
  - √ Short half-lives.
  - √ Rapid metabolism in the liver by conjugation.
  - √ No active metabolites.
- Triazolo compounds
  - √ Active and inactive metabolites.
  - √ Short (or ultrashort) half-lives.
  - √ Metabolized by oxidation in the liver.

Table 3.1. Antianxiety and Sedative/Hypnotic Agents*

Generic Name (Brand Name)	High Potency	Low Potency	Antianxiety Dose (mg/day)	Hypnotic Dose (mg/day)	Comments
	SHORT- AND INTERMEDIATE-ACTING BENZODIAZEPINES*				
alprazolam (Xanax)	√		0.125–1.5 daily (bid or tid)	0.25–1	Dose of 2 mg or more produces increased sedation; usual range 0.25–0.5; interdose rebound anxiety may be a problem in some patients; interdose anxiety and withdrawal syndrome often problematic

(*cont.*)

Continued

Generic Name (Brand Name)	High Potency	Low Potency	Antianxiety Dose (mg/day)	Hypnotic Dose (mg/day)	Comments
lorazepam** (Ativan)	√		0.25–2 (divided doses)	0.25–2	Intermediate onset of action; commonly prescribed, well tolerated.
midazolam (IV or IM only) (Versed)	√				For perioperative sedation and sometimes anesthetic induction; not for routine anxiolytic or sedative use; sedative doses should be avoided outside the ICU because of the danger of respiratory and CNS depression.
oxazepam** (Serax)		√	10 (od-tid)	10–30	Slower penetration into brain may reduce utility as hypnotic (although still clinically useful); recommended for elders.
SEDATIVES/HYPNOTICS					
chloral hydrate		√		250–500	Not suggested and rarely used anymore for sleep; low therapeutic index—fatalities at double the maximum recommended therapeutic dose; tolerance develops quickly; withdrawal syndrome sometimes severe (e.g., delirium and occasionally fatal).
estazolam** (ProSom; intermediate-acting)	√			0.5 (0.5–2)	Rapid onset of action (15–30 min.), daytime sedation; not suggested for elders.
nitrazepam (Mogadon, Nitrazadon)		√		2.5 mg hs; some may require 5 mg but increased risk of adverse effects	Elimination half-life is 40% longer in elders because of larger volume of distribution; metabolizing capacity declines in alcoholic liver cirrhosis; renal insufficiency- clearance unimpaired; long half-life; accumulates with long-term dosing; not suitable for maintenance anxiety control in elders, although single dose well tolerated.

(cont.)

Continued

Generic Name (Brand Name)	High Potency	Low Potency	Antianxiety Dose (mg/day)	Hypnotic Dose (mg/day)	Comments
temazepam** (Restoril; intermediate acting)		√		15 (7.5–30)	Relatively slower absorption rate; onset of action 20–40 min.; low dose may be used in elders for time-limited sleep therapy; side-effect risks increase with higher doses.
triazolam (Halcion)*	√			0.125–0.25	Onset of action 20 min.; may provoke early A.M. awakening; ultrashort acting; not suggested for elders.
zaleplon** (Sonata; short-acting nonbenzodiazepine)		√		5–10 hs	Immediately before bed for sleep induction; short acting—not as useful for sleep maintenance.
zolpidem** (Ambien; short–intermediate-acting nonbenzodiazepine)		√		5–10 hs	Give immediately before bed; useful sleep induction and maintenance drug; little rebound.
zopiclone** (Imovane; short–intermediate-acting)		√		3.75–7.5	Rebound potential; profile similar to benzodiazepines but weaker muscle relaxant properties.
flurazepam (Dalmane; long-acting)		√		15–30	Not suggested for elders; prolonged action due to metabolite; onset of action about 30 min.; chronic administration leads to daytime sleepiness and residual impairment because of drug accumulation.
quazepam (Doral; long-acting)		√		7.5–15	Not suggested for elders; slower absorption rate; onset of action 30 min.; next-day sedation, ataxia; not typically associated with withdrawal or rebound effects.

(*cont.*)

Continued

Generic Name (Brand Name)	High Potency	Low Potency	Antianxiety Dose (mg/day)	Hypnotic Dose (mg/day)	Comments
		LONG HALF-LIFE BENZODIAZEPINES			
chlordiazepoxide (Librium)		√	5–30	5–30	Not suggested for elders; initial daily dose 5 mg and only gradually increase, with caution, to 20–30 mg/day.
clonazepam** (Klonopin, Rivotril)	√		0.25–1	0.25–2	Useful in elders; long-half life, so potential for accumulation.
clorazepate (Tranxene)		√		3.75–15	Long-acting agent not suggested for routine use in elders; little amnesic effect in normal elders (i.e., compared to lorazepam); no data on impaired or physically frail elders; combined use with primidone leads to depression, irritability, aggressive behavior.
diazepam (Valium)		√		2–5	Long-acting; accumulates with prolonged use; tolerated in single doses for acute uses but not for longer-term use; short time to onset of action in single dose.

* High-potency short half-life drugs may be associated with more severe discontinuation syndromes if stopped abruptly; also appear to carry a higher risk of dependence, although not clearly demonstrated.
** Useful for elders.

- 7-nitro compounds.
  - √ Active compound.
  - √ Long half-life.
  - √ Liver metabolism by nitroreduction and oxidation.
  - √ Metabolites inactive.

Propranolol

- Useful for control of physiological symptoms associated with anxiety.
  - √ Palpitations, tachycardia, GI upset, tremors, sweating.
    - 30–120 mg/day, po tid.
- Only marginally effective for panic and social phobia.
  - √ Rapid onset of action (Tmax 2–4 hours, general adult data).
    - Initiate at 10 mg bid po.
    - Increase in 10 mg increments, tid–qid dosing, as necessary, to dose range of 30–60 mg.

- √ Among beta-blockers, highest rates of CNS side effects.
- √ Monitor cardiovascular, respiratory, and endocrine functioning during use.
  - Monitor heart rate—<55 beats per minute is the limiting end point.
  - Diabetes—masks symptoms of hypoglycemia and increases risk of unrecognized severe insulin reaction.
  - Cardiovascular disorders
    - Contraindicated with bradyarrhythmias, asthma, CHF.
  - Caution in pulmonary insufficiency and endocrine disorders.

PHARMACOLOGY

- GABA
  - √ Inhibitory brain neurochemical that inhibits neural excitation.
  - √ $GABA_A$ receptor
    - 3 subtypes—omega 1, 2, 3
  - √ Omega 1 (Type I)
    - Mediates sedation/hypnotic effects of benzodiazepines; less likely to induce memory disturbance, tolerance, dependance.
  - √ Omega 2 (Type II)
    - Mediates anxiolytic, anticonvulsant effects
  - √ Classical benzodiazepines are GABAergic substances that interact with receptors nonselectively.
    - In contrast to selective agents (e.g., the nonbenzodiazepine zolpidem) that works only at one type of receptor site.
  - √ Benzodiazepines dampen or interfere with prefrontal dopaminergic function through their GABAergic activity and indirectly by inhibition of serotonergic and noradrenergic prefrontal influences.
  - √ Hence they decrease the acute stress response.

Relevance to elders

- Dopaminergic activity progressively declines with age.
  - √ Manifested in some as dulling of alertness, attention, memory, intellectual performance, and sexual activity.
- This dopaminergic (and, to an extent, 5HT) involution may explain why elders are less tolerant of stress and more susceptible to the side-effects of benzodiazepines.
  - √ Cognitive impairment has been associated with reduced function of both dopamine and serotonin, which can be exacerbated by benzodiazepines.

Table 3.2. Pharmacokinetics of Antianxiety and Sedative/Hypnotic Agents

Generic Name (Brand Name)	Bioavailability (%) (range)	Plasma Protein Binding (%)	Volume of Distribution (range)	Elimination Half-Life in Hours (range)	Speed of Onset of Action—T-max in Hours (range)	Absorption	Excretion	Metabolism
alprazolam (Xanax)		65–75 (mostly to albumin; general adult data)	1–1.2 l/Kg (increased in men but not women)	21 (9–37) (prolonged, especially in men)	0.8 (0.5–2.1)	Delayed by food/antacids; intermediate speed of distribution	Oral clearance 0.86 (0.4–1.84) ml/min/kg; 80% renal, 7% fecal; clearance delayed in elderly men	Oxidative metabolism mediated by CYP3A4; active metabolite alpha-hydroxy-alprazolam less active than parent compound; hydroxy-alprazolam further metabolized to the active compound demethylalprazolam; both have low plasma levels and are renally excreted after glucuronidation

(*cont.*)

Continued

Generic Name (Brand Name)	Bioavailability (%) (range)	Plasma Protein Binding (%)	Volume of Distribution (range)	Elimination Half-Life in Hours (range)	Speed of Onset of Action—T-max in Hours (range)	Absorption	Excretion	Metabolism
buspirone (BuSpar)	4 (general adult data)	> 95 to both albumin and alpha-1 acid glycoprotein (general adult data)	5.3 l/kg (general adult data)	11 (men) 7 (women)	Rapid onset—0.6–1	Rapidly absorbed; time to steady state 1 day; food may decrease absorption but improve hepatic extraction and overall, increases bioavailability; rapid speed of distribution	< 1% excreted unchanged	Presystemic extraction, hydroxylation and oxidative cleavage produce active metabolite 1-pyrimidinylpiperazine (may account for psychostimulant effect); CYP3A4 thought to mediate metabolism, but evidence is indirect
chloral hydrate		94 chloral hydrate; 70–80% trichloroethanol		8 (4–12) (general adult data) but probably longer in elders	Rapid onset—sedation in 0.5–1	Rapidly absorbed	Duration of action 4–8 hours in general adults	Alcohol dehydrogenase to active metabolite trichloroethanol

chlordiazepoxide (Librium)	100	Free fraction in males not altered by age; higher in elderly females	Significantly increased with age	30 (18–45) (up to 200) especially prolonged in males; long half-life metabolites	Intermediate—0.5–4 (general adult data)	Delayed by food/antacids; slowly distributed	Clearance reduced—0.35 ml/min.	Oxidative metabolism; active metabolites desmethylchlodiazepoxide (half-life similar to parent compound), demoxepam (half-life double parent compound), desmethyldiazepam (very prolonged half-life triple parent compound)
clobazam (Frisium)			Increased with age	48 (23–77) especially prolonged in men		Delayed by food/antacids		n-demethylation to desmethylclobazam (half-life longer than parent compound)
clonazepam (Klonopin, Rivotril)		85 (some data give lower number in the 48% range)		19–50	Intermediate speed—1–2 hours (general adult data)	Intermediate speed of distribution	Renal	Nitro-reduction; inactive metabolite

(*cont.*)

Continued

Generic Name (Brand Name)	Bioavailability (%) (range)	Plasma Protein Binding (%)	Volume of Distribution (range)	Elimination Half-Life in Hours (range)	Speed of Onset of Action—T-max in Hours (range)	Absorption	Excretion	Metabolism
clorazepate (Tranxene)			Increased with age	82; parent drug inactive; metabolites long-acting and up to 120–200 hours (general adult data)	Rapid—1–2; (general adult data)	Delayed by food/antacids; rapidly distributed in the body		Oxidation to active metabolites, including desmethyl-diazepam
diazepam (Valium)			Increased with age	90 (up to 200 for metabolite)	Rapid—1.4 (0.5–2)	Delayed by food/antacids		CYP2C19 oxidative demethylation yields active metabolite desmethyl-diazepam (half-life double parent compound); hydroxylation forms temazepam
estazolam (ProSom)		93		18 (10–34)	Rapid onset of action in 15–30 min	Rapid absorption; delayed by food/antacids;	< 5% excreted unchanged in urine	Extensively metabolized to 4-hydroxyestazolam (and 1-oxo-estazolam, to a lesser extent); neither clinically significantly active

flurazepam (Dalmane)				120–160 (mostly the result of prolonged half-life of long acting metabolite)	0.5–1	Delayed by food/antacids		Oxidation to active metabolites hydroxyethylflurazepam (short half-life) desalkylflurazepam (major metabolite, very long half-life), and desmethyldiazepam
lorazepam (Ativan)	100	89	Unchanged with age 0.99 l/kg	16 (7–37)	Intermediate speed—1–6	Delayed by food/antacids; intermediate speed of distribution	Lower clearance 0.77 ml/min/kg	Glucuronidation
midazolam (Versed) (injectable and syrup only)	Bioavailability incomplete; absolute availability in men higher than young adults	97; free fraction not affected by age	0.8–1.7 l/kg	5.6 (1–10) (shorter in women)			Clearance 1–4.4 ml/min/kg	Oral administration: Significant first-pass metabolism with intestinal extraction by 3A isoenzymes; liver metabolism—metabolized by CYP3A4 to l-methylhydroxymidazolam; active, but half-life shorter than parent compound and therefore does not prolong drug action

(cont.)

Continued

Generic Name (Brand Name)	Bioavailability (%) (range)	Plasma Protein Binding (%)	Volume of Distribution (range)	Elimination Half-Life in Hours (range)	Speed of Onset of Action—T-max in Hours (range)	Absorption	Excretion	Metabolism
nitrazepam (Mogadon, Nitrazadon)			1.96 l/kg; increased with age	38 (26–64) 40% prolonged because of larger volume of distribution		Rapidly absorbed; delayed by food/antacids	0.84 ml/min/kg; clearance unchanged by age but 30% lower with cirrhosis	Nitro-reduction, metabolite not active
oxazepam (Serax)		96	Unchanged with age	8–10 (5–25) (unchanged in elders)	Slow—2–4 hours	Delayed by food/antacids; intermediate speed of distribution	70–80% excreted by kidneys; clearance unchanged in elders	Glucuronide conjugation; inactive metabolite
propranolol (Inderal, Ipran)				3.6				Metabolite 4-OH-propranolol (very short half-life of 20 min.)
quazepam (Doral)				53 (40–140 for active metabolite)	Rapid onset of action 30 min	Delayed by food/antacids;		Oxidation to active metabolites N-desalkyl-2-oxoflurazepam and 2-oxoquazepam; accumulates overnight; associated with CNS depression

temazepam (Restoril)			Unchanged with age	Biphasic; short half-life about 1 hour; terminal half-life in healthy elderly men 8; women 13–30; elderly inpatients 16 (8–38)	Rapid onset of action in 20–40 min	Delayed by food/antacids;	Elimination not affected by age in men but increased in women; clearance spared in liver disease	Principally metabolized by glucuronide conjugation
triazolam (Halcion)		75–80		1.7–5 (ultrashort-acting)	Males 0.5–6 hours; females 0.5–1.5			CYP3A oxidative metabolism to inactive methylhydroxytriazolam and 4-hydroxytriazolam
zaleplon (Sonata; nonbenzodiazepine)	30		1.27 l/kg (large)	1–2	Rapid—1	Fatty food with, or immediately after, a dose delays absorption by about 1 hour; maximum concentrations reduced by 35%	Total clearance 194–266 l/h	CYP3A4 and aldehyde oxidative metabolism; inactive metabolite 5-oxo-zaleplon

(*cont.*)

Continued

Generic Name (Brand Name)	Bioavailability (%) (range)	Plasma Protein Binding (%)	Volume of Distribution (range)	Elimination Half-Life in Hours (range)	Speed of Onset of Action—T-max in Hours (range)	Absorption	Excretion	Metabolism
zolpidem (Ambien; nonbenzodiazepine)	70	92 (slightly less in cirrhosis and renal failure but clinical significance unlikely)	Low (0.54–0.68 l/kg)	2.9 (geriatric) (1.5–3.2 range—general adult data)	Rapid—2 (range 0.75–2.6)	Maximum concentrations somewhat higher in elderly women compared to men; food increases absorption time and delays onset of sedative effects	Oral clearance 0.24–0.27 ml/min/kg (general adult data); clearance of metabolites largely renal; < 1% excreted unchanged	CYP3A4, 2C9, and 1A2 (2D6 and 2C19 minor contributors) oxidative metabolism to inactive metabolites; carboxylic acids and hydroxylation to metabolite X
zopiclone (Imovane) (Nonbenzodiazepine)	94	45 (general adult data)	Widely distributed	7–8	0.5–3.0 (general adult data)	Well absorbed	Metabolites cleared in urine, feces (7–10% unchanged) and lungs (50% as CO_2)	CYP 3A4 and 2C8; active metabolite-N-oxide-zopiclone has lower pharmacological activity but similar half-life as parent compound; other metabolite, n-desmethyl-zopiclone inactive

Table 3.3. Metabolism of Benzodiazepines

Drug	Comments on Metabolism
	Long-acting Benzodiazepines
bromazepam chlordiazepoxide clobazam clonazepam clorazepate diazepam flurazepam loprazolam lormetazepam prazepam quazepam	Metabolized by phase 1 *oxidative metabolism in liver.* • Not suggested for elders. • This system produces active metabolites of some drugs (although not all are clinically relevant). • Is more affected by age-related reduction in efficiency. √ Reduced clearance and prolonged half-lives. • Plasma levels of long-acting drugs higher in elders; highly protein bound and therefore free fraction increases with reduction in plasma proteins with age. • Effects of age on prolonging metabolism and increasing plasma levels are especially pronounced in males.
	Intermediate-acting Benzodiazepines
lorazepam oxazepam temazepam	Metabolized by phase II *glucuronidation.* • Does not produce active metabolites. • Is not affected by age-related changes. • Plasma levels of short- or intermediate-acting drugs not higher in elders. • Generally do not accumulate over time. • Renal disease impairs excretion and requires dose reduction. • Obesity: increased volume of distribution and clearance but half-life unchanged.
alprazolam estazolam halazepam	Metabolized by oxidative metabolism subject to age-related changes. • Active metabolites (except estazolam) • alprazolam—severe withdrawal and dependency • estazolam—highly lipid soluble (not suggested for elders)
	Short-acting Benzodiazapines
midazolam triazolam	Metabolized by oxidative metabolism

In single-dose treatments, do not confuse duration of action with half life (i.e., short half-life drugs do not necessarily have short duration of action and long half-life drugs do not necessarily have long duration of action).

Key determinants of rate of onset and duration of action

- Rate of absorption
- Rate of distribution
  - √ Highly lipophilic drugs (diazepam, flurazepam, quazepam)
    - ▫ Reduced duration of action because of distribution into adiposetissue
      - ◦ With prolonged use drug accumulates in body tissue leading to prolonged effects.
    - ▫ Cross blood-brain barrier more quickly leading to more rapid onset of action
    - ▫ Have higher brain clearance rate
  - √ Less lipophilic drugs (e.g. lorazepam)
    - ▫ Slower onset of action

- longer duration of action of *single* dose
  - Effective brain concentrations persist longer because of reduced peripheral tissue distribution

Clinical characteristics and efficacy of benzodiazepines

- All benzodiazepines exert five major actions (to slightly varying degrees):
  - √ Hypnotic
  - √ Anxiolytic
  - √ Anticonvulsant
  - √ Muscle relaxant
  - √ Amnesic
    - Effects proportional to amount of receptor occupancy of drug.
    - Elders more sensitive to effects at receptor sites, especially in the presence of brain disease (e.g., dementia, Parkinson's disease, CVA).
- All benzodiazepine agents are equally effective anxiolytics.
  - √ Rapid onset
    - Immediate effects are sedative rather than antianxiety effect per se.
  - √ Highly effective
  - √ Selection of a drug is based on elimination half-life, with shorter-acting agents preferred.
  - √ Panic disorder
    - High-potency drugs preferred (e.g., alprazolam, clonazepam).
    - Low-potency drugs too sedating.
  - √ Generally have low level of toxicity.
- All benzodiazepines act on all subtypes of benzodiazepine receptors.
  - √ Explains broad spectrum of action (i.e., myorelaxant, antianxiety, anticonvulsant, and sedative).

Note: Data on dosing and effects in elders are often extrapolated from younger populations.

GERIATRIC ISSUES

Prescription Patterns

- Elders (especially women) are overrepresented by as much as 2:1 as users of benzodiazepines.
- 40–50% of benzodiazepine prescriptions are written for elders, especially women.

- 33% of long-term benzodiazepine users are elderly.
- In one study, majority of elderly benzodiazepine users took the drug daily, with the proportion increasing with advancing age.
  - √ Many elders take more than the manufacturer's suggested therapeutic dose.
- Elders tend to use benzodiazepines for longer duration than younger adults.
- 6–16% of community-dwelling elders report taking benzodiazepines.
  - √ Three-quarters for > 1 year; women > men.

Self-reported use not always reliable; many patients prescribed benzodiazepines do not take them or do so intermittently; conversely, some deny or do not report use when they are taking benzodiazepines (general adult data).

- Long-term use more common in elders, despite guidelines recommending shorter courses of treatment with benzodiazepines.
  - √ In one study 30% of elders prescribed benzodiazepines took them for > 30 consecutive days.
- Figures are higher in nursing homes/institutions, where benzodiazepines may be overprescribed.
  - √ Higher rates in residents admitted from hospital.
- Prescribing patterns reflect shift to shorter-acting drugs (alprazolam, lorazepam).
- Elders receive large amounts of drug in each prescription (in one study 180 or more in 36% of prescriptions) compared with younger groups.
  - √ Creates problems with prolonged use, overuse because of availability, and poor monitoring due to infrequent reevaluation of prescribed dose.
- Anxiolytics often prescribed inappropriately for depressive symptoms, rather than more appropriate antidepressant regimens.

Using Anxiolytics in Elders

Managing anxiety disorders in elders begins with careful assessment and differential diagnosis, especially for causes of secondary anxiety (see Table 3.6, p. 398).

- History taking
  - √ Past illnesses (e.g., relapsing panic)
  - √ Medication
  - √ Substance use
    - ▫ Especially alcohol, which is a marker of abuse potential for benzodiazepines and potentiates adverse effects.

- √ Family history
  - ▫ Especially for panic and depressive disorders.
- Symptoms and signs of anxiety include
  - √ Subjective experience of dread, demoralization, depression
  - √ Motor tension/tremor
  - √ Restlessness
  - √ Irritability
  - √ Fatigue
  - √ Tension headache
  - √ Swallowing difficulty ("lump" in throat)
  - √ Sweating/flushing/chills
  - √ Tachycardia
  - √ SOB
  - √ Dry mouth
  - √ Dizziness
  - √ GI problems (i.e., nausea, vomiting)
  - √ Urinary frequency
  - √ Hyperalertness
  - √ Increased startle reflex
  - √ Insomnia
- Require full physical examination, especially for causes of secondary anxiety.
- Order laboratory tests
  - √ CBC, urinalysis Vitamin B_{12}, folate, ECG, TSH, FBS, electrolytes, adrenal, liver and kidney function tests, sometimes blood gases if indicated, toxicology screen as indicated.
- Assess impact of symptoms to determine if medication therapy is indicated.
- Identify and correct underlying causes of secondary anxiety.
- Identify and address psychosocial stressors.
  - √ Often requires specific psychotherapeutic interventions (e.g., counseling, support, CBT, IPT, or insight-oriented therapy).
    - ▫ Psychotherapy commonly indicated as primary or adjunctive intervention for anxiety associated with adaptational issues, external stresses, or vulnerability to anxiety rooted in personality disorder.
  - √ Implement environmental and psychosocial changes.
    - ▫ Provide sleep hygiene education, and clear information about procedures and what to expect.
    - ▫ Encourage family support, predictable routines, and strong therapeutic relationships.
    - ▫ Teach relaxation techniques.
- Some data indicate that psychotherapeutic approaches (e.g., CBT) are the most effective treatments for generalized anxiety.
  - √ Benzodiazepines may *reduce* its efficacy.

- A range of drugs is indicated, including antidepressants (usually SSRIs, venlafaxine XR, or bupropion), buspirone, benzodiazepines, propranolol, anticonvulsants (gabapentin), and sometimes antipsychotics for severe anxiety states and agitation associated with cognitive impairment.
  - √ Panic disorder may require ongoing treatment, especially with SSRIs.
    - ▫ Clinical reports in 60-year-olds of use of imipramine and alprazolam in panic suggest equal effectiveness of both.
    - ▫ Good studies of benzodiazepines in older adults for this indication lacking.

Benzodiazepine Therapy

- Use of benzodiazepines depends on patient factors and the indication for which the drug is prescribed.
- Advantages of this class are its
  - √ Rapid onset of action
  - √ Effectiveness
  - √ Relative nontoxicity compared to many other agents
    - ▫ Although there are significant problems that need to be avoided.
- Oral drugs of choice in elders
  - √ Lorazepam, oxazepam, temazepam, and alprazolam
  - √ Observe for interdose anxiety and rapid development of tolerance.
- Parenteral drugs of choice in elders
  - √ Midazolam or lorazepam
  - √ Use IV-IM
    - ▫ Painful and absorption unpredictable
- *Note:* Many guidelines for benzodiazepine use in younger adults recommend longer-acting agents (diazepam, nitrazepam, flurazepam, clorazepate) for next-day sedation and anxiolysis.
  - √ Inadvisable for elders, although not many studies of this form of acute use.
- Buspirone
  - √ Safe and well tolerated in anxiety and mixed anxiety–depression disorders
    - ▫ Little adverse effect on cognition and psychomotor performance.
- Beta-blockers—nonselective blockers (propranolol, pindolol, timolol) and cardioselective beta-1 agents (atenolol, acebutolol, metoprolol)
  - √ Do not address anxiety per se but blunt autonomic physiological responses, especially tachycardia and sweating.

- √ Avoid in cardiovascular disease, and avoid nonselective blockers in asthma and COPD.
- √ Cardioselective beta-1 agents preferred in pulmonary disease and diabetes.
  - ▫ Less interference with glycogenesis and physiological symptoms of hypoglycemia.
  - ▫ Such interference may be dangerous if patient remains unaware of problem until BS levels are very low.

- Usually treatment with benzodiazepines is short term.
  - √ Recommended for 2–4 weeks.
    - ▫ Longer therapy often required for states of chronic anxiety or refractory states (e.g., depression, personality disorders).
    - ▫ Duration of therapy is short for stress-induced anxiety (precise guidelines scarce; 4 months maximum suggested, followed by gradual taper) or when used as adjunct for depression (4 weeks).
  - √ Treatment is indicated if daily performance is impaired by anxiety or internal dysphoria is excessive.
- Long-term treatment is sometimes necessary.
  - √ Chronic primary anxiety (e.g., GAD) often treated with long-term benzodiazepine therapy.
    - ▫ Discontinuation very difficult because of patients' psychological dependence and fear of rebound anxiety.
  - √ Patients often continue to benefit from long-term use.
  - √ Best strategy is to reduce dose to minimum tolerated and continue, often in combination with other agents such as antidepressants.
  - √ Usually safe, but regular monitoring is essential part of safe management.
    - ▫ Look for cognitive change, gait instability.
    - ▫ Reduce dose as necessary.
  - √ Consider a nonbenzodiazepine alternative such as buspirone.
  - √ With repeated doses, long-acting agents accumulate in lipid tissue with increased adverse effects.
  - √ Despite cautions, evidence suggests tolerance to side effects develops over time.
    - ▫ Many elders who take sedatives chronically do not suffer from theoretically expected side effects.
  - √ Although the clinical significance is unclear, chronic benzodiazepine administration produces immunological changes (i.e., changes in lymphocytes and cytotoxicity) similar in direction to the natural changes that occur with aging (as well as those that occur during unresolved stress situations).
  - √ During chronic use, sometimes over years, the health and metabolic status of elders can decline.

- Requires ongoing monitoring for gradual or sudden changes in tolerance to drug and dose reduction or discontinuation, as necessary.

Table 3.4. Guidelines for Using Benzodiazepines for Antianxiety

1. Use for shortest time possible.
2. Use lowest effective dose.
3. Short-acting agents preferred, but *avoid* ultrashort-acting agents (e.g., triazolam).
4. Monitor adverse effects, especially sedation, falling, and cognitive impairments.
5. Be cautious with concurrent psychotropics, especially those with sedative actions.
6. Use caution in patients with history of alcoholism or other substance abuse.
7. Caution in hospitalized patients; increased risk of delirium/cognitive impairment.
8. Discontinue as soon as feasible.
9. Taper slowly to avoid discontinuation syndromes.
10. Long-term, maintenance use sometimes necessary, with careful monitoring.

Dosing

See Table 3.1 on pages 372–375.

- Begin at lowest effective and tolerated dose.
  - √ Most elders require reduced doses.
  - √ Consider reduced dose in elderly men (compared with women) until patients' response to drug known.
- Increase dose slowly, with careful side-effect monitoring, until desired therapeutic effects attained.
- When intermediate-acting agents used, patients who metabolize drugs more quickly (i.e., similar to general adults) may require bid or tid dosing to produce day-long antianxiety effects.
- Dose increase may be necessary to achieve anxiolysis in patients taking concurrent antiseizure medication (e.g., barbiturates, phenytoin).
- Drug effects begin after first dose and may increase until steady state.

Table 3.5. Advising Patient and Family about Benzodiazepines

1. Educate re target symptoms of treatment.
2. Describe dosing schedule, including maximum daily doses, importance of not doubling up on dose, and of taking sedatives on empty stomach.
3. Explain potential benefits as well as limitations of expectations—for example, drug may reduce lag time to sleep but does not eliminate it; it may add to sleep duration but the increase in total sleep time may be modest.
4. Explain risks (cognitive impairment [usually mild], daytime sedation, falls, impaired reflexes and performance [driving car or crossing streets].
5. Explain risks of abrupt withdrawal—for example, seizures.
6. Warn re drug interactions, especially alcohol ("One drink feels like three").
7. Describe expected course of treatment—time-limited, depending on symptom course, emerging tolerance, and reduced effectiveness.
8. Inform who to call, and when, if adverse effects occur.
9. Monitor the schedule by seeing patient regularly.

Efficacy and Tolerability

Effectiveness of benzodiazepines in elders

- All benzodiazepines are equally effective for anxiety states.
  - √ Base choice of drug on side-effect profile.
- Effective in panic disorder, GAD, anxiety symptoms associated with social phobia, acute situational anxiety.
  - √ Panic best addressed by alprazolam or clonazepam.
- Alprazolam may be preferred for anxiety associated with depression.
- Social phobia amenable to a variety of treatments, including clonazepam or alprazolam, but SSRIs, phenelzine, or buspirone are more effective (general adult data).

Tolerability in elders

- Studies of utility versus adverse-effect potential do not exist.
  - √ Commonly stated positions re overprescription seem to be more presumptive than evidence-based.
- When given in the presence of comorbid dementia, benzodiazepines are a common cause of excess morbidity.
- Sensitivity to adverse effects are a function of age and dose.
  - √ Controlled trial evidence of age-related decline in adaptive capacity to inhibit adverse drug effects and of increased drug-sensitivity in elders.
- Increased sensitivity to clinical and toxic effects of benzodiazepines in elders probably related to
  - √ Less ability than younger adults to overcome drug-induced impairments in problem solving and other tasks, even at low doses.
    - ▫ Impairments become evident much earlier than they do with younger adults.
  - √ Less reserve capacity for dealing with cognitive tasks requiring psychomotor speed.
  - √ Impairment more long-lasting than it is in younger adults, especially at higher doses.
    - ▫ Impairment becomes more evident as task demands increase.
  - √ Altered pharmacokinetics/dynamics.
    - ▫ Cerebral end organ sensitivity.
    - ▫ Prolonged half-lives of those anxiolytics metabolized by hepatic oxidation.
  - √ Presence of disease states (e.g., hepatic, neurological).
  - √ Drug interactions
    - ▫ Polypharmacy common in elders.
    - ▫ Example: interference of hepatic metabolism by fluoxetine,

antineoplastic drugs, H_2-blocking drugs, steroids, additive effects of other CNS depressant/sedating drugs.

- √ Increased sensitivity cannot be explained on the basis of prolonged metabolism rates, increased half-life, or higher plasma levels alone.
  - ▫ May be associated with changes in the benzodiazepine-$GABA_A$ receptor.

- Long-term treatment may induce benzodiazepine sensitization process that worsens progression of disease over time.
- Fairly well documented that the best tolerated drugs for longer duration of use are shorter-acting agents (e.g., lorazepam, oxazepam, and possibly alprazolam), but this is no guarantee they will not produce a hangover effect or be associated with increased risks (e.g., hip fracture).
  - √ Oxazepam especially indicated in the most sensitive patients.
  - √ For single dose, may use long-acting agents.
    - ▫ Diazepam or quazepam probably safe and effective.
    - ▫ They accumulate over time and are not suggested for routine longer-term use.

Compliance

- Otherwise well elders seem to use benzodiazepines responsibly, tolerate them well, and do not escalate doses.
- Poor compliance usually underdosing.
  - √ Cognitive impairment may lead to forgetting to take prescribed doses or, less commonly, to make up for missed doses by taking a few at a time.
  - √ Sometimes elders will take an extra middle-of-the-night dose if they cannot sleep.
    - ▫ Best to warn patients about the dangers of doing this, since peak plasma levels at night are associated with increased psychomotor impairment and risk of falls.

Cognitive effects

- Some tolerance to chronic treatment develops in elders, but less so than in younger adults.
- Clinical relevance of impairment not uniform; it is more problematic in already cognitively impaired elders, whereas others may tolerate effects better.
- Reliability of elders self-rated sedation is questionable.
  - √ External observers tend to rate sedation effects higher than patients themselves.
- Relationship of performance to plasma drug levels.
  - √ Plasma levels and half-life measures do not correlate well with drug-induced memory impairments (see Table 3.2, p. 377).

ANXIETY DISORDERS

- Anxiolytic agents are indicated if symptoms are significant and not controlled by addressing precipitating or underlying factors or disorders.
- Anxiety disorders are often hidden or do not come to clinical attention, especially in community-dwelling elders.
- Anxiety disorders usually begin in early adulthood, often becoming chronic in a pattern of remission and relapse, continuing into old age.
- Unusual for a new-onset primary anxiety disorder to present in late life, except for agoraphobia.

Panic Disorder (With and Without Agoraphobia)

See also page 39.

- In elderly samples, < 0.5% period prevalence.
  - √ 0.9% prevalence in geriatric patients in inpatient and outpatient clinic settings.
- Depression often comorbid and may be associated with new-onset panic in late-life.
- Late onset panic associated with more SOB, COPD, medical disorders.
- One-third to one-half of patients with chest pain in presence of normal coronary arteries have panic symptoms.
  - √ Often associated with prior history of depression (mixed age data).
  - √ Occurs in 5–8% of patients with mitral valve prolapse.
  - √ Typical anginal pain and coronary artery disease not associated with panic disorder.
- Clinical reports suggest new-onset panic also may emerge associated with stroke, hip fracture, COPD, bereavement, retirement.
- Complications of inadequately treated panic disorder include
  - √ Suicide
  - √ Depression
  - √ Alcohol abuse
  - √ Increased cardiovascular mortality in males (general adult data)

Treatment

- SSRIs are treatment of choice.
  - √ Nortriptylene also effective.
- Most benzodiazepines ineffective in blocking panic.

- √ Alprazolam and Clonazepam are exceptions.
  - ▫ Alprazolam effective over a range of doses 1–5 mg/day.
    - ◦ Short duration of action may induce inter-dose panic.
    - ◦ Severe withdrawal symptoms including panic.
    - ◦ Discontinue very slowly 0.125 mg q 1–2 weeks.
  - ▫ Clonazepam
    - ◦ Dose 1–2 mg/d hs
    - ◦ Sedating
    - ◦ May be depressogenic
- √ Buspirone ineffective.
- Benzodiazepine may be combined with SSRI.
  - √ If effective, the anxiolytic is tapered while SSRI is continued for 1.5–2 years.
  - √ CBT is integrated into the overall treatment plan.
- High-potency drugs preferred for panic.
  - √ Alprazolam and clonazepam are effective.
  - √ Low-potency drugs too sedating.
- Clonazepam preferred as an adjunct to SSRIs.
  - √ Shows little interdose rebound, faster onset of action, less severe withdrawal, and favorable dosing schedule (bid instead of tid or qid).

Phobias (Agoraphobia, Specific, Social)

- 6-month prevalence of 10–19%.
- Commonly comorbid with depression.
- Social phobia remains chronic and persistent in old age.
- Higher psychiatric and medical comorbidity in elders.
- Elders rarely seek help.

Phobias may emerge acutely, secondary to other age-related disorders and problems, such as

- Physical attack/mugging
- Falls
- Sense of danger in the environment (e.g., changing quality of the neighborhood, weather)
- Physical frailty

Agoraphobia

- Prevalence of 8%.
- Rarely associated with panic in elders.
- Fears often realistic.
  - √ Fear of going out at night.
  - √ Fear of victimization.
- Associated with significant social impairment.
- Early parental loss may be predisposing factor.

- Not generally responsive to medication.
  - √ Acute anxiety associated with agoraphobia may respond to alprazolam.
    - ▫ SSRIs sometimes effective.
- Psychotherapy, including exposure and deconditioning, better than medication in general adults but utility in elders not well investigated yet.

Social phobia

- SSRIs effective.
- Clinical data suggest utility for clonazepam 0.5 mg/day and buspirone 15 mg tid (general adult data).
  - √ Data are sparse and best viewed as anecdotal.
- MAOIs (irreversible and reversible) may be effective.
- Propranolol may be useful adjunct in more refractory situations, with appropriate caution.
  - √ Not recommended in physically frail elders
  - √ Administer about 2 hours before stressful event or known anxiety trigger.
- CBT or other psychotherapy usually important in treatment.

Specific phobia

- Benzodiazepines generally not useful.

Obsessive–Compulsive Disorder (OCD)

- Incidence in elders 0.8%.
  - √ 1.5% 6-month and 2–3% lifetime prevalence reported.
- Onset usually in younger years, persisting into late life.
- Symptoms include contamination fears, self-doubts (fear of harming others), rituals (checking, counting, washing).
- Comorbidities common with OCD.
  - √ Obsessional ruminations associated with depression.
  - √ Risk of anxiety disorder (panic, GAD, phobia).
  - √ Treatment is with SRI, often in high dose (see p. 38).
  - √ Alcohol abuse.
- Management
  - √ Complete medical evaluation.
  - √ SSRIs are drugs of choice.
    - ▫ Clomipramine if SSRI fails. Increase dose to target range of 100–200 mg/day.
  - √ Case reports of response to
    - ▫ ECT for OCD with depression
    - ▫ Venlafaxine
    - ▫ TCA
  - √ Benzodiazepines alone not effective for this indication.

Posttraumatic Stress Disorder (PTSD)

See also page 41.

- May emerge de novo in old age or persist for many years into old age (e.g., Holocaust, war, torture, combat, or personal-injury survivors).
- Benzodiazepines may be useful for managing discrete situations of anxiety or hyperarousal, but they are adjunctive medications for this condition.
- Many drugs have been tried for PTSD: for repetitive trauma, GABAergic agents (e.g., tiagabine, valproate, topiramate, carbamazepine); for single episode trauma, SSRIs.
- Partial successes, but none definitive.

Generalized Anxiety Disorder (GAD)

See also page 40.

- Sometimes starts after age 65; may be more common in women.
- Symptoms include excessive anxiety/worry, plus at least three additional symptoms (e.g., restlessness, fatigue, impaired concentration, irritability, sleep disturbance).
  - √ New-onset anxiety in late life usually associated with depression or dysthymia.
  - √ 35% of elders with major depression have at least one lifetime diagnosis of anxiety disorder.
    - ▫ 20–36% have current diagnosis. May be mimicked by anxiety associated with medical conditions (CVS, pulmonary, thyroid, neurological disorders).
- Treatment
  - √ Benzodiazepines are not recommended as first-line therapy because of need for long-term treatment and dangers of side effects, as well as dependence, in elders. However, they are often necessary and are used commonly. If used, try
    - ▫ Lorazepam 0.5–1 mg bid–tid
    - ▫ Clonazepam 0.5–1 mg/day
    - ▫ Buspirone 5–20 mg (tid especially effective in benzodiazepine-naïve patients).
      - ◦ May also address comorbid depressive symptoms, if present.
- When used for anxiety associated with depression
  - √ Benzodiazepines improve speed of onset of response in first few weeks of therapy by reducing anxiety (general adult data but relevant to elders).
    - ▫ The benefit is not better than placebo after 4 weeks.
    - ▫ When an anxiolytic is used in depression, best to tapered it as soon as possible.

- Effective agents include
  - √ Paroxetine
  - √ Mirtazapine (early general data).
  - √ Gabapentin may be useful adjunct (no geriatric data).
  - √ CBT

Anxiety Disorder Due to a General Medical Condition

See Table 3.6.

Substance-Induced Anxiety Disorder

See Table 3.6.

Secondary Anxiety

Table 3.6. Causes of Secondary Anxiety

Primary Condition Leading to Secondary Anxiety	Comments
Neurological • Dementia—BPSD; reversal of diurnal cycle • Small stroke • TIA • Parkinson's disease • Catatonia • Akathisia • Encephalopathy • Mass lesion • Postconcussion syndrome	• Anxiety disorder occurs frequently with dementia in a sporadic manner and is often associated with concurrent depression. • BPSD often presents as agitation/sleep disturbance. • Dementing disorders in the presence of unmanageable, challenging tasks may induce panic and anxious uncertainty.
Depressive disorders	• Commonest comorbid condition in new-onset late life anxiety; anxiety usually resolves with treatment of depression, but may persist (ongoing anxiety is a prognostic marker for increased rate of relapse or recurrence of depression); anxiolytics are used as adjunctive or augmenting agents of antidepressants.
Psychotic disorders	• Anxiolytics are adjunctive to antipsychotic drugs.
Personality disorders	• Benzodiazepines are adjunctive therapy for sleep and intermittent situational anxiety/panic; heightened potential for abuse; may induce behavioral disinhibition.
Age-related psychological factors and reactions that induce anxiety	• Poor physical health. • Economic worries. • Abandonment, fears of loss of spouse, family, or other supports. • Death anxiety. • Overwhelming day-to-day tasks that exceed cognitive or physical capacity. • Relocation to long-term care setting.

(cont.)

Continued

Primary Condition Leading to Secondary Anxiety	Comments
Grief	• Anxiety associated with psychological factors and/or emergence of depression.
Delirium	• See p. 252.
Substance use, abuse, and withdrawal	• Increased risk of benzodiazepine abuse in this group, although few geriatric data.
Endocrine disorders • Hyperthyroidism • Less commonly √ Hypothyroidism √ Hypoglycemia √ Pheochromocytoma √ Hypoparathyroidism	• Anxiety-like symptoms include trembling, increased startle, tachycardia or hyperreflexia; high rates in diabetics.
Metabolic conditions • Hyperkalemia • Hyperthermia • Hyponatremia • Hypoxia • Porphyria	
Immunologic conditions • Anaphylaxis • SLE	
Cardiovascular and pulmonary disorders • Silent MI • CHF • Cardiac arrhythmia- VPCs, atrial tachycardia • Pulmonary embolus • Pneumothorax • Pulmonary edema • COPD • Asthma • Angina pectoris • Valvular disease	• Anxiety in 70–80% of ICU patients, especially monitored or ventilated patients; symptoms include dread, bewilderment, weakness, dizziness, respiratory distress, sweating; rate of panic disorder high (34%) in patients with chest pain and normal coronary arteries, idiopathic cardiomyopathy, asthma, and COPD (general adult data) IV lorazepam or midazolam suggested.
Gastrointestinal disorders • Peptic ulcer disease • Irritable bowel syndrome	• High rates of association between anxiety and GI disease (e.g., irritable bowel syndrome), but cause and effect not yet clarified.
Drugs and stimulants • Anticholinergics • Antidepressants • Antihypertensives (reserpine, hydralazine) • Antipsychotics (akathisia) • Antitubercular agents (isoniazid, cycloserine) • Benzodiazepines • Bronchodilators/sympathomimetics (isoproterenol, theophylline) • Digitalis toxicity • Calcium channel blockers (verapamil, nifedipine, diltiazem) • L-dopa • Lidocaine • MAOIs • Methyldopa	• Drug use/misuse/withdrawal (e.g., alcohol/amphetamines/nicotine/excess caffeine/cocaine, marijuana, narcotics) may induce anxiety. As little as 1.5 cups of coffee (150 mg of caffeine) can induce anxiety or even panic; cocaine, marijuana, narcotics use rare in elders. However, some drug use is culturally determined and may be more common in elders from those groups (e.g., khat buds and leaves contain excitatory ephedrine-like substance; chewing common in many African and Arabic societies and practiced by immigrants to North America).

(*cont.*)

Continued

Primary Condition Leading to Secondary Anxiety	Comments
• Methylphenidate • Methysergide • Monosodium glutamate • Nicotinic acid • Nonprescription drugs (containing adrenergic agents such as ephedrine, amphetamines, pseudoephedrine, phenylpropanolamine) • Procarbazine • Quinidine • Sedative/hypnotic withdrawal effects • SSRIs • Steroids • Thyroid hormone • Tricyclics	

OTHER CONDITIONS WHERE BENZODIAZEPINES MAY BE USED

- Mania
  - √ Clonazepam, lorazepam effective (general adult data).
  - √ Used for early tranquillization before primary treatment (i.e., valproate or lithium) takes effect.
- Sleep disorders (see p. 411)
  - √ Insomnia
  - √ REM sleep disorder.
  - √ Sleep-related abnormal periodic limb movements (e.g., nocturnal myoclonus).
- Perioperative sedation/anesthesia induction
  - √ Lorazepam 1–2 mg IV/IM
  - √ Midazolam 1 mg infused over 2 min. with additional 1 mg increments to a maximum of 3–3.5 mg (lower doses may be necessary in physically frail elders).
- Nonpsychotropic uses
  - √ Tinnitus (alprazolam)
  - √ Nausea/vomiting associated with chemotherapy (e.g., lorazepam).
  - √ Phantom limb pain.
  - √ Restless leg syndrome.
  - √ Motor symptoms associated with
    - ▫ NMS
    - ▫ Neuroleptic-induced catatonia
    - ▫ Catatonia associated with schizophrenia, affective disorders, alcoholism, combined cerebellar and brainstem atrophy (lorazepam 2 mg IM).
    - ▫ Akathisia

SIDE EFFECTS

- Benzodiazepines and benzodiazepine-receptor agonists generally safe and well tolerated if
  - √ The correct drug is used judiciously.
  - √ The patient is accurately diagnosed.
  - √ Indications are clearly defined.
  - √ Doses are appropriate.
  - √ Drug is used for appropriate lengths of time.
  - √ End points are clearly defined.
- Clinical monitoring especially advisable with long half-life agents.
  - √ Side effects may emerge only after steady state achieved.
  - √ Short half-life agents also pose increased risks of side effects, such as hip fracture due to falling.
  - √ Dose and duration of use more than half-life may be more critical.
- Commonest side effects of benzodiazepines include
  - √ Sedation
  - √ Fatigue
  - √ Weakness
  - √ Headache
  - √ Confusion
  - √ Dizziness
  - √ Impaired coordination
  - √ Agitation
  - √ Tremor
  - √ Ataxia
  - √ Hypotension

Toxicity

Acute toxicity

- Daytime sedation.
- Increased susceptibility to falls, especially in first week of therapy
- Psychomotor incoordination.
- Memory impairment (usually reversible on discontinuation).
- Impaired concentration.
- Excitement
- Delirium

Chronic toxicity

- Cognitive decline resembling dementia.
- Increased mortality risk associated with chronic daily use (general adult data).

Tolerance

- Develops rapidly (sometimes in a few days, especially with short-acting agents).

- Changes in sleep pattern induced by benzodiazepines tend to return to baseline after a few weeks on the drugs.
- Benzodiazepines alter normal sleep architecture.
  - √ Reduce non-REM-1 and 3/4 (slow wave) sleep, increase non-REM-2 sleep, and delay first period of REM sleep.
- Some evidence that effective sedative effects continue for a longer time with long-acting agents such as flurazepam.
- Tolerance to anxiolytic effects probably takes much longer to develop, if it does so at all.
- Duration of anxiolytic efficacy not well determined for elders but probably measured in months or even years.
  - √ Effectiveness of very long-term, continuous therapy over years not well studied.
  - √ Some suggest it may not be very effective and may exacerbate anxiety in some cases.
    - ▫ Issue remains somewhat controversial.
- Data conflict on the development of tolerance to cognitive and psychomotor effects (i.e., memory, visuospatial, and learning inhibition).
  - √ Some studies and clinical data show that no tolerance develops, whereas other data show tolerance and improved task performance after about 1 week (general adult data).
- Short-term memory impairment probably persists over time.

Rebound Insomnia

- There is increased total wake time after withdrawal of a hypnotic.
- Onset is usually within 1–3 nights after abrupt discontinuation.
- Related to
  - √ Dose
    - ▫ Control by using lowest effective dose.
  - √ Abrupt discontinuation
- Occurs especially with short- (triazolam, midazolam) and intermediate-acting (lorazepam, temazepam) benzodiazepines but not as apparent with estazolam, zolpidem, or zaleplon.
  - √ Long-acting agents unlikely to produce immediate rebound but may lead to delayed rebound.
  - √ With ultrashort-acting triazolam, rebound may occur during the course of one night, with early A.M. awakening and daytime anxiety.
    - ▫ One reason it is not suggested for elders.
  - √ Symptoms are generally short-lived over several nights (3–7 days) but sometimes more.
    - ▫ Prolonged sleep latency.
    - ▫ Increased REM duration and intensity.

- Increased caution in patients sensitive to stress states (e.g., angina patients).
- Increased problem in patients sensitive to dream states (e.g., trauma survivors).

- Rebound effects are dose-related (i.e., more likely at higher doses).
- Tapering regimen reduces rebound effects.
- Effects occasionally may last weeks, especially with long-acting agents such as diazepam and nitrazepam.
- Occurs especially after prolonged use but arises as early as 1 week after use.

Hangover Effects

- Some residual impairment next day.
- Varies among drugs and according to rapidity of metabolism, dose, and duration of treatment.
  - √ More likely in elders with less cognitive capacity.
  - √ Especially evident with nitrazepam, producing impaired performance on psychomotor tasks.
    - □ Clinical relevance unclear, as some patients can compensate with reduced speed and increased caution.

Dependence

Physical dependence is present when discontinuation of a medication results in a withdrawal syndrome that has a predictable onset, duration, and course and can be suppressed by readministering the medication.

- Occurs even at therapeutic doses and may make withdrawal problematic.

Management requires patient education, motivation, and support.

- May take many weeks and several attempts before success.
- Easier to manage in a hospital or long-term care institution where medication can be controlled.
- Occasionally cannot be managed on an outpatient basis and may require use of hospital.
  - √ Taking advantage of a hospitalization for other reasons is one strategy to alter drugs in the context of a controlled environment.

Respiratory Depression

- Mechanisms of effect on respiration include
  - √ Reduced hypoxic/hypercapnic drives.
    - □ May decrease ventilatory response and induce hypercapnea.

- √ Impaired arousal induced by airway obstruction.
- √ Change in pattern of sleep—increasing proportion of sleep where respiratory abnormalities are most common.

Benzodiazepine use

- May worsen or induce sleep apnea.
- May increase mortality.
  - √ Cause unknown but may be a respiratory mechanism.
- Requires increased caution in patients with sleep apnea, snoring, hypertension, or obesity.
  - √ Generally safe in small doses in asthma and COPD if used with caution.
  - √ Avoid use in patients with measurable chronic carbon dioxide retention.

Falls

- Leading cause of injury-related mortality and hospitalization in those > 75 years.
- High rates (44%) of falls associated with benzodiazepine use in nursing homes.
  - √ Rates increase with increasing doses.
- Risk factors include
  - √ Advanced age.
  - √ Impaired motor control.
  - √ Variety of illness states.
  - √ Multiple medication regimens.
  - √ History of alcohol/drug abuse.
  - √ Gender: 2:1 male:female risk ratio.
  - √ Benzodiazepine use
    - ▫ Risk may be greatest in first 2 weeks after prescription.
    - ▫ Declines and then increases again after 4 weeks of treatment.
    - ▫ Short and long half-life agents create about equally great risk of falls.
    - ▫ Rapid dose increases.
    - ▫ High or excessive dosages (> 3 mg diazepam equivalents) increase risk.
  - √ Hypnotic regimens and drugs may be more likely to induce falls than anxiolysis, although data not conclusive.

Driving

- Increased accident risk.
- Longer half-life agents may be more problematic.
  - √ Promote residual daytime cognitive impairment.

- Increased risk with concurrent use of two or more agents (including antidepressants).
- Newer hypnotics such as zopiclone have some adverse effects on some driving skills but seem less intense than benzodiazepines.

Inhibited Rehabilitation

- Psychomotor impairment worsens performance during rehabilitation therapy, especially with multiple doses of longer-acting drugs.

Incontinence

- Increased risk.
- Especially with oxidatively metabolized benzodiazepines and long acting agents.
- Increases risk of falls at night when patient gets up to void.

Cognitive Impairment

- Sometimes persists to next day.
- Anterograde amnesic syndrome especially with triazolam and less often lorazepam.
  - √ May be desirable in some situations (e.g., sedation for medical/surgical procedures).
- Amnestic effects include impairment of information acquisition and consolidation and storage of memory.
  - √ May be worse with alcohol abuse.
  - √ May resemble, and even meet criteria for, dementia.
- New evidence that chronic benzodiazepine use may be associated with accelerated cognitive decline in elders.

Table 3.7. Psychomotor and Cognitive Effects of Anxiolytics and Sedative/Hypnotics

Psychomotor/Cognitive Effects	Comments
ALPRAZOLAM	
• Effects vary in studies; generally well tolerated but may lead to some alterations in performance. • Impaired psychomotor performance with acute high oral doses. • Acute performance effects of single doses. √ Significant dose-dependent impairments of memory and performance, with variable tolerance developed over time. √ Acute treatment produces impaired memory function comparable to diazepam; impairments still evident 5 hours after dose ingestion.	• Chronic tolerance to alprazolam develops more slowly in elders than in younger adults; low doses and caution while titrating dose are indicated; impairment is somewhat more evident with alprazolam than with lorazepam.

(*cont.*)

Continued

Psychomotor/Cognitive Effects	Comments
√ *Chronic treatment* (i.e., > 21 days): 0.25 mg bid does not produce residual impairment in performance next day but higher doses (0.5 mg bid) do (although not as great as diazepam). √ Little self-rated sedation associated with measured declines in function.	
CLORAZEPATE	
• Little impairment of immediate or delayed recall in elders, despite longer action at doses of 3.75–7.5 mg.	
DIAZEPAM	
• 2.5 mg produces significant next-day decline in function.	• IV route is 2–3 times more potent in elders; phase 1 oxidative metabolism and clearance are affected by age and liver status.
ESTAZOLAM	
• Minimal effects on next-day performance in otherwise healthy elders at dose of 1 mg.	
FLURAZEPAM	
• Performance impairment next day and impaired capacity to participate in rehabilitation activities.	
LORAZEPAM	
• Impaired memory with acute high doses, and impaired memory after prolonged treatment. √ Some tolerance develops to this effect. • Acute performance effects of single doses. √ Dose-dependent significant impairments of (explicit) memory and perceptual priming. √ Impairments still evident 5 hours after dose ingestion. √ Impairment in performance tasks (variable tolerance to this effect develops over time). • *Chronic treatment* (i.e., > 21 days): In 0.5 and 1 mg doses bid, does not produce residual impairment in performance the next day. • *Acute treatment:* Produces impaired memory function comparable to diazepam.	• Relatively short elimination half-life; little risk of cumulative toxicity. • No active metabolite √ No oxidative metabolism (metabolism unaffected by age) • Induces greater impairment of recall than alprazolam.
OXAZEPAM	
• Hangover effects √ Some reduction in next-day performance. √ Anterograde impairment of long-term verbal memory (not as great as lorazepam) (general adult data).	• Relatively short elimination half-life. • Little risk of cumulative toxicity. • No active metabolite.
TEMAZEPAM	
• Decreased daytime performance (reaction time) after first dose. √ Effect increases with prolonged administration.	
TRIAZOLAM	
• Elders more sensitive to cognitive effects. • Ultrashort-acting action associated with amnesic syndromes next day.	• Not generally suitable for elders.

Table 3.8. Side Effects of Anxiolytics and Sedative/Hypnotics

	Most Common*	Most Serious and Less Common	Comments	Management
Body as a whole		• Impaired acute stress response. • Immunological disturbance.		
Cardiovascular	• Dizziness 13% • Hypotension 5% • Palpitations 8%	• Bradycardia • Fainting 3%	• Worse if combined with opiates. • Severe cardiovascular collapse can occur if coadministered with clozapine.	• Monitor BP/heart rate as indicated
Central and peripheral nervous system	• Somnolence/drowsiness 35% • Headache 9% • Hypokinesia • Ataxia 17% • Abnormal coordination 20% • Fatigue • Confusion 10% • Weakness 18% • Increased postural sway • Vertigo • Syncope • Paradoxical excitation/disinhibition (aggression, assaultiveness, excessive extroversion) • Hiccups	• Prolonged reversible dementia. • Impaired intellectual/psychomotor function. • Amnestic effects (usually mild anterograde). • Bizarre/abnormal behavior. • Delirium • Dysarthria/stuttering • Sleep disorders √ Vivid dreams √ Sleepwalking • Rare case reports of dystonia, parkinsonism, and tardive dyskinesia. √ Most often with diazepam, but also reported with bromazepam.	• Gait and balance disturbance leads to high risk of falls. √ Risk of hip fracture about 5% √ Falls more likely on day of drug • Disinhibition may be more evident in patients with brain damage (e.g., stroke, dementia trauma). • Longer-term use does not seem to affect immediate recall. • Warn patients about operating machinery and driving at least until they are used to the effects of the drug. √ Ask family to monitor if concerned √ Review driving ability regularly with patient and/or family √ Statutory notifications where necessary • Warn about avoiding concurrent alcohol or other CNS depressants (e.g., sedative antihistamines, sedative antidepressants or antipsychotics).	• Tolerance to common effects usually develops within 2 weeks. • Mange by titrating dose slowly, monitoring carefully, especially at night and patient/family education.

(cont.)

Continued

	Most Common*	Most Serious and Less Common	Comments	Management
Eye	• Blurred vision 11% • Dryness	• Rare worsening narrow-angle glaucoma		• Bethanechol 5–10 mg p.o. BID-TID for blurred vision although rarely necessary to intervene pharmacologically.
Gastrointestinal	• Dry mouth 13% • Nausea/vomiting 7% • Diarrhea 7% • Constipation 7%	• Bitter taste		• Reduce dose
Psychiatric		• Anxiety • Depression and rarely suicidality • Mania √ Especially with alprazolam • Depersonalization • Drug dependence • Behavioral disturbances associated with dementia or brain injury √ Agitation, aggression, hyperactivity • Paradoxical reactions √ Stimulation √ Agitation √ Panic √ Rage √ Increased muscle spasticity √ Sleep disturbances √ Hallucinations √ Confusion	• Depression reported associated with benzodiazepines. √ Causal relationship not clearly demonstrated, but seems related to relatively higher dose ranges. √ Monitor for this effect, especially with preexisting neurological impairment. • Behavioral disturbance more likely in early stages of treatment. √ May resolve spontaneously as treatment continues.	• Gradually reduce dose or discontinue. • Stimulants have been used to treat behavioral disturbances.

		• ECT √ Longer-acting drugs may decrease duration of seizure activity the next morning and treatment response may be compromised. √ This effect not seen with single doses of shorter-acting agents. √ Age also reduces seizure duration.		
Renal		• Hesitancy or retention		
Reproductive		• Impotence with clorazepate		• Change drug
Respiratory	Nasal congestion 7%	• Respiratory depression • Worsened sleep apnea, especially central type but also obstructive type, may induce hypoxia and occasionally death.	• Respiratory depression occurs with high doses, especially IV. • Controversial at therapeutic doses √ In COPD use low-dose therapy only • Avoid benzodiazepines in patients with either form of sleep apnea.	• Respiratory depression is usually brief. • Exacerbated by narcotic coadministration.
Skin and appendages	Rash/itch 5%			

* Percentages are general adult data.

DRUG–DRUG INTERACTIONS

Table 3.9. Drug–Drug Interactions

Anxiolytic/Sedative	Interacting Drug	Effect and Comments
All	CNS depressants—opiates, narcotics, sedative/hypnotics, sedative antihistamines, other CNS depressants (benzodiazepines, barbiturates droperidol, alcohol, clonidine)	Increased CNS depression; increased mortality risk in suicide when taken concurrently with anxiolytic/sedative overdose
Benzodiazepines	Alcohol	Potentiates action, especially with longer-acting agents; prolongs half-life of drug by competing for microsomal enzymes
	Anticholinergic drugs (including phenothiazines, some SSRIs tricyclic antidepressants)	Cognitive impairment
	Caffeine	Antagonizes benzodiazepines
	Cimetidine	Impairs clearance and increases plasma concentration of oxidatively metabolized benzodiazepines; use ranitidine or famotidine instead
	Clozapine	Hypotension, including circulatory collapse, sedation, increased danger of respiratory depression
	Digitalis	Increases plasma concentration of benzodiazepines
	Disulfiram	Increases most benzodiazepine levels
	Ephedrine theophylline (and other sympathomimetics and stimulants)	Reduces effect of benzodiazepines; may require higher dose
	Food and antacids (aluminum/magnesium hydroxide)	Delay absorption; may not be clinically important, unless patient needs rapid effect (e.g., sleep induction)
	Flumazenil	Competitively inhibits CYP3A4; prolongs half-life of triazolam and alprazolam
	Isoniazid	Increased benzodiazepine levels
	L-dopa	Effect of l-dopa antagonized; may exacerbate Parkinson's disease; oxazepam less likely to cause this effect
	MAOIs	Increased benzodiazepine levels
	Nefazodone and fluvoxamine	Increases half-life of diazepam
	Phenytoin	May increase 3-hydroxy compounds (lorazepam)
	Probenecid	Reduces effect of benzodiazepines (but not 3-hydroxy agents such as lorazepam)
	Rifampin	Antagonizes benzodiazepines, requiring increased dose in some patients
	Theophylline	Antagonizes benzodiazepine action

(cont.)

Continued

Anxiolytic/Sedative	Interacting Drug	Effect and Comments
Drugs oxidatively metabolized by CYP3A4 (long-acting and some short-acting benzodiazepines, such as midazolam, triazolam) plus zolpidem, zaleplon, and possibly zopiclone	Azole antifungal agents Antidepressants (nefazodone, fluvoxamine, fluoxetine valproic acid) Antibiotics (erythromycin, clarithromycin, cyclosporin, isoniazid) cimetidine disulfiram amiodarone ritonavir grapefruit juice antifungal agents propoxyphene	Inhibit 3A4 oxidative metabolism; increase plasma concentration of anxiolytic/sedative
	carbamazepine rifampin phenytoin dexamethasone	Induce 3A4 metabolism; reduce plasma concentration of anxiolytic/sedative

SLEEP DISORDERS

Sleep disorders may be classified as

- Initial insomnia
  - √ Difficulty falling asleep; prolonged sleep latency of > 1 hour.
- Impaired sleep maintenance
  - √ Frequent awakenings; 1–2 periods of wakefulness lasting longer than 1 hour each, or more than 2 periods of any length.
- Terminal insomnia
  - √ Early morning awakenings; no further sleep after 5 A.M.
- Other components of classification include
  - √ Nonrefreshing sleep.
  - √ Duration of disorder.
    - ▫ May be transient (one to several nights), short term (few days up to a month), or chronic (> 1 month).
  - √ Excessive daytime sleepiness.
    - ▫ Common in elders.
  - √ Primary (not due to another disorder or substance-induced) vs. secondary.

Epidemiology

- Sleep disorders are very common.
- Rates vary by study, location, and definition.
  - √ 15% (range 15–35%) of general population and 25% (range 10–60%) of community elders.
    - ▫ Higher incidence in women.
  - √ > 50% in nursing homes.

- Relationship to age not consistent; some studies find increased rates in elders, others do not.
  - √ Increased rate of physical disorders, rather than age per se, is key reason for differences in rates of sleep disturbance in the elderly.
- Usually not reported spontaneously to physicians (general adult data).
- Associated with
  - √ Depressive/anxiety symptoms.
  - √ Alcohol misuse.
  - √ Increased nocturnal voiding.
  - √ Pain
  - √ Poor self-rated health and increased number of physical disabilities (respiratory complaints, cardiovascular disease such as angina and arrhythmia, arthritis).
  - √ Recent use of medical services.
  - √ Use of sedative hypnotics.
  - √ Nonprescription medication use (e.g., nondrowsy cold/sinus medications).
  - √ Sedentary lifestyle (as opposed to aerobically fit).
  - √ Institutionalization.
- Elders consume 40% of all sedative/hypnotic agents.
- 4% of general population and 14–22% of elders (women > men) take sleep medications.
  - √ Especially those who consulted a physician or other health professional within past 6 months.
- Rates of intermittent drug use (as opposed to continuous) rise with increasing age, although sleep disorders do not seem to increase.

Sleep changes in those over 50 years old include

- Longer sleep latency.
- Non-REM (restorative) sleep, especially delta-wave sleep, diminished.
  - √ Early awakening and more frequent and increased duration of night awakenings lead to relative sleep deprivation.
- Decreased total sleep time in some studies, but finding varies from study to study.
- Depth and efficiency of sleep decreased.
- Circadian rhythm altered.
  - √ Increased daytime sleeping and naps.
  - √ Reduced night sleeping.
  - √ May impair alertness when driving.

Causes of Sleep Disorder

- Acute sleep problems.
  - √ Acute stress or adjustment disorder, medication effects, medical illness, bereavement, acute psychological trauma, acute relationship discord.
  - √ Usually lasts days to weeks.
  - √ May herald psychiatric disorder.
- Persistent insomnia.
  - √ Treat underlying disorders.
  - √ May persist after successful treatment of primary psychiatric disorder.

Table 3.10. Causes of Sleep Disorders

Impairment	Comments
	PHYSICAL/PHYSIOLOGICAL
Age-related sleep changes	Sleep fragmentation, disturbed circadian rhythm, disrupted sleep architecture
Pain-related conditions	Arthritis, cancer, disc disease, duodenal ulcer, coronary artery disease
Sleep-disordered breathing	Apneic episodes: cessation of airflow for at least 10 seconds; often related to weight gain or obesity • Types of sleep apnea: √ Obstructive (repetitive upper airway obstruction, snoring associated) √ Central (failure in central regulation of breathing associated with cerebrovascular or cardiac disease) √ Mixed • Found in 5–20% of general elders and up to 40–50% of institutionalized elders. • Often leads to daytime somnolence and nocturnal insomnia. • Managed with weight loss, avoidance of sedative drugs, sleeping on one's side, treatment of associated conditions, C-PAP (continuous positive airway pressure); occasionally requires tracheostomy.
Medical disorders	Hypertension, CHF, hypothyroidism Secondary sleep disturbances (e.g., cough, urinary frequency, gastroesophageal reflux, COPD, cerebrovascular disease, renal dialysis)
Restless legs syndrome/ nocturnal myoclonus	Associated with sleep disturbance in 70–80% of patients; various types of myoclonic and/or hypnic jerks may be released with relaxation, drowsiness, and sleep and cause severe insomnia. • Restless legs syndrome occurs in 5% of geriatric subjects: √ Symptoms are usually nocturnal and include unusual, indescribable, deep creeping/crawling sensation in the legs and an irresistible urge to move legs. √ Occurs only at rest and is relieved by movement. √ Aggravated by caffeine, diuretics, antihistamines, antidepressants, antipsychotics, bronchodilators, electrolyte imbalance, anemia, and uremia. √ Clonazepam is effective treatment but caution with benzodiazepines is advised since they may aggravate sleep apnea. √ l-dopa/carbidopa is often helpful.

(*cont.*)

Continued

Impairment	Comments
	• Periodic leg movements of sleep (nocturnal myoclonus) occurs in 30–50% of elders. √ Repetitive, sometimes violent, movements every 20–40 seconds during non-REM sleep. √ Aggravated by similar medications as restless leg syndrome, and treatment similar.
Parasomnias	REM sleep behavior disorder or sleepwalking. • Characterized by loss of normal atonia during REM and unusual sleep behaviors associated with aggressive or violent dreams. √ May be injurious to patient or bed partner.
Neurological disorders	Parkinson's disease, dementia (including Alzheimer's disease, Lewy body and vascular), olivopontocerebellar degeneration, Guillaine–Barre syndrome, subarachnoid hemorrhage (abnormal REM sleep behavior disorder may occur)
	ENVIRONMENTAL
Life situations that disrupt sleep rhythms	Example: admission to an institution; travel across time zones
Housing conditions	Example: noise; inappropriate temperature regulation (especially too hot)
	PSYCHOLOGICAL*
Psychiatric disorders	Presence of depression, anxiety, panic, psychosis, dementia, PTSD, sleep cycle reversal, sundowning. For example, in depression: • Higher REM density • Longer first REM episode • Shorter REM latency • Shift of slow waves to second non-REM episode
Alzheimer's disease	Loss of REMs, multiple awakenings, loss of spindles and K complexes, reduction of all slow-wave sleep
Poor sleep habits	Lack of sleep routine, leaving lights on, avoidance of going to bed, sleeping in inappropriate places (e.g., sofa, chairs), daytime napping, stimulant bedtime drinks
Substance use	Alcohol, smoking, caffeine, sedative/hypnotics, illicit drugs
	IATROGENIC
	• Adrenergic bronchodilators • Anticholinergics (may cause agitation/confusion) • Antidepressants • Antihypertensives • Antiparkinsonian agents • Beta-adrenergic blockers (cause nightmares) • Caffeine in coffee, tea, cola, and some OTC drugs (e.g., ASA or acetaminophen preparations) • Cardiac agents—quinidine-like agents • Cimetidine (associated with agitation) • Corticosteroids • Diltiazem • Diuretics • Levodopa • Methyldopa • Nifedipine • Phenytoin • Sympathomimetics, including decongestants • Thyroid hormone

* In 37–67% of insomnias; general adult data.

Indications for Sedative/Hypnotics

The most conservative guidelines advise use of benzodiazepines when sleep disturbance is severe, disabling to the patient or family, causing severe stress, and when other measures have failed. Often a more liberal threshold for prescription is appropriate.

- Elders often find shortened sleep cycle very distressing.
  - √ Being awake and lonely at night, especially when sleep disorder is associated with depression or other anxiety symptoms.
    - ▫ Short-term adjunctive therapy for depression is often necessary and prudent.
- Tolerance of sleep disturbance varies, so threshold for prescription of sleep medication should be tailored to patient's need.
- Tolerance to sedative effects develops relatively rapidly, especially with shorter-acting agents typically recommended for elders.
  - √ Some patients assert, however, that they get a major benefit from the sedative effect during prolonged treatment.
    - ▫ Likely the result of an anxiolytic or subjective belief, rather than sedative effect.

Situationally-induced sleep disturbance

- Treat with a brief course of sedative/hypnotic in lowest effective dose for 1–2 weeks, followed by reassessment.
- Cognitively impaired patients very sensitive to side effects and require monitoring for instability and danger of falls at night.

Chronic insomnia

- Challenging to manage.
- Some patients who fail to respond to array of other interventions require long-term sedative therapy administered intermittently (for about 2-week periods), with trials of dose reduction and discontinuation.
  - √ Restrict drugs to an as-needed basis up to 3–4 times a week, if possible.
- Some patients need long-term maintenance.
  - √ Monitoring is essential.

Periodic limb movements in sleep, restless leg syndrome

- May be associated with sleep apnea, so treat with caution.
  - √ Consider sleep-laboratory study for diagnosis.
- Reduce/discontinue aggravating medications. (see Table 3.10, p. 413)
- Treat underlying conditions (e.g., iron deficiency anemia; responds to iron repletion).

- Pergolide or levodopa (may be effective in the long term).
- Clonazepam 0.5–1 mg/day effective.
  - √ Often used adjunctively with folate, vitamins B_{12}, C, and E (high doses of 800–1200 IU/day), iron, magnesium.
  - √ Other drugs include ropinirole, mirtazapine, nefazodone, bromocriptine.

Management of Sleep Disorders

Improved sleep may increase daytime alertness and reduce side effects of sleep disturbance.

- Side effects of sleep disturbance include
  - √ Excessive daytime sleepiness
  - √ Headaches
  - √ Nocturnal GI reflux
  - √ Depressive symptoms
  - √ Sexual dysfunction
  - √ Irritability
  - √ Reduced concentration
  - √ Impaired mental function
  - √ In the extreme, increased mortality

Table 3.11. Checklist for Taking a Sleep History

- Quality of and satisfaction with sleep—refreshed on awakening?
  24-hour sleep log—bedtime, routines, time to fall asleep, number of awakenings, interference with sleep (e.g., pain, dreams, dyspnea).
- Collateral information from sleep partner re. snoring, movements, restlessness, apnea.
- Duration of sleep complaint.
- Transient versus persistent, acute versus chronic.
- Activity levels—exercise, light exposure.
- Physical health system review/physical examination.
- Mental health—review presence of psychiatric disorder or incomplete response to its treatment.
- Drug use review—prescription, nonprescription, alcohol, other substances.
- Meals—timing and type.
- Environmental factors—temperature (heat), noise, light.
- Laboratory investigation—routine blood work, electrolytes, calcium, renal function, ECG, thyroid, respiratory function.

- Obtain a thorough history.
- Treat underlying causes of sleep disturbance first.
  - √ Sleep laboratory evaluation may be useful if sleep apnea or abnormal sleep (e.g., muscle movement abnormalities, narcolepsy) is suspected.

Behavioral/nonpharmacological therapies should be used routinely in all sleep disorders, with or without sedative/hypnotics. These therapies are very useful but require considerable motivation and supportive follow-up by the therapist. Key components are

- Identify sleep pattern and potential problems.
  - √ If possible, have patient use a 2-week sleep diary noting bedtime, awakening time, time to fall asleep, number of awakenings at night, total sleep time, sleep quality, time in bed, and daytime naps; level of well-being next day; exercise patterns; alcohol, caffeine, nicotine, and other substance use patterns; stimulus reduction patterns (leaving TV off at night).
  - √ Ask bed partner for history.
- Introduce stimulus control techniques (e.g., shutting out light and noise).
- Restrict/avoid daytime naps.
- Provide general education of both patient and family regarding sleep needs.

Table 3.12. Sleep Hygiene Checklist

- Establish regular sleep routines around retiring and rising.
- Avoid daytime napping.
- Establish conducive environment—comfortable mattress, comfortably warm ambient temperature, noise reduction (e.g., use earplugs if necessary, turn off lights and television).
- Engage in regular daily exercise, especially in A.M.; avoid heavy exercise/physical activity before bed.
- Avoid stimulants/alcohol at night; carbohydrate snack at bedtime acceptable.
- Manage separation anxieties e.g., reluctance to disengage by turning off comforting T.V.
- Bladder control training, as necessary.
- Limit time spent in bed to sleeping activities; avoid long periods of lying in bed attempting to sleep; do relaxation exercises out of bed if unable to sleep.

Behavioral/nonpharmacological methods include

- Avoid stimulating substances before bed, such as alcohol, caffeine, nicotine.
- Alter work habits.
  - √ For elders, managing personal care and daily chores may be time consuming and complex causing a delayed bed time and interfering with sleep, especially if impaired cognition reduces efficiency and increases anxiety about getting tasks completed.
  - √ May require external support to organize environment and carry out some of the tasks for the patient.
- Cognitive therapy (e.g., blocking unwanted thoughts, countering anxiety-provoking thought patterns) may accompany treatment of sleep disorder.
- Relaxation exercises.
- Bright light therapy in A.M. for initial insomnia and in evening for middle and terminal insomnia.
  - √ Caution re. possible retinal damage (consider pretreatment retinal examination).

- Positive pressure airway device/laser surgery for sleep apnea.
- Promote daytime functioning.

Pharmacological intervention

Sedative/hypnotics are useful for sleep induction and maintenance, but all studies in elders are relatively short term (not longer than 1 month).

- In sleep disorder associated with depression, definitive therapy is antidepressant, but sedatives are useful adjunct.

Effectiveness of benzodiazepines on some parameters of sleep (e.g., sleep induction) beyond that of placebo is still uncertain; data on benzodiazepine-receptor agonists (zaleplon, zolpidem) are still accumulating; higher quality trials show only modest effectiveness outcomes.

Current data suggest the following effects of sedative/hypnotics

- Reduced sleep latency (faster onset of sleep).
  - √ General adult data, variable effects on sleep latency: Meta-analytic data indicate no significant shortening of sleep latency; other data show sleep latency reduced by about 30% with pharmacology (and by 43% with behavioral interventions).
  - √ Elders, fewer data.
    - ▫ Some studies show 30 minutes reduction in sleep latency (zopiclone sometimes performs better but overall no advantage shown).
- Reduced nocturnal awakenings.
  - √ 46% with pharmacotherapy and 56% with behavioral therapies (general adult data).
- Increase in total sleep time.
  - √ General adult data: 12% with pharmacotherapy and 6% with behavioral therapy.
  - √ Elders: Increased total sleep time 47–81 minutes for first few nights (no advantage with zopiclone on meta-analytic data).
- Sometimes sedative/hypnotics improve the subjective quality of sleep.
  - √ Elders perceive greater benefit from benzodiazepines used for insomnia than that perceived by the prescribing physician. This issue is directly discussed with patients when planning duration and monitoring of treatment.
- Benzodiazepines alter normal sleep pattern.
  - √ Prolong stage 2 sleep (light sleep).
  - √ Decrease slow-wave and REM stages
    - ▫ Temazepam the exception.

- √ Prolong REM latency—delayed onset of first REM episode and diminished dreaming (may be an advantage in patients who have disturbing dreams when using antidepressants).
  - Flurazepam the exception.
- Naturalistic community studies suggest that overall sleep benefit from hypnotics may be slight; possible reasons include
  - √ Inadequate doses of hypnotics, leading to limited duration of action.
  - √ Development of drug tolerance with prolonged use.
  - √ Drug-withdrawal insomnia in patients attempting to limit drug use.
  - √ Short duration of drug action.
  - √ Unrecognized sleep disorders unresponsive to hypnotics (e.g., sleep apnea).

Basic sedative/hypnotic prescribing principles

- Educate patient regarding reasons for using drugs and treatment approach.
- Discontinue ineffective drug regimens, including other prescription hypnotics and OTC drugs.
  - √ Patients often resist this step and need support and education to enlist their cooperation and that of their families.
- Use lowest effective dose.
- Prescribe before bedtime.
  - √ Unwise to manage interrupted sleep with hypnotic during the middle of the night.
    - Dangers of falls and next-day psychomotor and cognitive impairment.
    - Zolpidem is a possible exception because of its short duration of action, but data for elders not available so this indication cannot be endorsed for elders.
- Use on as-needed basis except when patient needs consistent sedation for a few days (e.g., after prolonged sleep impairment).
- Use for short time periods of 1–4 weeks, if possible.
  - √ In chronic psychiatric disorders, may be impossible to adhere to this guideline.
- Discontinue by gradual tapering.
- Monitor patients when adjusting dose up or down (e.g., for rebound insomnia).
- Evaluate patients regularly, at least every 3–6 months for cognitive and psychomotor side effects, compliance, misuse, and use of concurrent substances, especially alcohol.
- Monitor changes in tolerance for agents whose pharmacokinetics are age-sensitive.

  - √ Alprazolam, chloral hydrate, chlordiazepoxide, clonazepam, diazepam, flurazepam, midazolam, quazepam, triazolam, zolpidem.
- Monitor patients whose cognitive capacity or brain reserve is compromised.
  - √ Tolerance for benzodiazepines and sedative/hypnotics is diminished, requiring downward dose adjustment.
- Plasma levels not very helpful clinically.
  - √ Possible exception is alprazolam.
    - ▫ Therapeutic range of 20–40 ng/ml in panic disorder (general adult data).

Choosing a Sedative/Hypnotic

- Drugs of choice: Rapid onset of action with medium duration is often best.
  - √ Lorazepam, temazepam, zopiclone, estazolam.
  - √ Zaleplon and zolpidem useful for sleep induction but less effective for sleep maintenance.
  - √ Goal is sleep induction and maintenance with the drug cleared by morning.
    - ▫ Elimination half-life (in elders) of more than 15 hours leads to drug accumulation.
    - ▫ Rapid absorption is an advantage to induce sleep rapidly so that the patient does not feel it is necessary to take a second dose and get unwanted additive side effects.
- Early A.M. awakening might be addressed with a longer-acting agent
  - √ With prolonged use, hangover effects are a major disadvantage, and *these agents generally are avoided in elders.*
- Oxazepam has slow onset of action.
  - √ Even so, may be used for sleep, but advise patient to take drug 1–2 hours before bed.
- Ultrarapidly metabolized agents (e.g., triazolam) *not* suggested for elders.
  - √ Rapid and sometimes intense rebound insomnia, significant next-day memory impairment or amnesia.
- Long-acting agents (e.g., diazepam, nitrazepam) eliminated slowly and generally not suitable for long-term nighttime sleep induction and maintenance in elders; however, the situation is not entirely clear.
  - √ Diazepam does not have prolonged action when used in single dose.
    - ▫ No demonstrated increased risk of falls with small doses of diazepam (1 mg).

- Diazepam may induce less tolerance to sedative effect.
- Hence, for longer-term therapy in otherwise well and robust elders, low-dose diazepam occasionally may be useful, despite general caution about its use in elders.

- REM sleep behavior disorder responds to low doses of clonazepam.
- Trazadone useful with appropriate cautions in elders (see p. 210).
- Melatonin
  - √ Dose 3–6 mg hs.
    - May rebalance low melatonin associated with aging.
    - Clinical data for utility in MCI sleep impairment.
  - √ Taper to avoid rebound insomnia.

Drugs usually not suggested for elders

- Little if any indication for long-acting hypnotic agents such as flurazepam.
- Quazepam not suggested because of accumulation of drug/metabolites over time.
  - √ However, lower dose (7.5 mg) does not accumulate substantially over first week and appears to be relatively safe and effective, so guidelines on this drug for healthy elders are flexible at this time.
- Chloral hydrate and antihistamines not very effective and tolerance develops rapidly.
  - √ Antihistamines have undesirable side effects.
    - Impaired cognition, decreased daytime alertness, anticholinergic effects.
    - Hospitalized patients are especially at risk of delirium and longer lengths of stay.
- L-tryptophan ineffective and danger of eosinophilia, myalgia.
- Barbiturates, ethchlorvynol, glutethimide, methprylon, methaqualone lethal in overdose, rapid tolerance, addictive, numerous drug interactions.

Precautions

- Evaluate drug interaction potential.
- Cautious prescribing of medication supplies for potentially suicidal patients who may overdose.
- Use lowest effective dose.
  - √ But also be careful not to underdose.
- Reduce dose of agents metabolized by oxidation in presence of severe liver disease.
- With prolonged use, periodic routine blood counts, chemistry, and urinalysis suggested.

Dealing with Nonresponse

- Reevaluate
  - √ Diagnosis
  - √ Tolerance for drug and dose.
  - √ Physiological tolerance to the drug.
    - ▫ Reduces effect.
  - √ Cognitive status and brain reserve.
    - ▫ May increase side effects.
- Investigate concurrent substance use (i.e., alcohol, other drug use, other psychotropic agents, other medications, OTCs).
- Reevaluate dose and increase/decrease as appropriate.
  - √ Advisable to increase dose of sedative in early stages of treatment if necessary but dose increases in a drug that has lost its effectiveness because of tolerance are not suggested.
- Switching drugs.
  - √ Switching among benzodiazepines not usually very useful.
    - ▫ Some patients occasionally respond better to a given agent, perhaps for psychological reasons.
  - √ Switching to a nonbenzodiazepine can improve sedative response if the benzodiazepine does not work or tolerance has developed.

Adverse Effects of Sedative/Hypnotics

In addition to the side effects noted for anxiolytics (see pp. 401–409), key concerns include

- Tolerance
- Rebound effects
- Impaired daytime performance
- Memory loss

If sleep is not induced by benzodiazepine

- Next-day drowsiness, confusion, agitation may result.

Warn patients about hazards; these are especially likely in patients with dementia, visual impairment, postural hypotension, and other neurological or musculoskeletal disability; general cautions include

- Ataxia and falls
- Cognitive changes
- Respiratory depression
- Sleep apnea
- Confusion
- Psychomotor impairment

- √ Impairments include reduced vigilance, divided attention, delayed speed of response, motor incoordination, all of which can be part of other age-related disturbances (e.g., early dementia).
- √ 1.5–4-fold increase in risk of accidents, especially during initial use (general adult data).

- Concurrent medications and alcohol
  - √ Commonly used OTC agents include diphenhydramine (e.g., Nytol, Sominex, Sleep-eze), diphenhydramine in combination (e.g., Anacin PM, Doan's PM, Extra Strength Excedrin PM, Tylenol PM), doxylamine (e.g., Unisom Nighttime), tryptophan, melatonin.
- Caution against adjusting dose without consulting physician.
  - √ Explain that increasing the dosage can encourage dependence and increase daytime impairment of alertness and concentration.

ALCOHOL ABUSE AND ALCOHOLISM

Alcoholism is defined as a primary chronic disease with genetic, psychosocial, and environmental factors influencing its development and manifestations. The disease is often progressive and fatal.

Benzodiazepines are cross-tolerant with alcohol and hence are the drugs of choice for management of alcohol withdrawal.

- Syndrome includes impaired control over drinking, preoccupation with alcohol, use of alcohol despite adverse consequences, denial, and other distortions in thinking.
- Prevalence (from various general and geriatric studies).
  - √ 1-year general community; prevalence in elders conservatively estimated at 3% for men and .5% for women.
  - √ Emergency room 14%
  - √ Inpatient psychiatry units 23–44%
  - √ General hospital setting 18%
  - √ Nursing home admissions to VA facilities 11%
- New-onset alcoholism emerges in late life.
  - √ Risk factors in elders include
    - ▫ Family history.
    - ▫ Opportunity, finances, and time to drink.
    - ▫ Increased CNS sensitivity to alcohol.
    - ▫ Diminished physiological tolerance to alcohol.
    - ▫ Chronic medical disorder with pain/insomnia.
    - ▫ Possibly psychosocial stressors such as bereavement.

Management

Conduct full assessment.

- Consider use of CAGE screening tool for alcoholism and Michigan Alcoholism Screening test—geriatric version (MAST-G).
- Complete physical and laboratory workup.
  - √ Elders more likely to suffer from complicating physical and cognitive comorbidities than younger alcoholics (e.g., polyneuropathy, cerebellar ataxia).
  - √ Elders more likely to manifest biochemical abnormalities than younger alcoholics.
  - √ Full laboratory screen
    - ▫ Blood and urine alcohol levels.
    - ▫ Liver function, CBC, electrolytes, urinalysis, B_{12} and folate, toxicology for concurrent substances.
    - ▫ Neuroimaging (CT, MRI) in the presence of cognitive impairment, neurological features.
- Complete psychosocial workup.
- Assessment of secondary factors.
  - √ Example: Ability to manage concurrent medical or psychiatric disorders, self-neglect, malnutrition, falls, abuse of other drugs including OTCs.
- Medication review for alcohol-related alterations in metabolism.
- Psychiatric assessment for depression, psychosis, withdrawal episodes, violence, suicidality.
- Cognitive assessment.
- Collateral information.

Hospitalization for detoxification

- Higher rate of morbidity and mortality in elders, especially from delirium tremens.
- Provide supportive therapy and creation of therapeutic alliance, patient education, treatment of concurrent depression or other disorders, pain management, grief work, intermittent monitoring of blood/urine alcohol.

Alcohol Withdrawal Syndrome

Pathophysiology

- Alcohol is GABAergic.
- GABA inhibits sympathetic (adrenergic) outflow.
- Cessation of alcohol releases sympathetic outflow by reducing GABA potentiation.
  - √ Requires careful monitoring for the sometimes intense withdrawal syndrome with hyperadrenergic features.

  - ▫ Sweating, anorexia, tachycardia, hypertension (systolic > 160 mm Hg, diastolic > 100 mm Hg), agitation, increased danger of MI or CVA, tremors, seizures, psychosis.
  - √ Onset as early as 6 hours after discontinuation.

Withdrawal

- May increase in severity with repeated episodes (kindling effect).
- May be more severe in elders.
  - √ Increased symptoms.
  - √ Possible increased cognitive impairment, daytime sleepiness, and hypertension.

Drug Treatment

Benzodiazepines are the drugs of choice.

- *Avoid* using benzodiazepines metabolized by CYP3A4 liver enzymes.
  - √ Metabolism may be impaired in cirrhosis associated with alcoholism.
  - √ Case reports of prolonged sedation requiring ventilation.
  - √ IM benzodiazepines (e.g., diazepam, chlordiazepoxide), if diluted in propylene glycol, have a twofold delay in achieving peak concentrations and erratic absorption.
    - ▫ Multiple doses within a short time may accumulate and reach peak concentrations at the same time (about 36 hours later in patients with reduced liver efficiency), inducing toxic reaction that includes respiratory depression.
- Suggest drug metabolized by glucuronidation.
  - √ Lorazepam a good choice.
    - ▫ 1 mg q 4 hours for alcohol withdrawal syndrome and 1 mg q 8 h for prophylaxis against emergence of syndrome.
    - ▫ Predictable absorption and half-life with IM route.
  - √ Oxazepam 15 mg q 4 hours a good choice if very rapid action not required.
    - ▫ Peak plasma concentrations 5.5 hours after oral administration.
- Benzodiazepines must be tapered slowly.
  - √ Sharp discontinuation may induce withdrawal syndrome.

Adjunctive therapy

- Balance fluid and electrolyte imbalances.
- Administer thiamine 50–100 mg IV for a least 3 days (to prevent Wernicke-Korsakoff syndrome).
- Administer multivitamin with a minimum of 1 mg of folate.

- Other medications
  - √ Clonidine (alpha-2 adrenergic agonist) has been used to control alcohol withdrawal.
    - ▫ Reduces adrenergic manifestations of alcohol withdrawal (e.g., hypertension, tachycardia, increased respiratory rate, tremor, diaphoresis, restlessness).
- Neuroleptic for psychosis (e.g., haloperidol).
- Atenolol for tremor, tachycardia, diaphoresis, hypertension.

DISCONTINUATION/WITHDRAWAL AND REBOUND SYNDROMES

Discontinuation of antianxiety and sedative hypnotic drugs may lead to withdrawal and rebound anxiety. These responses differ from each other.

Withdrawal

- Withdrawal symptoms occur in about 35% of patients on benzodiazepines longer than 4 weeks (general adult data).
  - √ Usually occur because of abrupt discontinuation (sometimes inadvertent because of forgotten doses or admission to hospital) but may emerge with gradual tapering of chronic usage, especially from higher-than-usual doses.
  - √ May emerge in the early morning following hs administration of an ultra-short–acting agent.
  - √ Occur because of physiological dependence.
    - ▫ May develop in as little as 2 weeks on therapeutic doses of some agents, including nonbenzodiazepines, especially agents with short half-lives.
  - √ Availability of supportive care often determines success of tapering and discontinuation.

Table 3.13. Risk Factors for Benzodiazepine Withdrawal Syndrome

- Long duration of treatment
- High doses
- History of addictive behavior
- Abrupt discontinuation
- Use of short half-life compounds
- Use of high-potency drugs

Short half-life agents are associated with earlier and more severe withdrawal symptoms, although long half-life is not a guaranteed protection against withdrawal. For example, minor symptoms of withdrawal may occur 4–6 weeks after discontinuation of diazepam.

- Symptoms are a function of patient's metabolism, properties of the drug (e.g., rate of elimination), dose, duration of dosage, rate at which dose is decreased or discontinued.
- Syndrome is usually mild but may include psychiatric, neurological, gastrointestinal, and other symptoms.

Table 3.14. Benzodiazepine Withdrawal Symptoms

Psychiatric Symptoms	Neurological Symptoms	GI Symptoms	Other
Agitation	Ataxia	Loss of appetite	Flushing
Anxiety	Bad dreams	Metallic taste	Hypertension
Apprehension	Blepharospasm	Nausea	Hypotension
Delirium	Catatonia	Vomiting	Perspiration
Depersonalization	Headache		Photophobia
Depression (sometimes quite severe)	Hyperacusis		Tachycardia
Dysphoria	Hyperosmia and partial complex seizures		Tinnitus
Hallucinations	Impaired concentration		Morning sweats
Irritability	Incoordination		
Paranoia	Memory impairment		
	Myoclonus		
	Paresthesias		
	Rebound insomnia		
	Seizures		
	Sensory hypersensitivity rebound		
	Shakes, muscle aches, twitches, and tremor		
	Unusual muscle movements (lip smacking, tongue movements, leg cramps)		

Seizures

- 4% of patients withdrawn from benzodiazepines (general adult data; may be higher in elders with predisposing brain injury/pathology).
- Especially occurs when
  - √ Short half-life agents are discontinued abruptly.
  - √ High-dose dependence present.
  - √ Predisposition present.
    - Head injury
    - Dementia
    - Dependence on multiple drugs
    - Alcohol addiction
    - Drugs that lower seizure threshold (e.g., tricyclics or neuroleptics)
    - Abnormal EEG that lowers seizure threshhold

Onset of symptoms

- Usually within 6–72 hours of stopping a shorter-acting drug (e.g., lorazepam, oxazepam) and 4–7 days with a longer-acting drug.

- √ Symptoms can emerge almost immediately in patients taking ultra-short–acting agents such as triazolam.
- √ Avoid rapid withdrawal in predisposed patients.
- Duration days to 2–4 weeks.
  - √ Note: Triazolam associated with daytime anxiety and withdrawal reaction during therapeutic use because of very rapid metabolism.
- Hallucinations may persist for several weeks (rarely).

Rebound Anxiety

- Defined as an increase in anxiety symptoms above pretreatment anxiety levels, following withdrawal of the drug.
- Common reaction in about 40–45% of patients.
- Symptoms include anxiety, restlessness, dysphoria, loss of appetite, nausea, insomnia.
- Usually transient but may last up to 3 weeks (general adult data).
- More evident with rapidly metabolized drugs (e.g., lorazepam, alprazolam).

Management

Success rates of withdrawal programs from chronic benzodiazepine use vary widely, from 15% to 73%.

- Minimize sleep and anxiety rebound by slow withdrawal schedule.
- Adjust speed of withdrawal to patient's tolerance.
- Most paticnts tolerate a weekly taper of 10–25%.
- Usually takes 2–3 months or longer.
  - √ First trial of withdrawal may be unsuccessful, requiring reinstitution of the drug.
    - ▫ Should not discourage second attempt.
    - ▫ Warn patient against demoralization.
    - ▫ Usually requires frequent contact with prescriber and at least supportive therapy, and often more formal psychotherapy, accompanying the withdrawal.
- Where appropriate, allow patient to adjust dose to own tolerance.
- Beware of too rapid "cold turkey" regimens sometimes desired by overly self-reliant or pseudoindependent personality types.

To buffer withdrawal in particularly difficult cases, during dose reduction consider

- Zopiclone substitution for the benzodiazepine, followed by tapering.
- Adding SSRI (e.g., paroxetine 10–20 mg) to the benzodiazepine

before reducing benzodiazepine dose in order to "cover" emergence of rebound anxiety and/or panic.
- Adding carbamazepine 200–800 mg/day.
- Adding gabapentin 300–900 mg/day.
- Adding propranolol (for autonomic symptoms).
- Switching to a longer-acting agent and then tapering that drug.

Note: None of these strategies has been well investigated in elders, and each strategy carries the risks associated with each agent. Side effects of substitution drugs carry their own risk of prompting failed withdrawal because of dropouts or intolerance.

OVERDOSE

Although generally considered to be less lethal in overdose than older agents such as barbiturales, benzodiazepines are still associated with lethality and safety in overdose should not be taken for granted. There is an increased risk of lethality when consumed in combination with alcohol, barbiturates, or other CNS depressants.

Table 3.15. Symptoms and Management of Overdose

Symptoms	Management
• Respiratory depression • Somnolence • Hypotension • Delirium/confusion/restlessness • Impaired coordination • Ataxia/falls • Immobility • Slurred speech • Incontinence • Coma • Fatalities (rare unless concurrent agents used)	• Consider toxicology screen for multiple agents. √ *Note:* alprazolam, lorazepam, temazepam, triazolam may not be detected in urine. • Induce emesis with caution re aspiration. • Administer gastric lavage. • Maintain airway. • Monitor vital signs. • Maintain close observation. • Administer IV fluids to maintain blood pressure and encourage diuresis. • Administer flumazenil (benzodiazepine-receptor agonist): √ 1 mg IV injected at rate of 0.1 mg/15 sec. √ Occasionally may be necessary to infuse IV at rates of 0.1–0.5 mg/hr, adjusted to patient's level of wakefulness over several days. √ Flumazenil has a short half-life of just under 1 hour. √ Sometimes administered rectally. √ Oral administration, when available, may be preferable once patient can swallow. √ Reverses sedation but continue monitoring for sedation and respiratory depression. √ Caution re. risk of seizures (especially in long-term benzodiazepine users) and cyclic antidepressant overdose; *case report of complete heart block with flumazenil.* • Hemodialysis, hemoperfusion, and exchange transfusion are ineffective. • For hypotension, administer norepinephrine or metaraminol.

INDIVIDUAL ANTI-ANXIETY AND SEDATIVE/ HYPNOTIC DRUG PROFILES

ALPRAZOLAM

Drug	Manufacturer	Chemical Class	Therapeutic Class
alprazolam (Xanax)	Pharmacia & Upjohn (Pfizer)	triazolobenzodiazepine	anxiolytic

Indications: FDA/HPB

- Short-term relief of symptoms of anxiety; generalized anxiety disorder.
- Panic disorder with or without agoraphobia.

Indications: Off label

- Anxiety associated with depression.
  - √ Some evidence for efficacy as antidepressant, but not commonly used for this indication in elders.
    - ▫ Case reports of effectiveness in OCD-related depressive states.
- Cognitively impaired agitated patients.
  - √ Used with moderate success in nursing home patients.
- Augmentation of antipsychotics in younger schizophrenics.
- Augmentation of antimanic treatment (general adult data) as alternative to neuroleptic.
- Adjunctive to propranolol or nitroglycerine in treatment of anxiety associated with angina pectoris (young-old age group).
- Anxiety associated with cancer treatment (mixed-age data).

Pharmacology

See also Table 3.2, page 377.

- Elimination primarily through oxidative metabolism and then renal excretion of glucuronidized metabolite.
- Renal insufficiency has little effect on pharmacokinetics.
- Reduced clearance in severe liver disease.
- Kinetics altered by age.
  - √ Single dose oral clearance reduced and half-life prolonged in healthy elderly men: about half that of younger men; not as marked in women; medical illness increases half-life; peak plasma levels in men not affected by age in one study.
  - √ Active metabolites (mainly alpha-hydroxy-alprazolam) do not form as rapidly in elders and are renally excreted after glucuronidation (the rate of which is not age dependent).
  - √ Smaller volume of distribution in elderly men.
  - √ Unbound free fraction not influenced significantly by age.

Mechanism of action

- $GABA_A$ receptor agonist

Choosing a Drug

- High-potency benzodiazepine
  - √ Used for elders in low dose ranges.
  - √ Requires multiple daily doses (to avoid interdose anxiety).
  - √ Increased withdrawal symptoms on discontinuation compared to other benzodiazepines (general adult data).
- Little impairment of psychomotor performance in otherwise healthy elders with acute low dosing.
- No build-up of impairment with regular dosing over a few days of drug use.
  - √ Probably indicates tolerance to effects.
- Sedation does not seem to build.
  - √ Tolerance develops rapidly, especially at lower doses of 0.25–0.5 mg.
- IV form: Onset of action more rapid than oral but pharmacokinetics otherwise similar.
- Sustained-release form not yet available, but application for approval has been submitted.
  - √ Offers reduced dose schedule, but premarketing experience with elders very limited.

Dosing

- Elders tolerate low doses well.
- Anxiety management: Start at 0.125–0.25 mg 1–3 times a day.
  - √ Increase dose by 0.125–0.25 mg q 4–5 days.
  - √ 2 mg dose produces greater sedation and impaired psychomotor performance than lower doses.
- Panic disorder
  - √ Dosing not studied in elders.
  - √ Double doses over those for general anxiety disorder may be required.
  - √ Determined by trial in each case.
  - √ Wide range of effective doses: 1–10 mg.
    - ▫ Doses over 2 mg not suggested for routine use.
- Dosing for off-label indications:
  - √ Depression: 2–3 mg/day.
  - √ Adjunct in angina: Reported dose of 1–2 mg/day in mixed-age population.

Increasing dose and reaching therapeutic levels

- Common daily dose-0.25 mg bid (range 0.25–2 mg/day).
- Usual maximum about 0.75–1 mg/day but wide individual variation.

Discontinuation and Withdrawal

See also, pages 426–429.

- Severe withdrawal reactions are thought to be uncommon, but overall rate not determined in elders.
- Withdrawal delirium may occur.

Possible withdrawal reactions include:

- Anxiety, panic attacks, fatigue, irritability, heightened sensory perception, impaired concentration and coordination, paresthesias, diarrhea, blurred vision, panic, tachycardia, diaphoresis, tremulousness, headache, insomnia, nausea, vomiting, dry mouth, poor appetite, weight loss, sweating, muscle spasms, weakness, dizziness.
- Occasionally hypertension and seizures and rarely bronchospasm and psychosis.
  - √ Onset of seizures reported within 20–72 hours (mixed-age population data).
- Generally associated with prolonged treatment at relatively high doses (above 4 mg/day in general adults but dosage levels this high in elders not suggested).
  - √ Even therapeutic levels have been associated with withdrawal syndrome upon abrupt withdrawal.
- Dose of alprazolam associated with withdrawal symptoms not established for elders.
- Safe rate of withdrawal also not established, but probably in the range of 0.25 mg/day q 5–7 days.
  - √ Withdrawal and/or rebound symptoms may emerge even with slow and small incremental dose reduction.

Manage by

- Reinstituting drug temporarily before attempting withdrawal again.
- Substitution of another benzodiazepine is largely unsatisfactory, but may be partially helpful.
- Concurrent drugs reported effective in reducing abstinence effects:
  - √ Carbamazepine 100 qid or 200 bid.
    - ▫ Carbamazepine suggested for inpatients only (general adult data).
  - √ Buspirone 5 mg tid, or dose as tolerated, while alprazolam is reduced.

Side Effects

See also pages 401–409 for full range of side effects common to all benzodiazepines.

- Overall well tolerated but withdrawal problematic in some patients.

Table 3.16. Side Effects of Alprazolam

Side Effects	Most Common	Most Serious and Less Common	Comment
Body as a whole	• Fatigue/ weakness • Drug dependence • Appetite increased • Weight gain	• Anorexia	• Dependence may occur after relatively brief period on therapeutic doses √ Risk greater at higher doses
Cardiovascular	• Hypotension	• Syncope • Tachycardia	
Central and peripheral nervous system	• Drowsiness/ sedation • Ataxia • Headache • Cognitive (memory impairment) √ Usually mild • Dysarthria	• Incoordination • Amnesia • Seizures (case report) • Delirium • Coma	• Seizures and delirium associated with abrupt discontinuation
Gastrointestinal	• Constipation • Diarrhea • Nausea • Dry mouth		
Liver and biliary		• Jaundice	
Psychiatric	• Interdose anxiety • Irritability	• Depression • Suicidality • Rapid mood changes in bipolar patients • Disinhibition with hs sedation • Rage reactions • Case reports of restlessness, agitation, and paranoid ideation	• Depression or suicidality not directly attributable to alprazolam, but issue remains somewhat controversial • Anxiety rebound may occur in the morning before first daily dose • Behavioral disinhibition not well documented • Risk of physical dependence √ Usually with high doses (general adult data) □ May occur even after short periods on relatively low doses
Reproductive	• Sexual dysfunction		
Respiratory	• Nasal congestion	• Respiratory depression	

(*cont.*)

Continued

Side Effects	Most Common	Most Serious and Less Common	Comment
Skin and appendages		• Pruritis	
Special senses	• Blurred vision	• Increased intraocular pressure (rare)	• Avoid in narrow angle glaucoma
Urinary		• Incontinence	

Monitoring

- Plasma levels sometimes helpful.
  - √ 20–40 ng/ml range in panic disorder.
- BP, until stabilized.

Drug Interactions

- Alprazolam potentiated, sometimes dramatically, by inhibitors of CYP3A4 (see p. 410 for more complete list).
  - √ Especially cimetidine, nefazodone, fluvoxamine, azole antifungal agents (e.g., itraconazole, ketoconazole), fluoxetine, and propoxyphene.
- Grapefruit juice may impede metabolism and increase plasma level.
- Carbamazepine reduces alprazolam plasma concetrations.
- Digoxin plasma levels significantly increased by 1 mg/day of alprazolam.
  - √ May be related to reduced renal clearance.
- Avoid alcohol.
- Caution with
  - √ All CNS depressants (e.g., sedating antihistamines, narcotic analgesics, opiates alone or in combination [e.g., with ASA or acetaminophen]).
  - √ Sedative/hypnotic agents, other benzodiazepines, central alpha-2 antagonists (e.g., clonidine).
  - √ Some antibiotics (e.g., clarithromycin, cyclosporine, erythromycins).
  - √ Phenytoins (theoretical interaction not observed clinically).
- Imipramine and desipramine concentrations are increased.

Disability Interactions and Contraindications

- Contraindicated in
  - √ Acute narrow angle glaucoma
  - √ CNS depression

- Caution in liver/renal dysfunction.
- Special caution in monitoring compliance in patients with history of alcohol or drug abuse.

Overdose, Toxicity, Suicide

- Generally, reasonably safe in overdose.
  - √ Fatalities reported with alprazolam alone, but usually occur with combination overdoses, including alcohol.
  - √ Geriatric data not available.

Symptoms

- CNS depression
- Lethargy
- Combativeness
- Uncooperativeness

Management (see also p. 429)

- Induce emesis (in conscious patient).
- Monitor vital signs.
- Provide general supportive measures (airway, oxygenation, fluids).
- Administer gastric lavage.
- Consider norepinephrine for severe cardiopulmonary collapse.
- Hemodialysis probably of little value.

Caregiver Notes

- Advise patient and family.
  - √ Avoid alcohol.
  - √ Be cautious with driving, until the patient becomes familiar with reaction to the drug.
  - √ Do *not* stop medication abruptly.

Clinical Tips

- Sedation effects may limit utility in the larger doses sometimes required for panic management.
- Monitor plasma digoxin levels when coadministered.
- Consider the possibility of interdose or morning rebound in patients who develop intermittent anxiety prior to next dose of drug.
  - √ Manage by shortening interval between doses while maintaining the same total daily dose.
    - ▫ Be cautious not to promote dependence by increasing the dose as a result of the development of tolerance, another reason for interdose rebound.

- Occasional reports of seizures, even with slow taper.
- Withdrawal schedule should be *very* gradual.
  - √ High doses are not usual in elders, but if used, taper at a rate of 10–15% q 2–3 weeks.
  - √ Low-dose therapy also should be tapered slowly.

BUSPIRONE

Drug	Manufacturer	Chemical Class	Therapeutic Class
buspirone (Buspar)	Bristol	azaspirodecanedione	nonbenzodiazepine anxiolytic

Indications: FDA/HPB

- Anxiety

Indications: Off label

- Depression
  - √ Overall, general adult data support the antidepressant properties, but the strength of the data varies from study to study.
  - √ Certainly not a first-line antidepressant, but may be a good choice for treating anxiety with comorbid depression.
  - √ Potentiates SSRIs (general adult data).
- BPSD—aggression/agitation/disinhibition.
- Report utility in augmentation of SSRIs in treatment of OCD.
- Levodopa-induced dyskinesia may improve with higher doses (clinical reports).
- May reduce alcohol craving.

Pharmacology

See also page 377.

- Metabolite 1-pyrimidinylpiperazine is an alpha-2 adrenoreceptor antagonist.
  - √ May account for psychostimulant properties of buspirone.
- May indirectly influence GABA receptor complex.
- Reduce dose in renal and hepatic impairment.
  - √ Increased plasma concentrations and half-life (with severe hepatic impairment).
- No significant age-related differences in Tmax, half-life, or plasma concentrations.
  - √ Marked interindividual variation in pharmacokinetics, but not age related.

Mechanism of action

- Complex and not well characterized.
  - √ Has been characterized as a mid-brain modulator.
  - √ Does not bind to GABA receptors.
- Acts on the dopaminergic system as both antagonist and agonist.
  - √ Partial antagonism at the D_2 receptor.
  - √ Increases striatal concentrations of dopamine, homovanillic acid, and dihydroxyphenylacetic acid.
- Antagonist and partial agonist at the presynaptic $5HT_{1A}$ receptors.
  - √ Down-regulates $5HT_2$ receptors.
  - √ Tends to "normalize" serotonin levels.
- Metabolite antagonizes alpha-2 adrenoreceptor.

Choosing a Drug

- Generalized anxiety
  - √ Suggested agent based on limited geriatric data.
  - √ Significant improvement after 2–4 weeks of treatment.
  - √ Most effective in patients who are benzodiazepine-free for 1 month.
  - √ Reportedly as effective as benzodiazepines without as much sedation or effects on vigilance, psychomotor speed, and memory.
    - ▫ Advantageous cognitive profile not evident when compared to oxazepam (general adult data) or alprazolam (geriatric data in otherwise healthy elders).
- Antidepressant properties make it useful for anxiety with comorbid depression.
- Little interaction with CNS depressants.
- Anxiolytic of choice for patients with pulmonary disease (clinical reports).
- Not suitable for prn use for acute anxiety symptom relief.
  - √ Delayed onset of anxiolytic action (1–2 weeks, up to 4–6 weeks for full effects).
  - √ Compliance sometimes a problem in patients used to, or demanding of, immediate effects seen with benzodiazepines.
- Ineffective in panic disorder.
- Some effectiveness demonstrated in BPSD.
- Multiple daily dosing required—bid–qid.
- Must be taken regularly.

Quality of the data

- Several general adult, double-blind, controlled trials but, other than uncontrolled, clinical data, little that is specific to elders.

Dosing

Initial dose

- Starting dose 5 mg/day bid.

Increasing dose and reaching therapeutic levels

- Increase by 5 mg q 3 days.
- Target dose 10 mg tid (range 5 mg bid–20 mg tid).
- For levodopa-induced dyskinesia: 20 mg/day.
- For agitation/aggression in dementia: 15–30 mg/day (range up to 60 mg/day) in divided doses tid.
  - √ Average effective dose 35 mg/day.

Discontinuation and Withdrawal

Discontinuation does not require long taper; minimal withdrawal symptoms (general adult data).

Side Effects

- Generally well tolerated, even in octogenarians.
- Little cognitive effect after a single acute dose.
- Most prominent side effects include dizziness, headache, nervousness, lightheadedness, sweating, and nausea.

Table 3.17. Side Effects of Buspirone

Side Effects	Most Common*	Most Serious and Less Common
Body as a whole	• Weakness • Sweating	• Fatigue • Allergic phenomena
Cardiovascular	• Tachycardia	• Syncope • Hypotension • Hypertension
Central and peripheral nervous system	• Dizziness (8%) • Nervousness • Headache (4%) • Drowsiness • Paresthesia • Decreased concentration • Insomnia	• Theoretical potential to induce EPS-like symptoms, but little clinical data to support idea √ Oral dyskinesia (uncertain; case report) • Seizure • Slurred speech
Eye	• Blurred vision	
Gastrointestinal	• Nausea • Vomiting • Dry mouth • GI complaints √ Abdominal pain (6%) √ Constipation	• Diarrhea • Hypersalivation • Burning tongue
Hematological		• Leukopenia • Eosinophilia • Thrombocytopenia

(cont.)

Continued

Side Effects	Most Common*	Most Serious and Less Common
Metabolic and nutritional		• Serotonin syndrome (rare clinical reports) • Possible hypothermia
Psychiatric		• Paradoxical anxiety, agitation, racing thoughts, pressured speech, nervousness/restlessness • Euphoria √ Especially in dementia and with concurrent SSRI (case report data)
Skin and appendages	• Rash	• Alopecia
Urinary		• Possible retention

* Percentages are general adult data.

Drug Interactions

Potentiation of buspirone

- Inhibitors of CYP3A4 (see p. 410): observe fluoxetine, fluvoxamine particularly; occasional seizures reported, clinically significant interaction with *erythromycin*, *fluconazole*, *ketoconazole*, *itraconazole*, and *nefazodone*.
  - √ Lower the dose and titrate more cautiously if used in combination.
- Verapamil
- Diltiazem
- Caution with
  - √ Barbiturates
  - √ Cimetidine (increases plasma concentration; mild increase in adverse effects)
  - √ MAOIs (hypertensive effect)
- Haloperidol (plasma levels increased by buspirone)
- Trazodone (possible increased hepatic transaminase)

Action of buspirone antagonized by

- Inducers of 3A4 (may reduce concentration of buspirone), barbiturates, dexamethasone, rifampin, ritonavir, phenytoin, carbamazepine, oxybutynin, St. John's wort.
- Recent benzodiazepine use: Patients are less likely to respond to buspirone.

Disability Interactions, Precautions, and Contraindications

- Clinical reports of safety and efficacy in treating anxiety in patients with COPD, without inducing respiratory symptoms.

- Caution in seizure disorders.
- Caution with liver/renal impairment.
- MAOI use within 3 weeks contraindicated.

Effect on Laboratory Tests

- AST/ALT: Occasionally, increased levels.
- WBC: Occasional increased or decreased levels.

Overdose, Toxicity, Suicide

Symptoms of acute overdose

- GI: Nausea, vomiting, gastric distress.
- CNS: Dizziness, drowsiness, ataxia, tremor, incoordination, insomnia, hallucinations.
- Mood: High, rushing sensation.
- CVS: Hypotension.
- Other: Miosis.

Management

- Hospitalize.
- Administer gastric lavage or induce emesis (in conscious patient)
- Monitor vital signs.
- Provide general supportive measures.
- Run toxic screen for concurrent agents.
- Not dialyzable.

Clinical Tips

- Trial of 30 days is necessary nurse to determine if buspirone effective.
- Does *not* prevent benzodiazepine withdrawal.
  - √ If switching from a benzodiazepine to buspirone, taper benzodiazepine gradually.
    - ▫ Leave patient drug free for a week, if possible, before starting buspirone to distinguish between rebound anxiety from benzodiazepine withdrawal and effectiveness of buspirone on anxiety symptoms.
    - ▫ If drug-free period not clinically possible, buspirone initiation may overlap the benzodiazepine withdrawal.
      - ◦ Coadminister buspirone at therapeutic level (gradually titrated) for 4–6 weeks, during which the benzodiazepine is gradually tapered (about 15–20%/week).
    - ▫ Overall, discontinuing a benzodiazepine is often difficult.
  - √ Tricyclic coadministration has been found more effective than buspirone.

- Prior recent treatment with benzodiazepine associated with reduced effectiveness of buspirone.
- Onset of "antidisruptive" (in contrast to anxiolytic) effect in dementia syndromes may be immediate or delayed.

CHLORAL HYDRATE

Drug	Manufacturer	Chemical Class	Therapeutic Class
chloral hydrate	Generic	halogenated alcohol	sedative/hypnotic

Indications: FDA/ HPB

- Insomnia—short-term treatment.
- Alcohol withdrawal.

Pharmacology

See Table 3.2, page 377.

- Rapidly absorbed and metabolized in liver.
  √ Active metabolite trichloroethanol.
- Fast-acting (onset of action 30 minutes) and relatively short half-life (4–14 hours).

Choosing a Drug

- Not suggested and rarely used.
- Effective hypnotic with few hangover effects.
- Little effect on REM sleep.
- Liquid and suppository forms; unpleasant taste and odor.
- Tolerance (to sedative effect in 5–14 days) and physical dependence develop.
- Reduce dose in significant hepatic and renal impairment.

Dosing

- For *short-term use only*, as premedication in surgery or brief periods of sleep therapy.
- Dilute with 120 ml water to reduce gastric irritation.
- Daily dose regimen 250–500 mg hs.

Discontinuation and Withdrawal

- Sudden withdrawal from chronic use may induce delirium, seizures, and occasionally death.
- Always taper gradually.

Side Effects

Commonest effects include

- Gastric irritation (nausea vomiting, diarrhea, stomach pain).
- Unpleasant taste.
- Induction of hepatic enzymes.

Table 3.18. Side Effects of Chloral Hydrate

Side Effects	Most Common	Most Serious and Less Common
Body as a whole	Malaise	Hypersensitivity reaction
Cardiovascular		In large dose: • Cardiac arrhythmias • Hypotension • Torsades de Pointes
Central and peripheral nervous system	• Somnolence/drowsiness • Lightheadedness • Vertigo/dizziness • Headache • Ataxia • Confusion	• Delirium (including during withdrawal) • Nightmares
Eye		• Allergic conjunctivitis
Gastrointestinal	• Gastric irritation • Nausea • Vomiting • Diarrhea • Flatulence	
Hematological	• Eosinophilia	• Leukopenia
Liver and biliary		• Hyperbilirubinemia
Metabolic and nutritional		• Acute porphyria
Psychiatric		• Paradoxical excitation • Paranoia reported
Respiratory		• Respiratory depression
Skin and appendages	• Rash • Irritates skin and mucous membranes on contact	• Angioedema • Urticaria • Purpura

Drug Interactions

- Displaces other protein-bound drugs (e.g., warfarin), increasing plasma concentrations and anticoagulant effects.
- Avoid concurrent barbiturates—CNS depression.
- Avoid alcohol—CNS depression, tachycardia, flushing.

Effect on Laboratory Tests

- Increases urinary 17-hyroxycorticosteroid.
- Sometimes increases vitamin B_{12} readings.

tihyperten-

itis, ulcer)
itis.

tic Class

anticonvulsant

effective

ke symp-
gorrhea,
mpulsive

es.

ontraindications

ant use
class
se history

ics with as little as 4 g.*

necrosis, GI hemorrhage

ic damage

vith resistant cardiac arrhythmias.
iously vulnerable patients.

nd cardiac support (i.e., airway, oxygena-
ng, body temperature regulation, circula-
l electrolyte balance).
charcoal and gastric lavage soon after in-

e or norepinephrine for hypotension.
lialysis.

n 30 minutes.
s with

- √ Cardiac impairment, hypotensive disorders, or a sive medication.
- √ Gastrointestinal disorders (e.g., gastritis, esopha
  - ▫ Use rectal suppository except in colitis or proc

CLONAZEPAM

Drug	Manufacturer	Chemical Class	Therape
clonazepam (Klonopin, Rivotril)	Roche	benzodiazepine	anxiolytic,

Indications: FDA/HPB

- Panic disorder
- Seizure disorders

Indications: Off label

- Panic disorder, as adjunct to SSRIs.
- Mania
  - √ Early tranquilization until primary therapy become (e.g., lithium or valproate).
  - √ Efficacy studies vary in outcome.
  - √ Case reports also suggest effectiveness in manic-l toms associated with dementia and delirium (e.g., hyperactivity, intrusiveness, agitation, grandiosity, violence, anxiety).
- Movement disorders (case reports of effectiveness).
  - √ TD
  - √ Restless leg syndrome (general adult data)
  - √ Nonparkinsonian tremor
    - ▫ Orthostatic tremor
  - √ Myoclonus
    - ▫ Palatal myoclonus
- REM sleep behavioral disorders.

Pharmacology

See also page 377.

- Clearance may be decreased in elders.
- Reduce dose in severe liver impairment.

Mechanism of action

- Highly specific for binding at benzodiazepine receptor si
- Increases serotonin levels.

Choosing a Drug

- Anxiety: Suggested drug but long half-life may lead to accumulation and requires caution in elders.
- Panic disorder: Suggested because longer half-life reduces chance of interdose anxiety that may emerge with alprazolam.
  - √ bid dosing effective for panic (general adult data).
- Onset of action in 20–60 minutes.

Dosing

- Anxiety
  - √ Begin with 0.125–0.5 mg/day; increase slowly (especially in frail elders) by 0.125–0.25 mg q 5–7 days.
    - ▫ Sedation or confusion are usually the limiting side effect.
  - √ Target dose 1 mg/day.
- Panic: Usually requires larger doses, up to double the anxiety doses; begin with 0.5 mg; increase by 0.25–0.5 mg q 4-5 days, as needed and tolerated; target dose 1–2 mg/day (range 1–4 mg/day).
- Other use dosing.
  - √ TD: 0.5 mg bid (up to 3 mg/day) used clinically; no trials.
  - √ Depression: When used as adjunct to antidepressant therapy, 3 mg/day (divided doses bid) more effective than 1.5 (mixed-age population data).
  - √ Agitation in dementia: 0.5–1 mg bid.
  - √ Tremor and myoclonus: 0.5 mg bid.

Discontinuation and Withdrawal

See pages 426–429.

- Taper slowly to withdraw, about 10% per week.

Side Effects

Table 3.19. Side Effects of Clonazepam

Side Effects	Most Common*	Most Serious and Less Common
Cardiovascular	• Hypotension	
Central and peripheral nervous system	• Ataxia • Dizziness • Sedation/drowsiness 50% • Headache • Memory impairment	• Seizures
Eye	• Visual blurring	

(cont.)

Continued

Side Effects	Most Common*	Most Serious and Less Common
Gastrointestinal	• Constipation • Diarrhea • Dry mouth	
Hematological		• Neutropenia/thrombocytopenia (rarely)
Liver and biliary		• Hepatotoxicity √ Increased LFTs
Musculoskeletal	• Hypotonia	
Psychiatric		• Psychosis (case reports) • Behavioral disturbances • May induce depression
Respiratory		• Respiratory depression
Skin and appendages	• Rash • Pruritis	
Urinary		• Incontinence (rarely)

* Percentages are general adult data.

Monitoring: LFTs at baseline and regular intervals.

Drug Interactions

- Caution in combination with lithium and neuroleptics: May increase neurotoxicity.
- Caution with other CNS depressants: Increased CNS depressant effects.
- Some suggestion that inhibitors (inducers) of CYP3A4 may increase plasma levels of clonazepam.
  √ Clinical risks not confirmed (see p. 410).

Effect on Laboratory Tests

- LFTs sometimes increased.

Clinical Tips

- Give most of the dose hs, with smaller dose during the day, to minimize daytime sedation.
- For severe myoclonus, case reports suggest that combination therapy may be most effective.
  √ Clonazepam with valproate, primidone, and piracetam in different combinations or together.

DIAZEPAM

Drug	Manufacturer	Chemical Class	Therapeutic Class
diazepam (Valium)	Roche	benzodiazepine	anxiolytic; sedative/hypnotic

Indications: FDA/HPB

- Anxiety disorders
- Seizure disorders (as adjunct)
- Muscle relaxant (skeletal muscle spasticity)
- Alcohol withdrawal

Indication: Off label.

- Insomnia

Pharmacology

See page 377.

- After acute dose, active metabolite (desmethyldiazepam) contributes little to pharmacodynamic action.
  - √ During long-term therapy, metabolite accumulates along with diazepam.
  - √ Steady-state concentration of desmethyldiazepam equals or exceeds parent compound.
  - √ Other metabolites (i.e., temazepam and oxazepam) clear faster and do not accumulate to same extent.
- Chronic dosing leads to drug accumulation.
  - √ Partially offset by development of tolerance.
- Volume of distribution (especially in women) and half-life increase with age, largely due to changes in body distribution.
  - √ 4 times greater at age 80 than age 20.
- Clearance decreases significantly for all routes of administration.
- Lower plasma protein binding in elders.
  - √ Free fraction increases (secondary to lower albumin levels), but little clinical relevance.
- Smoking induces hepatic enzymes and increases metabolism.
- Cirrhosis: Reduce dose because of lowered rate of plasma clearance.

Choosing a Drug

- Not suggested for elders.
- Highly sedative in the day after administration.
  - √ Fatigue levels remain high for weeks after last dose.
- Sedation not greater than oxazepam but persists much longer after drug discontinuation.

Dosing

Daily dose regimen

- Once a day or every second day.

Initial dose

- 1–2 mg/day
- Therapeutic range 1–10 mg

Side Effects

See pages 401–409.

Drug Interactions

See page 410.

- Fluoxetine inhibits elimination of diazepam.
- Isoniazid increases diazepam (caution).
- Digitalis is increased by diazepam.
- Gallamine and succinylcholine: Diazepam prolongs intramuscular blockade.
- Theophylline antagonizes sedative effect.

Overdose, Toxicity, Suicide

See page 429.

ESTAZOLAM

Drug	Manufacturer	Chemical Class	Therapeutic Class
estazolam (Prosom)	Abbott	benzodiazepine	sedative/hypnotic

Indications: FDA

- Not available in Canada.
- Insomnia

Pharmacology

See page 377.

- Intermediate half-life (10–30 hours); clearance increased in smokers.

Mechanism of action: $GABA_A$ receptor agonist.

Choosing a Drug

- Not suggested for elders because of duration of action, although reasonably well-tolerated in robust elders.
- Rapidly absorbed.

- Intermediate half-life.
- Maintains efficacy in increasing total sleep time over 4 weeks of therapy.
  - √ Tolerance appears to develop slowly (geriatric data).
  - √ Up to 12 weeks in other studies (general adult data).
- Reduces sleep latency.
- Total sleep time increases about an hour on average.
- Rebound increased wakefulness transient on first night after discontinuation of drug.
- Daytime performance and anterograde memory unimpaired in healthy elders.
- Does not accumulate to produce carryover effects.

Dosing

- 1 mg hs usual dose (range 0.5–2 mg).
  - √ Start at 0.5 mg in frail or impaired elders.
- Increase gradually by 0.5 mg to 2 mg, if necessary and tolerated.

Side Effects

Well tolerated in otherwise well elders.

See pages 404–409.

Drug Interactions

- Similar to other benzodiazepines.
  - √ 3A4 inhibitors potentiate action (see Table 3.9, p. 410).
- Caution with CNS depressants.

Disability Interactions and Contraindications

- Respiratory depression
- Impaired renal/liver function
- Sleep apnea
- Caution with substance abuse history

Overdose, Toxicity, Suicide

See page 429.

LORAZEPAM

Drug	Manufacturer	Chemical Class	Therapeutic Class
lorazepam (Ativan)	Wyeth-Ayerst	benzodiazepine	anxiolytic; sedative/ hypnotic; anticonvulsant

Indications: FDA, HPB

- Short-term relief of anxiety symptoms.
  - √ Useful as adjunct to SSRIs for treatment of panic disorder (general adult data).
- Seizure disorder (indicated only in Canada).

Indications: Off label

- Management of alcohol withdrawal syndrome.
- Management of acute catatonia.
  - √ About 80% remission rate reported in suspected neuroleptic-induced catatonia.
- Management of mania: as adjunctive therapy (with mood stabilizer).
- Insomnia.

Pharmacology

- Unclear if age affects metabolism (data conflict).
- Lorazepam may continue to be detectable in the plasma weeks after discontinuation.
  - √ May be especially relevant in men.
- Renal disease does not appear to impair clearance or require dose reduction.
- Liver cirrhosis prolongs half-life.
  - √ Due to larger volume of distribution than other hydroxylated benzodiazepines (e.g., oxazepam, temazepam).

Mechanism of action

- GABA receptor agonist.
- Structural analogue of oxazepam but about 10 times its potency.

Choosing a Drug

- Anxiety: A drug of first choice.
- Anxiety associated with depression.
  - √ May enhance antidepressant response as well as reduce concurrent anxiety.
- May induce somewhat greater memory impairments in elders than some other benzodiazepines.
- Some data suggest slow absorption delays onset of action and reduces efficacy as sleep-induction agent.
- Variety of administration forms (oral, sublingual, IM, IV) available.
  - √ Parenteral route an advantage, especially for patients unable or unwilling to cooperate with oral therapy.
  - √ No potency/efficacy differences in oral vs. sublingual.
  - √ Data a little conflicting on speed of action (general adult data).

- Predictable IM absorption half-life of 20 minutes.
  - √ Time to onset of action 20–30 minutes.
  - √ Time to peak concentration 2 hours.
- Duration of effect 6–8 hours (general adult data).
  - √ May be too short to maintain sleep throughout the night in some patients.

Dosing

Initial dose

- Anxiolytic dose: initial 0.25–0.5 mg/day.
  - √ Increase by 0.25–0.5 mg q3–5 days, as needed and tolerated.
  - √ Target range 0.25–4 mg/day in divided doses bid or tid.
- Sedative dose: 1–2 mg hs.

Off-label indications dosing

- Catatonia 2 mg IM
  - √ Repeat as necessary if symptoms reappear.

Side Effects

- Abuse potential and withdrawal reaction (see pp. 401–409).

Table 3.20. Side Effects of Lorazepam

Side Effects	Most Common	Most Serious and Less Common	Comments
Body as a whole	• Increased body sway • Sleep disturbance		
Cardiovascular			• Cardiovascular collapse in overdose
Case reports		• SIADH • Transient global amnesia (TGA)	• TGA may last several hours in susceptible patients
Central and peripheral nervous system	• Sedation • Dizziness • Weakness • Ataxia • Headache • Subjective sleepiness • Impaired coordination • Impaired vigilance • Impaired capacity to divide attention • Reduced speed of response • Variable but sometimes impaired visual and verbal memory after single dose	• Anterograde amnesia • Myoclonic jerks • Nystagmus	• Functions associated with driving may be impaired despite subjective sense of normality • Clinical relevance of amnesic effects in healthy elders is unclear, more relevant to brain impaired with dementia. • Appears more likely than other benzodiazepines to induce memory impairment. √ Clinical relevance not clear, since lorazepam is generally well tolerated by elders.

(*cont.*)

Continued

Side Effects	Most Common	Most Serious and Less Common	Comments
Eye	• Diplopia		
Gastrointestinal	• Nausea		
Hematological			• Blood dyscrasias
Psychiatric		• Depression • Agitation	
Respiratory			• Respiratory depression
Urinary		• Incontinence	

Monitoring

- Plasma drug levels do not correlate with dose of drug.
  - √ Occasionally drug not detectable by standard assay methods, despite full-dose therapy.
    - ▫ Some data suggest therapeutic plasma level range is 20–80 ng/ml.

Drug Interactions

See also, page 410.

- Loxapine: Avoid concurrent use—may induce respiratory depression.
- Probenecid: Increases plasma levels and adverse effects.
- General cautions relevant to all benzodiazepines.
  - √ Inhibitors/inducers of CYP 3A4 enzyme.

Special Precautions

- Narrow angle glaucoma
- Alcohol consumption
- CNS depression
- Impaired liver function
- Impaired respiratory function
- Sleep apnea

Overdose, Toxicity, Suicide

See page 429.

Clinical Tips

- Cautions about driving impairment are important when using benzodiazepines, including lorazepam.

√ With increasing tolerance to the drug, impairments continue after subjective sleepiness diminishes.

- Caution patient to avoid alcohol.
- Dosing schedule not always clear and requires some clinical experimentation with the individual patient.
  √ Sometimes it is important to address daytime tension/anxiety that often accompanies insomnia as well as nocturnal sedation.
    - Consider spreading dose out during the day.
    - Rebound anxiety periods may emerge, especially in the morning after a reduced nocturnal dose.
- Tolerance seems to develop more rapidly than with some other benzodiazepines (e.g., temazepam).

MIDAZOLAM

Drug	Manufacturer	Chemical Class	Therapeutic Class
midazolam (Versed)	Roche	benzodiazepine	sedative

Indications: FDA, HPB

- Preoperative sedation/anxiolysis/amnesia

Pharmacology

- Ultra-short half-life (less than triazolam).
  √ Clearance somewhat slower and half-life longer in elders, but significant only for men.
- Parenteral route very rapid absorption.
  √ Onset of action in 3–6 minutes.
- Duration of action 2–4 hours.
- Onset of sedative effects in 15 minutes after IM injection (peak at 30–60 minutes) and 3–6 minutes after IV injection.
- Recovery may take 2–6 hours.

Choosing a Drug

- Use with extreme caution in elders; not for routine sedative/hypnotic use because of danger of serious cardiorespiratory events.
- Concomitant CNS depressants, especially narcotics, are usually contraindicated.
- Available in parenteral and syrup formulations.
  √ Suitable for hospital settings where it is used for patients

mechanically ventilated and continuously observed for respiratory depression.
  - √ Short elimination half-life, water soluble, well tolerated.
- May cause respiratory depression with prolonged use.

Dosing

- Lower doses of midazolam required for elders, based on increased pharmacodynamic sensitivity (pharmacokinetics are not changed in elders).
- Requires deep IM injection in large muscle mass.

Initiating therapy

- Administer immediately hs.
- IV dose: Unpremedicated patients use 1–1.5 mg IV by slow (30–60 seconds) injection for sedation.
- IM dose: 1–3 mg administered slowly over 30–60 seconds.
- To keep the patient asleep when intubated/mechanically ventilated.
  - √ Give initial intravenous bolus injection and wait 2–3 minutes to evaluate sedative effect before giving additional doses.
  - √ Then use continuous infusion rate of 0.025–0.03 mg/kg/hr.
    - ▫ May need faster rate in some patients, but danger of inducing very high plasma levels.
  - √ Change the flow rate only q 30 minutes and use alterations of 25–50% of the original dose.
  - √ Lower the dose appropriately for more frail or otherwise compromised patients.

Side Effects

See pages 401–409.

- Common side effects include fluctuations in vital signs.

Table 3.21. Side Effects of Midazolam

Side Effects	Most Common	Most Serious and Less Common
Cardiovascular disorders	• Hypertension • Hypotension • Tachycardia • Bradycardia	
Central and peripheral nervous system	• Anterograde amnesia • Headache • Excessive sedation • Dizziness • Hallucinations • Agitation • Confusion	• Acute agitation and combativeness reported

(*cont.*)

Continued

Side Effects	Most Common	Most Serious and Less Common
Gastrointestinal	• Hiccups • Nausea/vomiting	
Respiratory disorders	• Respiratory depression √ Significant and dangerous in COPD • Tachypnea • Decreased respiratory rate • Apnea	
Skin and appendages	• Pain at injection site	

Drug Interactions

- Narcotic premedication potentiates midazolam.
- Pancuronium may be potentiated by midazolam.
- Plasma concentration of midazolam altered by coadministration of inhibitor/inducers of CYP3A4 (see p. 410).

OXAZEPAM

Drug	Manufacturer	Chemical Class	Therapeutic Class
oxazepam (Serax)	Generic	benzodiazepine	anxiolytic

Indications: FDA/HPB

- Anxiety disorders
- Alcohol withdrawal

Indications: Off label

- Insomnia

Pharmacology

- Little age-related effects on metabolism.
- Mechanism of action: GABA receptor agonist.

Choosing a Drug

- Suggested for elders.
  √ No accumulation of active metabolites.
  √ Washes out after about 3 days.
- Absorbed slowly.
  √ May be less effective for acute anxiety.
  √ Delay in inducing sleep (although still effective in many patients, based on clinical responses).

Dosing

- Frequency of administration varies.
  - √ Some patients require tid administration for control of anxiety.
- Anxiety: starting dose 5–10 mg q day.
- Sleep: If used for sedation, advise patient to take drug 1–2 hours prior to bed (prolonged time to peak plasma levels).
  - √ Use the time for implementing nonpharmacological sleep hygiene measures.

Increasing dose and reaching therapeutic levels

- Anxiety: Increase by 5–15 mg q 4–5 days.

Maintenance dose

- Anxiety: 10 mg tid (range 10–45 mg).
- Alcohol withdrawal: 15–30 mg tid–qid.
- Insomnia: 10–30 mg hs.

Side Effects

See pages 401–409.

Special monitoring

- Therapeutic plasma level 0.2–1.4 μg/ml.

Drug Interactions

See Table 3.9 on page 410.

Disability Interactions

- Renal insufficiency: Reduce dosage or increase time between doses.

Overdose, Toxicity, Suicide

- Not dialyzable
- See page 429.

Clinical Tips

- Acute delusional state and rare status petit mal epilepsy may occur on withdrawal from higher dose therapy (case report).
- Delayed absorption time with capsule (as opposed to tablet) form of the drug.

TEMAZEPAM

Drug	Manufacturer	Chemical Class	Therapeutic Class
temazepam (Restoril)	Novartis	benzodiazepine	hypnotic

Indications: FDA/HPB

- Insomnia (transient and short term)

Indications: Off label

- Premedication before surgery

Pharmacology

See also page 377.

- Little age-related effects in men but prolonged half-life (18 hours) in women.
- Metabolized by glucuronidation, which is less sensitive to age-related changes in metabolism.
- Produces no active metabolites.
- Less lipid soluble than other benzodiazepines.

Choosing a Drug

- Suggested for insomnia in elders.
- Seems well tolerated in low doses in healthy elders.
- Readily absorbed orally in soft gelatin capsule form (45 minutes).
  - √ Hard capsule absorption is slower.
    - ▫ Mean peak time 1–2 hours—not suitable to induce sleep.
  - √ Newer smaller particle formulation improves rate of absorption and shortens Tmax.
- Half-life is fairly long (especially in women and elderly inpatients), suggesting potential for accumulation and caution in long-term usage.
  - √ Data inconsistent.
    - ▫ Some studies show no increased half-life or accumulation in elders.
- Some deterioration of daytime performance (e.g., hypersomnolence and decreased performance on tests of neurological function).
  - √ Similar extent to that induced by longer-acting nitrazepam, but here too data inconsistent.
  - √ May be related to its relatively low lipophilicity (and hence slower penetration into the brain).

- Evidence for tolerance and decreased effectiveness during relatively short-term use (2–3 weeks).
  - √ Data conflict.

Quality of the data

- Several randomized controlled studies (mostly general adult data).

Dosing

Initial dose

- 7.5 mg hs (*Note:* Only 15 and 30 mg *hard capsule* versions available in Canada).
  - √ Hard capsule form: 1–2 hours before bed.
  - √ Soft capsule form: 30–60 minutes before bed.
- Increase 7.5 mg q 4–5 days, as needed.
  - √ Many patients do well on 7.5 mg.
  - √ Target dose for those needing higher dose is 15 mg about 1 hour before bed.
    - ▫ Avoid higher dose in frail elders.

Discontinuation and Withdrawal

- Higher doses (15–30 mg) associated with more withdrawal effects.
  - √ Fewer effects if lower dose (7.5 mg) is withdrawn, even if abruptly.

Side Effects

See also pages 401–409.

Table 3.22. Side Effects of Temazepam

Side Effects	Most Common*	Most Serious and Less Common
Cardiovascular	• Hypotension √ Usually modest (10 mm Hg) and dose dependent √ Occasionally clinically important • Tachycardia (associated with hypotensive effect)	
Central and peripheral nervous system	• Drowsiness • Dizziness • Lethargy • Confusion • Ataxia • Hangover (dose-related)	• Agitation √ Sleepwalking √ Anger √ Panic

(*cont.*)

Continued

Side Effects	Most Common*	Most Serious and Less Common
Gastrointestinal	Bitter taste (5%)	
Musculoskeletal		• Increased risk of hip fractures
Psychiatric	• Euphoria	
Skin and appendages		• Skin rash

* Percentages are general adult data.

Special monitoring

- Therapeutic serum level 26 ng/ml.
- Women may be more sensitive to clinical and adverse effects than men.

Drug Interactions

See also page 410.

- Caution with azole antifungals.

Overdose, Toxicity, Suicide

See page 429.

TRIAZOLAM

Drug	Manufacturer	Chemical Class	Therapeutic Class
triazolam (Halcion)	Pharmacia and Upjohn (Pfizer)	triazolobenzodiazepine	hypnotic

Indications: FDA/HPB

- Short-term treatment of insomnia.

Indications: Off label

- Restless leg syndrome: report of efficacy in elders.
  - √ Increases total sleep time and efficiency, although leg movements not reduced.
  - √ Well tolerated.

Pharmacology

See page 377.

- Oxidative metabolism; principle metabolite oxazepam.

- Clearance lower in elders.
  - √ Outcome not uniform in all studies.
  - √ Some evidence that triazolam may accumulate in some patients after prolonged use.
- Peak plasma levels.
  - √ Higher in female elders than younger subjects.
  - √ Some data indicate peak levels are 2 times higher in elders.
- Tmax earlier than in younger subjects.

Choosing a Drug

- Not suggested for elders.
  - √ Early studies suggesting geriatric indications not supported by clinical experience and postmarketing trials.
    - ▫ Increased rate of confusion, amnesia, agitation, and bizarre behavior in elders 22–99 times greater than with temazepam (as an example of a reference benzodiazepine).
  - √ Probably best to avoid even in low doses of 0.125 mg, based on overall weight of evidence.
  - √ Caution especially relevant in frail elders with comorbid conditions (e.g., congestive heart failure).
  - √ Amnesic and confusional states when the drug wears off.
  - √ Drug has been delisted in Britain and New Zealand, temporarily delisted in Netherlands, and cautions released widely about its use.
- Ultra-short acting agent that induces sleep but does not maintain it for long periods.
  - √ Ultra-short half-life leads to daytime withdrawal effects.
- Tolerance develops rapidly.
- Greater difficulty falling back to sleep if awaken in night (e.g., because of nocturia).
- Greater sedation and psychomotor impairment in elders compared to younger patients.
- *Note:* Has been used in Alzheimer's disease but with poor sedative effect in the 0.125 mg dose (and increased side effects in higher dose).

Quality of the data

- Well studied in randomized placebo-controlled trials.

Dosing

Daily dose regimen

- Dosing for elders unclear.
  - √ Dose is 0.125 mg po hs.

  - Even 0.0625 mg in very sensitive patients—however, efficacy of that dose not well established.
  - Dose of 0.125 mg found ineffective for sedation in one group of patients with Alzheimer's disease.
  - √ Do not repeat during the night.
- Use for shortest time possible (1–2 weeks).

Side Effects

- Rates of side effects 3–13 times that of temazepam or flurazepam (general adult data).
  √ Doses used in comparisons are not clearly comparable.
- Daytime hyperexcitability and withdrawal difficulties much worse with this agent.
- Side effects less with lower dose range.

Table 3.23. Side Effects of Triazolam

Side Effects	Most Common	Most Serious and Less Common	Comments
Body as a whole	• Rebound insomnia (60%)		• Rebound may occur even after 1–2 nights of treatment
Central and peripheral nervous system	• Daytime confusion • Oversedation • Amnesic states • Motor incoordination 2 hours after dosing √ Danger of falls • Increased postural sway and instability. • Cognitive/perceptual impairment including confusion, disorientation. • Memory impairment evident especially at peak blood levels.	• Agitation (sleepwalking, anger, panic)	• Motor incoordination most evident in older patients with poor baseline coordination prior to drug. • Amnesic states in as many as 40%. • Sedation reported, even at low dose, in very old patients with congestive heart failure. • Many reports of more severe reactions √ Paranoid delusions at higher doses in general adults.
Gastrointestinal	• Dry mouth and xerostomia		
Psychiatric		• Early A.M. awakening • Anxiety • Hallucinations • Paranoid delusions	

Overdose, Toxicity, Suicide

See page 429.

Clinical Tips

- Although drug is not recommended, if it must be used (e.g., no other alternatives).
  - √ Use low doses (up to 0.25 mg) and avoid abrupt changes in dose to decrease likelihood of rebound phenomena.
- Monitor mental status the day after each dose.
  - √ Ask collateral sources for periods of memory gaps or confusional states.
    - ▫ The patient may not remember because of amnesic effects of drug.

ZALEPLON

Drug	Manufacturer	Chemical Class	Therapeutic Class
zaleplon (Sonata)	Wyeth-Ayerst Servier—Canada	pyrazolopyrimidine nonbenzodiazepine	sedative/hypnotic

Indications: FDA/HPB

- Short-term treatment of insomnia.

Pharmacology

- Disposition unaffected by age or sex.
- Clearance
  - √ Reduced in liver disease.
  - √ Unaffected in renal impairment.

Mechanism of action

- $GABA_A$-selective agent
  - √ Binds to omega-1 subunit.
  - √ Does not affect omega-2 receptors.

Choosing a Drug

- Rapid onset of action useful for sleep induction, but shorter duration of action makes it less effective for sleep maintenance and early A.M. awakening.
  - √ May be useful for middle-of-the-night use in some patients, but no geriatric studies for this indication and caution is advised.
- Short duration of side effects (< 5 hrs.; general adult data).
- Said to induce less memory impairment than zolpidem, but more than lorazepam.

√ Geriatric data scarce and clinical relevance not established.
- Psychomotor and memory function less affected, even at peak plasma levels, than with comparable hypnotic agents.
- May be slightly less sedative than zolpidem.
  √ Produces little hangover effect.
- Tolerance appears slow to develop.
  √ May continue to be effective for some months (or longer) while drug is in continuous use.
  √ Studies are poorly controlled and data should be viewed as preliminary.
- Abuse potential not determined but indirect evidence indicates similar potential as benzodiazepines.

Race/ethnicity

- Asian patients have slower metabolism.
  √ Maximum concentration 37% higher.

Dosing

Daily dose regimen

- 5 mg qhs po immediately before bed.
- 10 mg sometimes necessary for robust young-old elders.

Discontinuation and Withdrawal

- Some rebound insomnia.
  √ Said to be reduced if drug only used intermittently when insomnia occurs.

Side Effects

Table 3.24. Side Effects of Zaleplon

Side Effects	Most Common*	Most Serious and Less Common
Central and peripheral nervous system	• Migraine headache (15–18%) • Dizziness • Ataxia • Drowsiness • Amnesia • Decreased concentration • Impaired coordination • Paresthesias • Hangover • Rebound insomnia • Nervousness	

(cont.)

Continued

Side Effects	Most Common*	Most Serious and Less Common
Eye	• Impaired visual focusing	
Gastrointestinal	• Dyspepsia • Abdominal pain • Bad taste	• Constipation • Dry mouth
Musculoskeletal	• Hypertonia • Myalgia	
Psychiatric	• Confusion • Depression	• Acute onset hallucinations (case reports)
Respiratory	• Rhinitis • Pharyngitis	
Skin and appendages		• Rash

* Percentages are general adult data.

Drug Interactions

CNS depressants—consider reduced dose in combination with the following

- Opiates, opiate agonists
- Propoxyphene
- Tramadol
- Antidepressants (i.e., tricyclics, trazodone, fluvoxamine, fluoxetine venlafaxine, mirtazapine, nefazodone)
- Antihistamine/decongestant combinations
- Sedating antihistamines
- Antipsychotics (i.e., all atypicals, phenothiazines, haloperidol, molindone, loxapine, thiothixene)
- Barbiturates
- Benzodiazepines
- Dronabinol
- Droperidol
- Ethanol
- Metoclopramide
- CYP3A4 inhibitors (see p. 410)
- Azole antifungal agents

Action antagonized by

- CYP inducers
  - √ Rifampin
  - √ Phenytoin
  - √ Phenobarbitol
  - √ Carbamazepine

Disability Interactions and Contraindications

- Impaired liver function—reduce dose.
- Sleep apnea—contraindicated.
- Caution with respiratory compromise (caution recommended on theoretical rather than clinical data basis).

Overdose, Toxicity, Suicide

No specific data available.

Clinical Tips

- Residual effects not well established for elders; little next-day effect (general adult data).
- Duration of use not well established.
  - √ Guidelines similar to benzodiazepines (i.e., brief therapy up to 4 weeks), but may be useful for longer-term therapy.
- Middle-of-the-night use not recommended for elders—increased risk of confusion and falls.
- Tolerance appears to develop slowly, if at all.
- Some abuse potential but this is an unusual problem in routine therapy of elders.
  - √ Increased caution if history of substance abuse.
- Avoid fatty meal before taking the drug—increases time to sleep onset.

ZOLPIDEM

Drug	Manufacturer	Chemical Class	Therapeutic Class
zolpidem tartrate (Ambien)	Searle	imidazopyridine	hypnotic

Indications: FDA/HPB

- Short-term treatment of insomnia

Indications: Off label

- Agitation in dementia

Pharmacology

See page 377.

- Clearance reduced with
  - √ Age, especially over 70.
  - √ Hepatic and renal disease.

- Plasma levels increased in women.
- Rapid absorption.

Mechanism of action

- Short-acting (6–8 hours) nonbenzodiazepine which interacts at the benzodiazepine binding site.
  - √ Binds with high affinity to alpha-1-containing $GABA_A$ receptor binding sites at the type I (omega-1) site that contains the $GABA_A$ receptor and chloride channel.
    - ▫ Almost no affinity for the type II (omega-2) site.
    - ▫ Binds with low affinity for certain alpha-2/3/5-containing $GABA_A$ receptor subtypes (generally located on omega-2 receptor sites).

Actions by indication

- Sedative hypnotic (type I GABA receptor).
- Maintains sedative action for prolonged periods without tolerance developing (6 months in one geriatric study), but tolerance data inconsistent.
  - √ Initially increases deep sleep (stages 3 and 4) and decreases REM.
    - ▫ These effects decline after a few (4) weeks and appear to be dose dependent above 10 mg (general adult data).
  - √ Improves all measures of sleep (i.e., sleep efficiency, slow-wave sleep, total sleep time, time awake, nocturnal awakenings, percentage of REM sleep [reduced]).
- Ineffective anxiolytic, muscle relaxant, or anticonvulsant (no binding at the type II GABA receptor) at therapeutic doses.
- Despite some different properties, behavioral pharmacology appears very similar to classic benzodiazepine agonists.

Choosing a Drug

- Suggested for geriatric use, based on controlled trials.
- Main action is to enhance onset of sleep.
  - √ Not very useful for sleep maintenance.
- Rapid onset of action (within 30 minutes).
- Duration of action about 6–8 hours.
- Purportedly little negative effect on sleep architecture (unlike benzodiazepines).
- Data (general adult) suggest little rebound insomnia after discontinuation following prolonged use (e.g., compared to triazolam).

- Abuse potential appears similar to triazolam but less than trazodone (general adult data).
  √ Case reports of abuse in elders.
- Agitation with dementia: Anecdotal report of utility.
- Has been safely administered with SSRIs.
- Safely administered to COPD patients with no adverse effects on pulmonary function (general adult data with some geriatric).
- Next-day memory impairment may be less than benzodiazepines, but danger of confusion and psychomotor impairment in the few hours after taking the drug.

Race/ethnicity

- Does not affect drug metabolism.

Dosing Decision-Making

- 5 mg qhs initially.
  √ Some patients with more severe insomnia and who metabolize the drug well may benefit from 10 mg, but this higher dose not suggested for frail elders.
- Rapid onset of action—administer just before bed.
- Off-label indications dosing.
  √ Geriatric case report of improved behavior in agitated demented patient at 2.5 mg.

Discontinuation and Withdrawal

- Withdrawal syndrome may occur.
  √ Tremor, tachycardia, tachypnea, sweating, GI symptoms (nausea, vomiting, and abdominal pain, which may be severe).
- Case reports of withdrawal seizures after abrupt discontinuation of high-dose intake.

Side Effects

- Geriatric data and data in impaired and frail elders still limited, but overall seems well tolerated in otherwise healthy elders.
  √ Vertigo and confusion more evident in elders.
- Overall incidence of side effects > 60%.
- Most common side effects include nausea, dizziness, malaise, nightmares, agitation, headache, hypotension, and drowsiness.
- Higher incidence of side-effects with 10 mg dose.
- Next-day performance not affected in healthy elders, but some impairments within a few hours after drug administration.

Table 3.25. Side Effects of Zolpidem

Side Effects	Most Common*	Most Serious and Less Common	Comments
Body as a whole	• Malaise	• Abuse potential • Rebound insomnia	• Abuse potential comparable to triazolam (general adult data).
Cardiovascular		• Hypotension (dose related)	
Central and peripheral nervous system	• Drowsiness (3%) • Dizziness (0.8%) • Headache (18%) • Agitation (0.8%) • Lightheadedness • Unsteady gait (possible falls) • Nightmares	• Hypnogogic hallucinations √ May be associated with concurrent serotonergic drugs. • Confusional episodes • Delirium (case report; general adult) • Rare anterograde amnesia	• Impaired short-term memory, psychomotor performance, and increased postural sway occurs at peak blood levels (1–4 hours). √ Wears off by end of therapeutic period of 6–8 hours.
Eye	• Diplopia		
Gastrointestinal	• Nausea (7%)	• Abdominal pain • Vomiting • Diarrhea	
Musculoskeletal	• Myalgia (9%)	• Leg cramps (case report)	
Psychiatric	• Nocturnal agitation	• Brief psychotic episodes • Depression	• Caution in patients with depression. • Avoid in patients with psychosis.
Respiratory		• Exacerbates sleep apnea	• Obstructive apnea may emerge after a few nights of treatment.
Skin and appendages		• Rash • Pruritis	

* Percentages are from general adult data.

Monitoring

- Therapeutic plasma level not established for elders (some suggest a range of 80–150 ng/ml).

Drug Interactions

- Pharmacodynamic interactions with other drugs that have sedative properties and with CYP3A4, 2C9, 1A2 enzyme inhibitors (see p. 95).

- √ Increased plasma concentrations with
- √ Ketoconazole.
- √ Sertraline (clinical significance uncertain).
- √ Flumazenil: Antagonized hypnotic effect.
- √ Paroxetine: Case report of hallucinations, disorientation.
- √ Fluoxetine.
- Alcohol: No significant interaction but avoid coadministration.
- Reduced plasma concentrations with rifampicin.

Case reports of interaction with desipramine, bupropion, venlafaxine (hallucinations), and warfarin (increased prothrombin levels).

Disability Interactions and Contraindications

- Severe hepatic insufficiency (may cause encephalopathy)
- Myasthenia gravis
- Obstructive sleep apnea
- Respiratory depression
- Avoid alcohol (general caution)

Overdose, Toxicity, Suicide

- Symptoms generally not life threatening.
- Many patients show few symptoms of intoxication after ingestion; these may include
  - √ Drowsiness (most common)
  - √ Vomiting
  - √ Agitation
  - √ Dizziness
  - √ Hypotonia
  - √ Mydriasis
  - √ Hypotension
  - √ Incoherent speech.
  - √ Coma (doses ranged from 140–400 mg [general adult data with some elders included]).
  - √ Occasional fatalities reported.
  - √ Respiratory
    - □ Occasional respiratory depression.
    - □ Tachypnea (in patient with COPD)
  - √ Cardiac
    - □ Bradycardia
  - √ Hematological
    - □ Leukocytosis
  - √ *Note:* This list is for mixed age group of patients and includes single case reports.

Management

- Provide full supportive measures.
  - √ Maintain airway, as necessary.
  - √ Monitor vital signs for 12–24 hours.
  - √ IV fluids, as necessary.
- Administer gastric lavage and/or induce emesis.
- Consider administering activated charcoal.
- Consider flumazenil (antagonizes CNS depression of zolpidem).
  - √ Use in serious cases and with caution re risk of seizure induction.
- Screen for concurrent drugs (usually found in suicide attempts) which increase toxicity.
- Run a toxicology screen.
- Full blood count.
- Serum chemistry.
  - √ Hypokalemia associated with gastric lavage.
  - √ Metabolic acidosis associated with concomitant drugs.
  - √ Enzymes
    - ▫ Elevated AST/ALT in patients with liver disease or ingestion of concurrent medications.
    - ▫ Elevated creatinine.
  - √ In general, laboratory abnormalities not associated with zolpidem per se.
- ECG monitoring necessary initially.
- Recovery is usually within a few hours in otherwise uncomplicated cases.

Clinical Tips

- Warn patient of rapid onset of action and avoidance of activities requiring coordination and alertness after ingestion.
- For rapid effect, avoid administering with or after food—slows absorption and delays onset of action.
- Expectations of effectiveness should be modest.
  - √ Usually induces sleep more rapidly than before drug, by about 15–30 minutes.
  - √ Initially increases total sleep time by only about 25 minutes to 2 hours.
  - √ Sleep may improve further after 3–4 weeks of treatment.
- Abuse potential not determined in elders.
  - √ Probably low risk, but use with caution in presence or history of comorbid substance abuse.
  - √ Case reports of abuse.
  - √ Gradual taper of zolpidem, since withdrawal effects not controlled with benzodiazepines.

- May not reverse rebound that may occur when benzodiazepine discontinued.
  - √ Gradual benzodiazepine taper usually necessary when switching from a benzodiazepine to zolpidem.
    - But some data suggest zolpidem as an alternative to benzodiazepine tapering.
- Not effective in abstinence syndromes.
- Monitor patients on SSRIs or other serotonergic agents (hallucinations reported).
- Does not appear to produce as much rebound insomnia on withdrawal of therapeutic doses of drug.
- Weigh cost benefit of this drug for specific patient circumstances.
  - √ Slow development of tolerance an advantage of zolpidem in longer-term sleep therapy.
  - √ Similar results often obtainable with cheaper benzodiazepines in short-term therapy.

ZOPICLONE

Drug	Manufacturer	Chemical Class	Therapeutic Class
zopiclone (Imovane)	Aventis Pharma	cyclopyrrolone	sedative/Hypnotic

Indications: HPB

- Available in Canada for short-term treatment of insomnia.

Indications: Off label

- Some data (general adult) suggest utility as substitute for benzodiazepine during withdrawal programs.
  - √ Zopiclone can reduce rebound from benzodiazepines and is less likely to lead to withdrawal symptoms on its own.

Pharmacology

See page 377.

Decreased rate of metabolism leads to increased plasma levels.

- Age-dependent factor: Clearance at age 65–68 similar to younger adults but slower clearance and higher plasma concentrations in older groups (i.e., 74–85 yrs.).
- Sensitive to reduced liver function in cirrhosis.
- Sensitive to severe levels of reduced renal function.

Pharmacodynamic activity

- Sedative/hypnotic/anxiolytic.

- Anticonvulsant.
- Muscle relaxant.

Mechanism of action

- GABA agonist.

Therapeutic actions by indication

- Some efficacy in generalized anxiety as well as sleep disorders.

Choosing a Drug

- Tolerated well by elders.
- Tolerance not observed in time-limited trials.
  - √ Sustained hypnotic efficacy up to 8 weeks.
- Overall, offers only slight advantage over recommended benzodiazepines, but in some patients the response to zopiclone is much better.
- Effectiveness equals or exceeds other recommended benzodiazepine sedative/hypnotics for elders.
  - √ Sleep continuity improved.
  - √ May be more effective for this effect than benzodiazepines.
- More expensive than benzodiazepines.
  - √ Not sufficient demonstrated additional benefit to suggest zopiclone for routine use if cost is an issue.
- Residual psychomotor and memory deficits.
  - √ May persist the next day but do not consistently emerge in clinical trials.
  - √ Psychomotor effects within a few hours of administration are more consistently found.
- Variable rebound insomnia on discontinuation.
  - √ May be slight, but significant reactions also reported.
- Most effective for more recent onset sleep disturbance (< 1 year; general adult data).

Dosing

- Begin with 3.75 mg hs. immediately before bed.
  - √ Higher dose of 5–7.5 mg may be appropriate in young-elders.

Discontinuation and Withdrawal

- Rebound insomnia occurs on discontinuation but is not as problematic after short-term use.
- Requires gradual tapering.

Side Effects

- Generally well tolerated by elders at recommended doses.
- Commonest side effect is bitter taste.

Table 3.26. Side Effects of Zopiclone

Side Effects	Most Common*	Most Serious and Less Common
Body as a whole	• Fatigue	
Cardiovascular	• Palpitations	
Central and peripheral nervous system	• Vertigo • Rebound insomnia on discontinuation • Increases postural sway • Sleepiness • Headache	• Difficulty awakening in the morning • Nightmares • Global amnestic syndrome (chronic use, case report data)
Eye	• Blurred vision	
Gastrointestinal	• Bitter aftertaste (3–8% but ranging up to 39%) at peak concentrations after about 25 minutes, may lead to treatment discontinuation. • Dry mouth • Sialorrhea	• Nausea/vomiting • Diarrhea • Anorexia
Liver and biliary		• Occasional reports of increased ALT/AST
Metabolic and nutritional		• Weight loss
Musculoskeletal	• Arthralgia	
Skin and appendages	• Sweating	• Rash

* Percentages are general adult data.

Drug Interactions

- Plasma concentration of zopiclone increased by
  - √ Metoclopramide
  - √ Carbamazepine (increased psychomotor impairments; concentration of carbamazepine decreases concurrently).
  - √ Itraconazole
  - √ Erythromycin (potentiates psychomotor effects of zopiclone).
  - √ Possibly nefazodone (geriatric case report of CYP3A4 inhibition).
- Plasma concentrations decreased by
  - √ Rifampin
  - √ Atropine
- Alcohol, benzodiazepines, and other CNS depressants potentiate effects of zopiclone.
  - √ Do not alter metabolism.

Disability Interactions

- Cirrhosis of liver: Reduce dose.

Overdose, Toxicity, Suicide

- Safety in overdose not established but reports indicate general safety.

- √ Deaths reported with ingestion of > 400 mg plus another agent (alcohol or benzodiazepine) but not with zopiclone alone.
- Lethal plasma level for zopiclone as a solo drug reported in a few geriatric cases: 1.4–3.9 mg/l (estimated dose of at least 200–350 mg of zopiclone).

Management

- Monitor vital signs.
- Administer gastric lavage.
- Provide fluid IV, airway, and other supportive measures, as indicated.
- Hemodialysis of no value.
- Run toxic screen for other concurrent drugs.
- Consider flumazenil.

Clinical Tips

- Taper slowly to discontinue as with benzodiazepines.
  - √ Despite claims of slight rebound on discontinuation, data are inconsistent.
- Hangover effect is dose related—use smallest effective dose.
  - √ Some patients have strong reactions to this agent.
    - ▫ Next day-heaviness, dizziness, poor concentration, psychomotor impairment.
- Abuse potential not well determined.
  - √ Indirect measures suggest low propensity for abuse, but case report evidence is accumulating that it is not benign in this regard.
- Tolerance and dependence described in case reports (general adult data), so this drug should not be viewed as entirely free of these potentials.
- Abrupt switch from benzodiazepine to zopiclone appears to be the best strategy (although some recommend gradual transition).
  - √ Data still scant and not age specific.
- Weigh cost–benefit of this drug—much more expensive than benzodiazepines with not much added benefit in many cases.

HERBAL REMEDIES

Kava

Marketed under various names, including kava, kava-kava, kava root, kavain, kava pepper, kavapipar, kawa, kawa pepper, ava (pepper or root), awa, gi, intoxicating pepper, intoxicating long pepper, kao, piper methysticum, malohu, maluk, meruk, milik, kew, sakau, tonga, wurzelstock, yagona, yangona, maori kava.

Labeled indications: None

Claimed indications (unproved):

- Anxiety disorders
- Depression
- Insomnia
- Muscle tension
- Pain
- Psychosis
- Stress

Mechanism of action: Unclear; may have GABA receptor binding capacity.

Choosing a Drug

- Included here for information because used as a alternative medicine option by many patients.
- Not recommended for use in elders.
- *Recent warnings* not to use kava or kava-containing substances because of reports of liver toxicity (European general adult data).
  - √ 24 reports of liver toxicity (one death and several cases requiring liver transplantation).

Dosing

- Not standardized and doses therefore unreliable.
- No geriatric data.
- 70% standardized extract: 100 mg po tid (range 300–600 mg/day).
- Kava lactones: 60–100 mg po daily.
- Root tea: 1 cup po daily to tid.

Side Effects

Table 3.27. Side Effects of Kava

Side Effects	Most Common	Most Serious and Less Common
Body as a whole	• Weight loss	• Facial puffiness (with prolonged use)
Central and peripheral nervous system	• Restlessness • Drowsiness • Tremor • Fatigue • Headache	• EPS √ Oral and lingual dyskinesias √ Torticollis √ Oculogyric crisis

(*cont.*)

Continued

Side Effects	Most Common	Most Serious and Less Common
Gastrointestinal	• Dyspepsia • Mouth numbness (if chewed)	
Hematological		• Hematological disturbances with chronic use • Lymphocytopenia • RBC volume increased • Thrombocytopenia
Liver and biliary	• Liver toxicity—acute hepatitis	• Liver failure
Metabolic and nutritional		• Decreased protein levels (chronic use)
Psychiatric	• Depression	
Respiratory		• Pulmonary hypertension (chronic use)
Skin and appendages	• Skin rash	
Special senses	• Enlarged pupils • Blurred vision	
Urinary		• Hematuria (prolonged use)

Monitoring

- Monitor LFTs

Drug Interactions

- Potentiates sedative and CNS depressant effects of alprazolam, barbiturates, benzodiazepines, ethanol, some antidepressants, antihistamines, and opiates.

Disability Interactions

- Parkinson's disease—exacerbation

Valerian

No labeled indications.

Included here for information, because it is used as a alternative medicine option by many patients.

- Sleep induction
  - √ Efficacy not established but appears to decrease stage-1 sleep and increase slow-wave sleep.
- Anxiety release
- Restlessness

Pharmacology: No good data on mechanism of action or pharmacokinetics.

Dose

- Nonstandardized dosage forms; purity and action unreliable.
- Usually taken in a dose of 300–450 mg hs.
- Extract (0.4–0.6% valerian): 2–3 g orally daily tid.
- Simple tincture: 1–3 ml orally daily tid.

Withdrawal: Taper; may be a withdrawal syndrome after chronic use.

Caution

- May be hepatotoxic
- Driving
- Concurrent CNS depressants
- Drugs metabolized by CYP 3A4

Side effects: Rates in elders not known.

Table 3.28. Side Effects of Valerian

Side Effects	Most Common	Most Serious and Less Common
Cardiovascular		• Cardiac disturbance
Central and peripheral nervous system	• Headache • Insomnia • Morning hangover • Sedation	
Liver and biliary		• Hepatotoxicity
Psychiatric	• Agitation	

4. Mood Stabilizers

OVERVIEW

This chapter deals with drugs that are primarily used for treating (1) bipolar disorder and other affective disorders as well as (2) mania secondary to medical conditions that are more common in elders and (3) some forms of agitation associated with dementia. Anticonvulsants not covered here may have utility but are not yet well-studied in elders. Antipsychotics and benzodiazepines are discussed briefly as they apply to treatment of bipolar disorders and secondary mania or depression, but they are reviewed most fully in their own chapters.

Perhaps more than other disorders, bipolar disorder frequently requires concurrent use of agents. Single agents often do not provide a full spectrum of effectiveness for a given patient and need to be used in combination with concurrent, augmenting drugs. This strategy is complicated for elders, who are more sensitive to side effects and drug-induced toxicity.

Lithium and valproate are the most commonly used drugs of this class in elders. Carbamazepine has been used in the past but less so now. Gabapentin, topiramate and lamotrigine have been used in general adult patients but there is very little empirical data for elders.

Other Drugs/Treatments Used in Treatment of Mood Disorders

Atypical antipsychotics

- Olanzapine
  - √ Approved for treatment of acute mania.
  - √ Controlled studies (general adult data) show positive response in manic, rapid-cycling, and mixed phases of bipolar disorder.

        - Results are statistically significant but only show about 20% advantage over placebo for this indication.
    - √ No geriatric data.
- Risperidone
    - √ Little controlled data.
    - √ Overall, promising indications of efficacy; similar to olanzepine (general adult data).
- Quetiapine
    - √ Limited uncontrolled data are promising.
- Ziprasidone
    - √ Very limited data but promising.

Antidepressants (see p. 23).

- Prolonged use of antidepressants without concurrent mood stabilizer increases rates of rapid cycling.
    - √ Best to avoid their use in rapid cycling whenever possible.
    - √ If they are needed, always use them in combination with a mood stabilizer.
    - √ Risk of induction of mood switch is greatest with TCAs (general adult data).

Benzodiazepines (see p. 371)

- Used as concurrent agents to address.
    - √ Acute behavior
    - √ Anxiety/sleep disorder states

Calcium channel blockers

- Verapamil
    - √ Caution in elders with cardiovascular disease.
        - Potential for hypotension, bradycardia, cardiac conduction prolongation.
            - Especially in combination with lithium.
        - Monitor B.P., heart rate, ECG.
        - Contraindicated after MI and in AV block, hypotension, or sick sinus syndrome.
        - Caution in combination with lithium or carbamazepine (increased neurotoxicity).

Bupropion

- May be effective prophylaxis for mania (and depression).
- Possible indications include
    - √ Rapid-cycling disorders.
    - √ Intolerance or lack of response to lithium.

- Data scant for elders.
- Cannot be recommended for routine use.

Nonpharmacological intervention

- ECT
  - √ Well-recognized effective intervention.
- Transcranial magnetic stimulation (TMS).
  - √ Very early investigational stages; no geriatric data.
- Vagus nerve stimulation.
  - √ May be useful in resistant depression and resistant bipolar disorder (general adult data).
  - √ Little data; still in early investigational stage, although the instrument is approved for use in Canada.

Other interventions

- Omega-3 fatty acids.
  - √ Very little data; still in early investigational stage.
  - √ Presumed mechanism of action: Inhibition of neuronal signal transduction by dampening phosphatidyl inositol and arachidonic acid-mediated signal transduction.
    - ▫ Action similar to lithium or valproate.
- Donepizil 5 mg/day.
  - √ Data still very preliminary.
- Choline bitartrate.
- Inositol.

Table 4.1. Pharmacology of Mood Stabilizers

Generic Name	Bioavailability (%) (range)	Plasma Protein Binding (%)	Volume of Distribution (range)	Elimination Half-Life, in Hours (range)	Tmax (hours) (range)	Absorption	Excretion	Metabolized (P450 system)	Pharmacokinetic Linearity
lithium carbonate	90–100 (80–100)		0.5–0.7 l/kg; increased fat/lean body mass ratio reduces volume of distribution by 23%	Estimated at 24 (30–50); (8–35 is general adult range); steady state in 8–10 days	Immediate release form-1–2 (general adult data); delayed release form peaks at 4–6 hours (general adult data)	Complete absorption within 6 hours (general adult data); sustained release form has delayed GI absorption—more from small intestine; lithium citrate is most rapidly absorbed within 15 min. –1 hour	95% by kidneys; rest in feces, sweat; ⅓–⅔ excreted within 12 hours; ⅓ retained and gradually excreted over 2 weeks (general adult data)		
carbamazepine	75–80	68–80, mostly to albumin; only unbound fraction is biologically active and subject to metabolism	0.8–1.6 l/kg	Initially 18–65; after multiple dosing, falls to 12–17 because of auto-induction of its own metabolism; steady state in 2–4 days (general adult data); epoxide half-life 5–8 (general adult data)	5 (4–8, but as late as 24–32; general adult data)	Slow, erratic, and somewhat unpredictable	Renal excretion 98% after metabolism	Metabolized by arene oxidase; active metabolite carbamazepine 10,11-epoxide; antiepileptic effect, but also toxic	Non-linear

divalproex/ valproate	100	> 80 mostly to albumin; only unbound fraction is biologically active and subject to metabolism	0.16 l/kg	15 (5–20); steady state in 2–4 days (general adult data)	2.5 (1–4; general adult data); 3–5 (divalproex)	Rapid: peak levels in 1–4 hours (general adult data) depakote takes 2–4 hours; delayed by food; syrup more rapid-peak levels in 15 min-2 hours	Clearance unaffected by age; < 3% in feces and urine of unmetabolized drug; metabolized drug mostly excreted in urine.	70% metabolized in liver through conjugation with glucuronic acid, P450, and beta oxidation systems; metabolites-2-en-valproic acid (antiepileptic) and 4-en-valproic acid (toxic)	Metabolism of unbound divalproex linear; but linear kinetics occur only after protein binding is saturated
gabapentin	May be reduced at high doses	Not protein bound	58 (general adult data)	5–9			Primarily renal clearance of unmodified drug; declines with age and renal impairment	Little hepatic metabolism; no metabolites detected	

(*cont.*)

Continued

Generic Name	Percentage of Bioavailability (range)	Plasma Protein Binding (%)	Volume of Distribution (range)	Elimination Half-Life, in Hours (range)	Tmax (hours) (range)	Absorption	Excretion	Metabolized (P450 system)	Pharmacokinetic Linearity
lamotrigine	98	55	0.9–1.2 l/kg (general adult data)	31 (24–37); some ranges as wide as 7–70; longer half-life when in combination with valproate and shorter with phenytoin, carbomazepine	1.5–5	Rapid absorption; unaffected by food	Reduced clearance in elders by 37%, and in Asians; mostly renal clearance; 10% unchanged	Glucuronidation; autoinduction of metabolism may lead to increased clearance; clinical relevance not known	
topiramate	80	13–17		21 (general adult data); steady state in 4 days (general adult data)	2 (general adult data)	Rapid; reduced by food	Predominantly excreted in urine unchanged; clearance 20–30 ml/min	Minimal liver metabolism by hydroxylata-tion, hydrolysis, and glucuronida-tion; few age effects; several metabolites probably not clinically important.	Linear

Note: carbamazepine and valproic acid: unbound biologically active portion of drug is increased as dose increases or if protein bound fraction of the drug is displaced when a highly protein-bound drug is coadministered (e.g., aspirin, warfarin, digoxin, SSRI).

INDICATIONS FOR MOOD STABILIZERS

Treatment of acute episodes, management of recurrence, maintenance care, and relapse prevention of

- Bipolar disorder (main indication) (see also p. 37).
  - √ Bipolar I.
  - √ Bipolar II.
  - √ Mixed mood disorder.
  - √ Rapid-cycling mood disorder.
- Secondary mania (more frequent indication in elders than younger patients).
  - √ Secondary to a general medical condition.
  - √ Substance-induced mood disorder.
    - ▫ Alcohol, sedative/hypnotic withdrawal (e.g., use gabapentin).
- Other
  - √ Unipolar major depressive disorder (see p. 23).
    - ▫ Mood stabilizers are usually adjunctive therapy.
    - ▫ May be used for acute treatment.
    - ▫ May be used prophylacticly.
  - √ BPSD (see p. 236)
  - √ Schizoaffective disorder.
  - √ Mood disturbances in personality disorders.
  - √ PTSD.
  - √ Clinical reports of trials in other syndromes, with varying results: pain, restless leg, trigeminal neuralgia, postherpetic neuralgia.

BIPOLAR DISORDER

The essential feature of bipolar disorder is occurrence of at least one episode of mania, hypomania, or mixed affective state with or without depressed phases. There are two main forms: bipolar I and bipolar II.

- Bipolar I criteria
  - √ One or more manic or mixed episodes, with or without history of major depressive episodes.
  - √ Specifiers for the most recent episode include
    - ▫ Hypomanic
    - ▫ Manic
    - ▫ Mixed
    - ▫ Major depressive
  - √ *Note:* Substance-induced mood disorder and mood disorder due to a general medical condition do not count toward a bipolar I diagnosis.
- Bipolar II

- One or more major depressive episodes accompanied by at least one episode of hypomania with no episodes of mania.
- Does not include patients who "switch" to hypomania while treated with antidepressants, ECT or atypical antipsychotics.
- Causes impairment in social or occupational functioning or clinically significant distress.

Definitions

Definition of mania

- At least 1 week of
  - √ Abnormally elevated, expansive, or irritable mood.
  - √ Duration may be shorter if hospitalization is required.
- Three (four, if mood is only irritable) or more of the following:
  - √ Grandiosity/inflated self-esteem.
    - ▫ May be delusional.
    - ▫ Overt psychosis may include hallucinations.
  - √ Decreased need for sleep.
  - √ Hypertalkativeness/pressure to talk.
  - √ Flight of ideas/racing thoughts.
  - √ Distractibility.
  - √ Increased goal directed activity/psychomotor agitation.
  - √ Reckless, unwise, sometimes self-destructive or uninhibited behavior, including inappropriate or impulsive sexuality.
- Symptoms sufficiently severe to impair social or occupational functioning or require hospitalization.
- Symptoms not due to direct physiological or medical causes.

Definition of secondary mania: Mood disorder secondary to the direct physiological effects of a general medical condition.

Mania induced by organic pathology

- Cerebral disorders
  - √ Cerebrovascular disease (e.g., stroke).
    - ▫ More risk factors for cerebrovascular disease.
    - ▫ Higher rates of silent cerebral infarctions (especially right sided) and subcortical hyperintensities on MRI.
    - ▫ Mood disorder associated with Binswanger's disease: vascular disorder of subcortical white matter evident on MRI.
  - √ Degenerative neurological disorders (e.g., Parkinson's disease).
  - √ Head trauma.
  - √ Brain tumor.
  - √ Basal ganglia calcification.
  - √ Surgical brain lesions.
- Endocrine disorders.
  - √ Hyper- or hypothyroid.

- √ Parathyroid disease.
- √ Adrenal disease.
- Infections
  - √ AIDS dementia complex.
  - √ Neurosyphilis.
  - √ Other CNS infections (e.g., cryptococcus).
  - √ Hepatitis.
- Metabolic disorders (e.g., vitamin B12 deficiency).
- Autoimmune disorders (e.g., SLE).
- Cancer (e.g., pancreatic).

Substance-induced mood disorder

- Due to direct physiological effects of a substance.
  - √ Includes switching to manic state during treatment with
    - Psychotropics (antidepressants, atypical antipsychotics, buspirone, benzodiazepines).
    - Other treatments for depression (ECT, light therapy).
    - Other medications (steroids, levodopa, amantadine, stimulants [amphetamine, bronchodilators], decongestants, procarbazine, baclofen, bromides, anticholinergics, estrogen, disulfiram, folic acid).
- Switching to manic state because of substance misuse (e.g., alcohol, cocaine).
  - √ Alcohol most commonly misused by elders, but other substances are also implicated (e.g., cocaine).
  - √ Bipolar disorder and substance misuse commonly coexist.
    - Each component needs separate evaluation and management.

Secondary mood disorder in elders

- DSM note: When depression alone occurs in the context of Alzheimer's disease or vascular dementia, those diagnoses take precedence, and the depression is recorded as a specifier.
  - √ A fine distinction not especially relevant to clinical practice.
- Generally does not follow an episode of depression.
  - √ In younger age groups 60–70% of mania follows a depressive episode.
- More common than primary mood disorder in elders (i.e., usually associated with another primary disorder, such as dementia).
- Has later age of onset than primary mood disorder.
- Has no past psychiatric history.
- Family history of bipolar illness among first-degree relatives less common than in primary mood disorder, although still quite high overall (50% in one study).
- Poor long-term prognosis and associated excess mortality.

Definition of hypomania

- At least 4 days of abnormally and persistently elevated, expansive, or irritable mood.
- Symptom picture similar to mania but does not
  - √ Impair functioning significantly.
  - √ Require hospitalization.
  - √ Include psychotic symptoms.

Definition of mixed episodes

- Period of at least 1 week during which criteria for both depression and mania are met nearly every day.

Definition of cyclothymic disorder

- Over a 2-year period, frequent hypomanic and depressive mood swings that do not cross the threshold for diagnosis of major depression or mania.
- Have not remitted for more than 2 months at a time.

Epidemiology of Bipolar Disorder

- Still unclear if frequency of mania increases, decreases, or remains the same in late life.
- Lifetime prevalence of bipolar disorder 1.6–1.8%.
  - √ Lifetime prevalence of subsyndromal mania is 6% (compared with bipolar I disorder rate of 1%).
  - √ Bipolar disorder is 5–19% of mood disorders in elders.
  - √ 10% of all patients with bipolar disorder are > 50 years.
- Late-life bipolar disorder may present as
  - √ First episode of mania with prior history of depression.
  - √ First affective episode.
  - √ Recurrence of episodes that first emerged in young adulthood.
- In elderly bipolars who have been diagnosed with the disorder for the first time.
  - √ The age of onset of the index (first) episode of mania is generally almost 60 years.
    - ▫ Onset of primary mania after age 70, with no prior history of affective disorder, is most unusual.
  - √ Less commonly, mania begins in early adult life and episodes continue to occur into old age.

    More commonly (rough estimates, 30–50% of elderly bipolars), depression present in earlier life; several episodes of depression often precede the first episode of mania that emerges for first time in old age.
    - ▫ Mood disorder can change polarity in late life.
    - ▫ Latency from index episode of depression to first manic episode emerging for first time in late life is often very prolonged: 10–25 years or longer.

- √ Significant subset of new-onset mania in elders presents with no history of prior mood disorder.
    - ▫ Most are secondary mania.
    - ▫ A small number, de novo mania.
- Prevalence of mania in elders not well studied.
  - √ Incidence of first admissions for mania appears to increase with age.
  - √ Estimated 5–10% of geriatric inpatients present for treatment of mood disorders.
  - √ 10–20% of patients in lithium clinics are over 65 (clinical estimates).
  - √ 25% of hospitalized geriatric patients with mania have secondary mania.
  - √ Incidence in nursing homes estimated at 10%.
- Rapid-cycling disorders (i.e., > 4 episodes in 1 year; an illness modifier, not a diagnostic subtype) may be more prevalent in old age.
  - √ Tendency for episodes to become more frequent over the life course of the illness.
    - ▫ Especially associated with bipolar II, in particular, the depressed phase.
- Comorbidities
  - √ In younger patients, substance abuse (especially alcohol) is the most frequent Axis I comorbid condition (geriatric data are lacking).
  - √ Often associated with increased frequency of medical disorders and drug treatments (e.g., vascular dementia, Huntington's chorea, endocrine disorders, tumors, infectious diseases, collagen vascular diseases, MS, traumatic brain injuries, delirium).
  - √ Elders demonstrate increased rates of comorbid neurological disorders (e.g., ataxia, soft signs) and cognitive disturbance, and may have increased mortality rates.
  - √ 36% of cases are associated with neurological disorder/lesion (e.g., periventricular white matter intensities on MRI).

Diagnosis of Bipolar Disorder in Elders

Making a diagnosis of bipolar disorder in elders requires accurate history taking, especially collateral history.

- Mania in elders.
  - √ No well-controlled data.
  - √ Clinical presentation shows marked interindividual variation.
    - ▫ Not necessarily age-related.
  - √ Overall presentation resembles that in younger patients.
    - ▫ Some distinguishing features observed by clinicians.

- Poorer prognosis in presence of comorbid conditions.
  - √ Greater risk of chronic mania.

Symptom characteristics of mania in elders

- Many symptoms are less intense, and patients may be more slowed down.
- Mood is more labile, irritable, hostile, and aggressive (rather than euphoric or infectious, although data are inconsistent).
  - √ Easily misdiagnosed as agitated depression.
- More confusion, disorientation, distractibility
  - √ Easily mistaken for delirium.
  - √ Occasionally may present as pseudodementia.
- Evidence of generally increased cognitive impairment in late-life bipolar disorder is conflicting.
  - √ Comorbid neurological symptoms associated with higher rate of hospitalization.
- Delusions tend to be persecutory (rather than grandiose) and may be more common in late-onset forms.
- Speech is often repetitious and may be impoverished, but has manic pressure, with flight of ideas.
- Vegetative features are present, including insomnia, restlessness, pacing.
- Other features include demandingness, intrusiveness, argumentativeness, and aggression.
- Greater incidence of dysphoric mood.
- Features of both depression and mania within a single episode may occur more commonly in elders than in younger patients.
- Increased mortality rate.
- Episodes are often close together.

Late-onset mania, compared to early-onset form graduating into old age, associated with the following:

- Lower overall dysfunction.
- May show less residual pathology on discharge from hospital.
- Less insight.
- Comorbid cerebral organic impairment predominantly cerebrovascular.
  - √ Structural changes in the brain not well defined.
  - √ Increased subcortical hyperintensities in both young and old bipolars.
- Increased rate of cognitive impairment compared to early-onset forms.
- Often associated with antidepressant therapy prior to index episode.

- Possibly greater risk of relapse.
- Poor prognosis for morbidity and mortality (50% over 6 years).

Features that suggest secondary mania include

- Obvious medical or neurological impairment.
- First episode of mania after age 70.
- Organic picture—confusion, distractibility, disorientation, impaired cognition.
- Rapid cycling.
- Unresponsive chronic course.
- Toxic response to low doses of medications, especially lithium.
- Subcortical MRI hyperintensities are suggestive but not diagnostic.

Differential diagnostic issues in elders include

- Correct diagnosis of bipolar disorder often missed in nursing home environments, where index of suspicion for this disorder is low.
  - √ Depression, delirium, and dementia are suspected and diagnosed more often.
- Because of the overlap in symptoms between bipolar disorder and schizophrenia, geriatric patients may carry a longstanding, incorrect diagnosis of schizophrenia made at a time when differential diagnostic criteria were not as refined and accurate.
  - √ Especially relevant for the 10–30% of manic patients who become chronic.
    - ▫ They need to be reevaluated and rediagnosed to avoid incorrect/ineffective management.

Table 4.2. Differential Diagnosis of Bipolar Disease in the Elderly

Bipolar vs. schizophrenia and schizoaffective disorder
- Schizophrenia characterized by chronic psychotic picture, usually from early life, with more inconsistent affective symptoms.
- Schizoaffective disorder rare in elders and not studied; affective symptoms superimposed on psychosis.

Mania vs. depression
- May resemble agitated depression in elders, including dysphoria, agitation, irritability, mixed or labile affect, depressive thought content.
- Differentiate by
  - √ History, including past psychiatric and family genetic.
  - √ Prior presentations of depressions.
  - √ Prior response to mood stabilizers.
  - √ Trial of therapy.

Bipolar II vs. unipolar depression
- Bipolar depression sometimes may be distinguished from unipolar disorders by symptom picture and history (data is not geriatric-specific and refers to early-onset primary disorder, not late-onset form).

(*cont.*)

Continued

In bipolar depression, compared to unipolar depression, there may be:

- Increased volitional inhibition ("paralysis of will").
- Increased reverse vegetative signs (weight gain and hypersomnolence).
- Earlier age of onset.
- More frequent episodes.
- More equal gender distribution.
- More psychotic features.
- Increased risk of completed suicides.
  - √ Rates as high as 15–20% (general adult data), but geriatric data unavailable.
- Lifetime history of substance abuse.
- Lower average life expectancy.

Mania vs. dementia

- Sometimes hard to distinguish and easily misdiagnosed.
  - √ Rate of misdiagnosis not known.
- Late-onset mania may resemble dementia because it is associated with high incidence of comorbid neurological and cognitive disorder.
  - √ Few actually develop progressive dementias, such as Alzheimer's disease.
- Dementia resembles mania because it has some manic-like features.
  - √ Irritability, restlessness, lability of affect, impaired concentration, sleep disorder, poor social judgment, impulsivity.
- Occasionally a trial of therapy is necessary to distinguish.
- Case reports of lithium resolving both mood and dementia symptoms in patients originally misdiagnosed as dementia.

Fronto-temporal dementia

- Differentiate based on presence of sleep disorder in mania.

Bipolar vs. disinhibition syndromes

Disinhibition syndromes

- Associated with frontal lobe disorders but not mood disorders, per se.
- Arise in old age.
- Have no genetic history of the disorder.
- Are highly associated with neurological disease.
- Rarely respond well to mood stabilizers.

Mania vs. delirium

- Restlessness, sleep disruption, impulsivity, irritability, labile affect, and distractibility may be present in both conditions. (Diagnosis of delirium is described on page 253.)

TREATMENT OF BIPOLAR DISORDER

- No controlled data for elders.
- 18 % receive monotherapy, 50% antidepressants, 40% benzodiazepines, 33% antipsychotics (general adult data).
- Geriatric bipolar disorders are often complex to manage because of concurrent illnesses that interact with the basic bipolar pathology.
- Symptom control is often suboptimal, with chronic pictures sometimes emerging that are only partially responsive to medication management.
  - √ Full symptom remission over the course of 1 year of therapy occurs in a minority of patients (about 25–30%).
  - √ Similarly discouraging results for return of full function (24% in one study; general adult data).
    - ▫ Geriatric data not available but similar results are probable, based on clinical experience.

- ◻ Suicide is a significant risk in younger patients (rates of 10–19%), but geriatric data not available.

Management begins with complete physical workup.

- To establish correct diagnosis and rule out differential diagnoses.
- To determine concurrent disorders.

Table 4.3. Checklist for Diagnostic Workup for New-Onset Mania

- Complete history.
  - √ Medical, including recent illness, such as infection
  - √ Psychiatric
  - √ Family
  - √ Personal
  - √ Psychosocial
  - √ Substance use
- Medication review.
- System review.
- Complete physical exam, including neurological exam.
- Detailed mental status exam (beyond the screening of the MMSE).
- Neuroimaging (MRI preferred).
  - √ Especially if focal neurological findings emerge.
- Laboratory tests.
  - √ CBC and differential
  - √ Full blood chemistry
    - ◻ Electrolytes
    - ◻ BUN
    - ◻ Creatinine clearance
  - √ Toxic screen
  - √ LFTs (AST, ALT, alkaline phosphatase)
  - √ Prothrombin time
  - √ Urine—routine and micro, plus drug screen, as necessary.
  - √ Kidney function
    - ◻ Serum creatinine
    - ◻ BUN
  - √ B12, folate
  - √ TSH(s), T3, T4
  - √ ECG
  - √ Possible EEG

Note: The history can be more useful if it charts the episodes of mania and depression chronologically and relates them to other life events and treatment interventions, noting response to specific interventions. This approach is especially helpful with elders, for whom long and complex histories are the norm. (See Table 4.4)

Acute Mania

Management of acute mania in elders is often complicated by

- Comorbid medical conditions.
- Intolerance of medication side effects.
- Tendency to lithium-resistance in old age.
- Secondary mania, generally less responsive to treatment.

Pharmacological management, especially for very severe or refractory cases, may involve a complex interplay of mood stabilizers, antipsychotics, and antidepressants, together with the full array of psychosocial nonpharmacological interventions.

- Consider levels of danger to self and others and hospitalize accordingly.

Table 4.4. Suggested Form for Tracking Bipolar Illness Course

Episode	Patient's Age and Approximate Date of Each Episode	Duration	Precipitants	Treatment	Response	Caregiver/ Therapist Notes
1. 2. 3. Etc.						
Specify: • Mania (M) • Hypomania (H) • Depression (D) • Mixed (Mx) • *Note:* > 4 episodes in 1 year, specify rapid cycling			Specify: • Concurrent life events (LE) • Illnesses (I)	Specify medications or other interventions: • Medication (Med) • Hospitalization (Hosp) • ECT • Psychosocial • Other (specify)	• Full remission (F) • Partial remission (P) • Nonresponse (N)	

- Involve family members, as appropriate.
- Maintain close collaboration with family physician and other supports in the family system.

Therapeutic alliance is a crucial element of successful pharmacotherapy and needs to be worked toward by establishing trust and mutual collaboration in the treatment process.

- Absent or compromised treatment alliance interferes with compliance.
- Often difficult to establish in presence of limited insight common in manic conditions.

Pharmacotherapy

Treatment is complex because agents often only provide partial benefit, and two or three agents with complementary action sometimes need to be combined. Agents should be started one at a time, with additional agents added as necessary, rather than instituting initial cotherapy. For elders especially, the polypharmacy that is sometimes necessary increases the risk of toxic side effects.

Lithium and divalproex are both effective antimanic agents in otherwise healthy young elders (early 70s).

- Opinion split on drug of choice.
  - √ Lithium is treatment of choice if tolerated.
    - ▫ Remarkably little controlled geriatric data on treatment response.
      - ◦ Accumulated clinical data strongly indicate a favorable response in elders.
    - ▫ Has the edge in effectiveness (67% vs. 38% in recent retrospective study).
    - ▫ But higher incidence of side effects, especially neurological, gastrointestinal, and cardiac.
    - ▫ Frail elders often intolerant of neurological side effects that may emerge even at relatively low doses.
    - ▫ Lowering the dose is one strategy for being able to continue or reintroduce lithium rather than abandoning it in the face of side effects such as delirium.
  - √ Advantages of anticonvulsants (especially divalproex).
    - ▫ More tolerable side-effect profile.
    - ▫ Divalproex not as effective as lithium for classic manic episode but equally effective in mixed states.
    - ▫ Especially effective in lithium-resistant patients (e.g., rapid-cycling bipolar disorder or significant comorbid dysphoria).
    - ▫ Lamotrigine may be useful but data are sparse, and topiramate is unstudied in elders.

    - Divalproex
      - Better tolerated and safer for long-term therapy that may continue into old-old years, when patient develops frailty and risk factors for lithium toxicity.
    - Wide therapeutic window.
    - Fewer CNS side effects.
- In older groups, decide course of treatment based on clinical picture (e.g., comorbid neurological disorder increases sensitivity to lithium side effects and kidney toxicity with long-term use is a clinical concern).

With secondary mania or physical frailty, anticonvulsants, especially divalproex, are a better choice (especially for mania secondary to renal disease). Lithium the preferred drug if mania is associated with or secondary to liver disease.

- Rapid cycling predominantly associated with depression in terms of duration of time spent in depressive vs. manic states.
  - √ Medications should be chosen to deal with the most prominent symptom.
    - Lithium effective for manic symptoms but less so for depression.
    - Lamotrigine appears to be more effective for depressive symptoms in bipolar II patients (while less so for bipolar I patients) and seems free of mood-destabilizing effects.
- Acute mania seems to respond well to divalproex, olanzepine, and risperidone.
  - √ Atypical antipsychotics also useful to regularize sleep patterns in rapid cycling.
- Mixed and rapid-cycling states probably respond better to divalproex.
  - √ Rapid-cycling states do not respond well to carbamazepine or lithium (general adult data).
    - Lithium is effective for manic states but associated with worse depressive symptoms.

Use of antipsychotics with mania

- Atypical antipsychotics
  - √ Most often used as adjunctive therapy and for rapid control of acute symptoms.
  - √ Less useful for maintenance phase. Use mood stabilizers (lithium or divalproex).
  - √ Olanzapine (labeled use) and risperidone.
    - Risperidone needs to be titrated to therapeutic levels, which restricts its utility in highly acute states.
    - Occasionally may induce mania as side effect.

- √ Other atypicals show promising results clinically (e.g., quetiapine; general adult data only).
- √ Clozapine effective, but side effects limit use to more severe, refractory situations.
- √ Olanzapine and divalproex show equal efficacy in acute mania (general adult data), but divalproex produces fewer side effects.

- Typical antipsychotics
  - √ Clinical experience suggests effectiveness in geriatric mania, but data are limited.
  - √ High risk of side effects, especially delirium, EPS and TD.

Indications for concurrent medication with primary mood stabilizer

- In elders combinations not suggested or to be used cautiously include
  - √ Lithium/carbamazepine.
    - ▫ Neurotoxicity
  - √ Divalproex/carbamazepine.
    - ▫ May be hard to titrate therapeutic levels.
  - √ Divalproex and lamotrigine.
    - ▫ Increases lamotrigine plasma levels.
  - √ Carbamazepine/calcium channel blockers.
    - ▫ Neurotoxicity especially verapamil or diltiazem.
  - √ Carbamazepine/clozapine-contraindicated.
- Severe mania with anxiety but without psychosis.
  - √ Benzodiazepines (lorazepam 0.5–2 mg/day or clonazepam 0.5–2 mg/d, orally or IM) often useful in acute stages.
    - ▫ May be necessary and effective during long-term maintenance.
    - ▫ Observe for ataxia, slurred speech, cognitive impairment.
- Mixed bipolar state may be optimally treated by adding olanzapine to a mood stabilizer (general adult data).
- Mania with psychotic symptoms.
  - √ Atypical antipsychotics (e.g., olanzapine or clozapine).
  - √ Plus or minus benzodiazepine, although differential efficacy in psychotic vs. nonpsychotic patients not shown consistently (general adult data).
- Depression
  - √ 50% of bipolar patients receive antidepressants (general adult data).
  - √ Patients who tolerate and remain on an antidepressant appear to do better in the long term than those who do not (general adult data).
  - √ For mild states of depression, use mood stabilizer alone.
  - √ More severe states, add bupropion, SSRI, or venlafaxine.

- √ *Best to avoid antidepressants* if there a history of rapid cycling or switch to a manic state with antidepressants.
- √ Lithium and lamotrigine combination may be useful in bipolar depression (general adult data).

Optimize thyroid function with T_4 supplementation as necessary.

Nonresponse

- No good geriatric data to guide us.
- Recommendations are extrapolated from protocols for younger patients.
- Caution advised in elders because of age-associated complications in using drug combinations.

General approaches include

- Switch to a different mood stabilizer.
- Consider antipsychotic (olanzapine or clozapine).
- Add a second mood stabilizer.
  - √ Carbamazepine (avoid concurrent regimens as above).
    - □ May precipitate acute confusion in combination with lithium.
  - √ Gabapentin
  - √ Lamotrigine
    - □ Use low doses with divalproex
      - ○ Increased lamotrigine levels and side effects.
    - □ Well tolerated with lithium.
- Consider calcium channel blocker.
  - √ Verapamil
    - □ Especially useful for elders with concurrent hypertension, supraventricular tachycardia, TD.
  - √ Possibly nifedipine.
  - √ Observe for side effects.
    - □ Drug interaction (increased toxicity) with lithium or carbamazepine.
    - □ Cardiac arrhythmia—bradycardia, AV block.
    - □ Hypotension.
    - □ Flushing, dizziness, nausea.

Table 4.5. Pharmacological Management of Bipolar Subtypes*

Initial Intervention	Managing Non- or Incomplete Response
ACUTE MANIC EPISODE	
• Divalproex or lithium (lithium preferred, based on effectiveness alone). • Carbamazepine side-effect profile is unfavorable. √ Use as second-line intervention. • Concurrent atypical antipsychotic often necessary until symptoms controlled.	• After 2–3 weeks, switch to different mood stabilizer. • If no or partial response, add concurrent mood stabilizer. √ Lithium plus divalproex preferred. □ Lower lithium levels permitted by this combination (i.e., 0.4–0.6 mEq/l).

(*cont.*)

Continued

Initial Intervention	Managing Non- or Incomplete Response
• Add clonazepam (1–2 mg/day), lorazepam (0.5–2 mg/day), or other appropriate. benzodiazepine for short-term control of agitation, insomnia. • Symptom control begins in 1–3 weeks with mood stabilizer and earlier with antipsychotic/benzodiazepine use. • Use ECT for severe, unmanageable states.	• A third concurrent agent (e.g. gabapentin, lamotrigine) is required in unusual circumstances. √ Reevaluate diagnosis. □ In secondary mania, correcting underlying precipitant is necessary, but antimanic medication also may be necessary. □ Depression nonresponse, add antidepressant (bupropion, venlafaxine). √ Use ECT, as necessary.
ACUTE MANIC EPISODE WITH PSYCHOSIS	
• Mood stabilizer regimen as for acute manic episode. • Add concurrent antipsychotic (e.g., olanzapine 2.5–5 mg, or risperidone 1 mg, or clozapine slowly titrated) during acute phase. √ May be discontinued once episode is brought under good control. • Also consider haloperidol. √ Monitor for EPS.	• Switch from atypical agent to mid-potency typical antipsychotic (e.g., loxapine, perphenazine).
SCHIZOAFFECTIVE DISORDER	
• Begin with atypical antipsychotic or divalproex. • Consider lamotrigine or carbamazepine as second-line choices.	• Add combination of mood stabilizers as above. • Add atypical antipsychotic (e.g., olanzapine) or haloperidol for acute control. • Judicious use of benzodiazepines.
MIXED STATES—DEPRESSION AND MANIA	
• Common in elders. • Best to begin with divalproex. √ Carbamazepine is second choice; geriatric data not available. • Concurrent antipsychotic or antidepressant necessary sometimes, but avoid antidepressants if possible.	• Reevaluate diagnosis if no response in 2–3 weeks. • Switch to different mood stabilizer. • Add concurrent second mood stabilizer (e.g., gabapentin). • Consider ECT in more severe cases.
BIPOLAR DEPRESSION	
• Initiate mood stabilizer. √ Lithium or lamotrigine is best choice. √ Divalproex is ineffective. √ For faster response, use lithium plus bupropion, an SSRI, an MAOI, or venlafaxine.	• Consider careful use of antidepressant (bupropion or SSRIs may be best), recognizing danger of mood switch. • Newer antidepressant may be tried concurrently. • Taper antidepressant once depressive episode has passed (2–3 months). • Evaluate thyroid function. • Consider ECT.
RAPID-CYCLING BIPOLAR DISORDER	
• Divalproex (or, less enthusiastically, carbamazepine) drug of choice. • Discontinue antidepressants (although may be unavoidable in some circumstances). • 20–40% do not respond to lithium as first-line agent (general adult data).	• Prime indication for adding lithium and/or second or third mood stabilizer. • Add thyroxine 100–200 μg/day and optimize thyroid function. √ Hypothyroidism is a risk factor for rapid cycling in bipolar disorder.

(*cont.*)

Continued

Initial Intervention	Managing Non- or Incomplete Response
SECONDARY MANIA	
• Divalproex preferred. • Withdraw offending medications. • If symptoms subside, taper mood stabilizer. • Continue maintenance, if indicated.	
MANIA IN DEMENTIA	
• Poor outcomes with lithium; divalproex more effective.	

* *Note:* most data in Table 4.5 are extrapolated from general adult data.

When switching drugs

- Taper the first before introducing the second.
- Take your time.
- Conduct dose changes in smaller increments with elders.
- If not possible to taper one drug before starting the next, cross-taper the medications (i.e., reduce the first while concurrently increasing the second).

Note: If ECT is initiated, discontinue mood stabilizer prior to treatment.

- May reinstitute mood stabilizer after ECT complete.
  - √ If patient requires uninterrupted mood stabilizer, reduce to minimum therapeutic plasma level.

Maintenance Stage

For relapse prevention, continue for 8–9 months after control of symptoms before gradual tapering of medication.

- Patients require close (q 2–3 weeks) monitoring and maintenance of therapeutic alliance until fully stabilized, because noncompliance is high in this group of disorders.
- Recurrence of mania in younger adults after a first episode is 90%.
  - √ Geriatric data unavailable.
  - √ Elders generally require long-term management and regular follow-up.
- Long-term maintenance therapy against recurrence should be instituted if the patient has had a second episode (especially within past 3 years).
  - √ Some recommend initiating long-term maintenance after first episode, especially if episode was severe, required hospitalization, or was life-threatening.

- Follow-up schedule.
  - √ At least every 6 months once fully stabilized, with appropriate laboratory tests.
  - √ Varies depending on
    - ▫ Prior pattern of relapse periods.
    - ▫ Where patient lives (closer monitoring in community vs. institutional settings).
    - ▫ Reliability of other caregivers.
    - ▫ Patient insight and compliance.
    - ▫ Medical comorbidities.

Choice of best agent for long-term maintenance

- Lithium is still the most reliable agent, followed by divalproex.
- Divalproex and lithium combination may be necessary for some patients.
  - √ Superior for prevention of manic relapse.
  - √ Also higher rate of adverse effects (general adult data).
- Atypical antipsychotics probably effective, but data limited.
- Depot typical antipsychotics have shown promise in younger adults, but use in elders has not been studied.
  - √ Should be tried if other alternatives are not effective or available.
- Monthly (sometimes less frequent) maintenance ECT may be effective prophylaxis.
  - √ Generally safe with elders, using appropriate caution regarding side effects.

Breakthrough of bipolar symptoms

- May be mild increase in irritability, hyperactivity, or expansive mood, or full-blown major recurrence.
- Specific recommendations are based on clinical experience; no geriatric data.
  - √ If a single agent is being used for prophylaxis (e.g., divalproex), add second mood stabilizer rather than increasing dose of first agent.
    - ▫ Unless it was at low or subtherapeutic levels.
  - √ Consider atypical antipsychotic (e.g., olanzapine, risperidone) or a second mood stabilizer (e.g., lithium, gabapentin).
- When using combination therapies in elders, observe usual increased cautions re. monitoring and emergence of side effects.

Discontinuation and Withdrawal

- Abrupt discontinuation of prophylactic therapy leads to high rate of relapse.

- √ 50% within 5 months; adult studies mostly with lithium.
- Discontinuation of lithium may lead to long-term loss of lithium responsiveness.
- Lithium resistance may develop over time.
- Tapering schedule for mood stabilizers not known.
  - √ Suggest taper mood stabilizers over 2–4 weeks and monitor.

INDIVIDUAL MOOD STABILIZER DRUG PROFILES

CARBAMAZEPINE

Drug	Manufacturer	Chemical Class	Therapeutic Class
carbamazepine (Tegretol and Tegretol-XR)	Novartis	iminostilbene	anticonvulsant

Indications: FDA/HPB

- Anticonvulsant
- Trigeminal neuralgia

Indications: Off label

- Bipolar disorder
  - √ Acute mania; mania prophylaxis; rapid-cycling disorders (evidence conflicting).
- Dementia
  - √ Agitation and aggression in both nursing home and community.

Pharmacology

See page 482.

- Epoxide metabolite of carbamazepine is toxic.
  - √ If metabolizing enzyme is inhibited, epoxide may build up.
    - ▫ Epoxide metabolized by epoxide hydroxylase (inhibited by divalproex and lamotrigine).
    - ▫ Epoxide is not measured routinely when blood levels of carbamazepine are measured.
    - ▫ Epoxide levels not directly proportional to plasma carbamazepine levels.
  - √ Hence toxicity may emerge even when carbamazepine levels are within the therapeutic range.
- Nonlinear pharmacokinetics.
  - √ Self-induction of 3A4 leads to reduced blood levels in 2–4 weeks, and higher doses may be required after several weeks to maintain plasma concentrations.

Mechanism of action

- Ill defined—therapeutic effect may relate to antikindling effect, including GABAergic, serotonergic, and dopaminergic properties.
  - √ Modestly GABAergic and antiglutamatergic.
- Inhibition of synaptic transmission.
- Clinical relevance of other effects not known (e.g., sedation, anticholinergic action, muscle relaxation).

Choosing a Drug

- Little geriatric-specific data.
- Second- or third-line agent only.
  - √ Multiple drug interactions.
  - √ Significant side-effect profile.
- Response rate slightly less than lithium for acute mania.
- Useful in lithium nonresponders and rapid cyclers.
- As effective as lithium in prophylaxis of mania (general adult data).
  - √ Combination of lithium and carbamazepine more effective (general adult data only).
  - √ Also more toxic hence not suggested.

Dosing

- Little dose-response data, and none for elders.
  - √ For aggression in dementia, see page 246.
  - √ For elders, clinical experience suggests levels < 38 mmol/L.
- Daily dose regimen.
  - √ Begin with once a day at low dose, then bid.
  - √ Take with food.
- Starting dose.
  - √ In physically frail elders, start at low once-a-day dose of 100 mg and increase slowly.
  - √ Others start at 100 bid.
- Increasing dose and reaching therapeutic levels.
  - √ Increase very slowly 100–200 mg/day every 2–3 weeks.
  - √ Target dose range 200–1200 mg/day.
    - ▫ Bipolar 400 mg/bid.
    - ▫ Aggression in dementia 100–300 mg bid.
  - √ Target plasma levels 4–8 μg/ml (range 2.5–12).

Combination therapy

- Avoid divalproex combination.

Side Effects

- Significant anticholinergic and CVS side effects.
- Common effects include sedation, ataxia, incoordination, dizziness, nystagmus/blurred vision, weakness, fatigue, nausea, leukopenia, and allergic skin reactions.

Table 4.6. Side Effects of Carbamazepine

Side Effects	Most Common	Most Serious and Less Common	Comments
Body as a whole		• Pseudolymphoma syndrome characterized by fever, lymphadenopathy, generalized rash • Serum sickness • Glandular fever-like syndrome • Kawasaki-like syndrome • SLE-like syndrome • Necrotizing granulomatous vasculitis	• Hypersensitivity syndromes occur rarely during first month
Cardiovascular	• Orthostatic hypotension	• Bradyarrhythmias • Sinus node dysfunction √ Prolonged atrioventricular conduction (quinidine-like effect) √ Depressed idionodal rhythms • Linked to heart failure	• Women at greater risk • May emerge at therapeutic levels • Reduce dose • Potentiated by lithium and TCAs • Caution in heart block • Monitor ECG
Case reports		• Rare idiosyncratic pancreatitis • Aseptic meningitis	
Central and peripheral nervous system	• Drowsiness • Horizontal nystagmus • Lassitude • Confusion • Dizziness • Weakness • Ataxia • Clumsiness • Dysarthria	• Delirium • Paroxysmal choreoathetosis • Alteration in cognitive functioning at higher doses • Tremor	• Effects are dose dependent and often occur at the higher range of treatment • Intoxication-like symptoms of confusion, ataxia, drowsiness usually during initiation of therapy and especially with rapid titration • Tremor—dose related; manage with beta blockers • Delirium may emerge at conventional plasma levels • Minimize neurological side effects with low doses and slow dosage increments
Endocrine		• Hypothyroidism • SIADH	• Monitor TSH and free T4
Eye	• Blurred vision • Diplopia	• Lenticular opacities • Increased intraocular pressure in glaucoma	• Transient, dose dependant • Opacities are idiosyncratic reaction

(cont.)

Continued

Side Effects	Most Common	Most Serious and Less Common	Comments
Gastrointestinal	• Nausea • Vomiting • Transient diarrhea • Sialorrhea • Dry mouth	• Pancreatitis (rare)	• Diarrhea; may use antidiarrheal agents
Hematological	• Transient leukopenia and thrombocytopenia	• Rare aplastic anemia, agranulocytosis, pancytopenia, eosinophilia purpura	• Leukopenia—idiosyncratic reaction √ Occurs during first weeks of therapy and rarely goes below 2500 WBCs √ Not related to rare aplastic anemia √ Associated with rapid dose escalation • Management—WBC level above 3500/mm^3 √ Reduce dose and monitor WBC weekly √ At 3500/mm^3 or below, discontinue drug √ Hold drug until count returns above 3500/mm^3 √ Observe for infections √ Recovery usually spontaneous when drug discontinued for 1 week
Liver and biliary		• Hepatotoxicity √ Elevated liver enzymes, bilirubin, alkaline phosphatase □ Not usually clinically important √ Rare cholestatic hepatitis and/or hepatic failure	• Clinical monitoring for hepatic toxicity—general malaise, nausea, anorexia, jaundice • Monitor high LFTs weekly until levels plateau √ If levels are over 2 times normal (or 3 times baseline), discontinue drug and reevaluate liver (consultation, as necessary) • Usually resolves when drug is withdrawn
Metabolic and nutritional		• Hyponatremia (5–25%) • Weight gain √ May be associated with hypothyroidism	• Hyponatremia √ Caused by vasopressin-like effect on sodium absorption in renal tubules √ Interacts unfavorably with lithium—raises lithium levels in plasma √ Mental confusion and lethargy below 125 mEq/l √ Usually not clinically significant, but treat with sodium supplements or demeclocycline if necessary • Weight gain; check TSH

(*cont.*)

- CBC, platelets, and liver enzymes every 2 weeks for first 8–12 weeks or until WBC dips and rebounds, and every 1–3 months thereafter.
- Serum sodium q 3–6 months.
- LFTs, especially serum bilirubin, monthly for 2–3 months and q 6–12 months thereafter.

Disability Interactions and Contraindications

Consider discontinuing carbamazepine if

- WBC $< 3500/\text{mm}^3$.
- Neutropenia $< 1500/\text{mm}^3$.
- Platelets drop below 100,000.
- Erythrocytes drop below $3.0 \times 106\ \text{mm}^3$.
- Liver enzymes increase by more than 100%.
- Signs of infection—fever, sore throat, pulmonary hypersensitivity (e.g., dyspnea, pneumonitis, or pneumonia).
- Bleeding (e.g., nosebleeds), bruising.
- Severe skin rash (exfoliative reaction, urticaria, Stevens–Johnson syndrome).
- Avoid with concurrent bone marrow suppression, narrow angle glaucoma, or MAOI use within 2 weeks.

Effect on Laboratory Tests

- Increases BUN, LFTs, albuminuria, glycosuria.
- Decreases thyroid function tests, RBC, WBC, platelets, serum sodium.

Overdose, Toxicity, Suicide

Symptoms of carbamazepine overdose include the following

- Gastrointestinal
  - √ Nausea/vomiting
  - √ Dry mouth
  - √ Diarrhea
  - √ Constipation
  - √ Glossitis
  - √ Abdominal pain
- Respiratory depression with larger overdoses.
- CVS
  - √ Arrhythmias—AV block
    - ▫ Clinically significant events uncommon in general adults, but more problematic in elders.
  - √ Hypotension
  - √ Tachycardia

- Neurological
  - √ Tremor, agitation, restlessness, confusion, ataxia, vertigo.
  - √ Involuntary movements (e.g., athetoid movements, twitching)
  - √ Stupor/coma (larger overdoses).
- Anticholinergic toxicity e.g., urinary retention, constipation, dry mouth, delirium [fluctuating level of consciousness and attention, visual hallucinations, hyperactivity, increased startle response].
- Vision blurred.

Management

- Manage in emergency room.
- Start IV.
- Dialysis is not as effective as hemoperfusion.
- Provide supportive care.
- Monitor ECG.
- In early stages of overdose
  - √ Induce vomiting.
  - √ Administer gastric lavage.
- Seizure control—caution re. aggravating respiratory depression.

Clinical Tips

- Be alert to carbamazepine side effects and reduce dose or discontinue drug.
- Antimanic effect begins in about 6 days and peaks in about 2 weeks.
- Antiaggression effect takes 1 month.
- More effective than lithium in the absence of positive family history of bipolar disorder.
- If dose increase is too rapid, common side effects include nausea, vomiting, ataxia, drowsiness, dizziness, diplopia, clumsiness.
  - √ If this occurs, reduce dose and raise more slowly.
- Manage sedation by smaller, slower dose increases and hs dosing.
- Confusion may arise from hyponatremia and, rarely, water intoxication.
- Withdrawal usually not a problem but taper anyway.
- Patient should report bruising or bleeding, which may indicate thrombocytopenia.

GABAPENTIN

Drug	Manufacturer	Chemical Class	Therapeutic Class
gabapentin (Neurontin)	Pfizer	cyclohexanacetic acid	anticonvulsant

Indications: FDA/HPB

- Partial seizures
- Postherpetic neuralgia

Indications: Off label

- Bipolar disorder
  - √ Recent placebo-controlled trials have been negative.
  - √ Small case series showed effectiveness in mania.
  - √ Cannot be recommended at this time for this indication except in trial as adjunctive therapy.
  - √ all general adult data
- Purported to improve impulsive aggressivity and agitation associated with dementia in some patients.
  - √ Overall, early data not encouraging.
- As adjunct to other antiparkinsonian medication, improves rigidity, bradykinesia, and tremor.
- Case reports only of efficacy in
  - √ Neuropathic pain relief
  - √ Anxiety
  - √ Insomnia
  - √ Orthostatic tremor
- Inadvisable to use in presence of renal impairment.

Pharmacology

See page 482.

- Not metabolised in liver.
- Renal excretion of unmodified drug.
  - √ Reduce dose in presence of diminished glomerular function.
  - √ Reduce dose in elders.
    - ▫ Greater dose reductions as age increases.

Mechanism of action

- Increases brain GABA levels by inhibition of GABA transporter.
  - √ Dose-dependant action.
- Modestly antiglutamatergic decreasing glutamate synthesis.

Choosing a Drug

- No propensity to induce dependence (unlike benzodiazepines).
- Most benign adverse-effect profile of the newer anticonvulsants (general adult data).
- Renal failure requires careful dose adjustments.

Dosing

Daily dose regimen

- Tid required (short half-life).

- Hs dosing for insomnia.
- Initial dose
  - √ 100 mg po tid.
- Off-label indications
  - √ Effective dose ranges not well determined; clinical practice data only.
  - √ Dementia 100 mg tid.
  - √ Postherpetic pain: Dose not determined for elders.
    - ▫ Suggest beginning at 100–200 mg daily.
    - ▫ Increasing by 100 mg per day, employing tid dosing (general adult range 300–600 mg po tid).
  - √ Neuropathic pain: Dose not determined for elders.
    - ▫ General adult dosing 300 mg day 1, increasing to 300 bid day 2, and 300 mg tid day 3.
    - ▫ Target dose 100–600 mg tid
    - ▫ Suggested geriatric range one-third to one-half general adult range.
  - √ Sedation: Begin at 100 mg every 12 hours.
    - ▫ Increase by 100 mg every 3–5 days, to 300 mg q hs (range 100–1800 mg/day) (general adult data).
  - √ Renal impairment: Reduce dose based on creatinine clearance rates.
    - ▫ Clearance 30–60 ml/min: maximum dose 300 mg bid.
    - ▫ Clearance 15–30 ml/min: maximum dose 300 mg daily.
    - ▫ Clearance < 15 ml/min: 300 mg every other day.
- Increasing dose and reaching therapeutic levels.
  - √ Increase by 100 mg q 3–5 days.
- Target dose 300–400 mg tid (range 300–1800 mg/day).

Discontinuation and Withdrawal

- Do not discontinue abruptly—taper required.

Side Effects

- Generally well tolerated.
- Side effects usually mild and self-limiting.
- Few cognitive effects in healthy elders, but few data in cognitively impaired elders.

Table 4.8. Side Effects of Gabapentin

Side Effects	Most Common	Most Serious and Less Common
Body as a whole	• Weight gain	
Cardiovascular	• Peripheral edema	
Case reports		• Hypersensitivity syndrome

(*cont.*)

Continued

Side Effects	Most Common	Most Serious and Less Common
Central and peripheral nervous system	• Fatigue • Lassitude • Somnolence • Dizziness/ataxia • Nystagmus • Dysarthria	• Tremor
Eye	• Blurred vision • Diplopia	
Gastrointestinal	• Nausea • Vomiting • Dry mouth • Constipation	
Hematological		• Leukopenia
Musculoskeletal	• Myalgia	
Psychiatric	• Nervousness	• Rapid-cycling bipolar states induced occasionally
Reproductive		• Possible sexual dysfunction (general adult data)
Respiratory	• Rhinitis • Pharyngitis	

Special monitoring: Serum creatinine prior to beginning.

Drug Interactions

- Antacids—reduced absorption.
  - √ Aluminum hydroxide—give gabapentin 2 hours before.
- Alcohol—avoid.

Disability Interactions

- Renal impairment—reduced clearance, increased plasma levels, and increased half-life.

Overdose, Toxicity, Suicide

Rate of absorption slower than other anticonvulsants; less toxic in overdose.

- Symptoms
  - √ Diplopia
  - √ Drowsiness
  - √ Slurred speech
  - √ Lethargy
  - √ Diarrhea

Management

- Provide supportive care.
- Use hemodialysis in severe cases (theoretical value—clinical experience not available).

LAMOTRIGINE

Drug	Manufacturer	Chemical Class	Therapeutic Class
lamotrigine (Lamictal)	Glaxo SmithKline	phenyltriazine compound	anticonvulsant

Indications: FDA/HPB

- Adjunctive agent for partial seizures.

Indications: Off label

- Treatment-resistant bipolar disorder (one controlled study in general adults with bipolar I disorder; most studies nonblinded but show efficacy; all general adult data).
  - √ May be effective in rapid-cycling disorders although data limited and somewhat conflicting.
  - √ Refractory mania (case reports only).
  - √ Open trial suggests efficacy in treatment-refractory depression, hypomanic, manic, and mixed bipolar phases.
  - √ Prophylactic efficacy uncertain but trends in the positive direction (general adult data).
- Some clinical reports of effectiveness in depression and schizoaffective disorders.
- Possible neuroprotective effect in Alzheimer's disease.
  - √ Preliminary data of improved word recognition, naming, and depressed mood in Alzheimer's disease.

Pharmacology

See page 482.

Note: Autoinduction of metabolism may reduce plasma levels and lower half-life by 25%.

- Age, per se, does not influence clearance.
- Caution needed with impaired renal or hepatic function.

Mechanisms of action

- Not well established.
- Inhibition of voltage-dependent sodium channels.

- Inhibition of excitatory amino acids (e.g., glutamate and aspartate).
- Calcium antagonism.
- May block $5HT_3$ receptors.
- May potentiate dopaminergic transmission.

Choosing a Drug

- Not suitable for acute mania—requires slow dose escalation.
- High incidence of dermatological side effects.
  - √ Some very serious make this a third-line agent.

Race/ethnicity

- Clearance reduced by 25% in non-Caucasians.

Dosing

- No geriatric-specific data.
- Increase dose gradually to reduce risk of Stevens–Johnson syndrome.
  - √ Especially when using concurrently with divalproex.
- Initial dose.
  - √ 12.5 mg/day/po.
  - √ Based on anecdotal experience and basic 50% rule and conservative regimen suitable for frail elders.
  - √ More aggressive dosing sometimes used but rate of dose increase associated with emergence of rash, so caution necessary.
- Increasing dose and reaching therapeutic levels.
  - √ Increase 12.5–25 mg/day q 1–2 weeks.
  - √ Target dose of 100 mg/day in divided bid doses (range 100–300 mg/day).

Discontinuation and withdrawal

- Do not stop abruptly.
  - √ Taper gradually over at least 2 weeks.

Side Effects

- Modest tolerance for drug in elders.
- Many adverse effects.
- Serious rash, including Stevens–Johnson syndrome, is the most important side effect.

Table 4.9. Side Effects of Lamotrigine

Side Effects (General Adult Data)	Most Common	Most Serious and Less Common
Body as a whole	• Fatigue • Pain	
Central and peripheral nervous system	• Dizziness/ataxia • Tremor • Somnolence • Headache • Insomnia	• Incoordination • Memory/concentration impairment • Aphasia • Confusion
Eye	• Double vision • Blurred vision	• Nystagmus
Gastrointestinal	• GI effects usually transient (general adult data) • Nausea • Vomiting • Constipation • Dyspepsia	• Hepatic failure • Diarrhea • Abdominal pain
Hematological		• Aplastic anemia • Hemolytic anemia • Thrombocytopenia • Pancytopenia
Liver and biliary		• Case reports: hepatic failure
Musculoskeletal	• Arthralgia	
Psychiatric	• Nervousness	• Induction of mania • Depression
Skin and appendages	• Rash (5–15%, general adult data)	• Severe, occasionally fatal, skin conditions may emerge (0.3%). √ Stevens-Johnson syndrome √ Toxic epidermal necrosis • Dose-related, especially if upper recommended range exceeded or administered with concurrent valproate. • *Discontinue at first sign of rash.*

Drug Interactions

- Enzyme-inducing agents reduce half-life to about 13 hours (general adult data).
  - √ Phenytoin
  - √ Phenobarbital
  - √ Methsuximide
  - √ Mephenytoin
- Carbamazepine increases toxic epoxide metabolite.
- Valproate doubles lamotrigine levels and toxicity.
- Other cautions
  - √ Ethosuximide
  - √ Lopinavir/ritonavir

- √ Methotrexate
- √ Oxcarbazine
- √ Primidone
- √ Pyrimethamine
- √ Rifampin
- √ Trimethoprim
- √ Trimetrexate

Overdose, Toxicity, Suicide

- Symptoms
  - √ Dizziness
  - √ Sedation
  - √ Headache
  - √ Coma
- Dangers
  - √ Lethality data not available for elders, but potential to induce coma warrants caution in significant overdose.
  - √ Occasional lethality reported in sporadic general adult reports.

Management

- Hospitalize.
- Induce emesis or gastric lavage.
- Monitor vital signs frequently.
- Provide supportive care.
- Hemodialysis of uncertain utility.

Clinical Tips

- If using valproate and lamotrigine together, increase dose of lamotrigine more slowly than usual and monitor tolerance.
  - √ Valproate increases plasma levels of lamotrigine.

LITHIUM

Drug	Manufacturer	Chemical Class	Therapeutic Class
lithium carbonate (Eskalith, Eskalith CR,* Lithobid) lithium citrate syrup (Cebalith-S)	Eskalith—Glaxo SmithKline Lithobid—Solvay Carbolith—Roxane	alkali metal	antimanic

* Controlled release.

Indications: FDA/HPB

- Treatment of manic episodes in bipolar I and II disorders

Indications: Off label

- Effective continuation and maintenance therapy for preventing relapse in bipolar mood disorders.
  - √ Unipolar depression may be responsive sometimes, but evidence is less clear.
- Secondary mania, if tolerated.
- Augmentation of antidepressant therapy in antidepressant-resistant patients, including unipolar disorders.
- Management of some BPSD (e.g., aggression).
- Treatment of bipolar depression.
- Schizoaffective disorders.

Pharmacology

See page 482.

- Clearance of lithium prolonged in elders because of age-related reductions in creatinine clearance and GFR.
  - √ Dose reductions of 35% required at ages 65–70, decreasing thereafter by 1–2% per year.
- Lithium and sodium compete at the proximal renal tubule.
  - √ Sodium depletion leads to lithium retention and toxicity.

Mechanism of action

- Unclear, and clinical relevance of specific actions undetermined.
- Affects neurotransmitter systems, including serotonergic, adrenergic, dopaminergic, cholinergic; increases GABA transmission.
- Influences cellular ion transport and second messenger systems.
- Effect on
  - √ Cyclic adenosine monophosphate formation.
  - √ Receptor g-protein coupling.
  - √ Phosphoinositol metabolism.
  - √ Alters distribution and kinetics of sodium, potassium, calcium, magnesium.
- Intracellular actions of lithium include
  - √ Delay of norepinephrine-sensitive adenylate cyclase.
  - √ Reversal or balancing of calcium-mediated processes.
  - √ Passage through sodium and potassium channels.
  - √ Reduction of neurotransmitter sensitivity.
- Stabilization effect on neurotransmission receptor systems.
- Polyurea secondary to inhibition of renal response to ADH.

Therapeutic Actions by Indication

- Mania
  - √ Effective in reducing affective and ideational symptoms in 2–3 weeks in early-onset bipolar patients.
    - Elevated mood, grandiosity, impulsivity, flight of ideas, aggression, irritability, anxiety.
    - May also improve pressured speech, paranoid delusions, insomnia, assaultiveness, hypersexuality.
  - √ Control of florid symptoms of mania in acute phase.
  - √ Effective in late-onset mania but greater toxicity, since higher incidence of comorbid organic pathology.
  - √ Maintenance during chronic phase.
    - Prevention of mood disorder relapse and recurrence.
    - May require concurrent integrated use of antidepressants, other mood stabilizers as required, and thyroid replacement as necessary.
- Depression
  - √ Occasionally depression responds best to lithium while unresponsive to antidepressants.
  - √ In elders who have been responsive to lithium for many years, be cautious about recurrence of depression when switching to another antidepressant agent.
  - √ Augmentation of antidepressants.
    - In 50–65% of antidepressant-resistant patients, symptoms partially or completely remit in 2–12 days.

Choosing a Drug

- Overall tolerance in elders not well defined.
  - √ Otherwise healthy elders usually tolerate well-monitored lithium therapy.
  - √ Elders more sensitive to central effects of lithium.
  - √ Medically/neurologically impaired or frail elders are less tolerant.
  - √ Neurological side effects may be intolerable even within accepted therapeutic plasma levels.
  - √ Concurrent neurological disorders a risk factor for increased sensitivity to side effects.
- Elders more likely to be taking multiple medications with potential interactions with lithium (e.g., diuretics, NSAIDs).
- Controlled-release lithium associated with
  - √ Less fluctuation in plasma levels than standard lithium.
  - √ Slightly higher plasma levels, which may be significant in some elders.
  - √ More diarrhea, (more lithium in small bowel).

- √ Consider slow-release form when acute fluctuations in lithium levels are a danger and need to be avoided.
- Prognostic indicators of response to treatment
  - √ Poor response predicted by
    - More severe manic symptoms.
    - Greater dysphoria.
    - Psychosis.
    - Schizoaffective symptoms.
    - History of rapid cycling (i.e., more than four cycles/year).
    - History of poor lithium tolerance and neurotoxicity.
    - Significant comorbid conditions, especially neurological (as in secondary mania) and kidney.
    - History of poor compliance.
    - Hypothyroidism.
      - Correction of thyroid level essential to optimal response.
      - May be aggravated or induced by lithium.
    - *Absence* of genetic history of bipolar disorder (in first-degree relative).
    - Inability of caregivers in patient's home setting to monitor side effects and adjust dosages.

Dosing

- General rule: Use one-third to one-half adult dose.
  - √ Marked interindividual variability in tolerance.
  - √ Always individualize therapy based on both clinical response and plasma level monitoring.
- Need for dose reduction begins at about age 50 and increases thereafter.
- Use smallest dose that produces therapeutic plasma levels.
  - √ 0.5–0.8 mEq/l in acute phase if responsive.
    - If unresponsive, increase very cautiously to 0.8–1 mEq/l if side effects tolerated.
  - √ Observe for neurotoxicity at higher plasma levels (>0.7 mEq/l).

Daily dose regimen

- Usually once daily at night if peak plasma levels are tolerated.
- Otherwise, divided doses (e.g., bid, with larger dose at night).
- Alternate-day dosing has been used successfully.
  - √ Give 150% of daily dose.
  - √ Reduced side effects and compliance but efficacy has been questioned (general adult data only).
  - √ Not a suggested strategy.
- *Note:* Controlled-release lithium is not a sustained-release form.

- √ Does not offer a slow release of lithium over time—simply delays release until later time after administration.
- √ Requires divided doses q 12 hours to minimize high peak plasma levels.

Initial dose

- Otherwise well and robust elders, begin at 300 mg qhs.
- Frail or neurologically impaired elders, begin at 75–150 mg qhs.
  - √ Starting with 75 mg is prudent in frail elders to avoid occasional hypersensitivity and toxic response, even at low starting doses.
  - √ Lithium citrate syrup is useful for flexible, ultralow dosing.
    - ▫ Most rapidly absorbed form of lithium.

Increasing dose and reaching therapeutic levels

- Increase in 150 mg increments (by breaking 300 mg tablet in half) about every 3–7 days.
  - √ Allow steady state to develop before increasing dose.
- Use smaller dose increments of 75 mg in frail, cognitively impaired, or physically ill (renal, CVS) patients.
- Usual target therapeutic dose 300–900 mg hs.
  - √ Some patients require higher doses of 900–1800 mg/day for very severe mania.
    - ▫ Upper end of range is riskier in elders and should be used rarely and with caution.
    - ▫ Advisable not to use high-dose range in frail, very old, or otherwise vulnerable elders.
- *Note:* Tolerance for lithium declines as symptoms come under control.
  - √ Often requires dose reductions.
  - √ Monitor plasma levels more closely during this phase.

Maintenance dose

- Optimum plasma levels for elders not well defined.
  - √ Recommended range: 0.5–0.8 mmol/l.
    - ▫ For many elders 0.5 mmol/l or even lower (0.2–0.4 mEq/l) is sufficient for relapse prophylaxis.
    - ▫ 0.8 mmol/l suggested for patients with more than two episodes of mania, if tolerated.
  - √ Lithium levels often attained with doses of 300 mg/day (range 150–600 mg/day) but sometimes higher doses up to 1200 (rarely, 1800) mg/day required.
  - √ Lower dose and plasma level ranges used for frail or very old patients.

- Do not use combination of valproic acid and carbamazepine.
  - √ Problematic because of toxic side effects.
- Synergistic mood-stabilizing effects between lithium and valproic acid, but monitor carefully for side effects.

Combination therapy: Augmenting lithium with antidepressants

- Little placebo controlled-data on effectiveness.
  - √ About 50% response rate (general adult data only).
  - √ Overall, lithium potentiation may be less effective and less well tolerated in elders.
  - √ Most effective for bipolar forms of depression, but unipolar are less or not repsonsive.
- Dose
  - √ Give low doses (300 mg/day, clinically effective) hs to obtain target blood levels.
- Target plasma level for augmentation not well established for elders.
  - √ May be lower than therapeutic range for lithium in mania (i.e., 0.2–0.4 mmol/L; range 0.3–0.7).
  - √ Some recommend full therapeutic levels.
  - √ Each patient is mini-clinical trial in these situations.
- Caution in elders, especially those over 75 years.
  - √ Augmentation often associated with high risk of side effects, especially
    - ▫ At higher blood levels (0.8+)—tremor, neurotoxicity, ataxia, EPS, sinus bradycardia, delirium.
    - ▫ With increased age (75 plus).
- Response time varies from 2–10 days to up to 6 weeks.
  - √ 3–6-week trial advised.
- Overall, augmentation modestly effective in elderly subjects.
  - √ Strongest support for effectiveness is with TCAs in delusional depression in elders.
  - √ Additional support for augmentation effects with fluoxetine, venlafaxine, and MAOIs (general adult and limited geriatric data).
  - √ Maintain lithium augmentation for full duration of maintenance therapy.
    - ▫ Some evidence for increased risk of relapse if lithium augmentation withdrawn after effect obtained.
    - ▫ Long-term studies of efficacy not available, but clinical experience suggests its effectiveness.

For rapid behavioral control, consider

- Antipsychotic (e.g., olanzapine 2.5–5 mg/day or, for short durations, haloperidol 1–4 mg/day) or

- Benzodiazepine (e.g., lorazepam 1–4 mg/day or clonazepam 0.5–2 mg/day orally or IM).

Discontinuation and Withdrawal

- Taper gradually over 2–4 weeks to discontinue lithium.
- Monitor closely.
  - √ Abrupt discontinuation leads to relapse in 50% of patients within 5 months (general adult data).
  - √ However, evidence of an actual withdrawal syndrome with lithium is not strong.
    - ▫ Relapse is more likely part of the natural course of the illness.

Side Effects

- Frequency of toxic side effects about 10–20%.
- Toxicity usually associated with high plasma levels.
- Toxicity may develop even when within therapeutic plasma levels associated with
  - √ Rapid dose escalation at time of peak plasma levels.
    - ▫ Reduce effect by.
      - ◦ Using CR preparation.
      - ◦ Larger dose H.S.
      - ◦ Using tid or qid doses.
  - √ Use of concurrent psychotropics or other interacting drugs.
  - √ Organic brain disease or EEG abnormalities.
  - √ Reduced GFR.
  - √ Conditions leading to hyponatremia.
    - ▫ Excessive sweating.
    - ▫ Diarrhea.
    - ▫ Anorexia and nutritional deficiencies.
    - ▫ Drugs—Na depleting diuretics.
    - ▫ Salt restricted diets.
  - √ Very old age.

Elders, especially frail, impaired, or physically ill, are more prone to some side effects than younger patients, but data are limited and proneness has not been shown conclusively for all side effects (e.g., polyuria/polydipsia not more frequent in elders).

Physically healthy elders tend to tolerate properly monitored lithium well.

Body as a Whole

- Weight gain
  - √ No geriatric data.
  - √ Advise patient re. diet and exercise.

- Peripheral edema
  - √ May be significant.
  - √ Consider potassium-sparing diuretic.
    - ▫ Eg., amiloride (Moduret) or loop diuretic furosemide (Lasix).

Cardiovascular

Inversion/flattening of T waves—low clinical significance.

Widening of QRS complex on ECG—benign.

- Sinus node dysfunction.
  - √ Often not clinically significant.
  - √ Bradycardia.
  - √ Sick sinus-conduction disturbances—prolonged PR interval
- Rare—ventricular arrhythmias (VPBs, tachycardia), AV block, BBB, sino-atrial block, myocardial damage, sudden death.
- Peripheral edema.

Management

- T-wave changes are dose dependent.
  - √ Monitor plasma potassium levels.
- Sinus node dysfunction occurs especially in patients with pre-existing cardiac disease and is aggravated by digitalis and beta-blockers.
- Ventricular arrhythmias may be more dangerous in patients with ischemic heart disease.
- Cardiac changes disappear within 2 weeks of discontinuation of lithium.
- Stabilized patients probably don't need frequent ECG monitoring specifically for the lithium component of treatment, but routine pulse monitoring for regularity is advised.
  - √ Arrhythmias may be episodic and require Holter monitoring.

Central and Peripheral Nervous System

- Complaints of feeling drugged.
- Fatigue.
- Ataxia/vertigo.
- Incoordination.
- Tremor.
  - √ If severe can be very limiting and distressing.
    - ▫ Eg., interfere with dressing or eating.
  - √ Characteristics—fine, resting, and intentional, irregular, fluctuates in intensity
  - √ Onset within first 2–3 weeks of treatment.

- √ Aggravated by concurrent TCAs, neuroleptics (especially typical), high peak serum lithium levels.
  - ▫ Reduce dose, spread out dose through the day, or use hs single dose.
- Mild cognitive change: subjective memory complaints, reduced concentration, disorientation, may progress to more significant levels.
  - √ Differentiate from progression of dementia.
    - ▫ Sudden decline in cognitive ability.
    - ▫ Neuromuscular symptoms.
    - ▫ Associated with initiation or dose escalation of lithium.
    - ▫ Associated with addition of concurrent drugs (eg., divalproex, neuroleptic).
  - √ Distinguish from hypothyroidism and correct thyroid function.
- Drowsiness/fatigue/lassitude.
- Muscle fasciculations/twitching.
- Slurred speech.
- Incontinence (urine/feces).

Most serious and less common

Neurotoxicity: Important to distinguish from dementia; vulnerability increased by high lithium levels (but may be present at therapeutic plasma levels) and presence of underlying neurological pathology.

- Delirium: Symptoms may persist weeks or months after plasma lithium has declined to low or undetectable levels.
  - √ May occur at plasma level below that normally considered toxic, especially in presence of comorbid neurological disorder or EPS.
  - √ Delirium may last for weeks after lithium becomes undetectable in plasma.
- Tremor is fine resting, not as coarse as in Parkinson's disease. Hand tremor, if severe, can be very distressing and limit function.
- Acute toxicity resembles delirium or encephalopathy.
  - √ Begins with disorientation, confusion, distractibility, fluctuating consciousness.
  - √ Progresses to slurred speech, delusions, hallucinations, somnolence/stupor, muscle weakness, increased muscle tone and reflexes, sialorrrhea, hyperpyrexia.
  - √ May lead to serotonergic syndrome or NMS.
  - √ Toxic levels occasionally may progress rapidly to coma/death.
- EPS may emerge.
  - √ Parkinsonism with cogwheeling.
  - √ Oculogyric crisis.

- Dyskinesia
- Akathiesia
  - √ TD—relationship to lithium treatment unclear.
  - √ Mild neuropathy.
- Seizures
- EEG changes—encephalopathy.
- Myoclonus.
- Worsening of Parkinson's disease.
- Symptoms of dementia worsen and BPSD-like picture can cloud the correct diagnosis if toxicity is not suspected.
  - √ Misdiagnosis of toxicity as dementia is an easy mistake to make in elders, especially in long-term care settings.

Irreversible toxicity is uncommon but possible in about 10% of severe cases. It includes choreoathetosis and cerebellar dysfunction (ataxia, dysmetria, dysarthria scanning speech, impaired rapid alternating movements).

Management

Coadministration of neuroleptics with lithium increases rate of emergence of EPS, delirium, and cerebellar symptoms.

Factors that increase tubular reabsorption of sodium may lead to neurotoxicity and should be corrected.

Antiparkinsonian agents have no effect on lithium-induced cogwheeling.

Duration of neurotoxic symptoms 2–3 weeks after dose reduction/discontinuation, but sometimes more prolonged and occasionally irreversible, especially when cerebellar signs present.

Management of neurotoxicity:

- Reduce dose or discontinue lithium.
  - √ In mild cases symptoms remit when plasma levels return to therapeutic range.
    - ▫ Therapeutic range for a vulnerable patient may be lower than expected (eg., presence of concurrent dementia).
- Review, reduce, or discontinue other medications that may contribute to or cause delirium.
- Administer propranolol 20 mg bid for tremor.
  - √ Caution re. contraindications to beta-blockers–CHF, hypotension, asthma.
- Correct fluid and electrolyte imbalance.
  - √ Attend to hydration, Na depletion, diuretic administration, nutrition, and primary disease processes.
- General supportive measures.

- Hemodialysis is advised in severe neurotoxicity to prevent permanent toxic effects.
  - √ Some recommend its use early in the course, even if mild.
- Forced diuresis has questionable efficacy.
- For prolonged states of neurotoxicity, physiotherapy, speech therapy, etc., helpful.
- Improvement can continue over 6–12 months.
  - √ Return of manic symptoms may occur prior to remission of delirium
    - ▫ May require management.
      - ◦ Use atypical anti-psychotic cautiously (eg., quetiapine).
      - ◦ Avoid typical anti-psychotics if possible.
  - √ Caution re. premature conclusion that continuing neurotoxicity is irreversible since recovery can be prolonged.
    - ▫ Prolonged symptoms easily mistaken for dementia.

Endocrine

- Nontoxic goiter 8–10%.
  - √ Presents with swallowing problems 1–2 years into therapy.
- Suppression of thyroid function.
  - √ Onset 6–18 months.
  - √ Inhibition of T4 conversion to T3.
  - √ Elevated TSH.
- Diminished thyroid reserve in elders increases vulnerability to hypothyroidism with lithium.
  - √ Increased TSH may emerge within < 6 months of treatment and persist for years in up to 40% of cases (general adult data).
  - √ More common in women (10:1).
  - √ May be hard to diagnose.
    - ▫ Mimics depression or drug side effects.
    - ▫ Suspect with bradycardia, neurotoxicity, or other signs (e.g., hoarse voice, pretibial edema, cold intolerance, cognitive impairment).
- Increased FBS.
  - √ May accentuate diabetes.

Most serious and less common

- Hyperparathyroidism with chronic lithium administration.
  - √ If mild increase of Ca and parathormone levels, continue lithium with monitoring.
- Case report: myxedema coma.
- Hyperthyroidism—rarely clinically significant.
  - √ Sometimes leads to mood and behavioral disturbance requiring withdrawal of lithium.

Management

- Hypothyroidism
  - √ Rule out hypothyroidism prior to treatment.
    - ▫ Not a contraindication, but thyroid function should be corrected before beginning therapy.
  - √ Monitor thyroid regularly, especially in women.
    - ▫ Toxicity can be severe and hard to diagnose.
  - √ Hypothyroidism usually reversible when lithium is discontinued, but occasionally long-term effects persist.
  - √ Discontinue lithium.
  - √ Add thyroid hormone replacement if patient is symptomatic and TSH < 10 mU/L otherwise monitor TSH.
  - √ Check thyroid function every 3–6 months if lithium reintroduced.
  - √ Distinguish from depression with trial of thyroxine for 3 months.
  - √ Add antidepressant as appropriate for symptom picture and prior response patterns.
- Hyperparathyroidism
  - √ Consider parathyroid hormone therapy.

Eye

- Blurred vision.
- Nystagmus.
- Case report of lenticular opacities.
  - √ Causal relationship to lithium not established.

Gastrointestinal

- Thirst (50%)
- Dry mouth
- Diarrhea
- Gastric irritation
- Nausea

GI effects may be particularly troublesome in elders; tolerance often develops.

Management

- Slow schedule of increasing lithium dose.
- Lower dose.
- Administer lithium with food or switch to CR preparation.
- For diarrhea try syrup form instead of CR.
  - √ Antidiarrheal treatment (eg., simethicone/loperamide [Imodium advanced]).
- Monitor for dehydration or electrolyte imbalance.

Hematological

- Leukocytosis.
  - √ Usually reversible, transient for several months.
- Not associated with serious blood dyscrasias or infection.

Metabolic and Nutritional

SIADH (rare; see also p. 82).

Musculoskeletal

- Bone demineralization.
- Secondary to reduced uptake of calcium, phosphate, magnesium.

Psychiatric

- Toxicity occasionally presents with manic-like picture.
- Reduce dose.

Respiratory

- Respiratory depression.
  - √ Associated with preexisting COPD.

Skin and Appendages

- May worsen psoriasis, acne, folliculitis, rash, hair loss.
  - √ Psoriasis may be severe and occasionally require lowering dose, discontinuation of lithium, or steroids.
  - √ Zinc ointment for mild rashes.
- Fungal lesions.
  - √ Rare.
  - √ D/C lithium.

Urinary

- Long-term lithium use has been associated rarely with dose-related *pathological changes in kidney functioning*, including sclerotic glomeruli, fibrosis, and atrophic tubuli.
  - √ These changes are still controversial in some reports.
  - √ Increased creatinine may be indication to discontinue lithium and substitute valproate.
- Lithium reduces tubular concentration, which may become irreversible—especially problematic for men with prostatic hypertrophy.
  - √ Increased risks with multiple daily dosing and episodes of lithium toxicity.
  - √ May lead to incontinence, progressive urinary retention, and urinary tract infections.
- Nocturia
  - √ Increases risk of falls.

- Polyuria occurs in 20-40% of patients on lithium.
  - √ Urine culture distinguishes from urinary tract infection.
  - √ Elders commonly show WBCs in urine, especially in nursing home settings.
  - √ Often requires no treatment.
- Nephrogenic diabetes insipidus
  - √ Caused by arginine–vasopressin nonresponse at the distal nephron.
  - √ May be associated with focal interstitial nephritis, distal renal tubular dilation, and microcyst formation.
  - √ Occurs in about 12% of patients on long-term lithium therapy.
  - √ Symptoms: polyuria, excessive thirst, tachycardia, hypotension, hypernatremia; in extreme cases, hyperosmolar coma.
    - ▫ Usually mild and partial with *low urine* osmolarity and polyuria but *normal plasma* osmolarity.
    - ▫ Occasionally severe.
  - √ Degree of impairment may correlate with duration of lithium treatment (hence more likely to arise in elders who have been on chronic lithium therapy) or total lithium dose.
  - √ Not as prevalent at plasma levels of 0.5–0.8 mmol/L.
  - √ Especially important to ensure adequate hydration.
    - ▫ Vulnerable patients are those with vomiting, diarrhea, fluid restriction for other reasons (e.g., frail elders in nursing home).
  - √ Usually reversible on reducing dose or stopping lithium.
  - √ Urine volumes > 4 liters/day, add thiazides or amiloride.
  - √ Use NSAIDS for refractory cases.
  - √ Prevention: Consider annual 24-hour urine measurement.
  - √ Single hs dosing has a kidney-sparing effect, especially with regard to fibrosis, polyuria.
  - √ Management
    - ▫ Single hs dose.
    - ▫ Avoid CR preparation.
    - ▫ Reduce dose.
    - ▫ Severe symptoms unresponsive to dose reduction.
    - ▫ Discontinue lithium.
    - ▫ Potassium supplement.
    - ▫ Monitor renal function.
      - ◦ Urinary-specific gravity and osmolarity, serum creatinine, or creatinine clearance.
- Very rarely *nephrotic syndrome.*

Case Reports

- Malignant hyperthermia with concurrent TCA.

Monitoring

- *Note:* Toxic effects may occur even within therapeutic plasma levels.

Routine monitoring

Pretreatment laboratory investigations

- Blood screen
  - √ CBC and differential.
  - √ ESR.
- Urinalysis (routine and microscopic).
- Kidney function tests (BUN, serum creatinine; creatinine clearance when renal disease or side effects suspected (eg., nephregenic diabetes insipidus or renal tubular fibrosis)).
  - √ Baseline renal function important.
  - √ *Note:* Serum creatinine level is an insensitive test for renal function in elders and cannot be fully relied on.
    - ▫ May be normal in presence of renal impairment.
  - √ *Note:* Lithium excretion depends on GFR, which is normally reduced in elders.
    - ▫ If practical, use 24-hour creatinine clearance to monitor GFR, especially in patients with elevated plasma creatinine.
- Thyroid screen.
  - √ TSH(s).
  - √ T_3 resin uptake.
  - √ T_4 radio immune assay.
  - √ T_4 free thyroxin index.
  - √ Antithyroid antibodies.
- Parathyroid.
  - √ Parathyroid harmone.
  - √ Serum Ca.
- FBS.
- Serum electrolytes.
- ECG.
  - √ Baseline, because of sick sinus syndrome risk.
- Cognitive MS baseline.
- ADL/IADL inquiry, especially re. nutrition, reliability in managing own medications and self-monitoring health.
- Involuntary movement assessment, especially fine tremor.
  - √ AIMS (Adult Involuntary Movement Scale).
- Systems review, especially
  - √ Gastrointestinal
    - ▫ Diarrhea
    - ▫ Nausea
    - ▫ Edema

- ✓ Genitourinary
    - ▫ Frequency
    - ▫ Urgency
    - ▫ Nocturia
- ✓ Nutrition and fluid intake.
- ✓ Dermatological conditions/diseases.
- ✓ CVS
    - ▫ Congestive heart failure.
- ✓ CNS
    - ▫ *Note:* Parkinson's disease, stroke, Alzheimer's disease, other dementias which may predispose to increased toxicity or confusion about side effects (eg., source of tremor or agitation).
    - ▫ Tremor.
    - ▫ Gait instability.
    - ▫ MMSE < 25.
- Medication review for possible drug interactions.

Special monitoring

- Lithium plasma level.
    - ✓ Every 3–7 days during dose escalations.
    - ✓ At least every 3 months during continuation and early maintenance phase; more often if necessary.
    - ✓ As needed thereafter, but at least every 6 months, depending on stability of results, reliability and compliance with medications, and health.
    - ✓ Because of long half-life and time to steady state in some elders, consider repeating plasma lithium levels 2–4 weeks after last dose increase to ensure blood levels have not risen.
        - ▫ Take blood 12 hours after last dose.
        - ▫ Wait at least 5–7 days between dose increases for steady state to be achieved before monitoring plasma levels.
    - ✓ Toxic levels in elders not well defined, but side effects increase above 0.8 mEq/l.
        - ▫ Treatment plasma level range for acute mania 0.6–0.8 mEq/l.
        - ▫ Generally accepted maintenance levels are lower: 0.4–0.8 mEq/l.
        - ▫ Some indication that levels above 0.8 mEq/l, if tolerable, will be more effective for relapse prevention for elders.
    - ✓ Saliva levels may be helpful if plasma levels cannot be taken.
        - ▫ Generally twice as high as plasma.
    - ✓ Reassess lithium levels within a week of starting a potentially interacting medication (e.g., ACE inhibitor).

- Monitor every 3–6 months until stabilized.
  - √ Thyroid (TSH and antibodies).
  - √ Kidney function tests.
  - √ CVS.
    - ▫ Consider ECG.
    - ▫ Pulse rate and rhythm.
  - √ Parathyroid hormone and serum Ca
- Monitor every 6–12 months once stabilized.
  - √ Thyroid.
  - √ Kidney function.
  - √ Pulse rate/rhythm, possibly ECG.
- Monitor serum calcium and observe for signs of hypercalcemia
  - √ Tremor, ataxia, apathy, depressed mood.

Drug Interactions

- Concurrent therapy with antidepressants.
  - √ Occasionally reported as associated with severe neurotoxic reactions.
    - ▫ EPS, memory impairment, gait disturbance, stroke-like symptoms (reversible).
    - ▫ Cautious observation recommended.
  - √ TCAs commonly associated with increased tremor.
- NSAIDS are available OTC; caution patients to consult physician before starting any new drug.

Table 4.10. Lithium Drug Interactions

Drugs That Increase Plasma Lithium Levels	Drugs That Reduce Plasma Lithium Levels	Other Interactions
Alcohol	Acetazolamide	Digitalis: cardiac arrhythmias from digitalis toxicity
Antibiotics (ampicillin, tetracycline)	Caffeine (coffee, caffeine-containing cola, Mountain Dew, green tea, caffeine-containing bottled water (believe it or not), tea	Neuromuscular blocking agents (decamethonium, succinylcholine, pancuronium): prolonged muscle paralysis
Antidepressants	High-sodium diets	Potassium iodide: increased risk of hypothyroidism (synergistic effect)
Antipsychotics	Sodium bicarbonate	Tramadol: increased risk of serotonin syndrome
Benzodiazepines		Vasopressin: may antagonize antidiuretic effect
Carbamazepine		
Cardiac drugs		
Diuretics		
Methyldopa		
NSAIDs		
Phenytoin		

Increased Plasma Lithium Levels

Diuretics

- Diuretics that do not affect plasma lithium levels.
  - √ Furosemide (distal loop diuretic).
  - √ Amiloride (potassium sparing diuretic).

- Thiazides—hydrochlorothiazide.
  - √ Decrease renal lithium clearance by 25%.
  - √ Reduce lithium dose.
  - √ May be given safely by experienced clinicians with close lithium monitoring and rapid dose adjustment.
    - ▫ Most easily done with patients in institutional care.
- Potassium-sparing diuretics (amiloride, spironolactone, triamterene).
  - √ Monitor, but not as problematic as thiazides.
  - √ May increase lithium levels.
- Loop diuretics (furosemide, ethacrynic acid, torsemide, bumetanide).
  - √ Monitor, but not as problematic as thiazides.

Antidepressants

- SSRIs—increased toxicity; case reports of serotonin syndrome.
- TCAs—increased tremor.

Antipsychotics

- Persistent reports in past of increased neurotoxicity in combination with antipsychotics (especially typicals).
  - √ Including haloperidol and thioridazine.
  - √ More recent general adult studies do not confirm the danger.

Benzodiazepines

- Possible sexual dysfunction with combination.
- Case report of hypothermia with diazepam.

Carbamazepine

- Increased lithium plasma concentration.
- Neurotoxicity.
- Sinus node dysfunction.

Cardiac drugs

- ACE inhibitors (captopril, enalapril).
  - √ Data remain anecdotal and not geriatric-specific.
  - √ May increase lithium level; avoid coadministration.
  - √ Monitor renal function carefully when unadjusted high-dose combinations are used.
  - √ Adjust dosages downward.
- Calcium channel blockers (verapamil, diltiazem).
  - √ May potentiate cardiac conduction defects in combination with lithium.
    - ▫ Verapamil combination can increase dopamine synthesis and produce choreoathetosis.
    - ▫ Nifedipine does not seem to cause neurotoxicity.

Methyldopa

- Neurotoxicity.

NSAIDs

- Include diclofenac, flurbiprofen, ibuprofen, indomethacin, ketoprofen, ketorolac, naproxen, phenylbutazone, piroxicam, sulindac, oxaprozin.
- Increased serum lithium levels may induce toxicity.
- Monitor lithium levels if combination is used.
- Sometimes used in younger patients to manage lithium-induced nephrogenic diabetes insipidus.
  - √ Increased caution in elders re. neurotoxicity.
  - √ Not a suggested strategy.

Phenytoin

- Cerebellar ataxia (case reports).

Reduced Plasma Lithium Levels

Caffeine

- Induces sodium excretion (inhibits antidiuretic hormone).
- Lowers plasma lithium levels.
- May be clinically relevant in heavy caffeine drinkers.
- Levels may increase if caffeine intake is reduced.
- Advise patient to avoid coffee tea, or use decaffeinated products.

Sodium

- High sodium diets, if habitual, will decrease plasma lithium levels significantly.

Interactions with Illnesses and Contraindications

Table 4.11. Interactions with Illnesses and Contraindications

Condition	Comments
Arthritis	• Lithium may exacerbate symptoms • Avoid NSAIDS
Cardiovascular disease	• Uncorrected CHF reduces renal clearance; increases lithium concentration
Diabetes	• Lithium increases FBS • Monitor BS of diabetics carefully when initiating lithium therapy
Dehydration, Severe debilitation	

(cont.)

Continued

Condition	Comments
Elective surgery	• Discontinue lithium 2–3 days prior to surgery and restart when fluid/electrolyte balance restored • Administer IV fluid to NPO patients who have been on lithium • Caution with muscle relaxants
Organic brain syndromes	• Predispose to increased lithium toxicity • Avoid lithium when possible
Renal: Conditions that induce renal tubular reabsorption of sodium, hemoconcentration and electrolyte imbalance, and elevate lithium concentrations	• May precipitate a toxic reaction; intercurrent illnesses, viral infections, fever, dehydration, vomiting, diarrhea may produce electrolyte imbalance
Renal impairment	• Reduce lithium dose substantially • Monitor levels carefully • Avoid lithium in glomerulonephritis and pyelonephritis
Sodium: Any condition that significantly decreases serum sodium	• Medications (e.g., diuretics, especially thiazide diuretics) • Low-sodium diet • Drastic slimming diets • IADH secretions • Water intoxication • Excessive sweating (e.g., travel or exercise in hot climate) (5% of lithium excretion is in sweat) • Management √ Reduce dose √ Temporarily discontinue lithium √ Increase salt and water intake √ Avoid exercise in not environments
Thyroid disease	• Correct thyroid imbalances before beginning treatment with lithium

Effect on Laboratory Tests

- Increases
  - √ RBC glycine and choline levels.
  - √ Serum calcium (possibly from stimulation of parathyroid gland).
  - √ Serum magnesium.
  - √ $Iodine^{131}$ uptake.
  - √ TSH.
  - √ Leukocytes.
  - √ Eosinophils.
  - √ Platelets.
  - √ Glycosuria.
  - √ Albuminuria.
- Decreases
  - √ Vitamin B12 levels.
  - √ T_3, T_4 levels.

- √ Lymphocytes.
- √ Plasma phosphates.
- √ Urine concentration.

Overdose, Toxicity, Suicide

Symptoms of lithium overdose include the following

- Earlier—nausea, vomiting, diarrhea.
- Later—lethargy, weakness, dysarthria, rigidity, ataxia, coarse tremor, cogwheeling, increased muscle tone, hyperreflexia, fasciculation, myoclonus, EEG abnormalities.
- Cardiac effects—sinus arrest, asystole if preexisting conduction tissue disease, hypotension.
- End stages—seizures, renal failure, delirium, coma, death.
  - √ Significant neurological sequelae may persist after recovery from coma.

Management

- Hospitalize.
- Correct metabolic disturbances.
  - √ Commonly dehydration, GI upset, infection, hypokalemia.
- Monitor
  - √ Lithium levels frequently.
  - √ Creatinine.
  - √ Electrolytes.
  - √ Urinalysis.
  - √ Blood glucose.
  - √ EEG for persistent symptoms.
    - ▫ Slowing in delirium.
- Discontinue or reduce dose of lithium.
- Discontinue or reduce dose of drugs that decrease lithium clearance (e.g., thiazide diuretics).
- Discontinue or reduce dose of drugs that have additive effects (e.g., antipsychotics).
- If caught early, administer repeated gastric lavage.
  - √ Not useful after absorption has occurred.
- Restore fluids/serum electrolyte balance, especially sodium balance.
  - √ For sodium depletion causing toxicity, give 1–2 liters of IV sodium solution in first 6 hours; caution re. fluid overload.
  - √ Saline infusion may enhance excretion of lithium, as will urea, mannitol, or aminophylline.
- Hemodialysis is very effective for severe intoxication.
  - √ Institute if trough lithium level (i.e., 12 hours after ingestion) is 2–2.5 mEq/l (may be lower in frail elders), especially if patient's

condition is deteriorating, or if patient is unresponsive to other measures.
  - √ Clears 50 ml/min.
  - √ Requires long runs of 12 hours until plasma lithium is < 1 mEq/l.
  - √ Follow lithium levels every 4 hours after dialysis—levels sometimes rebound.
  - √ Expect lag time in recovery from neurotoxicity until intracellular lithium clears.
  - √ Irreversible neurotoxicity occasionally occurs.
- Activated charcoal of no value.

Caregiver Notes

- Warn patients and families about
  - √ Excessive sweating or dehydration, especially in summer or hot climates when traveling or exercising.
  - √ Need for adequate salt intake.
  - √ Need to avoid salt-restricted diets.
- Reinforce need for blood tests and the procedure for drawing trough levels.
- Consider medic alert card/bracelet for community dwelling elders.
- Do not double dose.
- Take with food/milk.
- Do not divide sustained release tablet.

Clinical Tips

- Lithium often used in elders.
  - √ Point prevalence of lithium use in patients over 65 years is 0.27%.
- Poorly tolerated in almost three-quarters of medically ill patients.
  - √ Dose and monitoring need to be adjusted.
- Lithium management almost always very long term.
  - √ Usually lithium continues to be necessary if the original diagnosis was correct and should not be discontinued, unless there are new age-related contraindications that emerge.
  - √ In elders, tolerance to lithium usually declines over time with age-related changes in physiological state and emergence of concurrent illnesses.
  - √ Important to monitor the patient's clinical state and review all routine lab tests in an ongoing manner and titrate the lithium dose to the new physical and metabolic realities of the patient's life (e.g., renal efficiency).

Some controversy remains about the possibility of structural kidney damage from lithium; best to manage patients with this potentially serious side effect in mind. If lithium level increases unexpectedly, assess renal function.

- Kidney damage sometimes occurs (perhaps commonly, but data not clear) in patients on long-term lithium therapy.
  - √ GFR occasionally declines somewhat, but capacity to recover after discontinuation appears to be preserved even after long-term therapy.
  - √ Urinary concentrating capacity is irreversibly impaired, sometimes progressing to nephrogenic diabetes insipidus.

ECT and lithium

- Discontinue lithium prior.
- ECT combined with lithium may
  - √ Increase post-ECT confusion, delirium, memory loss, and seizure prolongation.
  - √ Prolong muscle blockade of succinylcholine.
- Discontinuation may be followed by lithium nonresponsiveness when reinstituted.
  - √ Caution necessary when considering discontinuing lithium therapy in elders.

Noncompliance

- May account for poor response to maintenance therapy with lithium.
- Psychotherapy and attention to the therapeutic alliance can help improve compliance.
- Hyperparathyroidism risk increases with prolonged therapy of 10–20 years and requires regular monitoring of serum calcium.

TOPIRAMATE

Drug	Manufacturer	Chemical Class	Therapeutic Class
topiramate (Topomax)	Ortho McNeil	sulphamate-substituted monosaccharide	anticonvulsant

Indications: FDA/HPB

- Adjunctive therapy for partial onset and generalized seizures.

Indications: Off label

- Bipolar disorder
  - √ Controlled data negative in recent study.

- ✓ Uncontrolled data promising, especially in rapid cycling and mania.
- ✓ Geriatric indications can only be inferred.
- ✓ Data not strong enough to recommend this agent in elders at this time.
  - ▫ Except as clinical attempts of last resort where other agents have failed.

Pharmacology

See Table 4.1 on page 482.

- Renal impairment.
  - ✓ Clearance reduced.
  - ✓ May require dose reduction.
- Hepatic impairment.
  - ✓ Clearance reduced (mechanism unknown).

Mechanism of action

- Augments GABAergic transmission.
- Antagonizes glutamate (excitatory agent).
- Inhibits some isoenzymes of carbonic anhydrase.
- May possess sodium channel-blocking properties in neurons.

Choosing a Drug

- Associated with weight loss (general adult data).
  - ✓ An advantage for some bipolar patients who have gained weight on other regimens but a problem for frail elders.
- May precipitate
  - ✓ Depression (about 1 in 6 or 7 at doses of 600–1000 mg/day; general adult data).
  - ✓ Psychosis (case reports, general adult data).

Race/ethnicity

- No effect on phamacokinetics.

Dosing

- Daily dose regimen.
  - ✓ bid dosing
- Initial dose.
  - ✓ 25 mg q hs
- Increasing dose and reaching therapeutic levels.
  - ✓ Increase 25 mg/day in once-a-week increments.
  - ✓ Target dose 50 mg bid (range 25–100 mg bid).

Side Effects

Most common

- Psychomotor slowing
- Somnolence
- Fatigue

Table 4.12. Side Effects of Topiramate

Side Effects	Most Common	Most Serious and Less Common
Body as a whole	• Fatigue • Anorexia • Weight loss	
Cardiovascular	• Palpitations	
Central and peripheral nervous system	• Reduced cognitive function/concentration/ speech disorder √ Word-finding difficulty on acute dosing • Somnolence/sedation (not dose related) • Headache • Dizziness • Ataxia • Tremor • Nystagmus	• Paresthesias
Eye	• Visual disturbance	• Acute myopia with secondary angle closure glaucoma
Gastrointestinal	• Nausea • Vomiting • Diarrhea • Gas • Abdominal pain	
Hematological	• Leukopenia • Thrombocytopenia	
Psychiatric	• Irritability • Nervousness • Anxiety	• Psychosis • Depression
Respiratory		• Dyspnea • Upper respiratory infection
Skin and appendages	• Alopecia	
Urinary		• Renal stones

Drug Interactions

- Carbonic anhydrase inhibitors—acetazolamide may predispose to renal stone formation.
- Ethanol—CNS depression.
- Phenytoin—decreased topiramate level, increased phenytoin level.

Disability Interactions and Contraindications

- Renal impairment (creatinine clearance < 60).
  - √ Reduce dose by half.
- Hypersensitivity to the drug.

Clinical Tips

- Remind patients and families to report sudden visual changes immediately.
  - √ May signal acute myopia and secondary angle closure glaucoma.

VALPROIC ACID, VALPROATE, DIVALPROEX

Drug	Manufacturer	Chemical Class	Therapeutic Class
valproic acid (Depakene) sodium valproate (Depakene capsules) divalproex sodium (Depakote; injectable, Depacon)	Abbott	carboxylic acid	anticonvulsant

Indications: FDA/HPB

- Treatment of acute mania.
  - √ May be especially useful for rapid cyclers, mixed manic states, and lithium nonresponders.
    - ▫ Effective in combination with lithium in elderly nonresponders.
    - ▫ Alternative to lithium when patients are intolerant of lithium, require concurrent medication (e.g., thiazide diuretics), or have serious disease (e.g., CHF, renal impairment).
- Migraine prophylaxis.
- Seizure disorder.
- Impulsive aggressivity and agitation.

Indications: Off label

- BPSD, especially aggression and impulsivity associated with dementia.
  - √ Including Alzheimer's disease and vascular dementia, especially if associated with mood instability.
- Charles Bonnet syndrome (i.e., complex visual hallucinations associated with CNS or visual disturbances, often with retained insight; case reports).
- Occasionally treat/prevent depression.
  - √ Effects doubtful.

- Schizoaffective disorders.
  - √ May dampen affective swings.

Pharmacology

See page 482.

- 4-en-valproic acid metabolite associated with hepatotoxicity.
- P450 pathway thought to produce the most toxic metabolites.
  - √ Concurrent medication that inhibits P450 system may increase toxic metabolites.
- Half-life and volume of distribution of total valproate similar in young and elders.
  - √ Studies of different populations (e.g., more frail elders or those on concurrent medications show higher values for half-life).
  - √ However, free valproate fraction (i.e., the pharmacologically active component) higher in elders than young patients because of lower protein binding in elders.
    - ▫ May be clinically relevant.
    - ▫ Total concentrations in plasma do not distinguish total valproate from free fraction.
    - ▫ Hence increased pharmacologically active free fraction can be present, despite normal total values, and induce toxicity.
- Sprinkles and ER forms produce reduced peak plasma levels and more level concentrations.

Mechanism of action

- Inhibits GABA breakdown: clinical relevance of this action not determined; strongly GABAergic and modestly decreases glutamate synthesis.

Choosing a Drug

- Divalproex sodium well tolerated in elders.
  - √ Preferred to lithium and carbamazepine because of better tolerance, especially in cognitively compromised elders where lithium toxicity is common.
  - √ Less anticholinergic than carbamazepine.
  - √ Preferred to valproic acid because of fewer gastrointestinal side effects.
- May be more useful than other mood stabilizers in mixed or rapid-cycling states.
- Different formulations offer advantages.
  - √ Sprinkles and ER forms—more advantageous blood levels.
    - ▫ Inflexible dosage forms (500 mg) available for ER form, limiting use in elders who may require more flexible dosing.
  - √ Slow-release useful for patients intolerant of peak plasma levels.

- √ Syrup useful for patients who cannot swallow or require very low doses.
- √ Intravenous route not reported for psychiatric care in elders (but case reports of utility in general adult patients).

- Effectiveness in geriatric mania established in many reports.
- May be effective
  - √ In patients who failed to respond to lithium (general adult data) when used alone.
  - √ Or in combination with lithium.

Prognostic Indicators of Response to Treatment

- Comorbid neurological disorders.
  - √ Responded significantly better to valproic acid, even when refractory to lithium.

Initiating Therapy

- Conduct routine physical exam prior to administering the drug.
  - √ System review, especially dermatological, neurological.
  - √ Cognitive examination.
  - √ Baselines.
    - ▫ ECG
    - ▫ TSH(s), T_3, T_4
    - ▫ CBC (with platelets)
    - ▫ Serum electrolytes
    - ▫ LFTs
    - ▫ Urinalysis

Dosing

- Very limited dose-response data for elders (based mostly on clinical reports).
- Daily dose regimen.
  - √ Usually tid dosing.
  - √ Administer with food.
  - √ Increase dose slowly to avoid nausea, vomiting.
  - √ Use enteric-coated form, especially for patients with GI upset.
  - √ IV form may be useful in extreme situations of noncompliance.
    - ▫ Case report data only available for elders.
- Initial dose.
  - √ 125–250 mg/day po.
  - √ IV form.
    - ▫ Begin conservatively (e.g., 3–4 mg/kg/day).
    - ▫ Infuse over 60 minutes for each dose (5–10 mg/min) in divided doses bid (or tid for larger doses).

    - More aggressive regimens sometimes necessary (e.g., 500 mg bid).
    - Convert to oral form as soon as patient settles and becomes cooperative with treatment.
- Increasing dose and reaching therapeutic levels.
  - √ Increase dose by 250 mg q 5 days (or longer interval, depending on tolerance).
  - √ Target therapeutic dose is 800–1000 (range 500–2000) mg/day in 2–3 doses (to reach a blood level of 65–100 μg/ml).
  - √ For aggression in dementia 750–1500 mg/day has been used; anecdotal case report data only.
- Maintenance dose.
  - √ Effectiveness of valproic acid as prophylaxis against mania not well studied, but conventional practice is to use it for maintenance therapy.

Discontinuation and withdrawal

- Withdrawal usually safe and uneventful.
  - √ Taper by 10% daily.

Side Effects

Side effects of valproate (nausea) increase above 100 μg/ml; well tolerated within the therapeutic range.

Table 4.13. Side Effects of Valproate

Side Effects	Most Common	Most Serious and Less Common	Comments
Body as a whole	• Weight gain • Asthenia		
Case reports		• Rare idiosyncratic hemorrhagic pancreatitis • Impairment in respiration	
Central and peripheral nervous system	• Excess sedation, especially in dementia, with rapid dose escalation and higher dose ranges • Tremor (common) • Ataxia	• Parkinsonism and possibly cognitive impairment √ Reversible on discontinuation √ Develop insidiously over months to years	• Tolerance to sedation develops over 1–2 weeks √ This property may be useful for agitated patients • Little impact on cognitive function in otherwise well elders
Endocrine		• Hypothyroidism	• Monitor free T_4 and TSH
Ear		• Hearing impairment reported	

(cont.)

Continued

Side Effects	Most Common	Most Serious and Less Common	Comments
Gastrointestinal	• Nausea • Vomiting • Dyspepsia	• Case report: fecal incontinence	• For nausea √ Use enteric-coated form √ Start at low dose and increase slowly √ Administer with food. • GI effects less evident with divalproex compared to valproic acid.
Hematological	• Transient leukopenia √ During first weeks of therapy, rarely below 2500 WBCs. • Transient thrombocytopenia common in elders √ More than 50% in one study	• Rare aplastic anemia • Agranulocytosis	• Leukopenia not related to rare aplastic anemia • Regular monitoring of platelets recommended in elders • Management of WBC 3000/mm^3 √ Reduce dose and monitor WBC √ 2500/mm^3 or below, discontinue drug and monitor WBC √ Reinstitute cautiously when WBC rises above 3000/mm^3
Liver and biliary		• Hepatotoxicity (rare) √ Elevated liver enzymes √ May be fatal • Pancreatitis (rare)	
Metabolic and nutritional	• Weight gain • Edema	• Hyperammonemia with lethargy • SIADH	• Weight gain secondary to appetite stimulation • For ammonia increase, use supplemental carnitine
Musculoskeletal		• Skeletal muscle dysfunction, weakness	• Reported to impair mobility and create sudden marked dependence
Skin and appendages	• Rash	• Transient hair loss—trace metal depletion in GI tract • Exanthematous rashes—benign • Exfoliative disorders • Stevens–Johnson syndrome • Lyell syndrome—rare but may be fatal	• For hair loss √ Zinc and selenium replacement □ Use multivitamin preparation
Urinary		• Renal failure (rare)	

Monitoring valproate

- Therapeutic plasma levels not well determined for elders.
  - √ Best estimate is 65–100 μg/ml (trough level drawn 12 hours after last dose); contrasts with apparent lower levels in younger patients of 45–100 μg/ml.
    - ▫ Mania associated with dementia may respond at lower levels of 13–50 μg/ml.
  - √ Draw plasma levels 3–4 days after dose change when steady state has been achieve.

Special monitoring

- CBC, platelets, and LFTs weekly for first 4 weeks, or until WBC dips and rebounds.
  - √ Discontinue if
    - ▫ WBC < 3000/mm^3.
    - ▫ Neutrophils drop below 500.
    - ▫ Platelets drop below 100,000.
    - ▫ Liver enzymes increase by more than 100%.
  - √ Monitor q 1–4 weeks for 6 months, then every 3–6 months.

Drug Interactions

- Drugs that decrease valproate levels.
  - √ Carbamazepine.
  - √ Phenytoin.
    - ▫ Two actions: Initially decreases phenytoin levels but then they increase significantly, and valproate levels may decrease.
- Drugs that increase valproate levels (danger of toxicity).
  - √ Aspirin.
    - ▫ Interferes with mitochondrial function and beta-oxidation; bleeding times may be prolonged.
  - √ Cimetidine.
  - √ Chlorpromazine.
  - √ Erythromycin.
  - √ Felbamate.
  - √ Fluoxetine.
  - √ Lithium.
- Benzodiazepines, alcohol, and other CNS depressants.
  - √ Additive CNS depressant effect.
  - √ Increased plasma levels of some benzodiazepines.
- Lamotrigine—half-life doubled by valproate, increased plasma levels of lamotrigine and increased risk of skin rash.
- Phenobarbital (and primidone).
  - √ Increased phenobarbital levels, possibly to toxic levels.

- TCAs—plasma levels increased by valproate.
- Warfarin—increases anticoagulant action.
- Zidovudine—increased zidovudine toxicity.

Effect on Laboratory Tests

- Elevation of liver enzymes.
  - √ Idiosyncratic, not dose related.
  - √ May be secondary to accumulation of 4-em valproic acid metabolite.
- WBC—reduced.
- Thyroid function—may be reduced.

Interactions with Illnesses and Contraindications

- Hypersensitivity to drug or class.
- Extra care in dementia or other brain discasc, rcduced renal function, prolonged bleeding times.
- Liver disease/dysfunction.
  - √ Observe for hepatotoxicity.
    - ▫ Increased liver enzymes
    - ▫ Anorexia
    - ▫ Nausea
    - ▫ Malaise
    - ▫ Abdominal pain
    - ▫ Bruising
- Discontinue aspirin.

Overdose, Toxicity, Suicide

- Majority have relatively minor effects from overdose, with benign outcomes (general adult data; good geriatric data not available).
- Serum levels: peaks of > 450 μg/ml associated with more severe outcomes.
- Symptoms
  - √ Neurological
    - ▫ Somnolence
    - ▫ Tremor
    - ▫ Ataxia
    - ▫ Seizures
    - ▫ Coma (at peak values of > 850 μg/ml).
  - √ CVS
    - ▫ Heart block
    - ▫ Hypotension
  - √ Gastrointestinal
    - ▫ Anorexia
    - ▫ Vomiting

- √ Respiratory
  - ▫ Depression (at peak values of > 850 μg/ml).
- √ Metabolic
  - ▫ Acidosis (at peak values of > 850 μg/ml).
  - ▫ Hyperammonemia
  - ▫ Hypernatremia
  - ▫ Possible hyperglycemia in terminal stages
- √ Liver/pancreatic toxicity
- √ Hematological (at peak values of > 850 μg/ml).
  - ▫ Thrombocytopenia
  - ▫ Leukopenia
- √ May be fatal.

Management

- Manage in emergency room.
- Observe frail elders more closely.
- Start IV, maintain renal output.
- Administer emesis or gastric lavage if caught right away or if delayed-release form ingested.
  - √ Rapid absorption of other forms limits utility of this intervention.
- Monitor
  - √ Valproate serum levels (peak levels may not occur until 10 hours or more after ingesting).
  - √ Vital signs/level of consciousness.
  - √ ECG
  - √ LFTs.
  - √ Urinary output.
  - √ CBC and platelets (especially during the 3–5-day period after the overdose).
  - √ Blood chemistry.
- Mechanical ventilation, as necessary.
- Hemodialysis.
  - √ Initiate early.
    - ▫ Outcome poor if initiated in late stages of toxic syndrome.
- Consider L-carnitine, vasopressor, as needed.
- For severe CNS depressant effects, consider naloxone but caution re. seizures.

Caregiver Notes

- Do not chew capsules—irritating.
- Take drug with food/meals to reduce gastrointestinal upset.

- Sprinkle capsules may be swallowed whole or opened carefully and sprinkled on small amount of soft food (e.g., apple sauce).
  - √ Mix well.
  - √ Do not chew capsules; simply swallow.
- Avoid aspirin.
  - √ Report bleeding or bruising to doctor.
- Do not take double dose if dose is forgotten.

Clinical Tips

- Valproate-induced parkinsonism and possible cognitive impairment may be a particular diagnostic problem in elders, unless suspected.
  - √ These disorders emerge frequently in the normative course of aging.

5. Cognitive Enhancers

OVERVIEW

This chapter addresses key drugs developed for, or used in treatment of, the primary (core) symptoms of dementia.

- Only those drugs approved for use or with demonstrated efficacy are discussed.
- Currently there are four cognitive enhancers, all cholinesterase inhibitors, which have FDA approval for treating the core symptoms of Alzheimer's dementia.
- Other aspects of dementia-related pharmacology are addressed in the other chapters.

Table 5.1. Drugs Approved as Cognitive Enhancers

Generic (Brand) Names	Chemical Class
tacrine (Cognex)	Acridine—Nonselective
donepezil (Aricept)	Piperidine—selective reversible inhibitor of AChE
rivastigmine (Exelon)	Carbamate—reversible inhibitor of AChE and BChE
galantamine (Reminyl)	Tertiary alkaloid—selective, reversible inhibitor of AChE; enhances response of nicotinic receptors; may increase release of ACh and glutamate

Table 5.2. Other Cognitive Enhancers

Drug/Substance	Comment
NEUROTRANSMITTER ENHANCERS	
physostigmine	• No convincing data for efficacy of this drug in dementia in any of its current formulations (oral, patch, CR preparation)
ergoloid mesylates mixture (Hydergine)	• A once popular drug, it has very limited demonstrated efficacy and is no longer used for dementia; it is not included in this chapter

(cont.)

Continued

Drug/Substance	Comment
nicotine	• Cholinergic agonist • Some presynaptic effect in releasing ACh • Some observational evidence for protective action against Alzheimer's disease, but data inconsistent and sometimes conflicting • No convincing evidence for nicotine being effective in improving either cognition or behavior in Alzheimer's disease
ginkgo biloba	• Uncertain therapeutic effects √ Data very limited and of variable quality
milameline xanomeline (patch form)	• Cholinergic agonists
NEUROPROTECTIVE AGENTS	
• vitamin E • selegiline • nonsteroidal anti-inflammatories, including the new cox-2 inhibitors • estrogen HRT • sabeluzole • alcar • vitamin C • lazabemide • nicergoline • idebenone (synthetic coenzyme of Q10)	• Conflicting data on clinical utility. √ NSAIDS appear to have limited prophylactic action against AD probably by inhibiting inflammatory component of AD cascade. √ Recent data on Vitamin E and estrogen not promising, although many prescribing guidelines continue to endorse Vit. E. √ NSAIDs do not slow progression of Alzhermer's disease. √ Combination estrogen/progesterone HRT appears to worsen risk of developing dementia.
PREPARATIONS UNDER DEVELOPMENT OR INVESTIGATION	
memantine	• NMDA antagonist, FDA approval pending; efficacy demonstrated; may work synergistically with AChEIs; reversibly blocks NMDA receptors and interferes with its excito-toxicity; side effects include dizziness, fatigue, headache, somnolence, similar effectiveness as AChEIs
vaccine	• To prevent or reverse amyloid development; trials discontinued because of induction of cerebral inflammation but may be resumed
gamma and beta secretases	• To prevent amyloid formation
eptastigmine	• Carbamate derivative of physostigmine; reversible inhibitor of AChE; dose 45–60 mg; associated with sinus bradycardia and granulocytopenia (the latter halted further trials)
biogenic amines	• No useful clinical data available yet.
nerve growth factors (e.g., cerebrolysin)	• No useful clinical data available yet.

Indications FDA/HPB

√ To date, all drugs approved for treatment of dementia are specified for mild to moderate Alzheimer's disease.

Indications: Off-label

- Effective for cognition, agitation, and psychosis of DLB.

- Promising results are emerging for utility in vascular and Parkinson's dementia.
  - E.g., rivastigmine for behavioral aspect of vascular dementia
  - Early studies show promising results in Parkinson's dementia.
  - Recent data show improvement with AChEIs in severe Alzheimer's Disease.
    - Improvement reflected in reduced use of neuroleptics, anxiolytics.
  - Not useful for cognitive function in frontotemporal dementias.

PHARMACOLOGY

Mechanism of action of cholinesterase inhibitors (AChEIs)

Increases concentration of acetylcholine at the neuronal synapse, thereby enhancing cholinergic transmission and the action of acetylcholine (ACH), which is depleted in Alzheimer's disease (and some other dementias).

All AChEIs enhance ACh metabolism mainly by inhibition of the action of the G1 isoform of acetylcholinesterase (AChE), the main enzyme that breaks down acetylcholine.

There are various isoforms of AChE. New-generation cholinesterase inhibitors (i.e., post-tacrine) demonstrate greater specificity in inhibiting isoforms of AChE to reduce side effects caused by less selective agents (i.e., physostigmine, tacrine).

- Rivastigmine and tacrine have the additional action of inhibiting butyrylcholinesterase (BChE, formerly pseudocholinesterase), a secondary metabolizer of ACh in the healthy brain.
  - √ Some evidence that while AChE declines in Alzheimer's disease, BChE remains stable or increases by up to 80%.
    - Rationale for use of a drug with BChE inhibitor activity.
- Galantamine has the additional property of stimulating presynaptic nicotinic receptors, thereby enhancing release of ACh.
- All may also enhance ACh and postsynaptic cholinergic receptor interaction.
- Peripheral action outside the brain.
  - √ AChEs also are present in skeletal, cardiac, and smooth muscle, hematopoietic cells, and erythrocytes.
  - √ BChE is contained in plasma.
- Emerging data suggest some disease-modifying effects (i.e., blocking amyloid precursor protein metabolism).

CLINICAL INDICATIONS: DEMENTIA

Data support the utility of

- AChEIs in DLB—control of psychosis, agitation.
- Galantamine in mixed vascular and Alzheimer's disease population.
- Donepezil in vascular dementia population.
- Rivastigmine in Parkinson's disease.

Definition of dementia: A syndrome of intellectual and functional decline caused by cognitive impairment severe enough to impair occupational/social/daily living function.

- Core features
  - √ Memory impairment, plus one of the following
    - ▫ Aphasia
    - ▫ Apraxia
    - ▫ Agnosia
    - ▫ Disturbance in executive functioning (i.e., abstraction, planning, initiation, sequencing, monitoring, ceasing complex behavior)
  - √ Order of onset of features varies with the specific type of dementia.
- Associated features
  - √ Disinhibition
  - √ Impulsive aggression
  - √ Suicidality
    - ▫ Occurs usually in milder forms of dementia.
  - √ Anxiety
  - √ Depression
  - √ Sleep disturbances
  - √ Psychosis
  - √ Misidentification
  - √ Agitation
  - √ Delirium
  - √ Vulnerability to psychosocial stresses.
  - √ Motor disturbances (e.g., seizures and myoclonus).
- Noncognitive symptoms common in dementia.
  - √ 17–38% prevalence rates reported, especially anxiety.
  - √ Depression (6–45% in VaD).
- Epidemiology
  - √ Overall prevalence
    - ▫ > 65 years: 5–8%
    - ▫ > 75 years: 15–20%

Table 5.3. Pharmacology of Cholinesterase Inhibitors (Cognitive Enhancers)

Generic Name	Bioavailability (%)	Peak Concentrations	Plasma Protein Binding (%)	Volume of Distribution (range)	Elimination Half-Life (hours)	Drug Clearance at Steady State	Duration of Action	Absorption	Excretion	Metabolized P450 System	Reversibility	Linearity
donepezil	100	3–4 hours	96	12 l/kg	50–70; steady state reached in 15 days	Similar in young and elders; clearance reduced by hepatitis, cirrhosis		Unaffected by food	Intact in urine as well as metabolized	Glucuronidation; metabolized by CYP2D6, CYP3A4; 2 active metabolites	yes	Linear up to doses of 3 mg but slightly hyperbolic at higher doses
rivastigmine	35		40	5 l/kg (1.8–8)	2; metabolite is 2.5–4		8–12 hours	Well absorbed; peak in 1–4 hours; slowed 90 mins. by food; plasma levels higher in males	Metabolites in kidneys; caution in renal disease	Minimal P450 metabolism; 100% by hydrolysis to decarbamylated metabolite (activity about 10% of rivastigmine) decarbamylated metabolite responsible for cholinergic adverse effects	Yes (pseudo-irreversible)	Nonlinear

(*cont.*)

Continued

Generic Name	Bioavailability (%)	Peak Concentrations	Plasma Protein Binding (%)	Volume of Distribution (range)	Elimination Half-Life (hours)	Drug Clearance at Steady State	Duration of Action	Absorption	Excretion	Metabolized P450 System	Reversibility	Linearity
galantamine	90–100		Low—18%	2.6 l/kg	5.5 (young adult data); 7–9 (single geriatric study)			Rapidly absorbed; Tmax 1 hour; Rate delayed by food but extent of absorption unaffected; maximum concentrations 30–40% higher in AD patients than healthy volunteers	Metabolized primarily in liver. Clearance 20% lower in females	Glucuronidation; CYP2D6 CYP3A4; Major metabolite is O-demethylgalantamine glucuronide; minor metabolites are N-demethylgalantamine, epigalantamine; clinical relevance of metabolites appears slight but not yet fully established	Yes	Linear
tacrine	17 (9.9–36.4)			5 l/kg	2–4			Food slows rate by 30–40%; Tmax—1–2 hours		1A2	Yes	Nonlinear

    - > 85 years: 25–50%
    - Incidence increases into the 10th decade, after which it appears to level out.
- Usually chronic, sensorium not clouded (as it is in delirium) but higher risk for delirium.

Differential Diagnosis

The availability of drugs for Alzheimer's disease and the need for specific drug management of other forms of dementia/BPSD make differential diagnosis of the dementia subtype an essential part of the workup for drug treatment.

Primary Degenerative Dementing Disorders

- Alzheimer's disease (AD): 50–75% of all dementias.
- Lewy Body Dementia (DLB)—7–26% of dementias.
  - √ Now considered second most prevalent form of dementia.
- Vascular dementia (VaD): third most prevalent form—accounts for 10–20% (range 4.5–39%) of dementia cases (previously called multi-infarct dementia).
- True incidence and prevalence of various dementias remains uncertain.

Characteristics

- Anxiety especially prevalent in VaD (prevalence as high as 70%) compared to AD.
- Depression common in both AD and VaD, but seems to be more common in VaD.
- Psychosis common in AD, DLB and VaD.
  - √ Visual hallucinations more evident in VaD than AD.
    - Often associated with disruptions in visuospatial processing.

Vascular dementia

- Diagnosis includes criteria for dementia plus
  - √ Focal neurological signs.
  - √ And/or laboratory evidence of cerebrovascular disease.
- Often coexists with Alzheimer's disease.
    - the two disorders share some vascular risk factors (eg. hyper-tension, cerebrovascular disease) and pathological features (eg. iacunae and white-matter lesions)
- Noncognitive symptoms are common.
- Onset less common after age 75 (compared to AD).
- Risk factors for VaD include
  - √ Hypertension; cardiac arrhythmia; hypoxic events; diabetes mellitus.

- √ Coagulopathy
- √ Vasculitis
- √ Pulmonary Disease (hypoxia)
- √ Substance abuse
- √ Hyperlipidemia

- Caused by one or more strokes each one usually subclinical.
  - √ Small stokes produce patchy cognitive deficits that gradually merge into diffuse impairment.
- Show on MRI but not always on CT.
- As disease progresses infarcts and cortical atrophy show on CT.
- Abrupt onset, stepwise progression (but pictures vary considerably) with other evidence of cerebrovascular disease.
- Laboratory investigation.
  - √ CBC
  - √ FBS
  - √ ESR
  - √ ECG
  - √ Occasionally blood gases or pulmonary function.
- Treatment of hypertension and vascular disease can halt or slow progress.

Treatment strategies include

- General dementia management.
- Stroke prevention
  - √ Antiplatelet agents
    - ▫ Enteric coated ASA 325 mg/day still first choice.
    - ▫ Use ASA/dipyridamole or clopidogrel as second-choice drugs if ASA not tolerated.
    - ▫ SSRIs reduce platelet aggregation.
  - √ Antioxidants: Vitamins E and C
  - √ Antihypertensives, as needed (treat if systolic BP is in the range of 135–150 mm Hg).
  - √ Treat cardiac arrhythmias.
  - √ Cholesterol control (statins).
  - √ Estrogen no longer recommended.
  - √ Optimize cerebral perfusion with anticoagulants, such as warfarin or ASA, only if thromboemboli implicated in etiology.
- Managing noncognitive symptoms: see page 240.

Lewy body dementia

- More prevalent than earlier believed; accounts for 7–26% of dementia cases.
- Diagnostic criteria for DLB.

- √ Progressive cognitive decline with social/occupational impairment.
  - ▫ Especially deficits of attention, frontal-subcortical skills, visuospatial ability.
- √ Two of
  - ▫ Fluctuating cognition (attention, alertness).
  - ▫ Visual hallucinations.
  - ▫ Parkinsonian features.
- √ Plus
  - ▫ Falls.
  - ▫ Syncope.
  - ▫ Transient loss of consciousness.
  - ▫ Neuroleptic sensitivity.
  - ▫ Delusions.
  - ▫ Other hallucinations.
- Pathology: Lewy inclusion bodies in neurons of cerebral cortex.
  - √ Markedly reduced levels of choline acetyltransferase (catalyzes synthesis of Ach).
- Similar to Alzheimer's disease, with
  - √ Prominent visual hallucinations, delusions, depression.
  - √ Parkinsonian features.
  - √ Dramatic symptom fluctuation.
  - √ Falls.
  - √ Frequent transient loss of consciousness.
  - √ More rapid course.
- AChEIs particularly indicated in this disorder.
  - √ For control of psychosis, agitation, dementia.
  - √ Functional status may be markedly improved.
- Quetiapine 25–150 mg improved psychosis and agitation (uncontrolled study)
- Typical neuroleptics are contraindicated.

Pick's and other frontol-temporal dementias (FTD).

- Clinical diagnostic features include
  - √ Core features.
    - ▫ Insidious onset.
    - ▫ Gradual progression.
    - ▫ Early social/interpersonal functional decline.
    - ▫ Early emotional blunting.
    - ▫ Early loss of insight.
  - √ Supportive features.
    - ▫ Behavioral—decline in personal hygiene, mental rigidity, distractibility, hyperorality, diet change, perseveration.
    - ▫ Speech/Language—pressure, asponteneity, stereotypy, echolalia, perseveration, mutism.

    - ▫ Physical—primitive reflexes, incontinence akinesia, rigidity, tremor, labile BP.
    - ▫ Other—impaired frontal lobe tests. Normal EEG, frontal/anterior temporal imaging abnormalities.
- Pick's makes up 20% of FTD's.
- Pathology: Pick's disease shows Pick inclusion bodies in neurons of cerebral cortex.
- Pick bodies not seen in other forms of FTD.
- Relatively rare.
- ACh depletion not part of the pathological picture, so AChEIs are not indicated.
- Partially effective treatment options include
  - √ Guanfacine (29 μg/kg)
  - √ Dopamine agonists pramipexole or ropinirole (0.5 mg hs).

Primary progressive aphasia

- Uncommon syndrome related to frontotemporal dementia.
- Characterized by initial isolated dissolution of language function (expressive word amnesia followed by receptive), followed by more generalized deterioration of cognitive function and ADL.
- No data on efficacy of AChEIs.

Subcortical dementias

- Dementia associated with Parkinson's disease
  - √ Occurs in 20–60% of cases, especially late in the course.
    - ▫ 6-fold increase in dementia after 4 years.
      - ◦ Risk factors—advanced age, increasing severity of PD, MMSE <29.
  - √ Associated with gait and balance impairment (rather than tremor).
  - √ Insidious onset and slow progression.

Huntington's disease

  - √ Autosomal dominant inherited disorder.
  - √ Affects subcortical structures.
  - √ Produces motor behavioral and cognitive symptoms.

Other dementias

- Normal pressure hydrocephalus.
- Temporal arteritis.
- Progressive supranuclear palsy.
- Creutzfelt-Jacob disease
  - √ Rapidly progressive spongiform encephalopathy.
  - √ Associated with slow virus and related to bovine form (Bovine Spongiform Encephalopathy [BSE]).
- HIV encephalopathy

Dementias Secondary to General Medical Conditions

- Structural brain lesions.
  - √ Brain tumor.
  - √ Subdural hematoma.
  - √ Normal pressure hydrocephalus.
- Head trauma.
- Endocrine conditions.
  - √ Hypothyroidism.
  - √ Hypercalcemia.
  - √ Hypoglycemia.
- Nutritional conditions.
  - √ Vitamin deficiencies—B12, thiamine, niacin.
- Infections.
  - √ HIV.
  - √ Neurosyphilis.
  - √ Cryptococcus.
- Renal/hepatic impairment.
- Neurological conditions (e.g., multiple sclerosis).
- Medication effects.
- Autoimmune disorders (e.g., SLE).
- Substance-induced persisting dementia.

Associated Features of Dementia

- For behavioral and psychological symptoms of dementia (BPSD), see page 236.
  - √ Cholinesterase inhibitors sometimes useful for the management of associated features, such as agitation, psychosis, and aggression.
  - √ Drugs used for BPSD are discussed in their respective chapters and include antidepressants, neuroleptics, mood stabilizers, and benzodiazepines.

Alzheimer's Disease (AD)

- The most common cause of dementia in old age.
- Onset insidious; true time of onset not known.
- First symptoms are memory deficits.
  - √ Often appear during a frequently long preclinical period commonly characterized as mild cognitive impairment (MCI).
- MCI converts to dementia at a rate of about 10% per year.
  - √ Use prevention/treatment measures similar to AD—AChEIs, vitamin E.
  - √ Emerging data suggests AChEIs may be useful in slowing conversion of MCI to dementia.

- Diagnosed AD may emerge as early as late middle age, but generally prevalence becomes most evident and severe in middle and old-old age (over age 75). Hence its drug management is often undertaken in the context of complex physical and social comorbidities.
- Course of disease.
  - √ Once a diagnosis is made, the disease progresses over 8–10 years, concluding in death.
  - √ Alzheimer's disease may be classified according to levels of severity (see following table).

Table 5.4. Classification of Severity of Alzheimer's Disease

MILD

- Duration 2–3 years
- Manifest impairment of attention
- Forgetting recent information
- Often associated with anxiety and depression
- Occasional confusion or disorientation for time/place
- Some help needed with everyday independant activities of daily life

MODERATE

- Duration 2 years
- Amnesia for recent events
- Reversal of sleep cycle
- Some disorientation to time/place
- Psychosis—delusions, visual hallucinations
- Severe impairment of reasoning and ability to understand events
  - √ Dependency on others for personal care and routine activities of living (IADL and ADL)

SEVERE AND PROFOUND

- Duration 2–3 years
- Incoherent speech
- Disorientation for time/place/person
- Failure to recognize close relatives
- Motor rigidity
- Incontinence of urine and feces
- Complete dependence on others for basic personal care

TERMINAL

- Bed bound
- Requires constant care
- Susceptible to fatal infections/accidents

Measures of severity of AD

- Many studies of drug efficacy for AD use the Mini-Mental Status Exam (MMSE) scale (mild-to-moderate range 10–26, profound 0–9) to define severity of patients' disease.
- Different criteria for establishing severity levels make comparisons between studies problematic at times.

Pathology

Alzheimer's disease is a complex neurodegenerative disorder.

Brain pathology

- Neuritic plaques made of beta-amyloid protein.
- Neurofibrillary tangles.
  - √ Intracellular bodies derived from microtubules.
  - √ Occurs secondary to excess phosphorylation of microtubular tau proteins.
- Synaptic degeneration.
- Loss of presynaptic cholinergic neurons in the cortex and hippocampus.
  - √ Loss of basal forebrain cholinergic system probably central to production of cognitive deficits.

Neurochemical deficits

- ACh is a key neurotransmitter for memory functions.
- Its synthesis decreases in Alzheimer's disease (and probably in other forms of dementia) associated with concurrent reduction in choline acetyl-transferase levels.
  - √ Especially in the prefrontal, parietal, and temporal cortex and hippocampus.
  - √ With associated cell loss in the nucleus basalis of Meynert, locus coeruleus, raphe.
- Concurrent biochemical changes include potassium and calcium channel disruption.

Cholinergic system deficiencies may not be the sole deficits in AD, especially in early stages. Reduction in other neurotransmitter levels may be involved in significant primary or secondary ways. These include

- Serotonergic
- Noradrenergic

To a lesser extent

- Glutamate
- Dopamine
- Substance P.

Associated pathology includes:

- Inflammatory changes.
- Free radical formation.
- Nerve growth factor deficiency.

Brain pathology, neurochemical deficits, and associated factors interact to produce a pathological cascade that appears to lead to Alzheimer's disease.

Each deficit category has been, or is being, addressed with drug therapy with varying but generally modest or no success, although promising agents are in development.

Diagnosis

- Definitive diagnosis of AD made only on postmortem brain autopsy.
- Pathological diagnosis conforms to clinical diagnosis 70–90% of the time.

Components of clinical diagnosis include

- Careful history.
  - √ Drug history.
  - √ Medication changes.
  - √ Nutritional, traumatic, genetic disorders.
  - √ Medical history and functional inquiry.
    - ▫ Specific inquiry about history of concussion.
  - √ Psychiatric disorders.
  - √ Substance misuse.
    - ▫ Quantify use of alcohol, tobacco, caffeine.
- Physical examination.
  - √ Systemic disease.
  - √ Other neurological conditions (e.g., stroke).
- Mental status assessment.
  - √ Includes baseline evaluation of cognitive function (using standard instruments).
- Laboratory/imaging studies.
  - √ CT routinely recommended
    - ▫ unless diagnosis is obvious.
- MRI for suspected small lesions.
- SPECT sometimes helpful.
  - √ Bilateral temporal—parietal decreased perfusion.

TREATMENT OF DEMENTIA

Successful pharmacotherapy requires a multidimensional approach, the components of which are used concurrently or sequentially.

Psychiatric and psychosocial management components

- Psychotherapy: Various modalities tailored to capacity and needs of patient and family.
- Establishing family alliance and providing education enhances outcome.
  - √ Improves knowledge and treatment of disease and capacity to tolerate change in patient's behavior.

- Environmental and social intervention.
  - √ Safety monitoring.
    - ▫ Intervene re. hazards (e.g., driving).
- Longitudinal approach essential to manage progressive disorders.

Legal/financial guidance

- Ensure patient's wishes are determined while person is still competent.
- Review need for will, assigning power of attorney, other substitute decision makers.
  - √ Discuss need for legal consultation, as appropriate.
- Living will—discuss need to document, as appropriate.
  - √ Treatment decisions—e.g., feeding tube, antibiotics, fluids, oxygen, cardiopulmonary resuscitation, intensive care units, hospital transfer from LTC facility.

See page 240 for more detailed description of nonpharmacological adjuncts to therapy.

Address reversible causes

- Stop all unnecessary medication.
- Decrease others, if possible.
- Where possible, discontinue anticholinergic, tranquilizing, and sedating agents (including OTC agents) and alcohol.
- Treat depression or other psychiatric disorders.
- Treat intercurrent illness (e.g., infection, such as in urinary tract).
- Manage pain (e.g., occult hip fracture, fecal impaction).
- Manage cardiorespiratory problems (e.g., MI, pulmonary embolism).
- Manage neurological problems (e.g., subdural hematoma, TIAs, mass lesions, normal pressure hydrocephalus).
- Address nutritional deficiencies.
- Manage endocrine/metabolic/renal/hepatic pathology.

Manage BPSD (see p. 240).

Pharmacotherapy with Cognitive Enhancers—Cholinesterase Inhibitors (AChEI)

- Trial of AChEI indicated for all patients with Alzheimer's disease, DLB, vascular and mixed dementia and Parkinson's disease, unless contraindicated for other reasons.
  - √ Not indicated for Picks or other fronto-temporal dementias.
- If one agent fails, or loses effectiveness switch to a second.
- Consider adding vitamin E (antioxidant effect) and folic acid (reduces homocysteine) supplementation.

- Treatment goals with AChEIs include
  - √ Improved memory and other cognitive functions.
  - √ Temporarily halting or slowing course of the disease.
    - Emerging data suggests that some agents (rivastigmine) not only slow AD progression but alter the disease process—mechanism unknown and data still very early stages.
  - √ Maintenance or improvement in
    - Self-care
    - Behavior
    - Mood
    - Quality of life and relationships
  - √ Improve psychotic symptoms and BPSD.
  - √ Maintenance of baseline cognitive function demonstrated up to 1 year, but when it occurs, probably persists longer. Hence, continue maintenance AChEI.
  - √ These goals often not met.
    - Practical clinical expectations for these drugs should be very modest, at best, at present time.

Predictors of nonresponse to cholinergic enhancers

- Increased atrophy.
  - √ Thickness of substantia innominata (reflecting atrophy of cholinergic neurons in nucleus basalis of Meynert) on MRI may be prognostic marker for poorer response to cholinergic enhancers.
- Gender.
  - √ Male gender may predict better initial response (first 3 months) for some agents.
- Clinical presentation.
  - √ Patients with AD who show greater severity of delusions, agitation, depression, anxiety, apathy, disinhibition, and irritability may be more treatment-responsive to AChEIs.
    - Studies are flawed, but trends are similar for several ChEI agents (e.g., donepezil, metrifonate, tacrine, physostigmine).
- Apolipoprotein E4 allele.
  - √ No evidence for effect on immediate response but perhaps affects longer-term outcome.
    - Data in this area should be viewed as preliminary at this stage and not yet useful in routine clinical decision making.

Therapeutic action of AChEIs

- In addition to primary effects on cognition, AChEIs show clinical promise in management of
  - √ Neurocognitive symptoms of dementia (BPSD; e.g., agitation, aggression).

- √ Treatment of symptoms of psychosis associated with Lewy body dementia.
- √ Management of delirium.
- √ Management of toxicity associated with substance abuse.
- √ Dementia associated with Parkinson's disease.

Many other drugs have been used alone or in combination to treat or enhance the treatment of AD; evidence for efficacy is preliminary, controversial, or unconvincing.

Measuring efficacy of pharmacotherapy with AChEIs

- In outcome studies of AChEIs, efficacy most often based on improvement in
  - √ ADAS-cog: the 70-point cognitive subscale of the Alzheimer's Disease Assessment Scale.
  - √ Clinicians Interview-Based Impression of Change scale (CIBIC).
  - √ MMSE—Mini Mental State Examination.

ADAS-cog is comprised of 11 test domains

- Spoken language ability.
- Comprehension of spoken language.
- Recall (of test instructions).
- Word-finding difficulty.
- Following commands.
- Object naming.
- Construction drawing.
- Ideational praxis.
- Orientation.
- Word recall.
- Word recognition.
  - √ A spread of 3–4 points in the ADAS-cog score between controls and treatment groups considered significant.
    - ▫ Spread is based either on improvement in measures of cognition or lack of decline in the treatment group compared to placebo.
    - ▫ Usually a 6-month period used initially to determine if drug effect present.
    - ▫ ADAS-cog generally declines by 7–11 points/year in untreated Alzheimer's disease.

More recently, FDA requires premarketing/licensing studies to demonstrate efficacy on a global assessment scale, such as the CIBIC and CIBIC-plus (information obtained from both patient and caregiver).

- These scales are clinical and observational but not highly quantitative and not standardized; they are made up of four domains
  - √ General
  - √ Cognitive

- √ Behavior
- √ ADL

A number of other scales have been added to some, but not all, studies

- Quality of life (QoL).
  - √ Patient-rated 7-item scale measuring patient well-being in the context of relationships, eating, sleeping, and social and leisure activities.
- Behavioral change.
- Mental status performance (e.g., MMSE).
- Activities of daily living.
  - √ Interview for Deterioration in Daily Functioning Activities in Dementia (IDDD).
    - ▫ A 33-item questionnaire assessing initiative and performance, with two main sections on self-care and complex tasks.
  - √ Progressive Deterioration Scale (PDS).
    - ▫ A 29-item ADL scale.
  - √ Computerized Neuropsychological Test Battery.
- Deterioration.
  - √ Neuropsychiatric Inventory (NPI).

Generalizability of studies to clinical populations: Applicability of these results is not yet clear. With some exceptions, studies are not naturalistic, excluding patients with endocrine disorders, asthma, COPD, or significant hepatic or cardiovascular disease, and concomitant medications (including anticholinergics, anticonvulsants, antidepressants, antipsychotics, and drugs with central nervous system effects).

- With all drugs in this class, the subtlety of change is a barrier to determining efficacy in clinical practice.
  - √ Most effective monitoring is based on use of clinical scales that are often impractical in clinical practice.
  - √ Hence evaluation is often impressionistic and based on clinician and caregiver judgment, evaluated at intervals of 6 months, once therapeutic levels have been reached.
  - √ Patient self-evaluation is not helpful generally.
  - √ MMSE decline is another measure—2–3 points annually in untreated AD.

Guidelines for Switching AChEIs

- Reasons to switch include
  - √ Nonresponse to an AChEI that was administered in therapeutic doses.

- A drop of > 2 points on the MMSE, or increased functional disability.
  - √ Intolerable side effects before efficacy could be determined.
  - √ Patient–family request for a switch.
    - Evaluate before responding.
      - Family may have unrealistic expectations of treatment.
    - Patient response may be subtle but evident (e.g., stabilization and nonprogression)—if so, advise against change.
- Switching agents.
  - √ Drugs in this class have somewhat differing mechanisms of action. Possible that a patient may respond to one drug when unresponsive to another in the class.
    - E.g., data for improved response to rivastigmine after failed trials of donepezil.
  - √ Indications.
    - Intolerance of side effects at therapeutic doses.
      - intolerance to one drug does not predict intolerance to an alternative agent.
      - Data suggest that switch from donepezil because of intolerable side effects) to rivastigmine can produce clinical improvement and better tolerance. No reason that similar results can not be obtained with other switches (e.g., donepezil/galantamine, rivastigmine to donepezil, etc.).
    - Ineffective after 3–6 months at therapeutic levels (probably shorter trial period necessary for BPSD or Lewy body dementia where response can be expected in first 2 weeks).

Strategies

- If tolerability to prior AChEI was poor, washout of 7 days (or until symptoms resolve) recommended.
  - √ Washout advisable because of risk of increased nausea and vomiting secondary to additive effects of AChEIs.
    - Case report of fatal aspiration pneumonia during transition.
    - But note that there is a risk of withdrawal effects during washout period, with symptom relapse and functional decline.
- Begin escalation of new drug, at its initial dosing levels, employing its standard dosing recommendations.
- Augmenting strategies have not been well investigated.
  - √ Inadvisable to use two drugs from this class concurrently.
  - √ Gabapentin may control behavioral side effects of AChEIs (see p. 509).
  - √ SSRIs and trazodone may augment effects in BPSD.

√ Antioxidants (Vit. E), folic acid, and ASA indicated as safe augmenting strategies.
  - NSAIDs have potentially dangerous side effects and evidence for benefit has been called into question.

Side Effects of AChEIs

Side effects of AChEIs are relatively self-limiting, transient, and dose related; slow titration of about 12 weeks needed to achieve tolerance to side effects.

More common if dosages are increased rapidly; reduced by introducing the drug in low dose and titrating it up slowly.

Thin, small patients (<45 kg) are more prone to side effects.

Table 5.5. Side Effects of Cholinesterase Inhibitors

System Affected	Side Effects	Comments
Gastrointestinal	• Anorexia • Nausea • Vomiting • Diarrhea • Hypersalivation	• Most common side effects; usually transient and reduced if drug is titrated. • Caution if drug is discontinued and reinstituted—reintroduce at low dose and titrate slowly. • Hypersalivation may be severe and very troublesome to some patients—may respond to antihistamines or anticholinergics. • Rank order of side effects: rivastigmine > galantamine > donepezil.
Neurological	• Tremor • Dizziness • Agitation • Sleep disturbance, possibly disrupted dreaming • EPS √ Pisa syndrome (case report) √ Gait disturbance • Occasionally delirium	• Shortened REM latency, increased REM density, and reduced slow-wave sleep in normal subjects, leading to abnormal dreaming (nightmares). • EPS emerges occasionally, especially in combination with antipsychotic medication. • Manage by reducing or discontinuing drug. √ Sometimes switching drugs improves tolerance. □ Rivastigmine and galantamine have more flexible dosing regimens than donepezil. • Caution in using benzodiazepine sedation. √ May induce worsening of cognitive functioning.
Whole body	• Fatigue • Dizziness • Headache • Malaise	
Psychological	• Agitation • Behavioral disturbance • Confusion • Delusions • Paranoid reaction	• Avoid anticholinergic antipsychotic agents. • Manage by reducing/discontinuing drug. • Distinguish from dementia–related psychosis.

(cont.)

- Continue the drug 3–6 months before deciding on its effectiveness.
- Best to continue the drug as long as patient remains clinically stable, including into more severe stages of AD.

Discontinuation can be considered when

- The disease has progressed to the point that an expensive drug can no longer be justified.
- It is judged that the patient's life expectancy is too short to justify use of an expensive drug.
- An additional serious illness has emerged.
- The clinician and family agree that there seems to be no beneficial effect.

Caveat: In the individual case, improvement is often subtle and the main effect may be in the prevention or slowing of symptom progression. Neither clinician nor family may be able to determine, with confidence, if this effect is operative.

- Limited data suggest that donepezil (and likely other drugs) maintains its effect in slowing progression of the disease for up to 5 years and possibly longer.
- One strategy is to discontinue the drug and follow the patient after discontinuation.
- Abrupt discontinuation may lead to an accelerated rate of decline and possibly increased associated symptoms.
- Rebound effects on discontinuation
  - ✓ Anecdotal evidence for increased disorientation, agitation, visual hallucinations, lowering of mood and anxiety.
  - ✓ Best to taper AChEI.
  - ✓ If cognitive or functional decline accelerates, the drug can be reinstated.
    - ▫ Retitrate slowly to avoid severe vomiting.

Other indications

- When effective for acute symptoms (e.g., delirium or agitation), medication appears to work within days.
  - ✓ For usually transient events like delirium, maintain for days or weeks before a trial of discontinuing medication.

Cost effectiveness

- A number of studies has demonstrated the cost effectiveness of cholinergic enhancers.
  - ✓ Improved cost outcomes by delaying admission to institution and reducing need for care through improvement in cognitive function.

Continued

System Affected	Side Effects	Comments
CVS	• Syncopal events reported • Myocardial infarction • Infrequent cardiac arrhythmias √ Bradycardia • Hypotension √ Postural hypotension	• Increased sensitivity to carotid sinus s DLB. √ May be part of the reason for increa with AChEI. • Special caution in √ Sick sinus syndrome. √ Other supraventricular conduction c √ Congestive heart failure. √ Active coronary artery disease. • Syncope reported even in absence of p cardiac history.
Hematological	Bruising	
Liver	Hepatotoxicity	• Only with tacrine. √ 54% develop elevated serum transa √ In some studies 30% developed ele hepatic enzymes > 3 times normal. √ *This side effect eliminates tacrine as therapeutic agent.*

CAUTIONS AND CONTRAINDICATIONS

Contraindicated in patients with disorders sensitive to choline inhibitors

- Sick sinus syndrome, other supraventricular conduction
- Active gastrointestinal tract bleeding.
- Bladder obstruction.
- Asthma, severe obstructive pulmonary disease.
- Hepatic and renal impairment.
- Proceed with caution in dose escalation in patients with
  - √ Seizure disorders.
  - √ Active cardiac disease.
  - √ Congestive heart failure.
  - √ GI bleeding, history of ulcer.
  - √ Frailty and weight loss.
  - √ Hepatic and renal impairments.
  - √ Asthma, obstructive pulmonary disease.
  - √ Urinary outflow impedence or postbladder or GI surge
- Caution in anesthesia.
  - √ Possible interaction with inhaled anesthetics.
  - √ Exaggeration of effect of succinylcholine-type muscle ants.

Discontinuation and Withdrawal

Evidence is accumulating slowly to guide decision-making abou tinuation.

  - Stabilization may be prolonged for up to 24 months in some patients.
  - Example of savings: $4,839 (U.S., year 2000 data) after 2 years on rivastigmine.
- Weigh cost of drug.
  - √ Bear in mind that the costs of drug may prevent other therapies from being purchased, so careful discussion of cost-benefit in individual cases is important.

Caregiver Notes

Improvement in cognition and function is usually subtle; monitor with written record of:

- √ Personal impressions of clinical change.
- √ Performance of patient in activities of daily life.
  - Obtain form from physician.
- Because the results are subtle, it is necessary to keep an open mind about the need for long-term use of the drug.
- Although improvement or slowing of the disease is hard to demonstrate, a long-term commitment to the use of the drug is necessary for maximum benefit.
- Caregivers, especially those who are isolated and unsupported, are at significantly increased risk of depression and other stress-related effects.
  - √ Suggest
    - Formal respite care.
    - Caregiver supportive therapy.
    - Practical management advice, education, and referral to supportive resources—e.g., Alzheimer's Society.

Clinical Tips

- Tacrine not recommended
  - √ No longer used clinically.
- Educate patients and families about nature and course of the disease.
- Formal documented baseline assessment
  - √ For cognition, ADL
  - √ Behavior is important before beginning therapy.
- Goal of improved cognition often not achieved.
  - √ Practical clinical expectations for drugs should be very modest, at best, at the present time.

DONEPEZIL

Drug	Manufacturer	Chemical Class	Therapeutic Class
donepezil (Aricept)	Pfizer, Esai	piperidine, selective reversible inhibitor of AchE	antidementia

Indications: FDA/HPB

- Symptomatic treatment of patients with mild and moderate dementia due to probable Alzheimer's disease.

Indications: Off label

- Advanced forms of dementia, including
  - √ Psychosis/cognitive decline associated with DLB.
  - √ Advanced stages of Alzheimer's disease—some evidence for efficacy
  - √ Non-Alzheimer dementia (e.g., cognitive impairment associated with Parkinson's disease, multiple sclerosis).
    - ▫ Evidence is preliminary and uncontrolled or clinical.
  - √ Cognitive and behavioral symptoms of VaD.
- BPSD—action of drug is independent of effects on cognition.
- Delirium associated with dementia (case reports).
- As adjunct to control anticholinergic side effects of psychotropic medications.
- Initial studies indicate that donepezil appears to be safe for demented patients in nursing homes, including those on concomitant medication use.
  - √ As effective as for outpatients.
- Head-to-head studies with other AChEIs—mixed results.
  - √ One study, donepezil more effective for improved cognition and ADL function.
  - √ Other data show superiority for rivastigmine over donepezil but study was industry-funded.
  - √ One year trial showed clear superiority for galantamine.

Pharmacology

See Table 5.3 on page 555.

- Hepatic cirrhosis: Clearance decreased because drug is metabolized in liver.

Mechanism of action

- Binds to AChE with 1,250 times the affinity for binding BChE.
  - √ Prevents formation of the enzyme–ACh complex.

- √ Extent of AChE inhibition uncertain but cortical inhibition studies in patients with AD suggest only partial inhibition of 27%.

Therapeutic Actions

Alzheimer's disease

- Cognitive symptoms
  - √ Modest symptomatic improvement (4% change in ADAS-cog placebo comparison and 6% decrease in CIBIC; see following section on measurement) in about 30% of patients.
  - √ About 2 points difference with placebo on the MMSE at end point of studies.
  - √ 4-point difference on the ADAS-cog; more marked improvement in a small subset of patients (7–11 points on the ADAS-cog).
    - ▫ Benefit is evident in the *difference* between the placebo response and the active drug. (i.e., even in the presence of minimal absolute improvement on ADAS-cog with active drug. decline on scores in the placebo group produces statistically significant difference between active drug and placebo groups).
  - √ Improvement evident on formal cognitive subtests.
    - ▫ Observable clinical improvement often less evident.
  - √ Improvement may occur as early as 3 weeks after beginning treatment but generally is not apparent until 9–12 weeks after initiation of treatment (usually 10 mg).
    - ▫ No evidence for patient-rated improvement in quality of life, but this is hard to measure in any condition.
  - √ No effect on underlying disease demonstrated yet.
    - ▫ New studies examining this issue.
  - √ May slow pace of disease progression; amount of benefit hard to quantify but appears to be about 1-year delay.
    - ▫ Thereafter, increased levels of care, including institutionalization, become necessary.
- Behavioral symptoms.
  - √ Reduced emergence of agitation, especially aggression and verbal intensity.
  - √ Reduced need for sedatives.

Dementia with Lewy bodies (DLB) (see also p. 249).

Management issues

- A few case reports and studies suggest efficacy of AChEIs when there is marked cholinergic deficit as in DLB.

- Symptoms include
  - √ Hallucinations and delusions
  - √ Confusion
  - √ Aggression
  - √ Agitation
  - √ Attentional deficits
  - √ Sleep disturbance
    - ▫ Daytime hypersomnolence and nocturnal sleep disturbance.
  - √ Apathy
- Dosing of donepezil the same as for AD.
  - √ donepezil 10 mg/day
  - √ Improvement usually within a few days in responsive patients.

Vascular dementia

- Variable improvement of cognitive function.
- Improvement of associated behavioral symptoms.
- Evidence for some improvement in caregiver burden.
  - √ Reduced hours of care, about 1 hour/day.

Frontotemporal dementias

- No effect.
- Serotonergic and noradrenergic agents more useful.

Choosing a Drug

- All newer AChEIs are safer than tacrine (and velnacrine) since there is no hepatotoxicity.
- Drugs in this class have similar but not identical side-effect profiles.
- Donepezil differs from
  - √ Rivastigmine (and physostigmine), in having no peripheral cholinergic adverse effects.
  - √ Galantamine, in having no effect on nicotinic receptors.
- Efficacy appears dose dependent (i.e., larger doses produce best effect, to maximum of 10 mg). Drug with best-tolerated side-effect profile at higher doses is best choice.

Prognostic indicators

- Less treatment responsive—increased atrophy of nucleus innominata.
- More treatment responsive—greater severity of delusions, agitation, depression, anxiety, apathy, disinhibition, and irritability (data still in early stages of development).

Quality of the data

- Efficacy data come from several controlled and uncontrolled studies, most supported by pharmaceutical companies.
- True clinical utility remains somewhat controversial among some but subset of patients clearly benefits over the longer term.
- Longest study
  - √ Followed patients for up to 4.9 years, most on a dose of 10 mg.
    - ▫ Relationship to daily clinical practice limited, since this population was healthy and ambulatory.
    - ▫ One study showed very minor improvement in a more representative clinical sample.

Race/ethnicity—little data.

Dosing

- Long half-life permits single daily dose regimen at either 5 or 10 mg.
- Efficacy has been shown at 5 mg but greater effect at 10 mg (although still generally modest).

Starting dose

- Start at 5 mg hs (to minimize GI side effects).
  - √ If insomnia is a problem, administer in the morning.
- Maintain at 5 mg for 6–8 weeks (or longer, if necessary) until patient fully accommodates to dose level.

Increasing dose

- Begin 10 mg dose after 6–8 weeks on 5 mg.
- Most side effects emerge at 10 mg but are minimized if patient has chance to accommodate to the drug first.

Therapeutic and maintenance dose

- For treatment of AD, optimal maintenance dose is 10 mg.
- For off-label indications, dosing is less clear but 10 mg dose is usually the target.
  - √ Patients seem to respond to the 5–10 mg dose range, using similar guidelines for reaching therapeutic levels.

Combination therapy

- Donepezil and gabapentin.
  - √ Case reports of behavioral side effects of donepezil controlled by gabapentin 100 mg tid.
  - √ Donepezil augmentation of neuroleptic may enhance antipsychotic effects (open study with perphenazine). May also improve tolerance to EPS side effects.

- SSRIs and trazodone.
  - √ Helpful in controlling agitation in AD, especially associated with symptoms of frontotemporal dementia where AChEI is ineffective.
  - √ Recent controlled study suggests that combining an SSRI (sertraline) with donepezil may offer some synergistic advantage in agitation in dementia.
- Psychosocial interventions.
  - √ Concurrent stimulation of cognitive abilities, such as memory training.
  - √ Use of memory aids.
  - √ Organizational strategies for daily routines.
  - √ Reality orientation programs.
- Treatment of comorbid depression and psychosis are strongly indicated.
  - √ Use both pharmacological and behavioral interventions for dementia-related psychiatric symptoms (see pp. 236–247).
    - ▫ Distinguish dementia-related symptoms from AChEI side effects.

Side Effects

- Generally well tolerated in study samples.
  - √ Related to rate of titration.
    - ▫ Slow increase of medication over 6 weeks produces fewer side effects.
  - √ Patients may be more vulnerable to side effects in naturalistic settings.
- Symptoms are generally mild and transient but can be more severe.
  - √ Especially evident at the 10-mg dose.
  - √ 9–16% of patients on 10-mg dose withdrew from studies because of side effects.

Most common side effects are related to cholinergic action and are often self-limiting within a few days.

- Nausea, vomiting, and diarrhea.
- Urinary frequency/incontinence may occur, especially if maximum dose is exceeded.
- Vertigo
- Anorexia
- Hypersalivation
  - √ May be severe and very troubling.
  - √ May respond to antihistamines or anticholinergics.

- Use with appropriate caution: anticholinergics not usually appropriate for patients with dementia—theoretically counter therapeutic action of cholinergic agents.

- Insomnia (14%)
- Fatigue
- Syncope
- Muscle cramps
- Bruising

Most serious and less common symptoms include

- Depression
- Psychological disturbance
- Agitation
- Aggressive behavior
- Anxiety
- Induction of mania
- Confusion
- Delirium
- EPS emerges occasionally, especially in combination with antipsychotic medication.
- Gait disturbance
- Headache
- Stupor
- Dyskinesia
- Abnormal dreams
- Occasional nightmares
- Cardiac arrhythmias
- Myocardial infarction
- Weight loss
- Arthritis/arthralgia
- Myalgia

√ May resolve with withdrawal of medication.

Isolated reports

- Severe syncope
- CVA
- Convulsions
- Pisa syndrome
- Cardiac fibrillation
- GI hemorrhage

Monitoring

- Routine liver function monitoring is unnecessary.
  - √ But patients with liver or kidney disease should be monitored carefully for adverse effects.

Drug Interactions

Data are still limited. Drugs that inhibit liver enzymes (CYP) 2D6 and 3A4 may increase plasma levels and side effects of donepezil, but clinical effects not yet well delineated (see pp. 95–96).

- Ketoconazol increases plasma concentrations 23–30%.
- Other possible interactions with enzyme inhibitors include nefazodone, quinidine, fluoxetine, paroxetine.

Potentiation possible with

- Neuromuscular blocking agents such as succinylcholine.
- Cholinergic agents such as bethanechol.
- Ophthalmic agents such as pilocarpine or carbachol.

Case reports

- Possible drug interactions producing increased side effects include
  - √ Diltiazem
  - √ Fluoxetine
  - √ Paroxetine
  - √ Sertraline
  - √ Risperidone
    - ▫ Single case report of severe EPS in combination.
    - ▫ Patients on a combination of antipsychotic and AChEI may be more vulnerable to this effect. *Combination should be avoided.*

Antagonism

- Theoretically, action may be antagonized by anticholinergic agents (e.g., certain psychotropics and antiparkinsonian agents).
- Hence avoid coadministration of anticholinergic drugs.

Caution in concurrent use of

- NSAIDs.
  - √ GI complications may be exaccerbated.
- Other cholinesterase inhibitors.
  - √ Exacerbation of side effects.
- Inhaled anesthetics.
  - √ May decrease neuromuscular blocking effects of anesthetic.

Because of limited data, close monitoring is recommended when donepezil is administered concurrently with other drugs.

Disability Interactions and Contraindications

See page 571.

Contraindicated in patients with known hypersensitivity to donepezil or piperidine derivatives.

Special precautions

- Risk of dizziness or syncope requires extra caution to prevent falls.
  - √ Attendant risk of hip or other fractures.
- Observe for increased risk of EPS when used concurrently with risperidone or other neuroleptics.
  - √ Not recommended.
- Potentiates succinylcholine during anesthesia.
  - √ Known hypersensitivity to donepezil or piperidine derivatives.

Overdose: Toxicity, Suicide, Management

- Very few reported cases of overdose.
- Doses up to 70 mg reported with easily controlled symptoms of transient.
  - √ Vomiting
  - √ Lethargy
  - √ Flushing
  - √ Diarrhea
- Theoretically may lead to cholinergic crisis.
  - √ Nausea, vomiting
  - √ Salivation
  - √ Diaphoresis
  - √ Bradycardia, hypotension
  - √ Respiratory collapse
  - √ Convulsions

Management

- Administer charcoal for severe symptoms and if time of overdose is less than 8 hours.
- Otherwise, provide supportive care and observation.
  - √ Administer atropine sulphate for bradycardia.
    - ▫ 1–2 mg IV initially, with additional doses based on treatment response.
  - √ Symptoms generally resolve spontaneously.

Clinical Tips

- Main cognitive action of this drug is to modestly slow the progression of Alzheimer's decline.
  - √ Its clinical value for associated symptoms of psychosis and agitation, together with its favorable side-effect profile, make it a useful drug to try in all patients with AD or BPSD.
- Monitor q 2–3 weeks initially (more often by phone with family if indicated) until stabilized.
  - √ Then every 3–6 months for effect.
- Maintain careful observational records to determine if there is therapeutic effect.
  - √ Use standard instruments (e.g., MMSE or ADL instrument).
- If in doubt about effect of drug, taper and discontinue and monitor for rapid deterioration of symptoms within 6 weeks.
- When increasing to 10 mg, prescribe two 5-mg tablets so that dose can be reduced from 10 to 5 mg if side effects occur.
- If morning diarrhea a problem at the 10 mg hs dose, try 5-mg bid instead.
  - √ Note that each 5-mg tablet is about same price as the 10 mg so using 5 mg size doubles cost.
- Integrated therapies are the most practical treatment approach at this time, including
  - √ Medications for the primary cognitive disorder.
  - √ Vigorous treatment of comorbid conditions.
  - √ Formal caregiver support.
- If clinical decline or no improvement evident in 6 months, best to discontinue drug and switch to another.

GALANTAMINE

Drug	Manufacturer	Chemical Class	Therapeutic Class
galantamine (Reminyl)	Janssen	benzazepine	cognitive enhancer acetylcholinesterase inhibitor (reversible, competitive)

Indications: FDA/HPB

- Treatment of mild to moderate Alzheimer's disease.

Indications: Off label

- Vascular dementia.
- Data for utility of drugs in this class for other indications suggest galantamine may be useful for

- √ Psychosis/cognitive decline associated with Lewy body dementia.
- √ Agitation and aggression associated with dementia.
- √ Delirium associated with dementia (theoretical basis and case reports).
- √ Non-Alzheimer forms of dementia—e.g., VaD and cognitive impairment associated with Parkinson's disease, multiple sclerosis (evidence preliminary and uncontrolled or clinical).

Pharmacology

See page 555.

- Metabolite o-demethylgalantamine more potent and selective AChEI than galantamine (but less potent action on butyrylcholinesterase).
- Many of the pharmacokinetic studies were conducted on young healthy adults.

Mechanism of action

- Dual mechanism of action.
  - √ AChE enzyme inhibition.
  - √ Allosteric potentiation at presynaptic nicotinic receptors increases release of ACh.
    - May enhance electrical signals and increase release of other neurotransmitters, such as glutamate.

Therapeutic actions

- Slows progression of AD and modestly improves cognition, ADL, and behavior in subset of patients.
- May show small advantage over other AChEIs in improving ADL, but data still preliminary.
- Phase 3 studies show similar effect on ADAS-cog and CIBIC-CI as other AChEIs.
  - √ About a 4-point difference between drug (at higher dose) and placebo at 6 months.
  - √ Most of the effect appears to come from stabilizing decline, compared to placebo, with only minimal improvement in ADAS-cog scores.
- Benefit to cognition more evident in more impaired group of subjects (7 points difference).
  - √ Appears to modestly reduce need for caregiver support compared to placebo group.
- Therapeutic actions of galantamine may
  - √ Improve instrumental and basic ADL.

- √ Prevent decline in ADL for at least a year (compared to placebo decline).
- √ Improve caregiver burden.
  - ▫ Slightly reduces time spent in caregiving (by 10–12%).
  - ▫ Improves or slows emergence of behavioral disturbances.

Choosing a Drug

- Preliminary evidence that galantamine may have some advantage in efficacy and tolerability (less GI side effect).
- Some evidence that poor response to galantamine (e.g., side effects) may not affect efficacy of another in the class.
  - √ Substitute another in the class as trial if one drug fails.
- Prognostic indicators.
  - √ Male gender may predict better initial (first 3 months) response.
  - √ No evidence for effect of apolipoprotein E4 allele on immediate response, but perhaps affects longer-term outcome.
  - √ Data in this area preliminary and not yet useful in routine clinical decision making.

Quality of the data

- Data on pharmacokinetics of galantamine are limited and mostly based on small studies with healthy volunteers and patients with uncomplicated AD.
- Data for patients with AD plus concurrent medical disorders and concurrent medications are unavailable.

Dosing

Starting dose

- Start at 4 mg bid, morning and evening with meals.
- Maintain for 4–8 weeks before increasing dose.
- In patients with moderate hepatic impairment.
  - √ Begin at 4 mg for 4–8 weeks

Reaching therapeutic dose

- Increase slowly in 4 mg increments to maximum daily dose of 16 mg.
- Titrate slowly (q 4–8 weeks) to 16 mg, based on tolerance.
- Observe for effect and tolerability over 4-week period at therapeutic dose.
- If no effect, or to see if greater effect is possible, increase to 24 mg.
  - √ Based on clinical evaluation of benefit plus tolerability.

Note: Although some effects occur at 16-mg dose, the greatest therapeutic effects are evident at higher dosages, so 24-mg dose may be the best target; but side effects are more evident at this dose.

Maintenance dose

- If effect seen at initial maintenance dose of 16 mg, maintain at this dose.
- Otherwise maintain at 24 mg, if tolerated, for several months, monitoring closely.
- If no effect at 6 months or if decline continues, consider tapering galantamine.
  - √ Monitor for decline in function.
    - ▫ Sometimes occurs precipitously.
    - ▫ If so, consider reintroducing the drug, gradually retitrating to therapeutic levels.
  - √ Switch to another AChEI.

Side Effects

- Most common
  - √ Headache
  - √ Tremor
  - √ Dizziness
  - √ Agitation
  - √ Somnolence
  - √ Sleep disturbance
    - ▫ Possibly disrupted dreaming.
    - ▫ Shortened REM latency, increased REM density, reduced slow-wave sleep in normal subjects.
  - √ Increased salivation
  - √ Anorexia
  - √ Nausea (about 20%); vomiting (about 15%)
  - √ Diarrhea (about 4%)
  - √ Weight loss, mild
  - √ Abdominal pain (about 4%)
  - √ Dyspepsia
  - √ Rhinitis
- Generally well tolerated.
- Adverse effects usually mild.
- Most serious and less common.
  - √ Depression
  - √ Seizures
  - √ Ulcers
  - √ May aggravate asthma, COPD
    - ▫ Respiratory depression
- Manage side effects by reducing drug dose.

Drug Interactions

Data limited on drug interactions, but overall risk is low.

- Caution in concomitant use of inhibitors of CYP3A4 or CYP2D6 (see pp. 95–96).
- Increased bioavailability of 40% when coadministered with paroxetine.
  - √ Ketoconazole and erythromycin also increase bioavailability.
- Combination therapy with other AChEI not recommended.

Caution in concurrent use of

- Succinylcholine (exaggeration/prolongation of effects).
- Cholinergic agonists (bethanechol or ophthalmic agents such as pilocarpine or carbachol).
- Other cholinergic agents.
- NSAIDs (GI complications may be exacerbated).
- Anticholinergics may interfere with action of galantamine (or visa versa).
  - √ Example: Antagonize anticholinergic effects of ophthalmic anticholinergic cyclopentolate/phenylephrine.
- Other cholinesterase inhibitors (exacerbation of side effects).
- Inhaled anesthetics (may decrease neuromuscular blocking effects of anesthetic).

Disability Interactions and Contraindications

See page 571.

Clinical Tips

- Side effects emerge more frequently during rapid dose escalation.
- Flexible dosing (4 mg dosage form) available, so slow titration possible and often advisable, based on tolerance and side effects.
- Slower dose increases improve tolerance of the drug.
- Liquid form offers advantages for uncooperative patients or those with swallowing difficulties.
  - √ Requires use of a calibrated pipette (similar to an insulin syringe) to draw up the medication.
- GI side-effects generally limited to 5 or 6 days.
  - √ Associated with dose increases, although some effects (e.g., diarrhea or nausea) may persist and become intolerable.
- No new side effects observed to emerge during prolonged use of drug.
- Side-effect profile similar when used for vascular dementia.

RIVASTIGMINE

Drug	Manufacturer	Chemical Class	Therapeutic Class
rivastigmine (Exelon)	Novartis	Carbamate	antidementia; acetylcholinesterase inhibitor (noncompetitive)

Indications: FDA/HPB

- Symptomatic treatment of mild to moderate Alzheimer's disease.

Indications: Off label

Advanced forms of dementia, including some non-Alzheimer forms

- Dementia with Lewy bodies (DLB).
  - √ Based on current data, the most potent of the AChEIs for this indication.
  - √ Improves psychotic features (e.g., visual hallucinations).
  - √ May be marked improvement in cognitive performance.
  - √ May improve score on NPI.
  - √ No increase in parkinsonism or depression.
- Behavioral and psychological symptoms of Alzheimer's and related dementias (BPSD).
  - √ Control of secondary symptoms of dementia includes
    - Agitation
    - Irritability
    - Disinhibition
    - Fluctuations in behavior, such as sundowning syndrome
    - Aberrant motor behavior
    - Apathy
    - Anxiety
    - Depression
  - √ In some cases, reduction of secondary symptoms may account for the greatest improvement with this class of drugs.
- Cognitive and behavioral symptoms of vascular dementia (preliminary evidence)
- Possible utility in Parkinson's dementia.
- May take several weeks to begin to show therapeutic effect.
  - √ Agitation and aggression associated with dementia.

Pharmacology

- Clearance is reduced in patients with hepatic impairment (although no CYP enzyme metabolism involved) and may be reduced or paradoxically increased in renal impairment.

Mechanism of action

- An intermediate-acting, reversible cholinesterase inhibitor.
- Structurally related to physostigmine but not to donepezil or tacrine.
- Inhibits breakdown of acetylcholine by two modes of action
  - √ Pseudo-irreversible inhibition of
    - ▫ G1 isoform of acetylcholinesterase.
    - ▫ butyrylcholinesterase (action in the glial cells).
  - √ Anticholinesterase activity is relatively specific for brain acetylcholinesterase and butyrylcholinesterase compared with that in peripheral tissues.
  - √ Selectivity for hippocampus and cortex.
  - √ Lacks binding affinity for other neuroreceptors, unlike tacrine.

Therapeutic actions

- Main effect is to delay progression of AD symptoms.
  - √ Does not appear to reverse the process.
  - √ New data suggest it may modify actual process of disease course—mechanism unknown and data are still presumptive.
- Improves or stabilizes scores on the cognitive subscale of the ADAS-cog in about 55% of patients by about 4–5 points overall in relatively brief studies of up to 26 weeks.
  - √ Statistically significantly fewer, though still substantial numbers of, placebo patients also improve during this time.
  - √ Over longer periods, maintenance of drug shows protective function through slowing of disease progression.
  - √ A subset of patients gain more substantial benefit.
- Reduces progressive deterioration of ADL and IADL scores.
  - √ Reports of caregivers indicate some functional improvement (e.g., medication taking, dressing, hygiene, meal preparation) which may delay need for admission to long-term care facility.
- Clinician global evaluations (CIBIC-Plus) indicate improvement.
- For many patients, overall clinical improvement very modest and may not be clinically evident at all.

Choosing a Drug

- Some indication that rivastigmine shows greater effect than donepezil in more advanced cases of AD but data not conclusive.
- Cost and insurance coverage are determining factors for some.

Quality of the data

- Several double-blind, placebo-controlled studies (most sponsored by pharmaceutical company).

- Clinical utility of results remains controversial, but there is growing support for efficacy.

Dosing

Initial dose

- Standard starting dose.
  - √ 1.5 mg once or twice daily.
  - √ Morning and/or evening with food.
  - √ Administer liquid form using oral dosing syringe.
- Most conservative regimen is to begin at 1.5 mg O.D. advisable for the very old (> 85, especially female) or very frail.
- Flexible dosing available, so slow titration possible and often advisable, based on tolerance and side effects.

Reaching therapeutic dose

- Fairly lengthy titration period of about 12 weeks.
- Increase to 3 mg bid after minimum of 2–4 weeks (often longer).
- Increasing above 6 mg/day should be done with careful regard to side effects and not more frequently than every 2 weeks.
- If patient experiences side effects, stop medication for a few days, then resume at a lower or the same dose.
- Evaluate every 2–4 weeks during this stage.

Maintenance dose

- Maintain at 6–12 mg.
  - √ Most benefit gained at 12 mg dose, if tolerated.
    - ▫ Includes treatment of DLB.
- Therapeutic drug effect may continue throughout the course of the disease.
- Some patients deteriorate when medication is discontinued.
- If therapeutic effect evident and medication well tolerated, advisable to maintain the medication into late stages of disease process.
- Evaluate every 3–6 months during this phase.

Side Effects

- Related to cholinergic action.
- Generally well tolerated.
  - √ Significant dropout rates in trials generally associated with anticholinergic side effects.
- *Note:* Administer with food to reduce adverse effects and possibly improve GI absorption.

- Some data suggest rivastigmine associated with more side effects (especially GI) than donepezil or galantamine.
- Relatively self-limiting, transient, and dose related.
- Slow titration of about 12 weeks needed to achieve tolerance to side effects.
- More common if dosages are increased rapidly.

Table 5.6. Side Effects of Rivastigmine

Side Effects	Most Common	Most Serious and Less Common
Body as a whole	• Weight loss, especially in women (24%) • Fatigue • Sweating • Malaise	• Hot flushes • Flu-like symptoms
Cardiovascular		• Syncopal events reported • Increased sensitivity to carotid sinus syndrome in DLB √ May be part of the reason for increased falls with AChEI • Bradycardia • Hypotension • Postural hypotension
Central and peripheral nervous system	• Dizziness • Headache • Tremor • Somnolence • Asthenia • Insomnia	• Abnormal gait • Cerebrovascular disorder • Ataxia • Convulsions • EPS • Paraesthesia
Ear		• Tinnitus
Gastrointestinal	• More common in women • Nausea and Vomiting • Diarrhea • Abdominal pain • Dyspepsia, Anorexia • Hypersalivation √ May be severe and very troubling √ May respond to antihistamines or anticholinergics • Trimetho-benzamide may be effective √ Use with appropriate caution: anticholinergics not usually appropriate for patients with dementia, and theoretically counter therapeutic action of cholinergic agents	• Fecal incontinence • Gastritis
Musculoskeletal		• Arthralgia • Myalgia
Psychiatric	• Confusion • Depression • Anxiety	• Agitation • Behavioral disturbance • Delusions • Paranoid reaction

(cont.)

Continued

Side Effects	Most Common	Most Serious and Less Common
Respiratory	• Rhinitis	• Aggravates asthma, COPD • Respiratory depression
Skin and appendages		• Rash √ Stevens-Johnson syndrome—case report
Urinary		• Urinary incontinence and nocturia √ May be very troublesome and require medication dose adjustment or sometimes discontinuation. • Possible urinary obstruction

Drug Interactions

- Data limited, on drug interactions but overall risk low.
- Caution in concurrent use of
  - √ Succinylcholine (exaggeration/prolongation of effects).
  - √ Cholinergic agonists (bethenachol or ophthalmic agents such as pilocarpine or carbachol).
  - √ Other cholinergic agents.
  - √ NSAIDs (GI complications may be exaccerbated).
  - √ Anticholinergics may interfere with action of rivastigmine (or vice versa—e.g., antagonize anticholinergic effects of ophthalmic anticholinergic cylopentolate/phenylephrine).
  - √ Other cholinesterase inhibitors (exacerbation of side effects).
  - √ Inhaled anesthetics (may decrease neuromuscular blocking effects of anesthetic).

Disability Interactions and Contraindications

See page 571.

Clinical Tips

- Swallow capsules whole.
- Best to administer at mealtime, with food, to reduce side effects.
- If a dose is missed, wait and take the next regular dose.
  - √ Do not take a double dose to make up for the missed one.
- Does not appear to affect quality of sleep.
- If drug is discontinued for any length of time, it is important to restart the drug at a low dose and increase gradually to avoid severe nausea and vomiting.
- Improvement in cognition and function is usually subtle; monitor with written record of
  - √ Personal impressions of clinical change.
  - √ Performance of patient in ADL.

- Because the results are subtle, it is necessary to keep an open mind about the need for long term use of these drugs.
- But improvement or slowing of the disease is hard to demonstrate, a long-term commitment is necessary for maximum benefit.
- A bid dose recommended, but if side effects are severe, they may be ameliorated by using a tid dose for those patients who have motivated, reliable caregivers.
- Trimethobenzamide 250 mg bid for first 3 days of dose increase may improve tolerance to achieiving higher dose of rivastigmine.
- If switching between AChEIs, instruct patients and families to watch for cholinergic GI side effects and call doctor.
- If restarting drug after a period of several days off treatment reintroduce at lowest daily dose and increase gradually, according to recommended titration schedule.
  - √ Rapid reintroduction, after interruption of several days to weeks, sometimes induces severe vomiting at single dose of 4.5 mg.

TACRINE

Drug	Manufacturer	Chemical Class	Therapeutic Class
tacrine (Cognex)	First Horizon	aminoacridine class—nonselective, reversible, AChEI	antidementia

Indications: FDA/HPB

- Treatment of mild to moderate Alzheimer's disease.

Indications: Off label

- Potential utility in dementia-related
  - √ Apathy
  - √ Anxiety
  - √ Hallucinations
  - √ Disinhibition
  - √ Aberrant motor behavior
- Intractable sleep disturbance (dose 80 mg hs).

Pharmacology

- Clearance reduced in hepatic disease.

Mechanism of action

Properties include

- Stimulation of cholinergic firing at high doses.
- Blocks pre- and postsynaptic muscarinic and nicotinic receptors.

- Increases release of serotonin, DA, NE, GABA.
- Promotes inhibitory action on MAOA and B activity.

Choosing a Drug

Tacrine is not recommended or used since other, less toxic drugs have become available. Unfavorable drug properties include

- Rapid metabolism.
- Need for qid dosing.
- Unfavorable side-effect profile.

Dosing

- Start at 10 mg qid.
  √ Very short half-life.
- Increase by 10 mg qid every 6 weeks.
- Maximum dose 40 mg qid.
- Increase to maximum level over 18 weeks to minimize side effects.
- Give with food if GI side effects are troublesome.

Discontinuation and withdrawal

- Discontinue therapy if AST/ALT levels exceed 3 times upper limit of normal range.
- Continue to monitor closely for signs of hepatitis.

Side Effects

- About 30% of patients experience significant or serious side effects.
  √ Most notably, hepatotoxicity.
- Cholinergic effects are dose dependent.
- Most common (percentages are general adult data).
  √ Agitation
  √ Confusion
  √ Ataxia
  √ Nausea, vomiting (28%)
  √ Diarrhea (14%)
  √ Dyspepsia/anorexia (9%)
  √ Weight loss
  √ Abdominal pain
  √ Worsening of asthma and COPD
  √ Rash
  √ Bradycardia
  √ Urinary flow obstruction
  √ Myalgia (7.5%)

- Most serious and less common.
  - √ Seizures.
  - √ Sudden worsening of cognition on discontinuation.
  - √ Worsening of peptic ulcers.
  - √ Hepatotoxicity.
    - ▫ 30% of patients (in some studies) developed elevated ALT. > 3 times normal; jaundice.
      - ◦ Onset around 4–7 (up to 16) weeks.
      - ◦ Generally reversible with discontinuation of drug.
      - ◦ Rate is higher in women.
  - √ Hepatocellular necrosis or granulomatous changes.
    - ▫ This side effect eliminates tacrine as a useful therapeutic agent.

Drug Interactions

Potentiators of tacrine: Caution in concurrent use of

- Succinylcholine (exaggeration/prolongation of effects).
- Cholinergic agonists (bethanechol or ophthalmic agents such as pilocarpine or carbachol).
- Other cholinergic agents.
- Cimetidine (may potentiate effects).
- NSAIDs (GI complications may be exacerbated).
- Anticholinergics may interfere with action (or vice versa—e.g., antagonize anticholinergic effects of ophthalmic anticholinergic cyclopentolate/phenylephrine).
- Other cholinesterase inhibitors (exacerbation of side effects).
- Inhaled anesthetics (may decrease neuromuscular blocking effects of anesthetic).
- Inhibits theophylline metabolism and increases plasma concentration.
- Fluvoxamine (potentiates action).

Monitoring

- LFTs q 1–2 weeks for 4–5 months.

Disability Interactions and Contraindications

Proceed with caution in dose escalation in patients with

- Seizure disorders.
- Active cardiac disease.
- Congestive heart failure.
- GI bleeding, history of ulcer.
- Frailty and weight loss.

- Hepatic and renal impairments.
- Asthma, obstructive pulmonary disease.
- Parkinson's disease.
- Potentially serious liver toxicity requires LFTs (AST/ALT) every 1–2 weeks.
- Caution in
  - √ Anesthesia (because of possible interaction with inhaled anesthetics and exaggeration of effect of succinylcholine-type muscle relaxants).
  - √ Asthma.
  - √ Obstructive pulmonary disease.
  - √ Gastrointestinal disease.
  - √ Seizures.
  - √ Certain cardiac conditions.
    - ▫ Sick sinus syndrome.
    - ▫ Other supraventricular cardiac conduction defect conditions.
    - ▫ Bradycardia.

Overdose: Toxicity, Suicide Management

Lethal dose estimated at 12 times therapeutic dose.

Overdose symptoms are of cholinergic crisis

- Severe nausea
- Vomiting
- Salivation
- Sweating
- Bradycardia
- Hypotension
- Respiratory depression
- Collapse and convulsions

Treatment

- Provide supportive measures.
- Administer 1–2 mg IV atropine sulphate initially, with additional doses based on treatment response.
- Symptoms generally resolve spontaneously.

Appendix A
Newly Approved Drugs

ARIPIPRAZOLE

Drug	Manufacturer	Chemical Class	Therapeutic Class
Aripiprazole (Abilify)	Bristol Meyers Squibb	Quinolone derivative	Atypical antipsychotic

Indications: FDA/ HPB

- Schizophrenia

Indications: Off label

- Psychosis of Alzheimer's Disease (unpublished data)

Pharmacology

No geriatric data available yet

- Does not affect CYP450 enzymes

Mechanism of action

- Partial D2 receptor blockade in limbic system
- Antagonizes 5HT2a receptor
- Partial agonist at 5HT1a receptor
- Moderate binding at alpha1 adrenergic and histaminic receptors, and little affinity for muscarinic receptors
- In areas of dopaminergic hyperactivity it acts as antagonist and in areas of hypoactivity it acts as agonist
  - √ Hence characterized as dopamine system stabilizer

Table A.1. Pharmacokinetics of Aripiprazole

Bioavailability	Plasma Protein Binding	Volume of Distribution	Elimination Half Life	T_{max}	Absorption	Excretion	Metabolized p-450 system	Reversible
87%	99% (mainly albumin)		75 hrs	3 hrs	Unaffected by food		Metabolized by CYP2D6 and 3A4: active metabolite dehydro-aripiprazole	

Therapeutic Actions by indication

- Both acute and chronic symptoms of schizophrenia appear to be responsive and efficacy is comparable to risperidone and haloperidol (limited general adult data only)
- Improved Brief Psychiatric Rating Scale scores for hallucinations and delusions associated with community living patients with Alzheimer's disease at average dose of 10 mg (randomized placebo controlled double blind data not peer reviewed published yet)

Choosing a Drug

- Early data suggest efficacy and tolerance in elders but it is too early to be able to suggest it be used routinely in elders

Dosing

- Daily dose regimen
  - √ No dose finding studies in elders
  - √ General adult dose 10-15 mg once daily (maximum 30 mg)
  - √ For dementia, trial used 10 mg daily (range 1-17 mg)

Discontinuation and Withdrawal by indication

- No drug specific data available

Side Effects

- Limited data suggest comparable tolerance to other atypicals
- Appears to have low level of EPS effects but data are still in the early stages
- Overall favorable profile for lipids, weight and QTc interval (early general adult data)

Drug Interactions

- Potentiated by inhibitors of 3A4 and 2D6
- Action antagonized by inducers of 3A4
- Reduce dose in presence of these drugs
- See Table 1.31, page 95

ESCITALOPRAM

Drug	Manufacturer	Chemical Class
Escitalopram (Lexapro)	Forest /Lundbeck	SSRI- bicyclic phthalane derivative(S-enantiomer of racemic citalopram)

Indications: FDA/ HPB

- treatment of major depressive disorder

Indications: Off label

- Clinical data in elders suggests utility for depression associated with dementia
- General adult data shows effectiveness for
  - √ Panic disorder
  - √ generalized anxiety disorder

Pharmacology

- 50% higher plasma concentrations in elders
- hepatic damage doubles half-life and reduces oral clearance requiring lower doses
  - √ Kidney function is less problematic since the drug is extensively metabolized and little is excreted unchanged in the urine
- Linear pharmacokinetics at therapeutic doses but interindividual variability in plasma levels not established for elders

Mechanism of action

- Inhibition of reuptake of 5-HT
  - √ 100 times more potent than racemic citalopram
- Highly selective—no effect on dopamine and norepinephrine reuptake
- Very little or no affinity for serotonergic, adrenergic, dopamine, histamine, muscarinic or benzodiazepine receptors

Therapeutic Actions by indication

- Effective in depression associated with dementia and may improve cognition in treatment responsive patients
- No specific data yet on efficacy in BPSD, post stroke depression, psychotic depression, or aggression but these syndromes are responsive to citalopram and so may also respond to escitalopram.

Choosing a Drug

- Little geriatric specific data
- Early clinical experience suggests it is well tolerated in elders, especially at the 10 mg dose
- Quality of the Data
  - √ Newly launched drug; little geriatric specific data

Table A.2. Pharmacokinetics of Escitalopram

Drug	Plasma Protein Binding	Volume of Distribution	T_{max}(Hrs)	Elimination Half Life	Absorption	Clearance	Excretion	Metabolism	Linearity
escitalopram (almost all general adult data)	56%	12 L/kg	5	27–32 hrs (General adult data) 40–48 (geriatric data)	unaffected by food	600 ml/min	Predominently liver	N-demethylation mainly by CYP3A4 and CYP2C19 to mildly active S-demethyl citalopram and S-didemethyl citalopram	linear

Dosing

Initial dose:

- starting dose for patients > 65 years is 10 mg daily in AM (may be given at night if daytime somnolence is a problem but watch for sleep disturbances such as insomnia)

Increasing dose

- no geriatric data. Overall 10 mg dose appears as effective as 20 mg in general adult and mixed age premarketing studies

Discontinuation and Withdrawal by indication

- See citalopram for guidelines
- Discontinue slowly over 2-3 weeks to avoid withdrawal symptoms
- Withdrawal syndromes
  - √ No strong withdrawal or rebound effects reported, but as with other SSRIs monitor for GI disturbance, anxiety, insomnia, dizziness, asthenia, impaired concentration, headache, migraine

Side Effects:

- See also citalopram (p. 144)
- Preliminary data indicate it is generally well tolerated by elders
- Significantly increased rates of side effects at the 20 mg dose
- Key side effects include: nausea, ejaculatory impairment, insomnia, diarrhea, somnolence, dizziness, sweating, dry mouth, constipation
- Non-geriatric report of SIADH, activation of mania/hypomania
- Other side effects are similar to citalopram but there is no geriatric data yet to guide the clinician specifically for the elderly

Laboratory monitoring

- Routine:
  - √ No special precautions
  - √ See citalopram (p. 144)

Drug Interactions

See also Table 1.27.

- Increased levels of Metoprolol
- Cimetidine- may increase concentration of citalopram.
- CYP2C19 (omeprazole).

- Anticoagualants and anti- platelet agents- may increase risk of bleeding
- Usual cautions with alcohol although no strong interaction with alcohol has been noted

Note danger of serotonin syndrome with coadministration of

- MAOIs—life threatening complications; coadministration contraindicated-
- HCAs—possible, (although combinations may be used with appropriate caution and monitoring)
- SRI drugs and serotonergic agents such as all SSRIs bupropion, lithium, clomipramine, mirtazapine, nefazodone, v
- Buspirone—case report
- triptans
- OTC/alternative medicines
  - √ cold preparations (dextromethorphan)
  - √ SAMe
  - √ St John's Wort
- meperidine

Special Precautions:

- General precautions as for all psychoactive agents with driving or hazardous machinery
- Monitor serum sodium and inquire periodically for signs of SIADH (see p. 82)

Contraindications

- History of adverse reaction to or intolerance of the drug.

Overdose: Toxicity, Suicide

- See citalopram (p. 149).

Table A.3. Profiles of Aripiprazole and Escitalopram

Drug	Color	Capsule	Tablet	Liquid	Other	Scored	Dosage Size (Official)	Available in Canada and cost (CDN $)	Available in U.S. and Cost (U.S. $)
Aripiprazole (Abilify)	Blue		Modified rectangular, debossed on one side with "A-007" and "5".				5 mg	No	Yes
	Pink		Modified rectangular, debossed on one side with "A-008" and "10".				10 mg	No	$10.3997 each
	Yellow		Round, debossed on one side with "A-009" and "15".				15 mg	No	$10.3997 each
	White		Round, debossed on one side with "A-010" and "20".				20 mg	No	$14.5997 each
	Pink		Round, debossed on one side with "A-011" and "30".				30 mg	No	$14.8997 each
Escitalopram (Lexapro)	White to Off-White		Round, scored, film coated. Imprinted on scored side with "f" on the left side and "l" on the right side. Imprinted with "10" on the non-scored side.			Yes	10 mg	No	$2.1997 each
	White to Off-White		Round, scored, film coated. Imprinted on scored side with "f" on the left side and "l" on the right side. Imprinted with "20" on the non-scored side.			Yes	20 mg	No	$2.233 each
				Peppermint flavor.			5 mg/5 ml	No	Yes

Appendix B

Profile of Psychotropic Drugs

Antidepressants

Drug (brand name)	Color	Capsule	Tablet	Liquid	Other	Scored	Dosage Size (official)	Available in Canada and Cost (CDN $)	Available in U.S. and Cost (U.S. $)
amitriptyline (Elavil)	Blue		Round, film coated. In Canada, imprinted with MSD; 23. In U.S., imprinted with ELAVIL; 40.				10 mg	$0.0059 each	$0.383 each
	Yellow		Round, film coated. In Canada, imprinted with MSD; 45. In U.S., imprinted with ELAVIL; 45.				25 mg	$0.0079 each	$0.633 each
	Beige		Round, film coated. In Canada, imprinted with MSD; 102. In U.S., imprinted with ELAVIL; 41.				50 mg	$0.0169 each (generic only)	$0.933 each
	Orange		Round, film coated. In Canada, imprinted with MSD; 430. In U.S., imprinted with ELAVIL; 42.				75 mg	Yes	$1.29 each
	Mauve		Round, film coated, imprinted with ELAVIL; 43.				100 mg	No	$1.65 each
	Blue		Capsule shaped, film coated, imprinted with ELAVIL; 47.				150 mg	No	$2.16 each
	Light red			Oral suspension			10 mg/5 ml	Yes	No
					Injection		10 mg/ml	Yes	$15.53 for 1 vial

(cont.)

Drug (brand name)	Color	Capsule	Tablet	Liquid	Other	Scored	Dosage Size (official)	Available in Canada and Cost (CDN $)	Available in U.S. and Cost (U.S. $)
amoxapine (Asendin)	Off-white		Round, imprinted with WATSON; 379.			Yes	25 mg	No	$0.4599 each for generic
	Salmon		Round, imprinted with WATSON; 380.			Yes	50 mg	No	$0.6499 each for generic
	Blue		Round, imprinted with WATSON; 381.			Yes	100 mg	No	$1.8079 each for generic
	Peach		Round, imprinted with WATSON; 382.			Yes	150 mg	No	$2.699 each for generic
bupropion (Wellbutrin)	Yellow-gold		Coated, round, biconvex, imprinted with WELLBUTRIN; 75.				75 mg	No	$0.9799 each for brand name $0.5699 each for generic
	Red		Coated, round, biconvex, imprinted with WELLBUTRIN; 100.				100 mg	No	$1.3299 each for brand name $0.7399 each for generic
wellbutrin SR	Blue		Sustained release, coated, round, biconvex, imprinted with WELLBUTRIN SR; 100.				100 mg	$0.5333 each	$1.833 each
	Purple		Sustained release, coated, round, biconvex, imprinted with WELLBUTRIN SR; 150.				150 mg	$0.80 each	$1.933 each
citalopram (Celexa)	Beige		Coated, oval, imprinted with FP; 10 MG.				10 mg	No	$2.0416 each
	White (Canada) Pink (U.S.)		Coated, oval. In Canada, imprinted with C; N. In U.S., imprinted with FP; 20 MG.			Yes	20 mg	$1.25 each	$2.128 each
	White		Coated, oval. In Canada, imprinted with C; R. In U.S., imprinted with FP; 40 MG.			Yes	40 mg	$1.25 each	$2.2206 each
				Oral solution			10 mg/5 ml	No	$52.06 for 120 units

clomipramine (Anafanil)	Cream		Triangular, sugar coated, imprinted with GEIGY; DK	10 mg	$0.1626 each (generic price)	No
	Cream		Round, biconvex, sugar coated, imprinted with GEIGY; FH.	25 mg	$0.2215 each (generic price)	No
	Off-white		Round, beveled edge, sugar coated, imprinted with GEIGY; LP.	50 mg	$0.4078 each (generic price)	No
	Ivory and melon yellow	Yes		25 mg	No	$1.82 each for brand name $0.4999 each for generic
	Ivory and aqua blue	Yes		50 mg	No	$2.63 each for brand name $0.60 each for generic
	Ivory and yellow	Yes		75 mg	No	$3.32 each for brand name $0.84 each for generic
desipramine (Norpramine)	Blue		Round, biconvex, imprinted with 67; 7.	10 mg	No	$0.783 each
	Yellow		Round, biconvex, imprinted with NORPRAMIN; 25.	25 mg	$0.2544 each (generic price)	$0.80 each
	Green		Round, biconvex, imprinted with NORPRAMIN; 50.	50 mg	$0.411 each (generic price)	$1.41 each
	Orange		Round, biconvex, imprinted with NORPRAMIN; 75.	75 mg	$0.6334 each (generic price)	$1.93 each
	Peach		Round, biconvex, imprinted with NORPRAMIN; 100.	100 mg	No	$2.47 each
	White		Round, biconvex, imprinted with NORPRAMIN; 150.	150 mg	No	$3.54 each

(*cont.*)

Drug (brand name)	Color	Capsule	Tablet	Liquid	Other	Scored	Dosage Size (official)	Available in Canada and Cost (CDN $)	Available in U.S. and Cost (U.S. $)
doxepin (Sinequan)	Pink and red	Yes					10 mg	$0.1185 each (generic price)	$0.4699 each for brand name $0.15 each for generic
	Pink and blue	Yes					25 mg	$0.143 each (generic price)	$0.5899 each for brand name $0.1665 each for generic
	Pink and flesh (Canada) Pink and white (U.S.)	Yes					50 mg	$0.2228 each (generic price)	$0.7699 each for brand name $0.3332 each for generic
	Flesh (Canada) White (U.S.)	Yes					75 mg	$0.4774 each (generic price)	$0.40 each for generic
	Flesh and blue (Canada) Blue and white (U.S.)	Yes					100 mg	$0.627 each (generic price)	$1.40 each for brand name $0.3331 each for generic
	Blue	Yes					150 mg	No	$0.75 each for generic
				Oral liquid concentrate			10 mg/ml	No	$25.99 for 120 ml (generic price)
escitalopram*									

fluoxetine (Prozac)	Green and grey	In Canada, imprinted with LILLY; 3104; PROZAC; 10 MG. In U.S., imprinted with DISTA; 3104.	10 mg	Yes	$2.966 each for brand name $1.399 each for generic
	Green and white	In Canada, imprinted with LILLY; 3105; PROZAC; 20 MG. In U.S., imprinted with DISTA; 3105; PROZAC; 20 MG.	20 mg	$1.0112 each (generic price)	$2.966 each for brand name $1.399 each for generic
	Green and orange	Imprinted with DISTA; 3107; PROZAC 40 MG.	40 mg	No	$5.933 each for brand name $4.333 each for generic

* For data see Table A.3 in Appendix A.

(*cont.*)

Drug (brand name)	Color	Capsule	Tablet	Liquid	Other	Scored	Dosage Size (official)	Available in Canada and Cost (CDN $)	Available in U.S. and Cost (U.S. $)
	Green		Elliptical shaped, imprinted with PROZAC; 10.			Yes	10 mg	No	$2.966 each for brand name $1.399 each for generic
	Clear, colorless			Oral solution			20 mg/5 ml	Yes	$144.99 for 120 ml for brand name $99.99 for 120 ml for generic
Prozac Weekly	Green and clear	Time released, imprinted with LILLY; 3004; 90 MG.					90 mg	No	$19.25 each
fluvoxamine (Luvox)	White		Coated, elliptical, imprinted with SOLVAY; 4202.				25 mg	No	$2.766 each for brand name $1.999 each for generic
	White (Canada) Yellow (U.S.)		In Canada, coated, round, biconvex, imprinted with 291 twice on one side; In U.S., coated, elliptical, imprinted with SOLVAY; 4205.			Yes	50 mg	$0.4952 each (generic price)	$3.166 each for brand name $2.333 each for generic
	White (Canada) Beige (U.S.)		In Canada, coated, oval, biconvex, imprinted with 313 twice on one side; In U.S., coated, elliptical, imprinted with SOLVAY; 4210.			Yes	100 mg	$0.8902 each (generic price)	$3.199 each for brand name $2.366 each for generic

imipramine (Tofranil)	Coral	Triangular, coated, imprinted with GEIGY; FT in Canada/32 in U.S.	10 mg	$0.0059 each (generic price)	$0.71 each for brand name $0.18 each for generic
	Coral	Round, coated, imprinted with GEIGY; CZ in Canada/140 in U.S.	25 mg	$0.0107 each (generic price)	$0.95 each for brand name $0.11 each for generic
	Coral	Round, coated, imprinted with GEIGY; LB in Canada/136 in U.S.	50 mg	$0.186 each (generic price)	$1.79 each for brand name $0.22 each for generic
	Coral	Round, coated, imprinted with GEIGY; ATA	75 mg	Yes	No
maprotiline (Ludiomil)	Cream	Coated, round, biconvex, imprinted with CIBA; CO.	10 mg	$0.1515 each (generic price)	No
	Orange-brown (Canada) White or peach (U.S.)	In Canada, coated, round, biconvex, bevel edge, imprinted with CIBA; DP. In U.S., coated, round, or oval, imprinted with M; 60 or WATSON; 373.	25 mg	$0.2065 each (generic price)	$0.3399 each
	Brown-yellow (Canada) Blue or peach (U.S.)	In Canada, coated, round, biconvex, bevel edge, imprinted with CIBA; ER. In U.S., coated, round, or oval, imprinted with M; 87 or WATSON; 374.	50 mg	$0.3910 each (generic price)	$0.4599 each
	Red-brown (Canada) White (U.S.)	In Canada, coated, round, biconvex, bevel edge, imprinted with CIBA; FS. In U.S., coated, round, or oval, imprinted with M; 92 or WATSON; 375.	75 mg	$0.5340 each (generic price)	$0.8399 each

(cont.)

Drug (brand name)	Color	Capsule	Tablet	Liquid	Other	Scored	Dosage Size (official)	Available in Canada and Cost (CDN $)	Available in U.S. and Cost (U.S. $)
mirtazapine (Remeron)	Yellow		Coated, oval, imprinted with ORGANON; TZ3.			Yes	15 mg	No	$2.511 each
	Red-brown		Coated, oval, imprinted with ORGANON; TZ5.			Yes	30 mg	$1.24 each	$2.585 each
	White		Coated, oval, imprinted with ORGANON; TZ7.			Yes	45 mg	No	$2.751 each
(Remeron SolTab)	White		Round, orally disintegrating, imprinted with TZ1.				15 mg	No	$2.104 each
	White		Round, orally disintegrating, imprinted with TZ2.				30 mg	No	$2.085 each
	White		Round, orally disintegrating, imprinted with TZ4.				45 mg	No	$2.221 each
moclobemide (Manerix)	Pale yellow		Oval, biconvex, imprinted with ROCHE; 150.			Yes	150 mg	$0.3654 each (generic price)	No
	White		Oval, biconvex, imprinted with ROCHE; 300.			Yes	300 mg	$0.7973 each (generic price)	No
nefazodone (Serzone)	Pink		Hexagonal. In Canada, imprinted with BMS 50; 31. In U.S., imprinted with BMS 50.			No	50 mg	Yes	$1.212 each
	White		Hexagonal. In Canada, imprinted with BMS 100; 32. In U.S., imprinted with BMS 100.			Yes	100 mg	$0.80 each	$1.275 each
	Peach		Hexagonal. In Canada, imprinted with BMS 150; 39. In U.S., imprinted with BMS 150.			Yes	150 mg	$0.80 each	$1.287 each

	Yellow		Hexagonal. In Canada, imprinted with BMS 200; 33. In U.S., imprinted with BMS 200.		No	200 mg	$0.9333 each	$1.299 each
	White		Hexagonal, imprinted with BMS 250.		No	250 mg	No	$1.311 each
nortriptyline (Aventyl)	White and yellow	Imprinted with H 17.				10 mg	$0.1260 each (generic price)	$0.5899 each for brand name $0.233 each for generic
	White and yellow	Imprinted with H 19.				25 mg	$0.2547 each (generic price)	$1.0699 each for brand name $0.2165 each for generic
				Oral Solution		10 mg/5 ml	No	$66.19 for 480 ml for brand name $56.59 for 480 ml for generic
paroxetine (Paxil)	Yellow		Coated, oval, imprinted with PAXIL; 10.		Yes	10 mg	Yes	$2.699 each
	Pink		Coated, oval, imprinted with PAXIL; 20.		Yes	20 mg	$1.59 each	$2.899 each
	Blue		Coated, oval, imprinted with PAXIL; 30.			30 mg	$1.69 each	$3.033 each
	Green		Coated, oval, imprinted with PAXIL; 40.			40 mg	No	$3.199 each
	Orange			Oral suspension		10 mg/5 ml	No	$134.99 for 250 ml
(Paxil CR)	Yellow		Coated, round, controlled release, imprinted with PAXIL CR; 12.5.			12.5 mg	No	$2.571 each
	Pink		Coated, round, controlled release, imprinted with PAXIL CR; 25.			25 mg	No	$2.682 each
	Blue		Coated, round, controlled release, imprinted with PAXIL CR; 37.5.			37.5 mg	No	$2.764 each
phenelzine (Nardil)	Orange		Coated, round, imprinted with P-D, 270 in the U.S.			15 mg	$0.2999 each	$0.5199 each

(*cont.*)

Drug (brand name)	Color	Capsule	Tablet	Liquid	Other	Scored	Dosage Size (official)	Available in Canada and Cost (CDN $)	Available in U.S. and Cost (U.S. $)
sertraline (Zoloft)	Yellow	Imprinted with PFIZER; ZOLOFT 25 MG.					25 mg	$0.80 each for brand name $0.5040 each for generic	No
	White and yellow	Imprinted with PFIZER; ZOLOFT 50 MG.					50 mg	$1.60 each for brand name $1.008 each for generic	No
	Orange	Imprinted with PFIZER; ZOLOFT 100 MG.					100 mg	$1.75 each for brand name $1.1025 each for generic	No
	Light green		Coated, capsular shaped, imprinted with ZOLOFT; 25 MG.			Yes	25 mg	No	$2.366 each
	Light blue		Coated, capsular shaped, imprinted with ZOLOFT; 50 MG.			Yes	50 mg	No	$2.366 each
	Light yellow		Coated, capsular shaped, imprinted with ZOLOFT; 100 MG.			Yes	100 mg	No	$2.366 each
	Clear			Oral concentrate			20 mg/ml	No	$58.39 for 60 ml
tranylcypromine (Parnate)	Red		Coated, round, biconvex. In Canada, imprinted with SKF; N71. In U.S., imprinted with PARNATE; SB.				10 mg	$0.3341 each	$0.6437 each
trazodone (Desyrel)	Orange		Coated, round, imprinted with DESYREL			Yes	50 mg	$0.2214 each	$1.786 each for brand name / $0.1366 each for generic
	White		Coated, round, imprinted with DESYREL			Yes	100 mg	$0.3956 each	$3.222 each for brand name / $0.155 each for generic

	Orange		Rectangular. In Canada, imprinted with BL BL; 50 50 50. In U.S., imprinted with MJ 778; 50 50 50.	Yes—trisected and bisected	150 mg	$0.5812 each	$2.776 each for brand name / $0.4039 each for generic
	Yellow		Rectangular, imprinted with MJ 776; 100100 100.	Yes—trisected and bisected.	300 mg	No	$4.9836 each
trimipramine (Surmontil)	Pink				12.5 mg	$0.0820 each for generic	No
	Pink		Imprinted with 25		25 mg	$0.1040 each for generic	No
	Pink		Coated; Imprinted with 50		50 mg	$0.1999 each for generic	No
	Pink		Coated; Imprinted with 100		100 mg	$0.3418 each for generic	No
	Blue and yellow	Imprinted with OP; 718.			25 mg	No	$0.95 each
	Blue and orange	Imprinted with OP; 719.			50 mg	No	$1.62 each
	Blue and white	Imprinted with OP; 720.			100 mg	No	$2.05 each
	Pink and peach	Imprinted with P; 75 MG.			75 mg	0.5197 each	No
venlafaxine (Effexor XR)	Grey and peach	Extended release, imprinted with W EFFEXOR XR; 37.5.			37.5 mg	$0.780 each	$2.019 each

(*cont.*)

Drug (brand name)	Color	Capsule	Tablet	Liquid	Other	Scored	Dosage Size (official)	Available in Canada and Cost (CDN $)	Available in U.S. and Cost (U.S. $)
	Peach	Extended release, imprinted with w EFFEXOR XR; 75.					75 mg	$1.560 each	$2.239 each
	Dark orange	Extended release, imprinted with w EFFEXOR XR; 150.					150 mg	$1.650 each	$2.432 each
(Effexor)	Peach		Shield shaped, imprinted with 25 w; 701.			Yes	25 mg	No	$1.194 each
	Peach		Shield shaped, imprinted with 37.5 w; 781.			Yes	37.5 mg	Yes	$1.23 each
	Peach		Shield shaped, imprinted with 50 w; 703.			Yes	50 mg	No	$1.266 each
	Peach		Shield shaped, imprinted with 75 w; 704.			Yes	75 mg	Yes	$1.343 each
	Peach		Shield shaped, imprinted with 100 w; 705.			Yes	100 mg	No	$1.423 each

Antipsychotics

Drug (brand name)	Color	Capsule	Tablet	Liquid	Other	Scored	Dosage Size (official)	Available in Canada and Cost (CDN $)	Available in U.S. and Cost (U.S. $)
aripiprazole*									
chlorpromazine (in Canada, Largactil; in the U.S., Thorazine)	Opaque orange with natural body	Extended release, imprinted with SKF and T63.					30 mg	No	$1.20 each
	Opaque orange with natural body	Extended release, imprinted with SKF and T64.					75 mg	No	$1.60 each
	Opaque orange with natural body	Extended release, imprinted with SKF and T66.					150 mg	No	$2.10 each
	White (Canada) Orange (U.S.)		In Canada, generic only. In U.S., round, imprinted with SKF and T73.				10 mg	$0.0080 each for generic	$0.43 each
	White (Canada) Orange (U.S.)		In Canada, generic only. In U.S., round, imprinted with SKF and T74.				25 mg	$0.0092 each for generic	$0.58 each
	White (Canada) Orange (U.S.)		In Canada, generic only. In U.S., round, imprinted with SKF and T76.				50 mg	$0.0141 each for generic	$0.72 each

* For data see Table A.3 in Appendix A.

(cont.)

Drug (brand name)	Color	Capsule	Tablet	Liquid	Other	Scored	Dosage Size (official)	Available in Canada and Cost (CDN $)	Available in U.S. and Cost (U.S. $)
	White (Canada) Orange (U.S.)		In Canada, generic only. In U.S., round, imprinted with SKF and T77.				100 mg	$0.0221 each (generic only)	$0.92 each
	Orange		Round, imprinted with SKF and T79.				200 mg	No	$1.155 each
	Clear			Syrup			5 mg/ml	$0.0238	$28.43 for 120 ml bottle
	Yellow			Syrup			20 mg/ml	$0.0346	No
	Brown			Oral drops			40 mg/ml	$0.2702	No
					Suppository, imprinted with SKF and T70.		25 mg	No	$44.24 for box of 12
					Suppository, imprinted with SKF and T71.		100 mg	$1.8050	$55.53 for box of 12
					Solution for injection (ampoules or multi-dose vials).		25 mg/ml	$0.9700	$104.99 for 10 ml
clozapine (Clozaril)	Pale yellow		Round, compressed, embossed, imprinted with CLOZARIL; 25 (MG in Canada only).			Yes	25 mg	$2.75 each	$1.5629 each
	Pale yellow		Round, compressed, embossed, imprinted with CLOZARIL; 100 (MG in Canada only).			Yes	100 mg	$2.75 each	$4.0959 each

fluphenazine hydrochloride, (Prolixin (U.S.))	White	Round, biconvex, imprinted with PPP and 863.			1 mg	No	$1.14 each
	Generic only (Canada) Blue (U.S.)	Round, biconvex, imprinted with PPP and 864.			2.5 mg	No	$1.57 each
	Green	Round, biconvex, imprinted with PPP and 877.			5 mg	No	$1.91 each
	Pink	Round, biconvex, imprinted with PPP and 956.			10 mg	No	$2.49 each
	Orange		Oral elixir		0.5 mg/ml	No	$26.48 for 60 ml bottle
	N/A		Oral liquid concentrate		5 mg/ml	No	$180.99 for 120 ml
				Solution for injection	2.5 mg/ml	No	Yes
modecate concentrate (Canada)				Solution for injection	100 mg/ml	$29.78	No
modecate (Canada)				Solution for injection	25 mg/ml	$23.16	No
moditen enanthate (Canada)				Solution for injection	25 mg/ml	$43.55	No
moditen hydrochloride (Canada)	Clear		Oral elixir		0.5 mg/ml	$0.0310	No
	Pink	Round, biconvex.			1 mg	$0.0899 each	No
	Coral	Round, biconvex.			2 mg	$0.1077 each	No
	White	Round, biconvex.			5 mg	$0.01618 each	No

(*cont.*)

Drug (brand name)	Color	Capsule	Tablet	Liquid	Other	Scored	Dosage Size (official)	Available in Canada and Cost (CDN $)	Available in U.S. and Cost (U.S. $)
haloperidol (Haldol, U.S.)	White		Horse-shoe shaped with "H" cut out on center. Imprinted with MCNEIL; 1/2; HALDOL.			Yes	0.5 mg	No	$0.05 each for generic price
	Yellow		Horse-shoe shaped with "H" cut out on center. Imprinted with MCNEIL; 1; HALDOL.			Yes	1 mg	No	$0.07 each for generic price
	Pink		Horse-shoe shaped with "H" cut out on center. Imprinted with MCNEIL; 2; HALDOL.			Yes	2 mg	No	$0.10 each for generic price
	Green		Horse-shoe shaped with "H" cut out on center. Imprinted with MCNEIL; 5; HALDOL.			Yes	5 mg	No	$0.16 each for generic price
	Aqua		Horse-shoe shaped with "H" cut out on center. Imprinted with MCNEIL; 10; HALDOL.			Yes	10 mg	No	$0.16 each for generic price
	Salmon		Horse-shoe shaped with "H" cut out on center. Imprinted with MCNEIL; 20; HALDOL.			Yes	20 mg	No	$0.16 each for generic price
haloperidol lactate (Haldol, U.S.)	Clear			Oral liquid concentrate			2 mg/ml	No	$36.29 for 15 ml
					Intramuscular injection		5 mg/ml	No	$106.09 for 10 ml
haloperidol decanoate (Haldol decanoate, U.S.)					Intramuscular injection		50 mg/ml	No	$48.19 for 1 ml
					Intramuscular injection		100 mg/ml	No	$84.99 for 1 ml

haloperidol (Haldol, Canada)	Yellow		Round, biconcave, with beveled edges. Imprinted with MCNEIL; 1.			Yes	1 mg	$0.0614 each for generic price	No
	Pink		Round, biconcave, with beveled edges. Imprinted with MCNEIL; 2.			Yes	2 mg	$0.105 each for generic price	No
	Green		Round, biconcave, with beveled edges. Imprinted with MCNEIL; 5.			Yes	5 mg	$0.1487 each for generic price	No
	Aqua		Round, biconcave, with beveled edges. Imprinted with MCNEIL; 10.			Yes	10 mg	$0.133 each for generic price	No
	Salmon		Round, biconcave, with beveled edges. Imprinted with MCNEIL; 20.			Yes	20 mg	$0.6304 each for generic price	No
	Clear			Oral solution			2 mg/ml	$0.1073	No
					Solution for injection		5 mg/ml	$2.490 for 1 ml	No
haloperidol decanoate (Haldol–LA, Canada)	Amber				Solution for injection		50 mg/ml	$29.5190 for 5 ml	No
	Amber				Solution for injection		100 mg/ml	$11.6648 for 1 ml	No
loxapine (Loxitane, U.S.)	Dark green	Imprinted with W; WATSON; LOXITANE; 5 MG.					5 mg	No	$1.12 each
	Dark green and yellow	Imprinted with W; WATSON; LOXITANE; 10 MG.					10 mg	No	$1.42 each

(cont.)

Drug (brand name)	Color	Capsule	Tablet	Liquid	Other	Scored	Dosage Size (official)	Available in Canada and Cost (CDN $)	Available in U.S. and Cost (U.S. $)
	Dark green and light green	Imprinted with W; WATSON; LOXITANE; 25 MG.					25 mg	No	$2.07 each
	Dark green and blue	Imprinted with W; WATSON; LOXITANE; 50 MG.					50 mg	No	$2.76 each
loxapine (Loxitane C, U.S.)				Oral concentrated solution (120 ml bottle with dropper)			25 mg/ml	No	$291.27 per bottle
loxapine (Loxitane IM, U.S.)					Intramuscular solution for injection		50 mg/ml	No	Yes
loxapine (Loxapac, Canada)	Yellow		Round, biconvex.			Yes	5 mg	$0.15 each	No
	Green		Round, biconvex.			Yes	10 mg	$0.2498 each	No
	Pink		Round, biconvex.			Yes	25 mg	$0.3872 each for generic price	No
	White		Round, biconvex.			Yes	50 mg	$0.5162 each	No
	Clear, colorless			Oral liquid concentrate			25 mg/ml	$0.5232 each for generic price	No
					Injection		50 mg/ml	Yes	No

molindone (Moban	Orange	Round, biconvex, imprinted with NDC 63481-072; MOBAN 5.		5 mg	No	$1.102 each
	Lavender	Round, biconvex, imprinted with NDC 63481-073; MOBAN 10.		10 mg	No	$1.578 each
	Green	Round, biconvex, imprinted with NDC 63481-074; MOBAN 25.		25 mg	No	$2.438 each
	Blue	Round, biconvex, imprinted with NDC 63481-076; MOBAN 50.		50 mg	No	$3.04 each
	Tan	Round, biconvex, imprinted with NDC 63481-077; MOBAN 100.		100 mg	No	$4.056 each
	Clear		Oral liquid concentrate	20 mg/ml	No	$237.95 for 120 ml bottle
olanzapine (Zyprexa)	White with blue ink	Coated, round, imprinted with LILLY; 4112.		2.5 mg	$1.6875 each	$5.133 each
	White with blue ink	Coated, round, imprinted with LILLY; 4115.		5 mg	$3.375 each	$5.833 each
	White with blue ink	Coated, round, imprinted with LILLY; 4116.		7.5 mg	$5.0625 each	$6.399 each
	White with blue ink	Coated, round, imprinted with LILLY; 4117.		10 mg	$6.75 each	$8.733 each
	Blue	Coated, round, imprinted with LILLY; 4415.		15 mg	No	$13.266 each
	Red	Coated, round, imprinted with LILLY; 4420.		20 mg	No	$15.977 each
(Zyprexa Zydis)	Yellow	Round, orally disintegrating, imprinted with 5.		5 mg	No	Yes
	Yellow	Round, orally disintegrating, imprinted with 10.		10 mg	No	Yes
	Yellow	Round, orally disintegrating, imprinted with 15.		15 mg	No	Yes
	Yellow	Round, orally disintegrating, imprinted with 20.		20 mg	No	Yes
perphenazine (Trilafon*)	Various—white or grey	Coated, round.		2 mg	$0.0158 each	$0.2799 each

* Only generic available

(*cont.*)

Drug (brand name)	Color	Capsule	Tablet	Liquid	Other	Scored	Dosage Size (official)	Available in Canada and Cost (CDN $)	Available in U.S. and Cost (U.S. $)
perphenazine (U.S.); Apo-perphenazine PMS, perphenazine (Canada)	Various—white or grey		Coated, round.				4 mg	$0.0168 each	$0.3699 each
	Various—white or grey		Coated, round.				8 mg	$0.0201 each	$0.4399 each
	Various—white or grey		Coated, round.				16 mg	$0.0291 each	$0.6499 each
	Clear			Oral concentrate			16 mg/5 ml or 3.2 mg/ml	$0.2201	Yes
quetiapine (Seroquel)	Peach		Coated, round, biconvex, imprinted with SEROQUEL 25 on one side.				25 mg	$0.48 each	$1.68 each
	Yellow		Coated, round, biconvex, imprinted with SEROQUEL 100 on one side.				100 mg	$1.28 each	$2.83 each
	Pale yellow		Coated, round, biconvex, imprinted with SEROQUEL 150 on one side.				150 mg	Yes	Yes
	White		Coated, round, biconvex, imprinted with SEROQUEL 200 on one side.				200 mg	$2.57 each	$5.15 each
	White		Coated, round, biconvex, imprinted with SEROQUEL 300 on one side.				300 mg	Yes	Yes
risperidone (Risperdal)	Dark yellow		Oblong, biconvex, imprinted with RIS; 0.25.				0.25 mg	$0.415 each	$2.46 each
	Brown-red		Oblong, biconvex, imprinted with RIS; 0.5.			Half-scored	0.5 mg	$0.695 each	$3.00 each

	White	Oblong, biconvex, imprinted with RIS; 1.		Yes	1 mg	$0.96 each	$3.00 each
	Orange	Oblong, biconvex, imprinted with RIS; 2.		Yes	2 mg	$1.9166 each	$4.83 each
	Yellow	Oblong, biconvex, imprinted with RIS; 3.		Yes	3 mg	$2.875 each	$5.65 each
	Green	Oblong, biconvex, imprinted with RIS; 4.		Yes	4 mg	$3.83 each	$7.35 each
			Oral solution		1 mg/ml	$1.104	$108.99 for 30 ml
thioridazine (Mellaril*)	Various—orange, yellow, beige, yellowish-green, green	Various—round or triangular.			10 mg	$0.0143 each	$0.1099 each
thioridazine, thioridazine HCL, thioridazine hydrochloride (U.S.)	Various—orange, blue, white	Round.			15 mg	No	$0.2899 each
APO—thioridazine, novoridazine,	Various—orange, yellow, brown	Round.			25 mg	$0.268 each	$0.1299 each
PMS—thioridazine (Canada)	Various—orange, pink, white, yellow	Various—round or triangular.			50 mg	$0.0486 each	$0.1599 each
	Various—orange, white, green, greenish-grey	Round.			100 mg	$0.0974 each	$0.2199 each

* Only generic available

(*cont.*)

Drug (brand name)	Color	Capsule	Tablet	Liquid	Other	Scored	Dosage Size (official)	Available in Canada and Cost (CDN $)	Available in U.S. and Cost (U.S. $)
	Various—orange or green		Round				150 mg	No	$0.9665 each
	Various—orange, light blue		Round				200 mg	Yes	$0.9165 each
	Clear			Oral Solution			30 mg/ml	$0.1044	$21.19 for 120 ml
	Clear			Oral Solution			100 mg/ml	No	$45.39 for 120 ml
				Oral Solution			2 mg/ml	$0.0184	No
thiothixene* (Navane)	Various—yellow; orange and yellow; white, orange, and gold; tan and blue	Yes					1 mg	No	$0.1999 each
	Various—light green; green and yellow; white, blue and gold; tan and yellow; white	Yes					2 mg	$0.1856 each	$0.2699 each

	Various—orange; orange and white; white, orange, and black; tan and white	Yes			5 mg	$0.3193 each	$0.3499 each
	Various—white; green and white; black and blue; tan and peach; orange	Yes			10 mg	$0.4111 each	$0.4099 each
ziprasidone (Geodon)	Blue and white	Yes			20 mg	No	$3.88 each
		Yes			40 mg	No	$3.88 each
		Yes			60 mg	No	$3.88 each
		Yes			80 mg	No	$3.88 each
zuclopenthixol (Clopixol)	Light red-brown		Round, biconvex, film coated.		10 mg	$0.40 each	No
	Red-brown		Round, biconvex, film coated.		25 mg	$1.00 each	No
	Dark red-brown		Round, biconvex, film coated.		40 mg	$1.59 each	No
(Clopixol Acuphase)				Injection	50 mg/ml	$154.00 for 10 ml vial	No
(Clopixol depot)				Injection	200 mg/ml	$15.40 for one 1 ml ampoule	
						$28.60 for one 2 ml ampoule	No

* Only generic available

APPENDIX B

Anxiolytics/Hypnotics

Drug (brand name)	Color	Capsule	Tablet	Liquid	Other	Scored	Dosage Size (official)	Available in Canada and Cost (CDN $)	Available in U.S. and Cost (U.S. $)
alprazolam (Xanax)	White		Oval. In Canada, imprinted with UPJOHN 29. In U.S., imprinted with XANAX 0.25.			Yes	0.25 mg	$0.076 each (generic price)	$0.867 each for brand name $0.12 each for generic
	Peach		Oval. In Canada, imprinted with UPJOHN 55. In U.S., imprinted with XANAX 0.5.			Yes	0.5 mg	$0.920 each (generic price)	$1.072 each for brand name $0.12 each for generic
	Lavender (Canada) Blue (U.S.)		Oval. In Canada, imprinted with UPJOHN 90. In U.S., imprinted with XANAX 1.0			Yes	1 mg	Yes	$1.378 each for brand name $0.12 each for generic
(Xanax TS (Canada) Xanax (U.S.))	White		Oblong, imprinted with XANAX; 2.			Tri-scored	2 mg	Yes	$2.425 each for brand name $0.19 each for generic
Buspirone (Buspar)	White		Ovoid-rectangular, embossed with company logo; BUSPAR; 5.			Yes	5 mg	No	$0.7843 each for brand name $0.5553 each for generic
	White		Ovoid-rectangular, embossed with company logo; BUSPAR; 10.			Yes	10 mg	Yes	$1.3514 each for brand name $0.8164 each for generic
	White		Ovoid-rectangular, embossed with 822; 5; 5; 5.			can be bisected or tri-sected	15 mg	No	$2.0433 each for brand name $0.896 each for generic
	Pink		Ovoid-rectangular, embossed with 824; 10; 10; 10.			can be bisected or tri-sected	30 mg	No	$3.731 each for brand name $1.491 each for generic

chloral hydrate		Yes		Yes		500 mg 100 mg/ml	$0.316 each Yes	$0.933 each $8.99 for 90 ml
clonazepam Rivotril; (Canada, Klonopin) (U.S.)	Orange		In Canada, cylindrical, biplane, beveled edges, imprinted with ROCHE 0.5. In U.S., round, K-shaped perforation, imprinted with ROCHE; 1/2 KLONOPIN.		Yes	0.5 mg	$0.1166 each for generic price	$0.848 each for brand name $0.221 each for generic
	Blue		Round, K-shaped perforation, imprinted with ROCHE; 1 KLONOPIN.		Yes	1 mg	No	$0.965 each for brand name $0.243 each for generic
	White		In Canada, cylindrical, biplane, beveled edges, imprinted with ROCHE 2. In U.S., round, K-shaped perforation, imprinted with ROCHE; 2 KLONOPIN.		Yes	2 mg	$0.2010 each for generic price	$1.33 each for brand name $0.265 each for generic
diazepam (Valium)	White		Round, flat-faced, V-shaped perforation, beveled edges, imprinted with 2 VALIUM; ROCHE.		Yes	2 mg	No	$0.583 each for brand name $0.12 each for generic
	Yellow		In Canada, cylindrical, biplane, beveled edges imprinted with ROCHE 5. In U.S., round, flat-faced, V-shaped perforation, beveled edges, imprinted with 5 VALIUM; ROCHE.		Yes	5 mg	$0.0061 each for generic price	$0.855 each for brand name $0.155 each for generic
	Blue		Round, flat-faced, V-shaped perforation, beveled edges, imprinted with 10 VALIUM; ROCHE.		Yes	10 mg	No	$1.45 each for brand name $0.155 each for generic
estazolam (Prosom)	White		Imprinted with UC; Abbott Logo.		Yes	1 mg	No	$1.3245 each for brand name $0.7813 each for generic

(*cont.*)

Drug (brand name)	Color	Capsule	Tablet	Liquid	Other	Scored	Dosage Size (official)	Available in Canada and Cost (CDN $)	Available in U.S. and Cost (U.S. $)
	Pink		Imprinted with UD; Abbott Logo.			Yes	2 mg	No	$1.4692 each for brand name $0.861 each for generic
lorazepam (Ativan)	White		In Canada, round, imprinted with 0.5; W. In U.S., 5-sided, with a raised "A," imprinted with WYETH; 81.				0.5 mg	$0.0467 each	$0.8453 each for brand name $0.3751 each for generic
	White		In Canada, oblong, imprinted with 1; ATIVAN. In U.S., 5-sided, with a raised "A," imprinted with WYETH; 64.			Yes	1 mg	$0.476 each	$1.0672 each for brand name $0.478 each for generic
	White		In Canada, ovoid, imprinted with 2; ATIVAN. In U.S., 5-sided, with a raised "A," imprinted with WYETH; 65.			Yes	2 mg	$0.0774 each	$1.579 each for brand name $0.672 each for generic
	Pale green		Sublingual, round, flat, imprinted with w; 0.5.				0.5 mg	$0.0395 each for generic price	No
	White		Sublingual, round, flat, imprinted with w; 1.				1 mg	$0.0447 each for generic price	No
	Blue		Sublingual, round, flat, imprinted with w; 2.				2 mg	$0.0699 each for generic price	No
					Solution for injection		2 mg/ml	No	Yes
					Solution for injection		4 mg/ml	Yes	Yes
midazolam (Versed)					Solution for injection		1 mg/ml	Yes	Yes
					Solution for injection		5 mg/ml	Yes	$50.19 for 10 ml
	Red			Oral syrup			2 mg/ml	No	$168.89 for 118 ml
Apo-oxazepam Oxazepam (Canada), Serax (U.S.)	Pale yellow		Round, flat-faced, with beveled edge.			Yes	10 mg	$0.01 each for generic price	No

	Orange-yellow (Canada)		In Canada, round, flat-faced, with beveled edge.	Yes	15 mg	$0.0105 each for generic price	$1.1939 each
	Yellow (U.S.)		In U.S., pentagonal, imprinted with S; 15; WYETH; 317.				
	White		Round, flat-faced, with beveled edge.	Yes	30 mg	$0.0135 each for generic price	No
	Pink and white	Imprinted with SERAX; 10; 51; WYETH.			10 mg	No	$0.9831 each for brand name $0.3303 each for generic
	Red and white	Imprinted with SERAX; 15; 6; WYETH.			15 mg	No	$1.2431 each for brand name $0.4153 each for generic
	Maroon and white	Imprinted with SERAX; 30; 52; WYETH.			30 mg	No	$1.7771 each for brand name $0.684 each for generic
temazepam (Restoril)	Blue and pink	Imprinted with RESTORIL 7.5 MG; FOR SLEEP.			7.5 mg	No	$1.164 each
	Maroon and pink	In Canada, imprinted with SANDOZ; RESTORIL 15.			15 mg	$0.1102 each for generic price	$1.0223 each

(cont.)

Drug (brand name)	Color	Capsule	Tablet	Liquid	Other	Scored	Dosage Size (official)	Available in Canada and Cost (CDN $)	Available in U.S. and Cost (U.S. $)
		In U.S., imprinted with RESTORIL 15 MG; FOR SLEEP.							
	Maroon and blue	In Canada, imprinted with SANDOZ; RESTORIL 30. In U.S., imprinted with RESTORIL 30 MG; FOR SLEEP.					30 mg	$0.1326 each for generic price	$1.164 each for brand name $0.353 each for generic
triazolam (Halcion)	White		Elliptical. In the U.S., imprinted with HALCION 0.125.				0.125 mg	$0.0556 each for generic price	$1.09 each
	Powder blue		Elliptical. In Canada, imprinted with Upjohn 17. In the U.S., imprinted with HALCION 0.25.			Yes	0.25 mg	$0.07 each for generic price	$1.193 each

zaleplon (Canada), Starnoc Sonata (U.S.)	Light brown and white (Canada)	In Canada, gold stripe on body.			5 mg	Yes	$1.7555 each
	Green and pale green (U.S.)	In U.S., imprinted with 5 MG; SONATA.					
	White (Canada)	In Canada, pink stripe on body.			10 mg	Yes	$2.1442 each
	Green and light green (U.S.)	In U.S., imprinted with 10 MG; SONATA.					
zolpidem (Ambien)	Pink		Tablet-shaped, film coated, debossed with AMB 5; 5401.		5 mg	No	$1.82 each
	White		Tablet-shaped, film coated, debossed with AMB 10; 5421.		10 mg	No	$2.2354 each
zopiclone (Imovane)	White		Round, marked IMOVANE 5.		5 mg	Yes	No
	Blue		Oval, marked IMOVANE.	Yes	7.5 mg	Yes	No

Mood Stabilizers

Drug (brand name)	Color	Capsule	Tablet	Liquid	Other	Scored	Dosage Size (official)	Available in Canada and Cost (CDN $)	Available in U.S. and Cost (U.S. $)
carbamazepine (Tegretol)	White with red speckles (Canada)		Round, chewable.			Yes	100 mg	$0.1223 each	$0.2723 each for brand name
	Pink with red speckles (U.S.)		In Canada, imprinted with GEIGY; M/R. In U.S., imprinted with TEGRETOL; 52.						$0.1652 each for generic
	White with red speckles		Oval, chewable, imprinted with GEIGY; P.U.			Yes	200 mg	$0.2413 each	No
	White (Canada) Pink (U.S.)		In Canada, round, imprinted with GEIGY. In U.S., capsule-shaped, imprinted with TEGRETOL; 27.			In Canada, quadri-sected. In U.S., single-scored.	200 mg	$0.0795 each	$0.5108 each for brand name $0.175 each for generic
	Orange			Oral solution			100 mg/ 5 ml	$0.0578	$66.20 for 900 units
tegretol CR (Canada)	Yellow		Extended release, round, imprinted with T, 100 MG.				100 mg	No	$0.2716 each
Tegretol-XR (U.S.)	Beige-orange (Canada) Pink (U.S.)		Extended release. In Canada, oval, imprinted with C/G; H/C. In U.S., round, imprinted with T; 200 MG.				200 mg	$0.1887 each	$0.5193 each

	Brown-orange (Canada) Brown (U.S.)		Extended release. In Canada, oval, imprinted with CG/CG; ENE/ENE. In U.S., round, imprinted with T; 400 MG.	Yes	400 mg	$0.3775 each	$1.0083 each
divalproex sodium/ valproic acid Epival; (Canada), Depakote (U.S.)	Salmon-pink		Enteric coated.		125 mg	$0.153 each for generic price	$0.4428 each
	Peach		Enteric coated.		250 mg	$0.2750 each for generic price	$0.8369 each
	Lavender		Enteric coated.		500 mg	$0.5503 each for generic price	$1.5179 each
Epival ER (Canada) Depakote ER (U.S.)	Grey		Extended release.		500 mg	Yes	$1.5892 each
gabapentin (Neurontin)	White	Imprinted with PD; NEURONTIN/ 100 MG.			100 mg	$0.40 each	$0.4418 each
	Yellow	Imprinted with PD; NEURONTIN/ 300 MG.			300 mg	$0.9730 each	$1.1046 each
	Orange	Imprinted with PD; NEURONTIN/ 400 MG.			400 mg	$1.1595 each	$1.3253 each

(cont.)

Drug (brand name)	Color	Capsule	Tablet	Liquid	Other	Scored	Dosage Size (official)	Available in Canada and Cost (CDN $)	Available in U.S. and Cost (U.S. $)
	White		Film-coated, elliptical, NEURONTIN 600 printed in black ink.				600 mg	Yes	$1.8226 each
	White (Canada) Orange (U.S.)		Film-coated, elliptical, NEURONTIN 800 printed in orange ink in Canada/in black ink in U.S.				800 mg	Yes	$2.187 each
	Pale yellow			Oral solution			250 mg/ 5 ml	No	$96.16 for 470 ml bottle
lamotrigine Lamictal (Canada); Lamictal CD (U.S.)	White		Round, chewable, dispersible, debossed with LTG; 2.				2 mg	Yes	Yes
	White		Chewable, dispersible, caplet-shaped.				5 mg	Yes	$3.0669 each
	White		Chewable, dispersible, super-elliptical-shaped, debossed with GX CL5.				25 mg	No	Yes
(Lamictal)	White		Shield shaped, debossed with LAMICTAL; 25.			Yes	25 mg	$0.3315 each	$2.1583 each
	Peach		Shield shaped, debossed with LAMICTAL; 100.			Yes	100 mg	$1.3260 each	$2.4988 each
	Cream		Shield shaped, debossed with LAMICTAL; 150.			Yes	150 mg	$1.9890 each	$2.6259 each
	Blue		Shield shaped, debossed with LAMICTAL; 200.			Yes	200 mg	No	$2.7524 each

lithium carbonate Carbolith, (Canada), Lithane; Eskalith, Eskalith CR, Lithobid (U.S.)	Various	Yes				150 mg	$0.633 each for generic price	Generic only
	Various	Yes				300 mg	$0.664 each for generic price	$0.2999 each
(Carbolith)	Aqua-blue	Imprinted with ICN C13.				600 mg	Yes	No
(Lithobid)	Peach		Slow release, imprinted with SOLVAY 4492.			300 mg	No	$0.382 each
(Eskalith CR)	Yellow		Round, biconvex, debossed with SKF and J10.		Yes	450 mg	No	$0.6099 each
(Lithium citrate)				Oral syrup		300 mg/ 5 ml	No	$20.58 for 480 ml
topiramate (Topamax)	White and clear	Sprinkle capsule, imprinted with TOP; 15 MG.				15 mg	$1.00 each	$1.16798 each
	White and clear	Sprinkle capsule, imprinted with TOP; 25 MG.				25 mg	$1.05 each	$2.0165 each
	White		Round, coated, imprinted with TOP; 25.			25 mg	$1.05 each	$1.262 each
	Yellow		Round, coated, imprinted with TOPAMAX; 100.			100 mg	$1.99 each	$2.9586 each
	Salmon		Round, coated, imprinted with TOPAMAX; 200.			200 mg	$3.15 each	$3.3184 each

Cognitive Enhancers

Drug (brand name)	Color	Capsule	Tablet	Liquid	Other	Scored	Dosage Size (official)	Available in Canada and Cost (CDN $)	Available in U.S. and Cost (U.S. $)
donepezil (Aricept)	White		Round, film coated, ARICEPT debossed on one side, and STRENGTH debossed on the other.				5 mg	$4.59 each	$3.97 each
	Yellow		Round, film coated, ARICEPT debossed on one side, and debossed on the other.				10 mg	$4.59 each	$3.97 each
galantamine (Reminyl)	Off-white		Round, coated, biconvex, imprinted with JANSSEN; G4.				4 mg	$2.30 each	$1.9332 each
	Pink		Round, coated, biconvex, imprinted with JANSSEN; G8.				8 mg	$2.30 each	$1.9332 each
	Orange-brown		Round, coated, biconvex, imprinted with JANSSEN; G12.				12 mg	$2.30 each	$1.9332 each
rivastigmine (Exelon)	Yellow	STRENGTH and EXELON printed in red on capsule.					1.5 mg	$2.2950 each	$2.1174 each

Orange	STRENGTH and EXELON printed in red on capsule.		3.0 mg	$2.2950 each	$2.1174 each
Red	STRENGTH and EXELON printed in white on capsule.		4.5 mg	$2.2950 each	$2.1174 each
Orange and red	STRENGTH and EXELON printed in red on capsule.		6.0 mg	$2.2950 each	$2.1174 each
Clear yellow		Oral solution (120 ml)	2 mg/ml	No	Yes

APPENDIX B

References

INTRODUCTION

General

American Psychiatric Association. *Diagnostic and Statistical Manual of Mental Disorders-IV.* Washington, DC: Anthor; 1994.

Aparasu R, Mort J, Sitzman S. Psychotropic prescribing for the elderly in office-based practice. *Clin therapeutics.* 1998;20:603–616.

Blazer D, Hybels C, Simonsick E, Hanlon J. Marked differences in antidepressant use by race in an elderly community sample: 1986–1996. *Am J Psychiatry.* 2000;957:1089–1094.

Dubovsky S, Maxmen J, Ward N. *Psychotropic Drugs: Fast Facts* (third edition). New York: Norton; 2002.

Golden A, Preston R, Barnett S, Llorente M, Hamdan K, Silverman M. Inappropriate medication prescribing in homebound older adults. *JAGS.* 1999;47:948–953.

Hesse K, Driscoll A, Jacobson S. Neuroleptic prescriptions for acutely ill geriatric patients. *Arch Int Med.* 1993;153:2581–2587.

Jacobson S, Pies R, Greenblatt D. *Handbook of Geriatric Psychopharmacology.* Washington, DC: American Psychiatric Publishing, Inc.; 2002.

Katz I, Oslin D, eds. *Annual Review of Gerontology and Geriatrics: Focus on Psychopharmacologic Interventions in Late Life.* New York: Springer; 1999.

Koenig H, Meador K. Dosing recommendations and prescribing patterns for depressed medically ill hospitalized older patients. *J Am Geriatr Soc.* 1997; 45:1409.

Lasser R, Sunderland T. Newer psychotropic medication use in nursing home residents. *JAGS.* 1998;46:202–207.

Medical Economics Staff, ed. *Physicians' Desk Reference.* Montvale, NJ: Medical Economics Company; 2002.

Salzman C, ed. *Clinical Geriatric Psychopharmacology.* Baltimore, MD: Williams and Wilkins; 1998.

Salzman C. *Psychiatric Medications for Older Adults: The Concise Guide.* New York: Guilford Press; 2001.

Taylor D, Lader M. Cytochromes and psychotropic drug interactions. *Br J Psychiatry.* 1996;168:529–532.

Turnnheim K. When drug therapy gets old: pharmacokinetics and pharmacodynamics in the elderly. *Exp Gerontol.* 2003;38 (8):843–53.

Verbeeck R, Cardinal J, Wallace S. Effect of age and sex on the plasma binding of acidic and basic drugs. *Eur J Pharmacol.* 1984;27:91–97.

Zimmerman M, Mattis J, Pasternak M. Are subjects in pharmacological treatment trials of depression representative of patients in routine clinical practice? *Am J Psychiatry.* 2002;159:469–473.

ANTIDEPRESSANTS

Abrams R, Alexopoulos G, Spielman L, Klausner E, Kakuma T. Personality disorder symptoms predict declines in global functioning and quality of life in elderly depressed patients. *Am J Geriatr Psychiatry.* 2001;9:67–71.

Altshuler L, Bauer M, Frye M, Gitlin M, Mintz J, Szuba M, Leight K, Whybrow P. Does thyroid supplementation accelerate tricyclic antidepressant response? A review & meta-analysis of the literature. *Am J Psychiatry.* 2001;158:1617–1622.

Anstey K, Brodaty H. Antidepressants and the elderly: Double-blind trials 1987–1992. *Int J Ger Psychiatry.* 1995;10:265–279.

Freund KM, Moskowitz MA, Lin TH, McKinlay JB. Early antidepressant therapy for elderly patients. *Am J Med.* 2003;114 (1):15–9.

Hubbard R, Farrington P, Smith C, Smeeth L, Tattersfield A. Exposure to tricyclic and selective serotonin reuptake inhibitor antidepressants and the risk of hip fracture. *Am J Epidemiol.*. 2003;158 (1):77–84.

Kaldyand J, Tarnove L. A Clinical Practice Guideline approach to treating depression in long-term care. *J Am Med Dir Assoc.* 2003;4 (2 Suppl):S60–8.

Lenze EJ. Comorbidity of depression and anxiety in the elderly. *Curr Psychiatry Rep.* 2003;5 (1):62–7.

Ramaekers JG. Antidepressants and driver impairment: Empirical evidence from a standard on-the-road test. *J Clin Psychiatry.* 2003;64 (1):20–9.

Sambamoorthi U, Olfson M, Walkup JT, Crystal S. Diffusion of new generation antidepressant treatment among elderly diagnosed with depression. *Med Care.* 2003;41 (1):180–94.

Sauer WH, Berlin JA, Kimmel SE. Effect of antidepressants and their relative affinity for the serotonin transporter on the risk of myocardial infarction. *Circulation.* 2003;108 (1):32–6.

Schatzberg A, Kremer C, Rodrigues H, Murphy G and the mirtazapine versus paroxetine study group. Double-blind, randomized comparison of mirtazapine and paroxetine in elderly depressed patients. *Am J Geriatr Psychiatry.* 2002;10:541–550.

Sommer BR, Fenn H, Pompel P, DeBattista C, Lembke A, Wang P, Flores B. Safety of antidepressants in the elderly. *Expert Opin Drug Saf.* 2003; 2 (4):367–83.

Thomas P, Hazif-Thomas C, Clement JP. Influence of antidepressant therapies on weight and appetite in the elderly. *J Nutr Health Aging.* 2003:7 (3):166–70.

Unutzer J, Patrick D, Marmon T, Simon G. Katon W. Depressive symptoms & mortality in a study of 2558 older adults. *Am J Ger Psychiatry.* 2002;10:521–530.

Vandel P. Antidepressant Drugs in the Elderly—Role of the cytochrome P450 2D6. *World J Biol Psychiatry.* 2003;4 (2):74–80.

Young RC, Jain H, Kiosses DN, Meyers BS. Antidepressant-associated mania in late life. *Int J Geriatr Psychiatry.* 2003;18 (5):421–4.

Tricyclic Antidepressants (HCAs)

Abernathy D, Greenblatt D, Shader R. Imipramine and desipramine disposition in the elderly. *J Pharmacol Exp Therap.* 1984;232:183–188.

Alexopoulos G, Shamoian C. Tricyclic antidepressants and patients with pacemakers. *Am J Psychiatry.* 1982;139:519–520.

Beydoun A. Postherpetic neuralgia: Role of gabapentin and other treatment modalities. *Epilepsia.* 1999;40 (Suppl 6):S52–S56.

Brown R, Kocsis J, Glick I, Dhar A. Efficacy and feasibility of high dose tricyclic antidepressant treatment in elderly delusional depressives. *J Clin Psychopharmacol.* 1984;4:311–315.

Burns M, Linden C, Gravdins A, et al. A comparison of physostigmine and benzodiazepines for treatment of anticholinergic poisoning. *Ann Emerg Med.* 2000;35:374–381.

Clayton A. Antidepressant–induced tardive dyskinesia: Review and case report. *Psychopharmacol Bull.* 1995;31:259–264.

Cuttler N, Zavadil A, Eisdorfer C, Ross R, Potter W. Concentration of desipramine in elderly women. *Am J Psychiatry.* 1981;138:1235–1237.

Dalack G, Roose S, Glassman A. Tricyclics and heart failure [letter]. *Am J Psychiatry.* 1991;148:1601.

Faulkner R, Senekjian H, Lee C. Hemodialysis of doxepin and desmethyldoxepin in uremic patients. *Artif Organs.* 1984;8:152–155.

Furlanut M, Benetello P, Spina E. Pharmacokinetic optimisation of tricyclic antidepressant therapy. *Clin Pharmacokinet.* 1993;24:301–318.

Furlanut M, Benetello P. The pharmacokinetics of tricyclic antidepressant drugs in the elderly. *Pharmacological Res.* 1990;22:15–25.

Georgotas A, McCue R, Cooper T. A placebo-controlled comparison of nortriptyline and phenelzine in maintenance therapy of elderly depressed patients. *Arch Gen Psychiatry.* 1989;46:783–786.

Georgotas A, McCue R, Freidman, et al. The response of depressive symptoms to nortriptyline phenelzine and placebo. *Br J Psychiatry.* 1987;151:102–106.

Georgotas A, McCue R, Hapworth W, et al. Comparative efficacy and safety of MAOIs versus HCAs in treating depression in the elderly. *Biol Psychiatry.* 1986;21:1155–1166.

Halaris A. Antidepressant drug therapy in the elderly: Enhancing safety and compliance. *Int J Psychiatry Med.* 1986–1987;16:1–19.

Katz I, Simpson G, Curlik S, Parmelee L, Muhly C. Pharmcologic treatment of major depression for elderly patients in residential care settings. *J Clin Psychiatry.* 1990;51:41–47.

Leinonen E, Ylitano P. The influence of ageing on serum levels of tertiary tricyclic antidepressants. *Human Psychopharmacol.* 1991;6:139–146.

Marcus J. Dosing of antidepressants: The unknown art. *J Clin Psychiatry.* 1995;15:435–439.

Max M, Lynch S, Muir J, Shoaf S, Smoller B, Dubner R. Effects of desipramine, amitriptyline, and fluoxetine on pain in diabetic neuropathy. *N Eng J Med.* 1992;326:120–1256.

McCue R. Using tricyclic antidepressants in the elderly. *Clinics Geriatr Med.* 1992;8:323–334.

Miller M, Curtiss E, Marino L, Houck P, Paradis C, Mazumdar S, Pollock B, Foglia J, Reynolds C. Long-term ECG changes in depressed elderly patients treated with nortriptyline. *Am J Geriatr Psychiatry.* 1998;6:59–66.

Mittman N, Hermann N, Einarson T, Busto U, Lanctot L, Liu B, Shulman K, Silver I, Naranjo C, Shear N. The efficacy, safety, and tolerability of antidepressants in late life depression: A meta-analysis. *J Affective Disorders.* 1997;46:191–217.

Moskowitz H, Burns M. Cognitive performance in geriatric subjects after acute treatment with antidepressants. *Neuropsychobiology.* 1986;15 (Suppl 1): 38–43.

Neis A, Robinson D, Freidman M, Green R, Cooper T, Ravaris C, Ives J. Relationship between age and tricyclic antidepressant plasma levels. *Am J Psychiatry.* 1977;134:790–793.

Neshkes R, Gerner R, Jarvik L, Hintz J, Joseph J, Linde S, Aldrich J, Conolly M, Rosen R, Hill M. Orthostatic effect of imipramine and doxepine in depressed geriatric outpatients. *J Clin Psychopharmacol.* 1985;5:102–106.

Rao M, Deister A, Laux G, Staberlock U, Hoflich G, Moller H-J. Low serum levels of tricyclic antidepressants in amitriptyline- and doxepin-treated inpatients with depressive syndromes are associated with non-response. *Pharmacopsychiat.* 1996;29:97–102.

Ray W, Thapa P, Shorr R. Medications and the older driver. *Clin Geriatr Med.* 1993;9:413–438.

Schiffman S, Graham B, Suggs M, Sattely-Miller E. Effects of psychotropic drugs on taste responses in young and elderly persons. *Ann New York Acad Sci.* 1998;855:732–737.

Small G. Tricyclic antidepressants for medically ill patients. *J Clin Psychiatry.* 1989;50 (suppl 7):27–31.

Sprung J, Schoenwald P, Levy P, Krajewsky L. Treating intraoperative hypotension in a patient on long-term tricyclic antidepressants: A case of aborted aortic surgery. *Anesthesiology.* 1997;86:990–992.

True B, Perry P, Burns E. Profound hypoglycemia with the addition of a tricyclic antidepressant to maintenance sulfonylurea therapy. *Am J Psychiatry.* 1987;144:1220–1221.

Vandel P, Bonin B, Leveque E, Sechter D, Bizouard P. Tricyclic antidepressant-induced extrapyramidal side effects. *European Neuropsychopharmacol.* 1997;7:207–212.

Warnock J, Knesevich J. Adverse cutaneous reactions to antidepressants. *Am J Psychiatry.* 1988;145:425–430.

Williams G. Management of depression in the elderly. *Primary Care.* 1989;16:451–474.

Wrenn K, Smith B, Slovis C. Profound alkalemia during treatment of tricyclic antidepressant overdose: A potential hazard of combined hyperventilation and intravenous bicarbonate. *Am J Emerg Med.* 1992;10:553–555.

Irreversible Monoamine Oxidase Inhibitors (*MAOIs*)

Davidson J, Giller E, Zisook S, Overall J. An efficacy study of isocarboxazid and placebo in depression, and its relationship to depressive nosology. *Arch Gen Psychiatry.* 1988;45:120–127.

Georgotas A, Friedman E, McCarthy M, et al. Resistant geriatric depressions and therapeutic response to monoamine oxidase inhibitors. *Biol Psychiatry.* 1983;18:195–205.

Georgotas A, McCue R, Cooper T. A placebo-controlled comparison of nortriptyline and phenelzine in maintenance therapy of depressed elderly patients. *Arch Gen Psychiatry.* 1989;46:783–786.

Georgotas A, McCue R, Cooper T, Nagachandran N, Chang I. How effective and safe is continuation therapy in elderly depressed patients? *Arch Gen Psychiatry.* 1988;45:929–932.

Georgotas A, McCue R, Cooper T, Nagachandran N, Friedhoff A. Factors affecting the delay of antidepressant effect in responders to nortriptyline and phenelzine. *Psychiatry Res.* 1989;28:1–9.

Georgotas A, McCue R, Friedman E, Cooper T. A placebo-controlled comparison of the effect of nortriptyline and phenelzine on orthostatic hypotension in elderly depressed patients. *J Clin Psychopharmacol.* 1987;7:413–416.

Georgotas A, McCue R, Friedman E, Cooper T. Electrocardiographic effects of nortriptyline, phenelzine, and placebo under optimal treatment conditions. *Am J Psychiatry.* 1987;144:798–801.

Georgotas A, McCue R, Friedman E, Cooper T. Prediction of response to nortriptyline and phenelzine by platelet MAO activity. *Am J Psychiatry.* 1987;144:338–340.

Georgotas A, McCue R, Friedman E, Cooper T. Response of depressive symptoms to nortriptyline, phenelzine and placebo. *Br J Psychiatry.* 1987;151: 102–106.

Georgotas A, McCue R, Friedman E, et al. Clinical predictors of response to antidepressants in elderly patients. *Biol Psychiatry.* 1987;22:733–740.

Georgotas A, McCue R, Hapworth, et al. Comparative efficacy and safety of MAOIs versus HCAs in treating depression in the elderly. *Biol Psychiatry.* 1986;21:1155–1166.

Georgotas A, Reisberg B, Ferris S. First results of the effects of MAO inhibition on cognitive functioning in elderly depressed patients. *Arch Gerontol Psychiatry.* 1983;2:249–254.

Giese A, Leibenluft E, Green S, Moricle L. Phenelzine—associated inappropriate ADH secretion [letter]. *J Clin Psychopharmacol.* 1989;9:309–310.

Jenike M. Monoamine oxidase inhibitors as treatment for depressed patients with primary degenerative dementia (Alzheimer's disease). *Am J Psychiatry.* 1985;142:763–764.

Lazarus L. Groves L, Gierl B, et al. Efficacy of phenelzine in geriatric depression. *Biol Psychiatry.* 1986;21:699–701.

McGrath P, Stewart J, Nunes E, Ocepek-Welikson K, Rabkin J, Quitkin F, Klein D. A double-blind crossover trial of imipramine and phenelzine for outpatients with treatment-refractory depression. *Am J Psychiatry.* 1993; 150: 118–123.

Pontos L, Perry P, Liskow B, Seaba H. Drug therapy reviews: Tricyclic antidepressant and monoamine oxidase inhibitor combination therapy. *Am J Hosp Pharm.* 1977;34:954–961.

Reggev A, Vollhardt B. Bradycardia induced by an interaction between phenelzine and beta blockers. *Psychosomatics.* 1989;30:106–108.

Remick R, Froese C, Keller D. Common side effects associated with monoamine oxidase inhibitors. *Prog Neuro-Psychopharmacol Biol Psychiatry.* 1989;13:497–504.

Teicher M, Cohen B, Baldessarini R, Cole J. Severe daytime somnolence in patients treated with an MAOI. *Am J Psychiatry.* 1988;145:1552–1556.

Teusink J, Alexopoulos G, Shamoian C. Parkinsonian side effects induced by a monoamine oxidase inhibitor. *Am J Psychiatry.* 1984;141:118–119.

Thase M, Trivedi M, Rush J. MAOIs in the contemporary treatment of depression. *Neuropsychopharmacol.* 1995;12:185–219.

Thompson D, Sweet R, Marzula K, Peredes J. Lack of interaction of monoamine oxidase inhibitors and epinephrine in an older patient [letter]. *J Clin Psychopharmacol.* 1997;17:322–323.

Zisook S. Side effects of isocarboxazid. *J Clin Psychiatry.* 1984;45:53–58.

Selective Serotonin Reuptake Inhibitors (SSRIs)

Andrews W, Parker G, Barrett E. The SSRI antidepressants: Exploring their "other" possible properties. *J Affective Dis.* 1998;49:141–144.

Barbey J, Roose S. SSRI safety in overdose. *J Clin Psychiatry.* 1998;59 (suppl 15):42–48.

Baumann P. Care of depression in the elderly: Comparative pharmacokinetics of SSRIs. *Int Clinical Psychopharmacology.* 1998;13 (Suppl 5):S35–S43.

Baumann P. Pharmacokinetic-pharmacodynamic realtionship of SSRIs. *Clin Pharmacokinet.* 1996;31:444–469.

Benazzi F. SSRI discontinuation syndrome treated with fluoxetine. *Int J Geriatr Psychiatry.* 1998;13:421–422.

Bonner I, Vanneste J. Complex movement disorder associated with fluvoxamine [letter]. *Movement Dis.* 1998;13:848–849.

Bouwer C, Stein D. Use of selective serotonin reuptake inhibitor citalopram in the treatment of generalized social phobia. *J Affective Dis.* 1998;49:79–82.

Brosen K. The pharmacogenetics of the selective serotonin reuptake inhibitors. *Clin Pharmacol.* 1993;71:1002–1009.

Dalfen A, Stewart D. Who develops severe or fatal adverse drug reactions to selective serotonin reuptake inhibitors? *Can J Psychiatry.* 2001;46:258–263.

Dalton SO, Johansen C, Mellemkjaer L, Norgard B, Sorensen HT, Olsen JH. Use of selective serotonin reuptake inhibitors and risk of upper gastrointestinal tract bleeding: a population-based cohort study. *Arch Intern Med.* 2003; 163 (1):59–64.

DasGupta K. Treatment of depression in elderly patients: Recent advances. *Arch Fam Med.* 1998;7:274–280.

De Abajo F, Jick H, Derby L, Jick S, Schmitz S. Intracranial hemorrhage and use of selective serotonin reuptake inhibitors. *J Clin Pharmacol.* 2000;50:43–47.

Dell'Agnello G, Ceravolo R, Nuti A, et al. SSRIs do not worsen Parkinson's disease: Evidence from an open label, prospective study. *Clin Neuropharmcol.* 2001;24:221–227.

De Jong JC, van den Berg PB, Tobi H, de Jong-van den Berg LT. Combined use of SSRIs and NSAIDs increases risk of gastrointestinal adverse effects. *Br J Clin Pharmacol.* 2003;55 (6):591–5.

Ekselius L, Von Knorring L. Changes in personality traits during treatment with sertraline or citalopram. *Br J Psychiatry.* 1999;174:444–448.

Fava M. Weight gain and antidepressants. *J Clin Psychiatry.* 2000;61 (11 Suppl):37–41.

Finkel S, Richter E, Clary C, Batzar E. Comparative efficacy of sertraline vs. fluoxetine in patients age 70 or over with major depression. *Am J Geriatr Psychiatry.* 1999;7:221–227.

Goodman W, McDougle C, Price L. Pharmacotherapy of obsessive compulsive disorder. *J Clin Psychiatry.* 1992;53 (Suppl 4):29–37.

Hosak L, Tuma I. Comparative study of three antidepressants: Preliminary results. *Homeostasis.* 1996;37:138–139.

Judge R, Plewes J, Kumar V, Koke S, Kopp J. Changes in energy during treatment of depression: An analysis of fluoxetine in double-blind, placebo-controlled trials. *J Clin Psychopharmacology.* 2000;20:666–672.

Keck P McElroy S. New uses for antidepressants: Social phobia. *J Clin Psychiatry.* 1997;58 (Suppl 14):32–36.

Kelly R, Robinson H, Beringer T. Hyponatremia in an older patient [letter]. *JAGS.* 1999;47:1037–1038.

Kurzthaler I, Hotter A, Miller C, et al. Risk profile of SSRIs in elderly depressive patients with co-morbid physical illness. *Pharmacopsychiatry.* 2001; 34:114–118.

Lee A, Chan W, Harralson A, Buffum J, Bui B. The effects of grapefruit juice on sertraline metabolism: An in vitro and in vivo study. *Clin Therapeutics.* 1999; 21:1890–1899.

Leinonen E, Koponen H, Lepola U. Delirium during fluoxetine treatment: A case report. *Ann Clin Psychiatry.* 1993;5:255–258.

Malt U, Robak O, Madsbu H-P, Bakke O, Loeb M. The Norwegian naturalistic treatment study of depression in general practice (NORDEP)-I: Randomized double-blind study. *BMJ.* 1999;318 (7192):1180–1184.

McCance E, Marek K, Price L. Serotonergic dysfunction in depression associated with parkinson's disease. *Neurology.* 1992;42:1813–1814.

Menting J, Honig A, Verhey F, et al. Selective serotonin reuptake inhibitors (SSRIs) in the treatment of elderly depressed patients: a qualitative analysis of the literature on their efficacy and side effects. *Int Clinical Psychopharmacology.* 1996;11:165–175.

Modell J, Katholi C, Modell J, DePalma R. Comparative sexual side effects of bupropion, fluoxetine, paroxetine, and sertraline. *Clin Pharmacol Ther.* 1997;61:476–487.

Mulchahey J, Malik J, Sabai M, Kasckow J. Serotonin-selective reuptake inhibitors in the treatment of geriatric depression and related disorders. *Int J Neuropsychopharmacol.* 1999;2:121–127.

Nahas Z, Arlinghaus K, Kotrla K, Clearman R, George M. Rapid response of emotional incontinence to selective serotonin reuptake inhibitors. *J Neuropsychiatry.* 1998;10:453–455.

Naranjo C, Bremner K. Lanctot K. Effects of citalopram and a brief psychosocial intervention on alcohol intake, dependence, and problems. *Addiction.* 1995;90:87–99.

Nemeroff C. Evolutionary trends in the pharmacotherapeutic management of depression. *J Clin Psychiatry.* 1994;55 (Suppl 12):3–15.

Potenza M, Wasylink S, Longhurst J, Epperson C, McDougle C. Olanzepine augmentation of fluoxetine in the treatment of refractory obsessive-compulsive disorder [letter]. *J Clin Psychiatry.* 1998;18:423–424.

Reynolds C. Depression: Making the diagnosis and using SSRIs in the older patient. *Geriatrics.* 1996;51:28–34.

Rosenbaum J, Zajecka J. Clinical management of antidepressant discontinuation. *J Clin Psychiatry.* 1997;58 (Suppl 7):37–40.

Skerritt U, Evans R, Montgomery S. Selective serotonin reuptake inhibitors in the elderly. *Drugs Aging.* 1997;10:209–218.

Small G, Salzman C. Treatment of depression with new and atypical antidepressants. In C Salzman (ed), *Clinical Geriatric Psychopharmacology.* Baltimore: Williams and Wilkins; 1998;245–261.

Spalletta G, Guida G, Caltagirone C. Is left stroke a risk-factor for selective serotonin reuptake inhibitor antidepressant treatment resistance? *J Neurol.* 2003;250 (4):449–55.

Van Walraven C, Mamdani M, Wells P, Williams J. Inhibition of serotonin reuptake by antidepressants and upper gastrointestinal bleeding in elderly patients: Retrospective cohort study. *BMJ.* 2001;323:655–657.

Wade A. Antidepressants in panic disorder. *Int J Clin Psychopharmacol.* 1999;14 (Suppl 2):S13–S17.

Buproprion

Amann B, Hummel B, Rall-Autenreith H, Walden J, Grunze H. Bupropion-induced isolated impairment of sensory trigeminal nerve function. *Int Clin Psychopharmacology.* 2000;15:115–116.

Ascher J, Cole J, Colin J, et al. Bupropion: A review of its mechanism of antidepressant activity. *J Clin Psychiatry.* 1995;56:395–401.

Ashton A, Rosen R. Bupropion as as antidote for serotonin reuptake inhibitor-induced sexual dysfunction. *J Clin Psychiatry.* 1998;59:112–115.

Bodkin J, Lasser R, Wines J, Gardner D, Baldessarini R. Combining serotonin reuptake inhibitors and bupropion in partial responders to antidepressant monotherapy. *J Clin Psychiatry.* 1997;58:137–145.

Canive J, Clark R, Calais L, Qualls C, Tuason V. Bupropion treatment in veterans with posttraumatic stress disorder: An open study. *J. Clin Psychopharmacol* 1998;18:379–383.

Davidson J, Connor K. Bupropion sustained release: A therapeutic overview. *J Clin Psychiatry.* 1998;59 (Suppl 4):25–31.

Dunner D, Zisook S, Billow A, Batey S, Johnston A, Ascher J. A prospective safety surveillance study for bupropion sustained-release in the treatment of depression. *J Clin Psychiatry.* 1998;59:366–373.

Fatemi S, Emamiam E, Kist D. Venlafaxine and bupropion combination therapy in a case of treatment-resistant depression. *Ann Pharmacotherapy.* 1999; 33:701–703.

Fogelson D, Bystritsky A, Pasnau R. Bupropion in the treatment of bipolar disorders: The same old story? *J Clin Psychiatry.* 1992;53:443–446.

Gardos G. Reversible dyskinesia during bupropion therapy [letter]. *J Clin Psychiatry.* 1997;58:218.

Harris C, Gaultieri J, Stark G. Fatal bupropion overdose. *Clin Toxicology.* 1997; 35:321–324.

Horst D, Preskorn S. Mechanisms of action and clinical characteristics of three atypical antidepressants: Venlafaxine, nefazodone, bupropion. *J Affective Dis.* 1998;51:237–254.

Howard W, Warnock J. Bupropion–induced psychosis [letter]. *Am J Psychiatry.* 1999;156:2017–2018.

Humma L, Swims M. Bupropion mimics a transient ischemic attack. *Ann Pharmacotherapy.* 1999;33:305–307.

Kales H, Mellow A. Ileus as a possible result of bupropion in an elderly woman [letter]. *J Clin Psychiatry.* 1999;60:337.

Ketter T, Jenkins J, Schroeder D, et al. Carbamazepine but not valproate induces bupropion metabolism. *J Clin Psychopharmacol.* 1995;15:327–333.

Labbate L, Grimes J, Hines A, Pollack M. Bupropion treatment of serotonin reuptake antidepressant-associated sexual dysfunction. *Ann Clin Psychiatry.* 1997;9:241–245.

Labbate L, Pollack M. Treatment of fluoxetine-induced sexual dysfunction with bupropion: A case report. *Ann Clin Psychiatry.* 1994;6:13–15.

Malesker M, Soori G, Malone P, Mahowald J, Housel G. Eosinophilia associated with bupropion. *Ann Pharmacother.* 1995;29:867–869.

Marshall R, Liebowitz M. Paroxetine/Bupropion combination treatment for refractory depression [letter]. *J Clin Psychiatry.* 1996;16:80–81.

Park-Wyllie LY, Antoniou T. Concurrent use of bupropion with CYP2B6 inhibitors, nelfinavir, ritonavir and efavirenz: A case series. *AIDS.* 2003; 17 (4):638–40.

Pollock B, Sweet R, Kirshner M, Reynolds C. Bupropion plasma levels and CYP2D6 phenotype. *Ther Drug Monit.* 1996;18:581–585.

Reimherr F, Cunningham L, Batey S, Johnston J, Ascher J. A multicenter evaluation of the efficacy and safety of 150 and 300 mg/d sustained–release bupropion tablets versus placebo in depressed outpatients. *Clin Therapeutics.* 1998;20:505–516.

Settle E. Bupropion sustained release: Side effect profile. *J Clin Psychiatry.* 1998;59 (Suppl 4):32–36.

Settle E, Stahl S, Batey S, Johnston J, Ascher J. Safety profile of sustained release bupropion in depression: Results of three clinical trials. *Clin Therapeutics.* 1999;21:454–463.

Shad M, Preskorn S. A possible bupropion and imipramine interaction [letter]. *J Clin Psychopharmacology.* 1997;17:118–119.

Spier S. Use of bupropion with SRIs and venlafaxine. *Depression Anx.* 1998; 7:73–75.

Spiller H, Ramoska E, Krenzelok E, et al. Bupropion overdose: A 3-year multi-center retrospective analysis. *Am J Emerg Med.* 1994;12:43–45.

Sweet R, Pollock B, Kirshner M, Wright B, Altieri L, DeVane L. Pharmacokinetics of single- and multiple-dose bupropion in elderly patients with depression. *J Clin Pharmacol.* 1995;35:876–884.

Szuba M, Leuchter A. Falling backward in two elderly patients taking bupropion. *J Clin Psychiatry.* 1992;53:157–159.

Trappler B, Miyashiro A. Bupropion—amantadine associated neurotoxicity [letter]. *J Clin Psychiatry.* 2000;61:61–62.

Weihs K, Settle E, Batey S, Houser T, Donahue R, Ascher J. Bupropion sustained release versus paroxetine for the treatment of depression in the elderly. *J Clin Psychiatry.* 2000;61:196–202.

Yolles W, Armenta W, Alao A. Serum sickness induced by bupropion. *Ann Pharmacotherapy.* 1999;33:931–933.

Zisook S, Shuchter S, Pedrelli P, Sable J, Deaciuc. Bupropion sustained release for bereavement: Results of an open trial. *J Clin Psychiatry.* 2001;62:227–230.

Citalopram

Andersen G, Vestergaard K, Lauritzen L. Effective treatment of post stroke depression with the selective serotonin reuptake inhibitor citalopram. *Stroke.* 1994;25:1099–1104.

Angalone S, Bellini L, Di Bella D, Catalano M. Effects of fluvoxamine and citalopram in maintaining abstinence in a sample of Italian detoxified alcoholics. *Alcohol Alcoholism.* 1998;33:151–156.

Baettig D, Bondolfi G, Montaldi S, Amey M, Baumann P. Tricyclic antidepressant levels after augmentation with citalopram: A case study. *Eur J Clin Pharmacol.* 1999;44:403–405.

Barak Y, Swzrtz M, Levy D, Weizman R. Age-related differences in the effect profile of citalopram. *Prog Neuropsychopharmacol Biol Psychiatry.* 2003;27 (3):545–8.

Bezchlibnyk-Butler K, Aleksic I, Kennedy S. Citalopram: A review of pharmacological and clinical effects. *J Psychiatry Neurosci.* 2000;25:241–254.

Bonomo V, Fogliani A. Citalopram and haloperidol for psychotic depression [letter]. *Am J Psychiatry.* 2000;157:1706–1707.

Bouchard J, Strub N, Nil R. Citalopram and viloxazine in the treatment of depression by means of slow drop infusion: A double-blind comparative trial. *J Affective Dis.* 1997;46:51–58.

Bryois C, Ferrero F. Mania induced by citalopram. *Arch Gen Psychiatry.* 1994;51:664–665.

Gottfries C, Karlsson I, Nyth A. Treatment of depression in elderly patients with and without dementia disorders. *Int Clin Psychopharmacol.* 1992;6 (Suppl 5):55–64.

Gram L, Hansen M, Sindrup S, et al. Citalopram: Interaction studies with levomepromazine, imipramine, and lithium. *Therapeutic drug monitoring.* 1993;15:18–24.

Holland S, Townley S, Summerfield R. Citalopram—a risk factor for postoperative hyponatraemia. *Anaesthesia.* 2003;58 (5):491–2.

Koponen H, Lepola U, Leinonen E, Jokinen R, Penttinen J, Turtonen J. Citalopram in the treatment of obsessive-compulsive disorder: An open pilot study. *Acta Psychiatr Scand.* 1997;96:343–346.

Kyle C, Petersen H, Overo K. Comparison of the tolerability and efficacy of citalopram and amitriptylene in elderly depressed patients treated in general practice. *Depress Anxiety.* 1998;8:147–153.

Lauerma H. Successful treatment of citalopram-induced anorgasmia by cyproheptadine [letter]. *Acta Psychiatr Scand.* 1996;93:69–70.

Lavretsky H, Kumar A. Methylphenidate augmentation of citalopram in elderly depressed patients. *Am J Geriatr Psychiatry.* 2001;9:298–303.

Leinonen E, Lepola U, Koponen H, Turtonen J, Wade A, Lehto H. Citalopram controls phobic symptoms in patients with panic disorder: Randomized controlled trial. *J Psychiatry Neurosci.* 2000;25:24–32.

Lepola U, Koponen H, Leinonen E. Citalopram in the treatment of social phobia: a report of three cases. *Pharmacopsychiat.* 1994;27:186–188.

Luo H, Richardson J. A pharmacological comparison of citalopram, a bicyclic serotonin selective uptake inhibitor, with traditional tricyclic antidepressants. *Int Clin Psychopharmacol.* 1993;8:3–12.

Navarro V, Gasto C, Torres X, Marcos T, Pintor L. Citalopram versus Nortriptyline in late life-life depression: A 12-week randomized single-blind study. *Acta Psychiatr Scand.* 2001;103:435–440.

Nyth A, Gottfries C, Lyby K, et al. A Controlled multicenter clinical study of citalopram and placebo in elderly depressed patients with and without concomitant dementia. *Acta Psychiatrica Scand.* 1992;86:138–145.

Nyth A, Gottfries C. The clinical efficacy of citalopram in treatment of emotional disturbances in dementia disorders: A Nordic multicenter study. *Br J Psychiatry.* 1990;157:894–901.

Personne M, Persson H, Sjoberg G. Citalopram toxicity [letter]. *Lancet.* 1997; 350:518–519.

Pollock B, Mulsant B, Rosen J, et al. Comparison of citalopram, perphenazine and placebo for the acute treatment of psychosis and behavioral disturbances in hospitalized, demented patients. *Am J Psychiatry.* 2002;159:460–465.

Pollock B, Mulsant B, Sweet R, et al. An open pilot study of citalopram for behavioral disturbances of dementia. *Am J Geriatr Psychiatr.* 1997;5:70–78.

Reis M, Lundmark J, Bengtsson F. Therapeutic drug monitoring of racemic citalopram: a 5-year experience in Sweden, 1992–1997. *Ther Drug Monit.* 2003;25 (2):183–191.

Salokangas R, Saarijarvi S, Taiminen T, et al. Citalopram as an adjuvant in chronic schizophrenia: A double-blind placebo-controlled study. *Acta Psychiatr Scand.* 1996;94:175–180.

Sidhu J, Priskorn M, Poulsen M, Segonzac A, Grollier G, Larsen F. Steady-state pharmacokinetics of the enantiomers of citalopram and its metabolites in humans. *CHIRALITY.* 1997;9:686–692.

Uehlinger C, Nil R, Amey M, Baumann P, Dufour H. Citalopram-Lithium combination treatment of elderly depressed patients: A pilot study. *Int J Geriatr Psychiatry.* 1995;10:281–287.

Vartiainen H, Tiihonen J, Putkonen A, et al. Citalopram a selective serotonin reuptake inhibitor in the treatment of aggression in schizophrenia. *Acta Psychiatr Scand.* 1995;91:348–351.

Voegeli J, Baumann P. Inappropriate secretion of antidiuretic hormone and SSRIs. *Br J Psychiatry.* 1996;169:524–525.

Wade A, Lepola H, Koponen H, Pedersen V, Pedersen T. The effect of citalopram in panic disorder. *Br J Psychiatr.* 1997;170:549–553.

Clomipramine

Alderman C, Atchison M, McNeece J. Concurrent agranulocytosis and hepatitis secondary to clomipramine therapy. *Br J Psychiatry.* 1993;162:688–689.

Allsopp L, Cooper G, Poole P. Clomipramine and diazepam in the treatment of agoraphobia and social phobia in general practice. *Curr Med Res Opinion.* 1984;9:64–70.

Allsopp L, Huitson A, Deering R, Brodie N. Efficacy and tolerability of sustained-release clomipramine (Anafranil SR) in the treatment of phobias: A comparison with the conventional formulation of clomipramine (Anafranil). *Int Med Res.* 1985;13:203.

Balant-Gorgia A, Ries C, Balant L. Metabolic interaction between fluoxetine and clomipramine: A case report. *Pharmacopsychiatr.* 1996;29:38–41.

Bocksberger J-P, Gex-Fabry M, Gauthey L, Balant-Gorgia A. Clomipramine therapy in the geriatric hospital: Experience with therapeutic drug monitoring. *Ther Drug Monit.* 1994;16:113–119.

Cassano G, Petracca A, Perugi G, et al. Clomipramine for panic disorder: I. The first ten weeks of a long-term comparison with Imipramine. *J Affect Disord.* 1988;14:123–127.

De Wilde J, Mertens C, Wakelin J. Clinical trials of fluvoxamine vs. clomipramine with single and three times daily dosing. *J Clin Pharmacol.* 1983;15:427S–431S.

Eberhard G, von Knorring L, Nilsson H, et al. A double-blind randomized study of clomipramine versus maprotiline in patients with ideopathic pain syndromes. *Neuropsychobiology.* 1988;19:25–34.

Gersten S. Tardive-dyskinesia like syndromes with clomipramine [letter]. *Am J Psychiatry.* 1993;150:165–166.

Guillibert E, Pelicier Y, Archambault J, et al. A double-blind, multicenter study of paroxetine versus clomipramine in depressed elderly patients. *Act Psychiatr Scand.* 1989;80 (Suppl 350):132–134.

Lejoyeux M, Rouillon F, Ades J. Prospective evaluation of the serotonin syndrome in depressed inpatients treated with clomipramine. *Acta Psychiatrica Scand.* 1993;88:369–371.

Papp L, Schneier F, Fyer A, et al. Clomipramine treatment of panic disorder: Pros and cons. *J Clin Psychiatry.* 1997;58:423–425.

Sommer B. Syndrome of inappropriate antidiuretic hormone (SIADH) in an 80-year-old woman given clomipramine [letter]. *Am J Geriatr Psychiatry.* 1997;5:268–269.

Szegedi A, Wetzel H, Leal M, Hartter S, Hiemke C. Combination treatment with clomipramine and fluvoxamine: Drug monitoring safety and tolerability data. *J Clin Psychiatry.* 1996;57:257–264.

Trappler B. Treatment of obsessive-compulsive disorder using clomipramine in a very old patient. *Ann Pharmacother.* 1999;33:686–690.

Desipramine

Alderman J, Preskorn S, Greenblatt D, et al. Desipramine pharmacokinetics when coadministered with paroxetine or sertraline in extensive metabolizers. *J Clin Psychopharmacol.* 1997;17:284–291.

Dugas J, Bishop D. Non-linear desipramine pharmacokinetics: A case study. *J Clin Psychopharmacol.* 1985;5:43–45.

Kitanaka I, Ross R, Cutler N, Zavadil A, Potter W. Altered hydoxydesipramine concentrations in elderly depressed patients. *Clin Pharmacol Ther.* 1982;31:51–55.

Kutcher S, Reid K, Dubbin J, Shulman K. Electrocardiogram changes and therapeutic desipramine and 2-hydroxy-desipramine concentrations in elderly depressives. *Br J Psychiatry.* 1986;148:676–679.

Kutcher S, Shulman K, Reed K. Desipramine plasma concentration and therapeutic response in elderly depressives: A naturalistic pilot study. *Can J Psychiatry.* 1986;31:752–754.

Lydiard R. Desipramine-associated SIADH in an elderly woman: Case report. *J Clin Psychiatry.* 1983;44:153–154.

Nelson J, Jatlow P. Nonlinear desipramine kinetics: Prevalence and importance. *Clin Pharmacol Ther.* 1987;41:666–670.

Escitalopram

Brancaccio RR, Weinstein S. Systemic contact dermatitis to doxepin. *J Drugs Dermatol.* 2003;2 (4):409–10.

Croom KF, Plosker GL. Escitalopram: A pharmacoeconomic review of its use in depression. *Pharmacoeconomics.* 2003;21 (16):1185–1209.

Gutierrez MM, Rosenberg J, Abramowitz W. An evaluation of the potential for pharmacokinetic interaction between escitalopram and the cytochrome P450 3A4 inhibitor ritonavir. *Clin Ther.* 2003;25 (4):1200–1210.

Harvard Mental Health Letter. There is a new antidepressant escitalopram (Lexapro) that is a cousin of citalopram (Celexa). How are these two different and does the newer drug have any advantages? *Harv Ment Health Lett.* 2003;20 (1):8.

Wade A, Michael Lemming O, Bang Hedegaard K. Escitalopram 10 mg/day is effective and well tolerated in a placebo-controlled study in depression in primary care. *Int Clin Psychopharmacol.* 2002;17 (3):95–102.

Fluoxetine

Altamura A, DeNovellis F, Guercetti G, Invernizzi G, Percudani M, Montgomery S. Fluoxetine compared with amitriptyline in elderly depression: A controlled clinical trial. *Int J Clin Pharmacol Res.* 1989;9:391–396.

Amsterdam J, Garcia-Espana F, Fawcett J, et al. Blood pressure changes during short-term fluoxetine treatment. *J Clin Psychopharm.* 1999;19:9–14.

Amsterdam J, Garcia-Espana F, Fawcett J, et al. Efficacy and safety of fluoxetine in treating Bipolar II major depressive episode. *J Clin Psychopharm.* 1998;18:435–440.

Beasley C, Masica D, Heiligenstein J, Wheado D, Zerbe R. Possible monoamine oxidase inhibitor-serotonin uptake inhibitor interaction: Fluoxetine clinical data and preclinical findings. *J Clin Psychopharmacol.* 1993;13:312–320.

Benazzi F. Venlafaxine-Fluoxetine interaction [letter]. *J Clin Pharmacol.* 1999; 19:96–98.

Benfield P, Heel R, Lewis S. Fluoxetine: A review of its pharmacodynalic and pharmacokinetic properties, and therapeutic efficacy in depressive illness. *Drugs.* 1986;32:481–508.

Berman R, Darnell A, Miller H, Anand A, Charney D. Effect of pindolol in hastening response to fluoxetine in the treatment of major depression: A double-blind, placebo controlled trial. *Am J Psychiatry.* 1997;154:37–43.

Blumenfield M, Levy N, Spinowitz B, et al. Fluoxetine in depressed patients on dialysis. *Int J Psychiatry Med.* 1997;27:71–80.

Brown K, Sloan R, Pentaland B. Fluoxetine as a treatment for post-stroke emotionalism. *Acta Psychiatr Scand.* 1998;98:455–458.

Brymer C, Hutner-Winograd C. Fluoxetine in elderly patients: Is there cause for concern? *JAGS.* 1992;40:902–905.

Buff D, Brenner R, Kirtane S, Gilboa R. Dysrhythmia associated with fluoxetine treatment in an elderly patient with cardiac disease. *J Clin Psychiatry.* 1991; 52:174–176.

Cherin P, Colvez A, DeVille de Periere G, Sereni D. Risk of syncope in the elderly and consumption of drugs: A case-control study. *J Clin Epidemiol.* 1997;50:313–320.

Cook I, Leuchter A, Witte E, et al. Neurophysiologic predictors of treatment response to fluoxetine in major depression. *Psychiatry Res.* 1999;85:263–273.

Demedts P, Franck F, Wauters A, Neels H. Fluoxetine: Is the syndrome of inappropriate secretion of antidiuretic hormone in elderly patients associated with elevated serum levels? *Clin Toxicology.* 1998;36:129–130.

Dent L, Orrock M. Warfarin-fluoxetine and diazepam-fluoxetine interaction. *Pharmacotherapy.* 1997;17:170–172.

Devanand D, Kim M K, Nobler M. Fluoxetine discontinuation in elderly dysthymic patients. *Am J Ger Psychiatry.* 1997;5:83–87.

Druckenbrod R, Mulsant B. Fluoxetine induced syndrome of inappropriate antidiuretic hormone secretion: A geriatric report and review of the literature. *J Geriatr Psychiatry Neurol.* 1994;7:255–258.

Evans M, Hammond M, Wilson K, Lye M, Copeland J. Placebo controlled treatment trial of depression in elderly physically ill patients. *Int J Geriatr Psychiaty.* 1997;12:617–824.

Fairweather D, Kerr J, Harrison D, Moon C. A double blind comparison of the effects of fluoxetine and amitriptyline on cognitive function in elderly depressed patients. *Human Psychopharmacol.* 1993;8:41–47.

Falk W, Rosenbaum J, Otto M, Zusky P, Weilberg J, et al. Fluoxetine versus trazadone in depressed geriatric patients. *J Geriatr Psychiatry Neurol.* 1989;2:208–214.

Feigner J, Cohn J. Double-blind comparative trials of fluoxetine and doxepin in geriatric patients with major depressive disorder. *J Clin Psychiatry.* 1985; 46 (suppl 2):20–25.

Fruehwald S, Gatterbauer E, Rehak P, Baumhackl U. Early fluoxetine treatment of post-stroke depression—a three-month double-blind placebo-controlled study with an open-label long-term follow up. *J Neurol.* 2003; 250 (3):347–51.

Goldstein D, Hamilton S, Masica D, Beasley C. Fluoxetine in medically stable depressed geriatric patients: Effect on weight gain. *J Clin Psychopharmacol.* 1997;17:365–369.

La Pia S, Giorgio D, Ciriello R, et al. Double-blind controlled study to evaluate the effectiveness and tolerability of fluoxetine versus mianserin in the treatment of depressive disorders among the elderly and their effects on cognitive-behavioral parameters. *New Trends Experimental Clin Psychiatry.* 1992;8:139–146.

La Pia S, Giorgio D, Ciriello R, et al. Evaluation of the efficacy, tolerability, and therapeutic profile of fluoxetine versus mianserin in the treatment of depressive disorders in the elderly. *Curr Therapeutic Res.* 1992;52:847–858.

Leibovitz A, Bilchinsky T, Gil I, Habot B. Elevated serum digoxin level associated with coadministered fluoxetine. *Arch Intern Med.* 1998;158:1152–1153.

Leo R, Lichter D, Hershey L. Parkinsonism associated with fluoxetine and cimetidine: A case report. *J Geriatr Psychiatry Neurol.* 1995;8:231–233.

Lustman P, Freedland K, Griffith L, Clouse R. Fluoxetine for depression in diabetes: A randomized double-blind placebo controlled trial. *Diabetes Care.* 2000;23:618–623.

Maes M, Libberecht I, van Hunsel S, Campens D, Meltzer H. Pindolol and mianserin augment the antidepressant activity of fluoxetine in hospitalized major depressed patients, including those with treatment resistance. *J Clin Psychopharm.* 1999;19:177–182.

Mander A, McCausland M, Workman B, Flamer H, Christophidis N. Fluoxetine-induced dyskinesia. *Aust NZ J Psychiatry.* 1994;28:328–330.

Mentre F, Golmard J-L, Launay J-M, Aubin-Brunet V, Bouhassira M, Jouvent R. Relationships between low red blood cell count and clinical response to fluoxetine in depressed elderly patients. *Psychiatry Res.* 1998;81:403–405.

Mesters P, Cosyns P, Dejaiffe G, et al. Assessment of quality of life in the treatment of major depressive disorders with fluoxetine, 20 mg, in ambulatory patients aged over 60 years. *Int Clin Psychopharmacol.* 1993;8:253–259.

Montastruc J, Pelat M, Verwaerde P, et al. Fluoxetine in orthostatic hypotension of Parkinson's disease: A clinical and experimental pilot study. *Fundam Clin Pharmacol.* 1998;12:398–402.

Nierenberg A, Farabaugh A, Alpert J, et al. Timing of onset of antidepressant response with fluoxetine treatment. *Am J Psychiatry.* 2000;157:1423–1428.

Nobler M, Devanand D, Kim M, et al. Fluoxetine treatment of dysthymia in the elderly. *J Clin Psychiatry.* 1996;57:254–256.

Orengo C, Kunik M, Molinari V, Workman R. The use and tolerability of fluoxetine in geropsychiatric inpatients. *J Clin Psychiatry.* 1996;57:12–16.

Paul K. Anticholinergic delirium possibly associated with protriptyline and fluoxetine [letter]. *Ann Psychopharmacotherapy.* 1997;31:1260–1261.

Perucca E, Marchioni E, Soragna D, Savoldi F. Fluoxetine-induced movement disorders and deficient CYP2D6 enzyme activity. *Mov Disord.* 1997;12:624.

Pillans P. Fluoxetine and hyponatremia: A potential hazard in the elderly. *NZ Med.* 1994;107:85–86.

Quitkin FM, Petkova E, McGrath PJ, Taylor B, Beasley C, Stewart J, Amsterdam J, Fava M, Rosenbaum J, Reimherr F, Fawcett J, Chen Y, Klein D. When should a trial of fluoxetime for major depression be declared failed? *Am J Psychiatry.* 2003;160 (4):734–40.

Roose S, Glassman A, Attia E, Woodring S, Giardina E, Bigger T. Cardiovascular effects of fluoxetine in depressed patients with heart disease. *Am J Psychiatry.* 1998;155:660–665.

Small G, Birkett M, Myers B. et al. Impact of physical illness on quality of life and antidepressant response in geriatric major depression. *J Am Geriatr Soc.* 1996;44:1220–1225.

Spier S, Frontera M. Unexpected deaths in depressed medical inpatients treated with fluoxetine. *J Clin Psychiatry.* 1991;52:377–381.

Stokes P, Holtz A. Fluoxetine tenth anniversary update: The progress continues. *Clin Ther.* 1997;19:1135–1250.

Strik J, Honig A, Lousberg R, Cheriex E, Van Praag H. Cardiac side-effects of two selective serotonin reuptake inhibitors in middle-aged and elderly depressed patients. *Internat Clin Psychopharm.* 1998;13:263–267.

Thompson C, Peveler R, Stephenson D, McKendrick J. Compliance with antidepressant medication in the treatment of major depressive disorder in primary care: A randomized comparison of fluoxetine and a tricyclic antidepressant. *Am J Psychiatry.* 2000;157:338–343.

Tollefson G, Holman S. Analysis of the Hamilton depression rating scale factors from a double-blind, placebo–controlled trial of fluoxetine in geriatric major depression. *Int Clin Psychopharmacol.* 1993;8:253–259.

Trappler B, Cohen C. Use of SSRI's in "very old" depressed nursing home residents. *Am J Geriatr Psychiatry.* 1998;6:83–89.

Trappler B, Cohen C. Using fluoxetine in "very old" depressed nursing home residents. *Am J Geriatr Psychiatry.* 1996;4:258–262.

Tsai W.-C., Lai J.-S., Wang T.-G. Treatment of emotionalism with fluoxetine during rehabilitation. *Scand J Rehab Med.* 1998;30:145–149.

Wiart L, Petiti H, Joseph P. A., Mazaux J. M., Barat M. Fluoxetine in early post-stroke depression: A double blind placebo-controlled study. *Stroke.* 2000; 31:1829–1832.

Mirtazapine

Bailer U, Fischer P, Kufferle, Stastny J, Kasper S. Occurrence of mirtazapine-induced delirium in organic brain disorder. *Int Clin Psychopharmacol.* 2000;15:239–243.

Benkert O, Szegeti A, Kohnen R. Mirtazapine compared with paroxetine in major depression. *J Clin Psychiatry.* 2000;61:656–663.

Bennazi F. Serotonin syndrome with mirtazapine-fluoxetine combination [letter]. *Int J Geriatr Psychiatry.* 1998;13:495–496.

Berigan T. Sexual dysfunction associated with mirtazapine: A case report [letter]. *J Clin Psychiatry.* 1998;59:319–320.

Boyarsky B, Haque W, Rouleau M, Hirschfeld R. Sexual functioning in depressed outpatients taking mirtazapine. *Depress Anxiety.* 1999;9:175–179.

Bremner J, Wingard P, Walshe T. Safety of mirtazapine in overdose. *J Clin Psychiatry.* 1998;59:233–235.

Bruijn J, Moleman P, Mulder P, van den Broek W. Depressed in-patients respond differently to imipramine and mirtazapine. *Pharmacopsychiatry.* 1999;32:87–92.

Carpenter L, Leon Z, Yasmin S, Price L. Clinical experience with mirtazapine in the treatment of panic disorder. *Ann Clin Psychiatry.* 1999;11:81–86.

de Boer T. The pharmacologic profile of mirtazapine. *J Clin Psychiatry.* 1996;57 (Suppl 4):19–25.

De Leon O. Mirtazapine-induced mania in a case of poststroke depression [letter]. *J Neuropsychiatry Clin Neurosci.* 1999;11:115.

Dunner D, Hendrickson H, Bea C, Budech C, O'Connor E. Dysthymic disorder: treatment with mirtazapine. *Depress Anxiety.* 1999;10:68–72.

Falkai P. Mirtazapine:other indications. *J Clin Psychiatry.* 1999;60 (suppl 17): 36–40.

Farah A. Relief of SSRI-induced sexual dysfunction with mirtazapine treatment. *J Clin Psychiatry.* 1999;60:260–261.

Fawcett J, Barkin R. A meta-analysis of eight, double-blind, controlled clinical trials of mirtazapine for the treatment of patients with depression and symptoms of anxiety. *J Clin Psychiatry.* 1998;59:123–127.

Gelenberg A, Laukes C, McGahuey C, et al. Mirtazapine substitution in SSRI-induced sexual dysfunction. *J Clin Psychiatry.* 2000;61:356–360.

Girishchandra B, Johnson L, Cresp R, Orr R. Mirtazapine-induced akathisia [letter]. *MJA.* 2002;176:242.

Goodnick P, Puig A, DeVane C, Freund B. Mirtazapine in major depression with comorbid generalized anxiety disorder. *J Clin Psychiatry.* 1999;60:446–448.

Gorman J. Mirtazapine: Clinical overview. *J Clin Psychiatry.* 1999;60 (Suppl 17):9–13.

Guelfi J, Ansseau M, Timmerman L, Korsgaard S, Mirtazapine-Venlafaxine Study Group. Mirtazapine versus venlafaxine in hospitalized severely depressed patients with melancholic features. *J Clin Psychopharmacol.* 2001; 21:425–431.

Halikas J. Org 3770 (mirtazapine) versus trazodone placebo-controlled trial in depressed elderly patients. *Human Psychopharmacology.* 1995;10 (Suppl 2):S125–S133.

Holm K, Markham A. Mirtazapine, A review of its use in major depression. *Drugs.* 1999;57:607–631.

Holzbach R, Jahn H, Pajonk F, Mahne C. Suicide attempts with mirtazapine overdose without serious complications. *Biol Psychiatry.* 1998;44:925–926.

Hoyberg O, Maragakis B, Mullin J, et al. A double-blind multicenter comparison of mirtazapine and amitriptyline in elderly depressed patients. *Acta Psychiatr Scand.* 1996;93:184–190.

Kasper S. Clinical efficacy of mirtazapine: A review of meta-analyses of pooled data. *Int Clin Psychopharmacology.* 1995;10 (Suppl 4): 25–35.

Kasper S. Efficacy of antidepressants in the treatment of severe depression: The place of mirtazapine. *J Clin Psychiatry.* 1997;17 (suppl 1):19S–28S.

Kasper S, Praschak-Rieder N, Tauscher J, Wolf R. A risk-benefit assessment of mirtazapine in the treatment of depression. *Drug Safety.* 1997;4:251–264.

Kasper S, Zivokov M, Roes K, Pols A. Pharmacological treatment of severely depressed patients: A meta-analysis comparing efficacy of mirtazapine and amitriptyline. *European Neuropsychopharmacol.* 1997;7:115–124.

MacCall C, Callender J. Mirtazapine withdrawal causing hypomania [letter]. *Br J Psychiatry.* 1999;175:390.

Meco G, Fabriizio E, Di Rezze S, Alessandri A, Pratesi L. Mirtazapine in L-dopa-induced dyskinesias. *Clin Neuropharmacol.* 2003; 6 (4):179–81.

Montgomery S, Reimitz P, Zivkov M. Mirtazapine versus amitriptyline in the long-term treatment of depression: A double-blind placebo-controlled study. *Int Clin Psychopharmacol.* 1998;13:63–73.

Montgomery S. Safety of Mirtazepine: A review. *Int Clin Psychopharmacol.* 1995;10 (Suppl 4):37–45.

Moustgaard G. Treatment-refractory depression successfully treated with the combination of mirtazapine and lithium [letter]. *J Clin Psychopharmacol.* 2000;20:268.

Nutt D. Care of depressed patients with anxiety symptoms. *J Clin Psychiatry.* 1999;60 (Suppl 17):23–27.

Nutt D. Mirtazapine: pharmacology in relation to adverse effects. *Acta Psychiatr Scand.* 1997;96 (suppl 391):31–37.

Pact V, Giduz T. Mirtazapine treats resting tremor, essential tremor, and levodopa-induced dyskinesias. *Neurology.* 1999;53:1154.

Puzantian T. Mirtazapine an antidepressant. *Am J Health Syst.* 1998;55 (Suppl. January 1):44–49.

Radhakishun F, van den Bos J, van der Heijden B, Roes K, O'Hanlon J. Mirtazapine effects on alertness and sleep in patients as recorded by interactive telecommunication during treatment with different dosing regimens. *J Clin Psychopharmacol.* 2000;20:531–537.

Raji M, Brady S. Mirtazapine for treatment of depression and comorbidities in Alzheimer disease. *Ann Pharmacother.* 2001;35:1024–1027.

Schatzberg A, Kremer C, Rodrigues H, Murphy G, Mirtazapine VS Paroxetine Study Group. Double-blind randomized comparison of mirtazapine and paroxetine in elderly depressed patients. *Am J Geriatr Psychiatry.* 2002; 10:541–550.

Stahl S, Zivkof M, Reimitz P, Panagides J, Hoff W. Meta-analysis of randomized, double-blind, placebo-controlled, efficacy and safety studies of mirtazapine versus amitriptyline in major depression. *Acta Psychiatr Scand.* 1997;96 (Suppl 391):22–30.

Stormer E, Von Moltke L, Shader R, Greenblatt D. Metabolism of the antidepressant mirtazapine in vitro: Contribution of cytochromes P-450 1A2, 2D6, and 3A4. *Drug Metab Dispo.* 2000;28:1168–1175.

Szegedi A, Muller MJ, Angheleescu I, Klawe C, Kohnen R, Benkert O. Early improvement under mirtazepine and paroxetine predicts later stable response and remission with high sensitivity in patients with major depression. 2003;64 (4):413–20.

Thompson C. Mirtazapine versus selective serotonin reuptake inhibitors. *J Clin Psychiatry.* 1999;60 (Suppl 17):18–22.

Ubogu EE, Katirji B. Mirtazepine-induced serotonin syndrome. *Clin Neuroopharmacol.* 2003;26 (2):54–7.

Waldinger M, Berendsen H, Schweitzer D. Treatment of hot flushes with mirtazapine: Four case reports. *Maturitas.* 2000;36:165–168.

Whale R, Clifford E, Cowen P. Does mirtazapine enhance serotonergic neurotransmission in depressed patients? *Psychopharmacol.* 2000;148:325–326.

Wheatley D, van Moffaert M, Timmerman L, Kremer C; Mirtazapine-Fluoxetine Study Group. Mirtazapine: Efficacy and tolerability in comparison with fluoxetine in patients with moderate to severe depressive disorder. *J Clin Psychiatry.* 1998;59:306–312.

Moclobemide

Amrein R, Stabl M, Henauer S, Affolter E, Jonkanski I. Efficacy and tolerability of moclobemide in comparison with placebo, tricyclic antidepressants, and selective serotonin reuptake inhibitors in elderly depressed patients: A clinical overview. *Can J Psychiatry.* 1997;42:1043–1050.

Bonnet U. Moclobemide: Therapeutic use and clinical studies. *CNS Drug Rev.* 2003;9 (1):97–140.

Chan-Palay V. Depression and senile dementia of the Alzheimer's type: A role for moclobemide. *Psychopharmacol.* 1992;106:S137–S139.

Fairweather D, Hindmarch I. The behavioral toxicity of reversible inhibitors of monoamine oxidase A: Laboratory and clinical investigations. *J Clin Psychiatry.* 1995;15 (Suppl 2):68S–75S.

Hawley C, Quick S, Ratnam S, Pattinson H, McPhee S. Safety and tolerability of combined treatment with moclobemide and SSRIs: A systematic study of 50 patients. *Int Clin Psychopharmacol.* 1996;11:187–191.

Hetzel W. Safety of moclobemide taken in overdose for attempted suicide. *Psychopharmacol.* 1992;106:S127–S129.

Joffe R, Bakish D. Combined SSRI-moclobemide treatment of psychiatric illness. *J Clin Psychiatry.* 1994;55:24–25.

Kerr J, Fairweather D, Hindmarch I. The effects of acute and repeated doses of moclobemide on psychomotor performance and cognitive function in healthy elderly volunteers. *Human Psychopharmacol.* 1992;7:273–279.

Korpelainen J, Hiltunen P, Myllyla V. Moclobemide-induced hypersexuality in patients with stroke and Parkinson's disease. *Clin Neuropharmacol.* 1998; 21:251–254.

Kruger M, Dahl A. The efficacy and safety of moclobemide compared to clomipramine in the treatment of panic disorder. *Eur Arch Psychiatry Clin Neurosci.* 1999;249:S19–S24.

Magder D, Aleksic I, Kennedy S. Tolerability and efficacy of high-dose moclobemide alone and in combination with lithium and trazodone [letter]. *J Clin Psychopharmacol.* 2000;20:394–395.

Maguire K, Pereira A, Tiller J. Moclobemide pharmacokinetics in depressed patients: Lack of age effect. *Human Psychopharmacol.* 1991;6:349–352.

Nair N, Amin M, Holm P, et al. Moclobemide and nortriptyline in elderly depressed patients: A randomized multicenter study against placebo. *J Affect Disord.* 1995;33:1–9.

Pancheri P, Delle Chiaie R, Dinnini M, et al. Effects of moclobemide on depressive symptoms and cognitive performance in a geriatric population: A controlled comparative study versus imipramine. *Clin Neuropharmacol.* 1994;17:S58–S73.

Roth M, Mountjoy C, Amrein R. Moclobemide in elderly patients with cognitive decline and depression. *Br J Psychiatry.* 1996;168:149–157.

Schoerlin M, Horber F, Frey F, Mayersohn M. Disposition kinetics of moclobemide, a new MAO-A inhibitor, in subjects with impaired renal function. *J Clin Pharmacol.* 1990;30:272–284.

Sieradzan K, Channon S, Ramponi C, Stern G, Lees A, Youdim M. The therapeutic potential of moclobemide, a reversible selective monoamine oxidase-A inhibitor in Parkinson's disease. *J Clin Psychopharmacol.* 1995;15:51S–59S.

Tiller J. Antidepressants, alcohol and psychomotor performance. *Acta Psychiatr Scand.* 1990 (Suppl 360):13–17.

Tiller J, Maguire K, Davies B, Dowling J, Tung L, Rand M. Tyramine-induced cardiac arrhythmias. *Human Psychopharmacol.* 1990;5:313–321.

Warrington S, Turner P, Mant T, et al. Clinical pharmacology of moclobemide, a new reversible monoamine oxidase inhibitor. *J Psychopharmacol.* 1991;5:82–91.

Nefazodone

Alderman C. Possible interaction between Nefazodone and pravastatin [letter]. *Annals Pharmacother.* 1999;33:871.

Barbhaiya R, Akshay B, Greene D. A study of the effect of age and gender on the pharmacokinetics of nefazodone after single and multiple doses. *J Clin Psychopharmacol.* 1996;16:19–25.

Barbhaiya R, Shukla U, Greene D. Single-dose pharmacokinetics of nefazodone in healthy young and elderly subjects and in subjects with renal or hepatic impairment. *Eur J Clin Pharmacol.* 1995;49:221–228.

Catalano G, et al. Nefazodone overdose: A case report. *Clin Neuropharmacol.* 1999;22:63–65.

Davis L, Nugent A, Murray J, Kramer G, Petty F. Nefazodone treatment of chronic posttraumatic stress disorder: An open trial. *J Clin Psychopharmacol.* 2000;20:159–164.

De Vane L. Nefazodone in diabetic neuropathy: Response and biology [letter]. *Psychosomatic Med.* 2000;62:599–600.

Ferguson J, Shrivastava R, Stahl S, et al. Reemergence of sexual dysfunction in patients with major depressive disorder: Double-blind comparison of nefazodone and sertraline. *J Clin Psychiatry.* 2001;62:24–49.

Greene D, Barbhaiya R. Clinical pharmacokinetics of nefazodone. *Clin Pharmacokinet.* 1997;33:260–275.

Hicks J, Argyropoulos S, Rich A, et al. Randomized controlled study of sleep after nefazodone or paroxetine treatment in out-patients with depression. *Br J Psychiatry.* 2002;180:528–535.

Rickels K, Schweizer E, Case G, et al. Nefazodone in major depression: Adjunctive benzodiazepine therapy and tolerability. *J Clin Psychopharmacol.* 1998;18:145–153.

Robinson D, Roberts D, Smith J, et al. The safety profile of nefazodone. *J Clin Psychiatry.* 1996;57 (Suppl 2):31–28.

Sajatovic M, DiGiovanni, Fuller M, et al. Nefazodone therapy in patients with treatment-resistant or treatment-intolerant depression and high psychiatric comorbidity. *Clin Therapeutics.* 1999;21:733–740.

Saper J, Lake A, Tepper S. Nefazodone for chronic daily headache prophylaxis: An open- label study. *Headache.* 2000;41:465–474.

Smith D, Wenegrat B. A case report of serotonin syndrome associated with combined nefazodone and fluoxetine [letter]. *J Clin Psychiatry.* 2000; 61:146.

Sussman N, Ginsberg D, Bikoff J. Effects of nefazodone on body-weight: pooled analysis of selective serotonin reuptake inhibitor- and imipramine-controlled trials. *J Clin Psychiatry.* 2001;62:256–260.

Van Laar M, van Willigenberg A, Volkerts E. Acute and subchronic effects of nefazodone and imipramine on highway driving, cognitive functions, and daytime sleepiness in healthy adult and elderly subjects. *J Clin Psychopharmacol.* 1995;15:30–40.

Zisook S, Chentsova-Dutton Y, Smith-Vaniz A, et al. Nefazodone in patients with treatment refractory posttraumatic stress disorder. *J Clin Psychiatry.* 2000;61:203–208.

Nortriptyline

Buysse D, Reynolds C, Houck P, et al. Does lorazepam impair the antidepressant response to nortriptyline and psychotherapy? *J Clin Psychiatry.* 1997; 58:426–432.

Conforti D, Borgherini G, Fiorellini L, Magni G. Extrapyramidal symptoms associated with the adjunct of nortriptyline to a venlafaxine-valproic acid combination. *Int Clin Psychopharmacol.* 1999;14:197–198.

Dawling S, Crome P, Braithwaite R. Pharmacokinetics of single oral doses of nortriptyline in depressed elderly hospital patients and young healthy volunteers. *Clin Pharmacokinet.* 1980;5:394–401.

Desai A, Chibnall J. Comparative efficacy and safety of sertraline versus nortriptyline in major depression in patients 70 and older [letter]. *Int Psychogeriatrics.* 1999;11:339–342.

Lustman P, Griffith L, Clouse R, et al. Effects of nortriptyline on depression and glycemic control in diabetes: Results of a double-blind, placebo-controlled trial. *Psychosomatic Med.* 1997;59:241–250.

Marraccini R, Reynolds C, Houck P, et al. A double-blind, placebo-controlled assessment of nortriptyline's side effect during 3-year maintenance treatment in elderly patients with recurrent major depression. *Int J Geriatr Psychiatry.* 1999;14:1014–1018.

Mulsant B, Foglia J, Sweet R, Rosen J, Lo K, Pollock B. The effects of perphenazine on the concentration of nortriptyline and its hydroxymetabolites in older patients. *J Clin Psychopharmacol.* 1997;17:318–321.

Nebes RD, Pollock BG, Houck PR, Butters MA, Mulsant BH, Zmuda MD, Reynolds CF 3rd. Persistence of cognitive impairment in geriatric patients following antidepressant treatment: A randomized, double-blind clinical trial with nortriptyline and paroxetine. *J Psychiatr Res.* 2003;37 (2):99–108.

Nierenberg AA, Papakossstas GI, Petersen T, Kelly KE, Iacoviello BM, Worthington JJ, Tedlow J, Alpert JE, Fava M. Nortriptyline for treatment-resistant depression. *J Clin Psychiatry.* 2003;64 (1):35–9.

Reynolds C, Buysse D, Brunner D, et al. Maintenance nortriptyline effects on electroencephalographic sleep in elderly patients with recurrent major depression: Double-blind, placebo- and plasma-level-controlled evaluation. *Biol Psychiatry.* 1997;42:560–567.

Reynolds C, Miller M, Pasternak R, et al. Treatment of bereavement-related major depressive episodes in later-life: A controlled study of acute and continuation treatment with nortriptyline and interpersonal psychotherapy. *Am J Psychiatry.* 1999;156:202–208.

Reynolds C, Perel J, Frank E, et al. Three year outcomes of maintenance nortriptyline treatment in late-life depression: A study of two fixed plasma levels. *Am J Psychiatry.* 1999;156:1177–1181.

Robinson R, Schultz S, Castillo C, et al. Nortriptyline versus fluoxetine in the treatment of depression and in short-term recovery after stroke: A placebo-controlled, double-blind study. *Am J Psychiatry.* 2000;157:351–359.

Roose S, Laghrissi-Thode F, Kennedy J, et al. Comparison of paroxetine and nortriptyline in depressed patients with ischemic heart disease. *JAMA.* 1998; 279:287–291.

Scalco M, Almeida O, Hachul D, Castel S, Serro-Azul J, Wajngarten M. Comparison of risk of orthostatic hypotension in elderly depressed hypertensive women treated with nortriptyline and thiazides versus elderly depressed normotensive women treated with nortriptyline. *Am J Cardiology.* 2000;85: 1156–1158.

Scalco MZ, Serro-Azul JB, Giorgi D, Almeida OP, Wajngarten M. Effect of nortriptyline on the day-night systolic blood pressure difference in hypertensive and normotensive elderly depressed women. *Am J Cardiol.* 2003; 91 (10):1279–1281.

Schneider L, Sloane B, Staples F, Bender M. Pretreatment orthostatic hypotension as a predictor of response to nortriptyline in geriatric depression. *J Clin Psychopharmacol.* 1986;6:172–176.

Streim J, Oslin D, Katz I, et al. Drug treatment of depression in frail elderly nursing home residents. *Am J Geriatr Psychiatry.* 2000;8:150–159.

Taylor M, Reynolds C, Frank E, et al. EEG sleep measures in later-life bereavement depression. *Am J Geriatr Psychiatry.* 1999;7:41–47.

Watson C, Vernich L, Chipman M, Reed K. Nortriptyline versus amitriptyline in post-herpetic neuralgia. *Neurology.* 1998;51:1166–1171.

Young R, Kalayam B, Nambudiri D, Kakuma T, Alexopoulos G. Brain morphology and response to nortriptyline in geriatric depression. *Am J Geriatr Psychiatry.* 1991;7:147–150.

Young R, Mattis S, Alexopoulos G, et al. Verbal memory and plasma drug concentrations in elderly depressives treated with nortriptyline. *Psychopharmacol Bull.* 1991;27:291–294.

Paroxetine

Baldwin D, Bobes J, Stein D, Scharwachter I, Faure M. Paroxetine in social phobia/social anxiety disorder: Randomized, double-blind, placebo-controlled study. *Br J Psychiatry.* 1999;175:120–126.

Benbow S, Gill G. Drug points: Paroxetine and hepatotoxicity [letter]. *BMJ.* 1997;314:1387.

Bourin M. Use of paroxetine for the treatment of depression and anxiety disorders in the elderly: A review. *Hum Psychopharmacol.* 2003;18 (3): 185–90.

Cassano G, Puca F, Scapicchio P, Trabucci M. Paroxetine and fluoxetine effects on mood and cognitive functions in depressed nondemented elderly patients. *J Clin Psychiatry.* 2002;63:396–402.

Chua T, Vong S. Hyponatremia associated with paroxetine [letter]. *BMJ.* 1993; 306:43.

Cotterchio M, Kreiger N, Darlington G, Steingart A. Antidepressant medication use and breast cancer risk. *Am J Epidemiology.* 2000;151:951–957.

Dunbar G. Paroxetine in the elderly: A comparative meta-analysis against standard antidepressant pharmacotherapy. *Pharmacology.* 1995;51:137–144.

Dunner D, Cohn J, Walshe T, et al. Two combined, multicenter double-blind studies of paroxetine and doxepin in geriatric patients with major depression. *J Clin Psychiatry.* 1992;53 (Suppl 2):57–60.

Dunner D, Kumar R. Paroxetine: a review of clinical experience. *Pharmacopsychiatr.* 1998;31:89–101.

Eke T, Bates A. Drug points: acute angle closure glaucoma associated with paroxetine. *BMJ.* 1997;314:1387–1388.

Geretsegger C, Bohmer F, Ludwig M. Paroxetine in the elderly depressed patient: Randomized comparison with fluoxetine of efficacy, cognitive and behavioural effects. *Int Clin Psychopharmacology.* 1994;9:25–29.

Geretsegger C, Stuppaeck C, Mair M, Platz T, Fartacek R, Heim M. Multicenter double-blind study of paroxetine and amitriptyline in elderly depressed inpatients. *Psychopharmacol.* 1995;119:277–281.

Gilmor M, Owens M, Nemeroff C. Inhibition of norepinephrine uptake in patients with major depression treated with paroxetine. *Am J Psychiatry.* 2002;159:1702–1710.

Guillibert E, Pelicier Y, Archambault P, et al. A double-blind multicenter study of paroxetine versus clomipramine in depressed elderly patients. *Acta Psychiatr Scand.* 1989;80 (Suppl 350):132–134.

Gunasekara N, Noble S, Benfield P. Paroxetine: An update of its pharmacology and therapeutic use in depression and a review of its use in other disorders. ADIS drug evaluation; *Drugs.* 1998;55:85–120.

Hutchinson D, Tong S, Moon C, et al. Paroxetine in the treatment of elderly depressed patients in general practice: A double-blind comparison with amitriptyline. *Int Clin Psychopharmacol.* 1992;6 (Suppl 4):43–51.

Johnsen C, Hoejlyng N. Hyponatremia following acute overdose with paroxetine. *Int J Clin Pharmacol Therapeutics.* 1998;36:333–335.

Joseph J. Treatment of poststroke pathological crying [letter]. *Stroke.* 1997; 28:2321.

Judge R, Parry M, Quail D, Jacobson J. Discontinuation syndromes: Comparison of brief interruption in fluoxetine and paroxetine treatment. *Int Clin Psychopharmacol.* 2002;17:217–225.

Lantz M, Buchalter E, Giambanco V. Serotonin syndrome following the administration of tramadol with paroxetine [letter]. *Int J Geriatr Psychiatry.* 1998;13:343–345.

Lecrubier Y, Judge R. Long-term evaluation of paroxetine, clomipramine and placebo in panic disorder. *Acta Psychiatr Scand.* 1997;95:153–160.

Lewis C, DeQuardo J, DuBose C, Tandon R. Acute angle-closure glaucoma and paroxetine [letter]. *J Clin Psychiatry.* 1997;58:123–124.

McMahon C, Touma K. Treatment of premature ejaculation with paroxetine hydrochloride. *Int J Impotence Res.* 1999;11:241–246.

Moretti R, Torre P, Antonello RM, Cazzato G, Bava A. frontotemporal dementia: paroxetine as a possible treatment of behavior symptoms. A randomized, controlled, open 14-month study. *Eur Neurol.* 2003;49 (1):13–9.

Nebes R, Pollock B, Mulsant R, Butters M, Zmuda M, Reynolds C. Cognitive effects of paroxetine in older depressed patients. *J Clin Psychiatry.* 1999;60 (Suppl 20): 26–29.

Nelson J, Kennedy J, Pollock B, et al. Treatment of major depression with nortriptyline and paroxetine in patients with ischemic heart disease. *Am J Psychiatry.* 1999;156:1024–1028.

Nemeroff C. The clinical pharmacology and use of paroxetine, a new selective serotonin reuptake inhibitor. *Pharmacotherapy.* 1994;14:127–138.

Odeh M, Seligmann H, Oliven A. Severe life-threatening hyponatremia during paroxetine therapy. *J Clin Pharmacol.* 1999;39:1290–1291.

Pae CU, Kim JJ, Lee SJ, Chui-Lee CL, Paik IH. Provoked bradycardia after paroxetine administration. *Gen Hosp Psychiatry.* 2003;25 (2):142–4.

Paul S, Sankaran S. An unusually rapid onset of hyponatremia following paroxetine [letter]. *Aust NZ J Med.* 1998;28:640.

Pinner A. Drug points: Postural hypotension induced by paroxetine [letter]. *BMJ.* 1998;316:595.

Pollock B, Mulsant B, Nebes R, et al. Serum anticholinergicity in elderly depressed patients treated with paroxetine or nortriptyline. *Am J Psychiatry.* 1998;155:1110–1112.

Ramasubba R. Minor strokes related to paroxetine discontinuation in an elderly subjects: emergent adverse events. *Can J Psychiatry.* 2003;48 (4): 281–282.

Schone W, Ludwig M. A double-blind study of paroxetine compared with fluoxetine in geriatric patients with major depression. *J Clin Psychopharmacol.* 1994;13 (Suppl 2):34S–39S.

Solai L, Pollock B, Mulsant B, et al. Effect of nortriptyline and paroxetine on CYP2D6 activity in depressed elderly patients. *J Clin Psychopharmacol.* 2002;22:481–486.

Szegedi A, Wetzel H, Angersbach D, Philipp M, Benkert O. Response to treatment in minor and major depression: Results of a double-blind comparative study with paroxetine and maprotiline. *J Affective Dis.* 1997;45:167–178.

Wagstaff A, Cheer S, Matheson A, Ormrod D. Paroxetine: An update of its use in psychiatric disorders in adults. *Drugs.* 2002;62:655–703.

Weber E, Stack J, Pollock B, et al. Weight change in older depressed patients during acute pharmacotherapy with paroxetine and nortriptyline. *Am J Geriatr Psychiatry.* 2000;8:245–250.

Williams J, Barrett J, Oxman T, et al. Treatment of dysthymia and minor depression in primary care: A randomized controlled trial in older adults. *JAMA.* 2000;284:1519–1525.

Sertraline

Bondareff W, Alpert M, Friedhoff A, Richter E, Clary C, Batzar E. Comparison of sertraline and nortriptyline in the treatment of major depressive disorder in late life. *Am J Psychiatry.* 2000;157:729–736.

Brady K, Pearlstein T, Asnis G, et al. Efficacy and safety of sertraline treatment of posttraumatic stress disorder: A randomized controlled study. *JAMA.* 2000;283:1837–1844.

Cohn C, Shrivastava R, Mendels J, et al. Double-blind multi-center study of sertraline and amitriptyline in elderly depressed patients. *J Clin Psychiatry.* 1990;51:28–33.

Devanand DP, Pelton GH, Marston K, Camacho Y, Roose SP, Stern Y, Sackeim HA. Sertraline treatment of elderly patients with depression and cognitive impairment. *Int J Geriatr Psychiatry.* 2003;18 (2):123–30.

George T, Theodoros M, Chiu E, Krapivensky N, Hokin H, Tiller J. An open study of sertraline in patients with major depression who failed to respond to moclobemide. *Aust NZ J Psychiatry.* 1999;33:889–895.

Haselberger M, Freedman L, Lois S, Tolbert S. Elevated serum phenytoin concentrations associated with coadministration of sertraline. *J Clin Psychopharmacol.* 1997;17:107–109.

Krishnan K, Doraiswamy P, Clary C. Clinical and treatment response characteristics of late-life depression associated with vascular disease: A pooled analysis of two multicenter trials with sertraline. *Prog Neuropsychopharmacol Biol Psychiatry.* 2001;25:347–361.

Kumar L, Mulsant B, Pollock B, et al. Effect of sertraline on plasma nortriptyline levels in depressed elderly. *J Clin Psychiatry.* 1997;58:440–443.

Lee M-S, Han C-S, You Y-W, Kim S-H. Co-administration of sertraline and haloperidol. *Psychiatry Clin Neurosc.* 1998;52 (Suppl):S193–S198.

Levsky M, Schwartz J. Sertraline induced hyponatremia in an older patient [letter]. *JAGS.* 1998;46:1582–1583.

Londborg P, Wolkow R, Smith W, et al. Sertraline in the treatment of panic disorder: A multi-site, double-blind, placebo-controlled, fixed-dose investigation. *Br J Psychiatry.* 1998;173:54–60.

Magai C, Kennedy G, Cohen C, Gomberg D. A controlled clinical trial of sertraline in the treatment of depression in nursing home patients with late-stage alzheimer's disease. *Am J Geriatr Psychiatry.* 2000;8:66–74.

Newhouse P, Krishnan R, Doraiswamy P, Richter E, Batzar E, Clary C. A double-blind comparison of sertraline and fluoxetine in depressed elderly outpatients. *J Clin Psychiatry.* 2000;61:559–568.

Pearlstein T. Antidepressant treatment of posttraumatic stress disorder. *J Clin Psychiatry.* 2000;61 (Suppl 7):40–42.

Rosen J, Mulsant B, Pollock B. Sertraline in the treatment of minor depression in nursing home residents: A pilot study. *Int J Geriatric Psychiatry.* 2000;15:177–180.

Schneider LS, Nelson JC, Clary CM, Newhouse P, Krishnan KR, Shiovitz T, Weihs K; Sertraline Elderly Depression Study Group. An 8-week multicenter, parallel-group, double-blind, placebo-controlled study of sertraline in elderly outpatients with major depression. *Am J Psychiatry.* 2003; 160 (7):277–85.

Shapiro P, Lesperance F, Frasure-Smith N, et al. An open-label preliminary trial of sertraline for treatment of major depression after acute myocardial infarction (the SADHAT trial). *Am Heart J.* 1999;137;1100–1106.

Varia I, Logue E, O'Connor C, et al. Randomized trial of sertraline in patients with unexplained chest pain of noncardiac origin. *Am Heart J.* 2000; 140:367–372.

Warrington S. Clinical implications of the pharmacology of sertraline. *Int Clin Psychopharmacol.* 1991;2 (Suppl):11–21.

St. John's Wort

Linde K, Mulrow C. St. John's wort for depression. Cochrane library, Cochrane database of systematic reviews, 2000; CD000448.

Linde K, Ramirez G, Mulrow C. St. John's Wort for depression: An overview and meta-analysis of randomized clinical trials. *BMJ.* 1996;313:253–258.

Trazodone

Altamura A, Mauri M, Colacurcio F, et al. Trazodone in late-life depressive states: A double-blind multicenter study versus amitriptyline and mianserin. *Psychopharmacol.* 1988;95:S34–S36.

Altamura A, Mauri M, Rudas N, et al. Clinical activity and tolerability of trazodone, mianserin, and amitriptyline in elderly subjects with major depression: A controlled multicenter trial. *Clin Neuropharmacol.* 1989;12 (Suppl 1): S25–S33.

Ather S, Ankier S, Middleton R. A double-blind evaluation of trazodone in the treatment of depression in the elderly. *Br J Clin Pract.* 1985;39:192–199.

Bayer A, Pathy M, Cameron A, Venkateswalu T, Ather S, et al. A comparative study of conventional and controlled-release formulations of trazodone in elderly depressed patients. *Clin Neuropharmacol.* 1989;12 (Suppl 1):S50–S55.

Burns M, Moskowitz H, Jaffe J. A comparison of the effects of trazodone and amitriptyline on skills performance by geriatric subjects. *J Clin Psychiatry.* 1986;47:252–254.

Gerner R, Estabrook W, Steuer J, et al. Treatment of geriatric depression with trazodone, imipramine, and placebo: A double-blind study. *J Clin Psychiatry.* 1980;41:216–220.

Gerner R. Geriatric depression and treatment with trazodone. *Psychopathology.* 1985;20 (Suppl 1):82–89.

Gershon S. Comparative side effect profiles of trazodone and imipramine: special reference to the geriatric population. *Psychopathol.* 1984;17 (Suppl 2): 39–50.

Greenwald B, Marin D, Silverman S. Serotonergic treatment of screaming and banging in dementia. *Lancet.* 1986;2:1464–1465.

Haria M, Fitton A, McTavish D. Trazodone: A review of its pharmacology, therapeutic use in depression and therapeutic potential in other disorders. *Drugs Aging.* 1994;4:331–355.

Hayashi T, Yokota N, Takahashi T, et al. Benefits of trazodone and mianserin for patients with late-life chronic schizophrenia and tardive dyskinesia: An add-on double-blind, placebo-controlled study. *Int Clin Psychopharmacol.* 1997;12:199–205.

Houlihan D, Mulsant B, Sweet R, et al. A naturalistic study of trazodone in the treatment of behavioral complications of dementia. *Am J Geriatr Psychiatry.* 1994;2:78–85.

Lawlor B, et al. A pilot placebo-controlled study of Trazodone and Buspirone in Alzheimer's disease. *Int J Geriatr Psychiatry.* 1994;9:55–59.

Mukherjee P, Davey A. Differential dosing of trazodone in elderly patients: A study to investigate optimal dosing. *J Int Med Res.* 1986;14:279–284.

Nierenberg A, Adler L, Peselow E, Zornberg G, Rosenthal M. Trazodone for antidepressant-associated insomnia. *Am J Psychiatry.* 1994;151:1069–1072.

Okamoto Y, Matsuoka Y, Sasaki T, Jitsuiki H, Horiguchi J, Yamawaki S. Trazodone in the treatment of delirium [letter]. *J Clin Psychopharmacol.* 1999;19:280–282.

Pinner E, Rich C. Effects of trazodone on aggressive behavior in seven patients with organic mental behaviors. *Am J Psychiatry.* 1988;145:1295–1296.

Rao R. Serotonin syndrome associated with trazodone [letter]. *Int J Geriatr Psychiatry.* 1997;12:129–130.

Spar J. Plasma trazodone concentrations in elderly depressed inpatients: Cardiac effects and short-term efficacy. *J Clin Psychopharmacol.* 1987;7:406–409.

Sultzer D, Gray K, Gunay I, Berisford A, Mahler M. A double-blind comparison of trazodone and haloperidol for treatment of agitation in patients with dementia. *Am J Geriatr Psychiatry.* 1997;5:60–69.

Teri L, et al. Treatment of agitation in AD: a randomized placebo-controlled clinical trial. *Neurology.* 2000;55:1271–1278.

Warner M, Peabody C, Whiteford H, Hollister L. Trazodone and priapism. *J Clin Psychiatry.* 1987;48:244–245.

Wilson R. The use of low-dose trazodone in painful diabetic neuropathy. *J Am Podiatr Assoc.* 1999;89:468–471.

Venlafaxine

Agelink MW, Klieser E. Prolonged bradycardia complicates antidepressant treatment with venlafaxine and ECT [letter]. *Br J Psychiatry.* 1998;173:41.

Agelink MW, Zitzelsberger A, Klieser E. Withdrawal syndrome after discontinuation of venlafaxine [letter]. *Am J Psychiatry.* 1997;154:1473–1474.

Albers L, Reist C, Vu R, et al. Effect of venlafaxine on imipramine metabolism. *Psychiatry Res.* 2000;96:235–243.

Amchin J, Albano D. Clinical considerations in managing nausea associated with venlafaxine [letter]. *J Clin Psychopharmacology.* 1997;17:489–490.

Amore M, Ricci M, Zanardi R, Perez J, Ferrari G. Long-term treatment of depressed geropsychiatric patients with venlafaxine. *J Affective Dis.* 1997;46:293–296.

Amsterdam J. Efficacy and safety of venlafaxine in the treatment of bipolar II major depressive episode. *J Clin Psychopharmacology.* 1998;18:414–417.

Amsterdam J, Garcia-Espana F. Venlafaxine monotherapy in women with bipolar II and unipolar major depression. *J Affective Dis.* 2000;59:225–229.

Amsterdam J, Hooper M, Amchin J. Once- versus twice-daily venlafaxine therapy in major depression: A randomized, double-blind study. *J Clin Psychiatry.* 1998;59:236–240.

Ansari A. The efficacy of newer antidepressants in the treatment of chronic pain: A review of current literature. *Harv Rev Psychiatry.* 2000;7:257–277.

Aragona M, Inghilleri M. Increased intraocular pressure in two patients with narrow angle glaucoma treated with venlafaxine. *Clin Neuropharmacology.* 1998;21:130–131.

Bader G, Hawley J, Short D. Venlafaxine augmentation with methylphenidate for treatment-refractory depression: A case report [letter]. *J Clin Psychopharmacol.* 1998;18:255–256.

Benazzi F. Anticholinergic toxic syndrome with venlafaxine-desipramine combination [letter]. *Pharmacopsychiatr.* 1998;31:36–37.

Benazzi F. Venlafaxine drug-drug interactions in clinical practice [letter]. *J Psychiatry Neuroscience.* 1998;23:181–182.

Benazzi F. Venlafaxine-fluoxetine-nortriptyline interaction. *J Psychiatry Neurosci.* 1997;22:278–279.

Bernardo M, Navarro V, Salva J, Aruffat F, Baeza I. Seizure activity and safety in combined treatment with venlafaxine and ECT: A pilot study. *J ECT.* 2000;16:38–42.

Blass D, Pearson V. SIADH with multiple antidepressants in a geriatric patient [letter]. *J Clin Psychiatry.* 2000;61:448–449.

Cardona X. Venlafaxine–associated hepatitis [letter]. *Annals Intern Med.* 2000;132:417.

Clerc G, Ruimy P, Verdeau-Pailles J on behalf of the Venlafaxine French Inpatient Study Group. A double-blind comparison of venlafaxine and fluoxetine in patients hospitalized for major depression and melancholia. *Int Clin Psychopharmacol.* 1994;9:139–143.

Cunningham L. Once-daily venlafaxine extended release (XR) and venlafaxine immediate release (IR) in outpatients with major depression. *Annals Clin Psychiatry.* 1997;9:157–164.

Dahmen N, Marx J, Hopf H C, Tettenborn B, Roder R. Therapy of early poststroke depression with Venlafaxine: Safety, tolerability and efficacy as determined in an open, uncontrolled clinical trial [letter]. *Stroke.* 1999;30:691–692.

Danjou P, Hackett D. Safety and tolerance profile of venlafaxine. *Int Clin Psychopharmacology.* 1995;10 (Suppl 2):15–20.

Davidson J, DuPont R, Hedges D, Haskins J. Efficacy, safety and tolerability of venlafaxine extended release and buspirone in outpatients with generalized anxiety disorder. *J Clin Psychiatry.* 1999;60:528–535.

De Montigny C, Silverstone P, Debonnel G, Blier P, Bakish D. Venlafaxine in treatment resistant major depression: A Canadian multi-center open-label trial. *Clin Psychopharmacol.* 1999;19:401–406.

Diamond S, Pepper B, Diamond M, Freitag D, Urban G, Erdemoglu A. Serotonin syndrome induced by transitioning from phenelzine to venlafaxine: Four patient reports. *Neurology.* 1998;51:274–276.

Dunner D, Hendrickson H, Bea C, Buldech C. Venlafaxine in dysthymic disorder. *J Clin Psychiatry.* 1997;58 (12):528–531.

Einarson T, Arikian S, Casciano J, Doyle J. Comparison of extended-release venlafaxine, selective serotonin reuptake inhibitors, and tricyclic antidepressants in the treatment of depression: A meta-analysis of randomized controlled trials. *Clin Therapeutics.* 1999;21:296–308.

Fava M, Mulroy R, Alpert J, Nierenberg A, Rosenbaum J. Emergence of adverse events following discontinuation of treatment with extended-release venlafaxine. *Am J Psychiatry.* 1997;154:1760–1762.

Garber A, Gregory R. Benztropine in the treatment of venlafaxine-induced sweating [letter]. *J Clin Psychiatry.* 1997;58:176–177.

Gasto C, Navarro V, Marcos T, Portella MJ, Torra M, Rodamilans M. Single-blind comparison of venlafaxine and nortriptyline in elderly major depression. *J Clin Psychopharmacol.* 2003;23 (1):21–6.

Gelenberg A, Lydiard R B, Rudolph R L, Aguiar L, Haskins J T, Salinas E. Efficacy of venlafaxine extended-release capsules in nondepressed outpatients with generalized anxiety disorder. *JAMA.* 2000;283:3082–3088.

Gupta A.K, Saravay S. Venlafaxine-induced hyponotremia. [letter]. *J Clin Psychopharmacology.* 1997;17:223–225.

Hackett D, Salinas E. Neurobiological basis of antidepressant safety profiles. *Eur Psychiatry.* 1997;12 (Suppl):301s–306s.

Harvey A, Rudolph R, Preskorn S. Evidence of the dual mechanisms of action of venlafaxine. *Arch Gen Psychiatry.* 2000;57:503–509.

Hellerstein D, Batchelder S, Little S, Fedak M, Kreditor D, Rosenthal J. Venlafaxine in the treatment of dysthymia: An open label study. *J Clin Psychiatry.* 1999;60:845–849.

Hoencamp E, Haffmans J, Dijken W, Huijbrechts I. Lithiium augmentation of venlafaxine: An open-label trial. *J Clin Psychopharmacol.* 2000;20:538–543.

Jaffe M, Bostwick J. Buspirone as an antidote to venlafaxine-induced bruxism. *Psychosomatics.* 2000;41:535–536.

Khan A, Rudolph R, Baumel B, Ferguson J, Ryan P, Shrivastava R. Venlafaxine in depressed geriatric outpatients: An open-label clinical study. *Psychopharmacol Bull.* 1995;31:753–758.

Kiayias J A, Vlachou E D, Lakka-Papadodima E. Venlafaxine HCl in the treatment of painful diabetic neuropathy [letter]. *Diabetes Care.* 2000;23:699.

Lederking W, Tennen H, Nackley J, Hale M, Turner R, Testa M. The effects of venlafaxine on social activity level in depressed outpatients. *J Clin Psychiatry.* 1999;60:157–163.

Licht R, Kassow P. Venlafaxine for the treatment of psychotic depression [letter]. *Eur Psychiatry.* 1998;13:276–277.

Mahapatra S, Hackett D. A randomized, double-blind, parallel-group comparison of venlafaxine and dothiepin in geriatric patients with major depression. *Int J Clin Pract.* 1997;51:209–213.

Masood G, Karki S, Patterson W. Hyponatremia with venlafaxine. *Annals Psychopharm.* 1998;32:49–50.

Mitchel P, Schweitzer I, Burrows G, Johnson G, Polonowita A. Efficacy of venlafaxine and predictors of response in a prospective open-label study of patients with treatment-resistant major depression. *J Clin Psychopharmacol.* 2000;20:483–487.

Perry N. Venlafaxine-induced serotonin syndrome with relapse following amitriptyline. *Postgrad Med J.* 2000;76:254–256.

Poirier M, Boyer P. Venlafaxine and paroxetine in treatment-resistant depression: Double-blind randomised comparison. *Br J Psychiatry.* 1999;175: 12–16.

Preskorn S. Pharmacotherapeutic profile of venlafaxine. *Eur Psychiatry.* 1997;12 (Suppl 4):285s–294s.

Quella S, Loprinzi C, Sloan J, et al. Pilot evaluation of venlafaxine for the treatment of hot flashes in men undergoing androgen ablation therapy for prostate cancer. *J Urol.* 1999;162:98–102.

Reynolds C F, Frank E, Kupfer D J, et al. Treatment outcome in recurrent major depression: A post hoc comparison of elderly ("young old") and mid-life patients. *Am J Psychiatry.* 1996;153:1288–1292.

Rickels K, Feiger A. A double blind randomized placebo-controlled trial of once daily venlafaxine extended release (XR) and fluoxetine for the treatment of depression. *J Affective Dis.* 1999;56:171–181.

Rickels K, Pollack M, Sheehan D, Haskins J. Efficacy of extended release venlafaxine in nondepressed outpatients with generalized anxiety disorder. *Am J Psychiatry.* 2000;157:968–974.

Rudolph R, Entsuah R, Chitra R. A meta-analysis of the effects of venlafaxine on anxiety associated with depression. *J Clin Psychopharmacol.* 1988;18:136–144.

Rudolph R, Fabre L F, Feighner J P, Rickels C, Entsuah R, Derivan A T. A randomized placebo-controlled dose-response trial of venlafaxine hydrochloride in the treatment of major depression. *J Clin Psychiatry.* 1998;59: 116–122.

Rudolph R, Feiger A. A double-blind, randomized, placebo-controlled trial of once-daily venlafaxine extended release (XR) and fluoxetine for the treatment of depression. *J Affective Dis.* 1999;56:171–181.

Schatzberg A, Cantillon M. Antidepressant early response and remission with venlafaxine or fluoxetine in depressed geriatric patients. *Int J Neuropsychopharmacol.* 2000;3 (Suppl 1):S191.

Schwartz T. Diaphoresis and pruritis with extended release venlafaxine [letter]. *Ann Pharmacother.* 1999;33:1009.

Silverstone P, Ravindran A. Once-daily venlafaxine extended release (XR) compared with fluoxetine in outpatients with depression and anxiety. *J Clin Psychiatry.* 1999;60:22–28.

Smith D, Dempster C, Glanville J, Freemantle N, Anderson I. Efficacy and tolerability of venlafaxine compared with selective serotonin reuptake inhibitors and other antidepressants: A meta-analysis. *Br J Psychiatry.* 2002;180:396–404.

Spier S. Use of bupropionwith SRIs and venlafaxine. *Depress Anxiety.* 1998;7:73–75.

Stoner S, Williams R, Worrel J, Ramlatchman L. Possible venlafaxine-induced mania [letter]. *J Clin Psychopharmacol.* 1999;19:184–185.

Tharmapathy P, Selheim F, Odegaard K, Lund A, Holmsen H. Venlafaxine treatment stimulates blood platelet activity [letter]. *J Clin Psychopharmacol.* 2000;20:589–590.

Thase M. Effects of venlafaxine on blood pressure: A meta-analysis of original data from 3744 depressed patients. *J Clin Psychiatry.* 1998;59:502–550.

Thase M. Efficacy and tolerability of once-daily venlafaxine extended release (XR) in outpatients with major depression. *J Clin Psychiatry.* 1997;58:393–398.

Zimmer B, Kant R , Zeiler D, Brilmyer M. Antidepressant efficacy and cardiovascular safety of venlafaxine in young vs. old patients with comorbid medical disorders. *Intl J Psychiatry Med.* 1997;27:353–364.

ANTIPSYCHOTIC AGENTS

Aakerlund L, Rosenberg J. Postoperative delirium: Treatment with supplementary oxygen. *Br J Anaesth.* 1994;72:286–290.

Achiron A, Melamed E. Tardive eating dystonia. *Mov Disord.* 1990;5:331–333.

Addonizio G, Alexopoulos G. Drug-induced dystonia in young and elderly patients. *Am J Psychiatry.* 1988;145:869–871.

Allison D, Mentore J, Heo M, et al. Antipsychotic-induced weight gain: A comprehensive research synthesis. *Am J Psychiatr.* 1999;156:1686–1696.

Ansari A, Maron BJ, Berntson DG. Drug-induced toxic myocardiitis. *Tex Heart Inst J.* 2003;30 (1):76–9.

Arevalo G, Gershanik O. Modulatory effect of clozapine on levodopa response in Parkinson's disease: A preliminary study. *Mov Disord.* 1993;8:349–354.

Arunpongpaisal S, Ahmed I, Aqeel N, Suchat P. Antipsychotic drug treatment for elderly people with late-onset schizophrenia. *Cochrane Database Syst Rev.* 2003; (2):CD004162.

Ballard C, Holmes C, McKeith I, et al. Psychiatric morbidity in dementia with

Lewy bodies: A prospective clinical and neuropathological comparative study with Alzheimer's disease. *Am J Psychiatry.* 1999;156:1039–1045.

Balllard C, O'Brian J. Treating behavioural disease and psychological sign in Alzheimer's disease. *BMJ.* 1999;319:138–139.

Barnes T, Kidger T, Gore S. Tardive dyskinesia: A 3-year follow-up study. *Psychol Med.* 1983;13:71–81.

Batra A, Bartels M, Wormstall H. Therapeutic options in Charles Bonnet syndrome. *Acta Psychiatr Scand.* 1997;96:129–133.

Buckley N, Sanders P. Cardiovascular adverse effects of antipsychotic drugs. *Drug Saf.* 2000;23:215–228.

Burke W, Pfeiffer R, McComb R. Neuroleptic sensitivity to clozapine in dementia with Lewy bodies. *J Neuropsychiatry Clin Neurosci.* 1998;10:227–229.

Burns A. The oldest patient with Capgras syndrome? *Br J Psychiatry.* 1985; 147:719–720.

Buse J, Cavazzoni P, Hornbuckle K, Hutchins D, Breier A, Jovanovic L. A retrospective cohort study of diabetes mellitus and antipsychotic treatment in the United States. *J. Clin Epidemiol.* 2003;56:164–170.

Caligiuri M, Lacro J, Jeste D. Incidence and predictors of drug-induced parkinsonism in older psychiatric patients treated with very low doses of neuroleptics. *J Clin Psychopharmacol.* 1999;19:322–328.

Caligiuri M, Rockwell E, Jeste D. Extrapyramidal side effects in patients with Alzheimer's disease treated with low-dose neuroleptic medication. *Am J Geriatr Psychiatry.* 1998;6:75–82.

Casey D. Tardive dyskinesia and atypical antipsychotic drugs. *Schizophr Res.* 1999;35:S61–S66.

Centorrino F, Price B, Tuttle M, et al. EEG abnormalities during treatment with typical and atypical antipsychotics. *Am J Psychiatry.* 2002;159:109–115.

Chandran GJ, Mikler JR, Keegan DL. Neuroleptic malignant syndrome: Care report and discussion. *Can Med Assoc J.* 2003;160 (5):439–442.

Chong S, Sachdev P, Mahendran R, Chua H. Neuroleptic and anticholinergic drug use in Chinese patients with schizophrenia resident in a state psychiatric hospital in Singapore. *Aust NZ J Psychiatry.* 2000;34:988–991.

Chouinard G, Bradwein J, Annable L, Jones B, Ross-Chouinard A. Withdrawal symptoms after long-term treatment with low-potency neuroleptics. *J Clin Psychiatry.* 1984;45:500–502.

Coccaro E, Kramer E, Zemishlany Z, et al. Pharmacologic treatment of noncognitive behavioural disturbances in elderly demented patients. *Am J Psychiatry.* 1990;147:1640–1645.

Cochrane Database Syst. Rev. Antipsychotic drug treatment for elderly people with late-onset schizophrenia. *Cochrane Database Syst. Rev.* 2003; (2) CD004162.

Cohen C, Cohen G, Blank K, et al. Schizophrenia and older adults: An overview: Directions for research and policy. *Am J Geriatr Psychiatry.* 2000;8:19–28.

Cohen-Mansfield J, Garfinkel D, Lipson S. Melatonin for treatment of sundowning in elderly persons with dementia: A preliminary study. *Arch Gerontol Geriatr.* 2000;31:65–76.

Cohen-Mansfield J, Lipson S, Werner P, Billig N, Taylor L, Woosley R. Withdrawal of haloperidol, thioridazine, and lorazepam in the nursing home. *Arch Intern Med.* 1999;159:1733–1740.

Conn D, Lieff S. Diagnosing and managing delirium in the elderly. *Can Fam Physician.* 2001;47:101–108.

Cummings J, Gorman D, Shapira J. Physostigmine ameliorates the delusions of Alzheimer's disease. *Biol Psychiatry.* 1993;33:536–541.

Daniel D. Antipsychotic treatment of psychosis and agitation in the elderly. *J Clin Psychiatry.* 2000;61 (Suppl 14):49–52.

Devanand D. Conventional neuroleptics in dementia. *Int Psychogeriatr.* 2000;12 (suppl 1):253–261.

Dewey R, O'Suilleabhain P. Treatment of drug-induced psychosis with quetiapine and clozapine in Parkinson's disease. *Neurology.* 2000;55:1753–1754.

Dolder CR, Jeste DV. Incidence of tardive dyskinesia with typical versus atypical antipsychotics in very high risk patients. *Biol Psychiatry.* 2003; 53 (12):1142–5.

Eastham J, Jeste D. Treatment of schizophrenia and delusional disorder in the elderly. *Eur Arch Psychiatry Clin Neurosci.* 1997;247:209–218.

Eberlein-Konig B, Bindl A, Przybilla B. Phototoxic properties of neuroleptic drugs. *Dermatology.* 1997;194:131–135.

Edell W, Tunis S. Antipsychotic treatment of behavioral and psychological symptoms of dementia in geropsychiatric in patients. *Am J Psychiatry.* 2001;9:289–297.

Ellis T, Cudkowicz M, Sexton P, Growdon J. Clozapine and risperidone treatment of psychosis in Parkinson's disease. *J Neuropsychiatry Clin Neurosci.* 2000;12:364–369.

Espinoza R. Assessing antopsychotic effectiveness in dementia: a factor analysis approach. *J Am Med Dir Assoc.* 2003;4 (2):113–4.

Finkel S. Managing the behavioral and psychological signs and symptoms of dementia. *Int Clin Psychopharmacol.* 1997;12 (Suppl 4):S25–S28.

Fink M. Treating neuroleptic malignant syndrome as catatonia [letter]. *J Clin Psychopharmacol.* 2001;21:121.

Fraser G, Prato S, Riker R, Berthiaume D, Wilkins M. Frequency, severity, and treatment of agitation in young versus elderly patients in ICU. *Pharmacother.* 2000;20:75–82.

Frenchman I. Risperidone, haloperidol and olanzapine for the treatment of behavioral disturbances in nursing home patients: A retrospective analysis. *Curr Therapeutic Res.* 2000;61:742–750.

Fricchione G, Cassem N, Hooberman N, Hobson D. Intravenous lorazepam in neuroleptic-induced catatonia. *J Clin Psychopharmacol.* 1983; 3:338–342.

Friedman J. Atypical anti-psychotics in the EPS-vulnerable patient. *Psychoneuroendocrinology* 2003: (Suppl 1):39–51.

Gaertner I, Altendorf K, Batra A, Gaertner H. Relevance of liver enzyme elevations with four different neuroleptics: A retrospective review of 7,263 treatment courses. *J Clin Psychopharmacol.* 2001;21:215–222.

Ganguli R. Weight gain associated with antipsychotic drugs. *J Clin Psychiatry.* 1999;60 (Suppl 21):20–24.

Ganzini L, Casey D, Hoffman W, Heintz W. Tardive dyskinesia and diabetes mellitus. *Psychopharmacol Bull.* 1992;28:281–286.

Gattera J, Charles B, Williams G, M Cavenagh J, Smithurst B, Luchjenbroers J. A retrospective study of risk factors of akathesia in terminally ill patients. *J Pain Symptom Manage.* 1994;9:454–461.

Gerding L, Labbate L. Use of clonazepam in an elderly bipolar patient with tardive dyskinesia: A case report. *Ann Clin Psychiatry.* 1999;11:87–89.

Geroldi C, Frisoni G, Bianchetti A, Trabucci M. Drug treatment in Lewy Body dementia. *Dement Geriatr Cogn Disord.* 1997; 8:188–197.

Gershanik O. Drug-induced parkinsonism in the aged. *Drugs Aging.* 1994;5: 127–132.

Gianfrancesco F. Diabetes and atypical neuroleptics. *Am J. Psychiatry* 2003;160:388–389.

Glassman A, Bigger J. Antipsychotic drugs: Prolonged QTc interval, torsades de pointes, and sudden death. *Am J Psychiatry.* 2001;158:1774–1782.

Goff D, Wine L. Glutamate in schizophrenia: Clinical and research implications. *Schizophre Res.* 1997;27:157–168.

Greendyke R, Berkner J, Webster J, Gulya A. Treatment of behavioral problems with pindolol. *Psychosomatics.* 1989;30:161–165.

Hagg S, Joelsson L, Mjorndal T, Spigset O, Oja G, Dahlqvist R. Prevalence of diabetes and impaired glucose tolerance in patients treated with clozapine compared with patients treated with conventional depot neuroleptic medications. *J Clin Psychiatry.* 1998;59:294–299.

Hagg S, Mjorndal T. Repeated episodes of hypothermia in a subject treated with haloperidol, levomepromazine, olanzapine, and thioridazine [letter]. *J Clin Psychopharmacol.* 2001;21:113–115.

Hanson L, Wilkinson D. Drug induced akathisia, suicidal ideation and its treatment in the elderly. *Int J Geriatr Psychiatry.* 2001;16:231–232.

Haupt D, Newcomer J. Hyperglycemia and antipsychotic medications. *J Clin Psychiatry.* 2001;62 (Suppl 27):15–26.

Herrmann N. Recommendations for the management of behavioural and psychological symptoms of depression. *Can J Neurol Sci.* 2001;28 (Suppl 1): S96–S107.

Hilger H, Quiner S, Ginzel I, Walter H, Jama L, Barnas C. The effect of orlistat on plasma levels of psychotropic drugs in patients with long-term psychopharmacotherapy. *J Clin Psychopharmacol.* 2002;22:68–70.

Howard R. Cognitive impairment in late life schizophrenia: A suitable case for treatment. *Int J Geriatric Psychiatry.* 1998;13:400–404.

Jeste D, Eastham J, Lacro J, Gierz M, Field M, Harris M. Management of late-life psychosis. *J Clin Psychiatry.* 1996;57 (Suppl 3):39–45.

Jeste D, Eastham J, Lohr J, Salzman C. Diagnosis of disordered behavior and psychosis. In Salzman C, ed. *Clinical Geriatric Psychopharmacology.* Baltimore, MD.: Williams and Wilkins; 1998;97–105.

Jeste D, Eastham J, Lohr J, Salzman C. Treatment of disordered behavior and psychosis. In Salzman C, ed. *Clinical Geriatric Psychopharmacology.* Baltimore, MD.: Williams and Wilkins. 1998;106–149.

Jeste D, Lacro J, Palmer B, Rockwell E, Harris J, Caligiuri M. Incidence of tardive dyskinesia in early stages of low-dose treatment with typical neuroleptics in older patients. *Am J Psychiatry.* 1999;156:309–311.

Jeste D, Rockwell E, Harris M, Lohr J, Lacro J. Conventional vs. newer antipsychotics in elderly patients. *Am J Psychiatry.* 1999;7:70–76.

Jeste D. Tardive dykinesia in older patients. *J Clin Psychiatry.* 2000;61 (Suppl 4):27–32.

Johnson J. Delirium in the elderly. *Emerg Med Clinics NA.* 1990;8:255–265.

Jones E, Dawson A. Neuroleptic malignant syndrome: A case report with post-mortem brain and muscle pathology. *J Neurology Neurosurg Psychiatry.* 1989;52:1006–1009.

Juncos J. Management of Psychotic aspects of Parkinson's disease. *J Clin Psychiatry.* 1999;60 (Suppl 8):42–53.

Kaneko K, Yuasa T, Miyatake T, Tsuji S. Stereotyped hand-clasping: An unusual tardive movement disorder. *Mov Disord.* 1993;8:230–231.

Kim K, Pae C, Chae J, Bahk W, Jun T. An open pilot trail of olanzepine for delirium in the Korean population. *Psychiatry Clin Neurosci.* 2002;55:515–519.

Kinon BJ, Stauffer VL, McGuire HC, Kaiser CJ, Dickson RA, Kennedy JS. The effects of antipsychotic drug treatment on prolactin concentrations in elderly patients. *J Am Med Dir Assoc.* 2003;4 (4):189–94.

Kiriakakis V, Bhatia K, Quinn N, Marsden C. The natural history of tardive dyskinesia. *Brain.* 1998;121:2053–2066.

Koch H, Szersey A, Vogel M, Fischer-Barnical D. Successful therapy of tardive dyskinesia in a 71-year-old woman with a combination of tetrabenazine, olanzepine, and tiapride. *Int J Clin Pract.* 2003;57:147–149.

Koshino Y, Wada Y, Isaki K, Kurata K. A long-term outcome study of tardive dyskinesia in patients on antipsychotic medication. *Clin Neuropharmacol.* 1991;14:537–546.

Kramer M, Vandijk J, Rosin A. Mortality in elderly patients with thermoregulatory failure. *Arch Int Med.* 1989;149:1521–1523.

Lacro J, Jeste D. Geriatric Psychosis. *Psychiatric Quarterly.* 1997;68 (3):247–260.

Lee H, Cooney J, Lawlor B. The use of risperidone, an atypical neuroleptic, in Lewy Body disease. *Int J Geriatr Psychiatry.* 1994;9:415–417.

Lemke M. Effect of carbamazepine on agitation in Alzheimer's inpatients refractory to neuroleptics. *J Clin Psychiatry.* 1995;56:354–357.

Lenox R, Newhouse P, Creelman W, Whitaker T. Adjunctive treatment of manic agitation with lorazepam versus haloperidol: A double-blind study. *J Clin Psychiatry.* 1992;53:47–52.

Lima A, Soares-Weiser K, Bacaltchuk J, Barnes T. Benzodiazepines for neuroleptic-induced acute akathisia. *Cochrane Database of Systematic Reviews.* 2002;1.

Lindenmayer J, Kotsaftis A. Use of sodium valproate in violent and aggressive behaviors: A critical review. *J Clin Psychiatry.* 2000;61:123–128.

Lindenmayer J, Nathan A, Smith R. Hyperglycemia associated with the use of atypical antipsychotics. *J Clin Psychiatry.* 2001;62 (Suppl 23):30–38.

Lonergan E, Luxenberg J, Colford J. Haloperidol for agitation in dementia. *Cochrane Database of Systematic Reviews.* 2002;1.

MacIntyre J, McCann S, Kennedy S. Antipsychotic metabolic effects: Weight gain, diabetes mellitus, and lipid abnormalities. *Can J Psychiatry.* 2001;46:273–281.

Magnuson T, Roccaforte W, Wengel S, Burke W. Medication-induced dystonias in nine patients with dementia. *J Neuropsychiatry Clin Neurosci.* 2000;12:219–225.

Maixner S, Mellow A, Tandon R. The efficacy, safety, and tolerability of antipsychotics in the elderly. *J Clin Psychiatry.* 1999;60 (Suppl 8):29–41.

Mamo D, Sweet R, Chengappa K, et al. The effect of age on the pharmacologic management of ambulatory patients treated with depot neuroleptic medications for schizophrenia and related psychotic disorders. *Int J Geriatr Psychiatry.* 2002;17:1012–1017.

Mamo D, Sweet R, Keshavan M. Managing antipsychotic-induced Parkinsonism. *Drug Saf.* 1999;20:269–275.

Masand P. Side effects of antipsychotics in the elderly. *J Clin Psychiatry.* 2000;61:43–49.

Mauri M, Bitetto A, Fabiano L, Laini V, Steinhilber C, Fornier M, Rafique F. Depressive symptoms and schizophrenic relapses: The effect of four neuroleptic drugs. *Prog Neuro-psychopharmacol and Biol Psychiatry.* 1999;23:43–54.

Mazurek M, Rosebush P. Circadian pattern of acute, neuroleptic-induced dystonic reactions. *Am J Psychiatry.* 1996;153:708–710.

McDonald W. Epidemiology, etiology, and treatment of geriatric mania. *J Clin Psychiatry.* 2000;61 (Suppl 13):3–11.

McGrath J, Soares K. Benzodiazepines for neuroleptic-induced tardive dyskinesia. *Cochrane Database of Systematic Reviews.* 2002;1.

McGrath J, Soares-Weiser K. Neuroleptic reduction and/or cessation and neuroleptics as specific treatments for tardive dyskinesia. *Cochrane Database of Systematic Reviews.* 2002;1.

Miller L, Jankovic J. Neurologic approach to drug-induced movement disorders. *Southern Med J.* 1990;83:525–532.

Mintzer J, Brawman-Mintzer O. Agitation as a possible expression of generalized anxiety disorder in demented elderly patients: Toward a treatment approach. *J Clin Psychiatry.* 1996;57 (Suppl 7):55–63.

Neil W, Curran S, Wattis J. Antipsychotic prescribing in older people. *Age Ageing.* 2003;32 (5):475–83.

Mintzer J. Underlying mechanisms of psychosis and aggression in patients with Alzheimer's disease. *J Clin Psychiatry.* 2001;62 (Suppl 21):23–25.

Narayan M, Nelson J. Treatment of dementia with behavioral disturbance using divalproex or a combination of divalproex and a neuroleptic. *J Clin Psychiatry.* 1997;58:351–354.

Nishiyama K, Momose T, Sugishita M, Sakuta M. Positron emission tomography of reversible intellectual impairment induced by long-term anticholinergic therapy. *J Neurological Sciences.* 1995;132:89–92.

Patkar A, Kunkel E. Treating delirium among elderly patients. *Psychiatr Serv.* 1997;48:46–48.

Paulson G. Visual hallucinations in the elderly. *Gerontology.* 1997;43:255–260.

Pijnennburg YA, Sampson EL, Harvey RJ, Fox NC, Rossor MN. Vulnerability to neuroleptic side effects in frontotemporal lobar degeneration. *Int J Geriatr Psychiatry.* 2003;19 (1):67–72.

Pollock B, Mulsant B. Behavioral disturbances of dementia. *J Geriatr Psychiatr Neurol.* 1998;11:206–212.

Pollock B, Mulsant B, Sweet R, Rosen J, Altieri L, Perel J. Prospective cytochrome P450 phenotyping for neuroleptic treatment in dementia. *Psychopharmacology Bull.* 1995;31:327–332.

Ramsay R, Millard P. Tardive dyskinesia in the elderly. *Age and Ageing.* 1985;15:145–150.

Raskind M, Risse S, Lampe T. Dementia and antipsychotic drugs. *J Clin Psychiatry.* 1987;48 (5, Suppl):16–18.

Ray W, Meredith S, Thapa P, Meador K, Hall K, Murray K. Antipsychotics and the risk of sudden cardiac death. *Arch Gen Psychiatry.* 2001;58:1161–1167.

Regan W, Gordon S. Gabapentin for behavioral agitation in Alzheimer's disease [letter]. *J Clin Psychopharmacol.* 1997;17:59–60.

Roane D, Rogers J, Robinson J, Feinberg T. Delusional misidentification in association with Parkinsonism. *J Neuropsychiatry Clin Neurosci.* 1998; 10:194–198.

Ruskin P, Bland W, Feldman S. Continuous vs. targeted medication in older schizophrenic outpatients. *Am J Geriatr Psychiatry.* 1994;2:134–143.

Sakauye K. Psychotic disorders: Guidelines and problems with antipsychotic medications in the elderly. *Psychiatric Annals.* 1990;20:456–465.

Schenck C, Bundlie S, Ettinger M, Mahowald M. Chronic behavioral disorders of human REM sleep: A new category of parasomnia. *Sleep.* 1986;9:293–308.

Schneider L. Efficacy of treatment for geropsychiatric patients with severe mental illness. *Psychopharmacology Bull.* 1993;29:501–524.

Schneider L. Pharmacologic management of psychosis in dementia. *J Clin Psychiatry.* 1999;60 (Suppl 8):54–60.

Shalev A, Hermesh H, Munitz H. Mortality from neuroleptic malignant syndrome. *J Clin Psychiatry.* 1989;50:18–25.

Shalev A, Munitz H. The neuroleptic malignant syndrome: Agent and host interaction. *Acta Psychiatrica Scand.* 1986;73:337–347.

Sheikh R, Prindiville T, Yasmeen S. Haloperidol and benztropine interaction presenting as acute intestinal pseudo-obstruction [letter]. *AJG.* 2001; 96:934–935.

Shulman L, Minagar A, Rabinstein A, Weiner W. The use of dopamine agonists in very elderly patients with Parkinson's disease. *Mov Disord.* 2000; 15 (4):664–668.

Sky A, Grossberg G. The use of psychotropic medication in the management of problem behaviors in the patient with Alzheimer's disease. *Med Clin North Am.* 1994;78:811–822.

Smeraski P. Clonazepam treatment of multi-infarct dementia. *J Geriatr Psychiatry Neurol.* 1988;1:47–48.

Soares K, McGrath J, Deeks J. Gamma-aminobutyric acid agonists for neuroleptic-induced tardive dyskinesia. *Cochrane Database of Systematic Reviews.* 2002;1 (1).

Stein D, Laszlo B, Marais E, Seedat S, Potocnik F. Hoarding symptoms in patients on a geriatric psychiatry inpatient unit. *South Afr Med J.* 1997;87: 1138–1140.

Stephen P, Williamson J. Drug-induced parkinsonism in the elderly. *Lancet.* 1984;2:1082–1083.

Stern R, Duffelmeyer M, Zemishlani Z, Davidson M. The use of benzodiazepines in the management of behavioral symptoms in demented patients. *Psychiatric Clin North Am.* 1991;14:375–384.

Stubner S, Padberg F, Grohmann R, et al. Pisa syndrome (pleurothotonus): Report of a multicenter drug safety surveillance project. *J Clin Psychiatry.* 2000;61:569–574.

Sunderland T. Treatment of the elderly suffering from psychosis and dementia. *J Clin Psychiatry.* 1996;57 (Suppl 9):53–56.

Sweet R, Pollack B, Mulsant B, et al. Association of plasma homovanillic acid with behavioral symptoms in patients diagnosed with dementia: A preliminary report. *Biol Psychiatry.* 1997;42:1016–1023.

Sweet R, Pollock B. Late-life psychosis: Advances in understanding and treatment. In Katz I, Oslin D, eds. *Annual Review of Gerontology and Geriatrics*, vol. 19. New York: Springer; 1999;225–248.

Sweet R, Pollock B, Rosen J, Mulsant B, Altieri L, Perel J. Early detection of neuroleptic induced Parkinsonism in elderly patients with dementia. *J Geriatr Psychiatry Neurol.* 1994;7:251–254.

Tandon R, Milner K, Jibson M. Antipsychotics from theory to practice: Integrating clinical and basic data. *J Clin Psychiatry.* 1999;60 (Suppl 8):21–28.

Targum S, Abbott J. Psychoses in the elderly: A spectrum of disorders. *J Clin Psychiatry.* 1999;60 (Suppl 8):4–10.

Tariot P, Gaile S, Castelli N, Porsteinsson A. Treatment of agitation in dementia. In HR Lambed. *New Directions for Mental Health Services*, no. 76. San Francisco: Jossey-Bass; 1997;109–123.

Tariot P. Treatment strategies for agitation and psychosis in dementia. *J Clin Psychiatry.* 1996;57 (Suppl 14):21–29.

Thorpe L. The treatment of psychotic disorders in late life. *Can J Psychiatry.* 1997;42 (Suppl 1):19S–27S.

Todd R, Lippmann S, Manshadi M, Chang A. Recognition and treatment of rabbit syndrome, an uncommon complication of neuroleptic therapies. *Am J Psychiatry.* 1983;140:1519–1520.

Tuisku K, Lauerma H, Holi M, Honkonen T, Rimon R. Akathisia masked by hypokinesia. *Pharmacopsychiatry.* 2000;33:147–149.

Tunel, Salzman C. Schizophrenia in late life. *Psychiatr Clin North Am.* 2003;26:103–13.

Tune L, Steele C, Cooper T. Neuroleptic drugs in the management of behavioral symptoms of Alzheimer's disease. *Psychiatric Clin North Amer.* 1991;14:353–373.

Van Putten T, Gelenberg A, Lavori P, et al. Antichholinergic effects on memory: Benztropine vs. amantadine. *Psychopharmacol Bull.* 1987;23:26–29.

Van Putten T, May P, Marder S. Akathesia with haloperidol and thiothixene. *Arch Gen Psychiatry.* 1984;41:1036–1039.

Verghese C, Kessel J, Simpson G. Pharmacokinetics of neuroleptics. *Psychopharmacology Bull.* 1991;27:551–563.

Verma S, Davidoff D, Kambhampati K. Management of the agitated elderly patient in the nursing home: The role of the atypical antipsychotics. *J Clin Psychiatry.* 1998;59 (Suppl 19):50–55.

Weisbard J, Pardo M, Pollack S. Symptom change and extrapyramidal side effects during acute haloperidol treatment in chronic geriatric schizophrenics. *Psychopharmacology Bull.* 1997;33:119–122.

Wershing W. Movement disorders associated with neuroleptic treatment. *J Clin Psychiatry.* 2001;62:15–18.

Yudofsky S, Silver J, Hales R. Pharmacologic management of aggression in the elderly. *J Clin Psychiatry.* 1990;51 (10 Suppl):22–28.

Yudofsky S, Silver J, Jackson W, et al. The overt aggression scale: An operationalized rating scale for verbal and physical aggression. *Am J Psychiatry.* 1986;143:35–39.

Zayas E, Grossberg G. The treatment of psychosis in late life. *J Clin Psychiatry.* 1998;59 (Suppl 1):5–10.

Zayas E, Grossberg G. Treating the agitated Alzheimer patient. *J Clin Psychiatry.* 1996;57 (Suppl 7):46–51.

Atypical Antipsychotics

Balant-Gorgia A, Balant A. Antipsychotic drugs: Clinical pharmacokinetics of potential candidates for plasma concentration monitoring. *Clin Pharmacokinetics.* 1987;13:65–90.

Berman I, Klegon D, Fiedosewicz H, Chang H. The effects of novel antipsychotics on cognitive function. *Psychiatric Ann.* 1999;11:643–646.

Blin O. A comparative review of new antipsychotics. *Can J Psychiatry.* 1999; 44:235–244.

Brown C, Markowitz J, Moore T, Parker N. Atypical antipsychotics: Part II: Adverse effects, drug interactions, and costs. *Ann Pharmacother.* 1999;33:210–217.

Centorrino F, Price B, Tuttle M, et al. EEG abnormalities during treatment with typical and atypical antipsychotics. *Am J Psychiatry.* 2002;159 (1):109–115.

Chan Y, Pariser S, Neufeld. Atypical antipsychotics in older adults. *Pharmacotherapy.* 1999;19:811–822.

Chouinard G. Effects of risperidone in tardive dyskinesia: an analysis of the Canadian multicenter risperidone study. *J Clin Psychopharmacol.* 1995;15 (Suppl 1):36S–44S.

David A, Quraishi S. Depot perphenazine decanoate and enanthate for schizophrenia. *Cochrane Database of Systematic Reviews.* 2002;1.

Farver DK. Neuroleptic malignant syndrome induced by atypical antipsychotics. *Expert Opin Drug Saf.* 2003;2 (1):21–35.

Friedman JH. Atypical antipsychotics in the EPS-vulnerable patient. *Psychoneuroendoocrinology.* 2003;28 (Suppl 1):39–51.

Gianfrancesco FD. Diabetes and atypical neuroleptics. *Am J Psychiatry.* 2003;160 (2):388-9; author reply 389.

Glick I, Murray S, Vasudevan P, Marder S, Hu R. Treatment with atypical antipsychotics: New indications and new populations. *J Psychiatry Res.* 2001; 35:187–191.

Henderson D. Atypical antipsychotic-induced diabetes mellitus. *CNS Drugs.* 2002;16:77–89.

Jann M, Ereshefsky L, Saklad S. Clinical pharmacokinetics of the depot antipsychotics. *Clin Pharmacokinetics.* 1985;10:315–333.

Kapur S, Remington G. Atypical antipsychotics: New directions and new challenges in the treatment of schizophrenia. *Annu Rev Med.* 2001;52:503–517.

Kapur S, Zipursky R, Remington G. Clinical and theoretical implications of 5-HT2 and D2 receptor occupancy of clozapine, risperidone, and olanzapine in schizophrenia. *Am J Psychiatry.* 1999;156:286–293.

Keck P, Strakowski S, McElroy S. The efficacy of atypical antipsychotics in the treatment of depressive symptoms, hostility, and suicidality in patients with schizophrenia. *J Clin Psychiatry.* 2000;61 (Suppl 3):4–9.

Kumar V, Brecher M. Psychopharmacology of atypical antipsychotics and clinical outcomes in elderly patients. *J Clin Psychiatry.* 1999;60 (Suppl 13): 5–9.

Lovett W, Stokes D, Taylor L, Young M, Free S, Phelan D. Management of behavioral symptoms in disturbed elderly patients: Comparison of trifluoperazine and haloperidol. *J Clin Psychiatry.* 1987;48:234–236.

Madhusoodanan S, Suresh P, Brenner R, Pillai R. Experience with the atypical antipsychotics: risperidone and olanzapine in the elderly. *Ann Clin Psychiatry.* 1999;11:113–118.

Markowitz J, Brown C, Moore T. Atypical antipsychotics: Part I: Pharmacology, pharmacokinetics, and efficacy. *Ann Pharmacother.* 1999;33:73–85.

Masand P. Atypical antipsychotics for elderly patients. *Psychiatric Ann.* 2000;30:202–208.

Meyer J. A retrospective comparison of weight, lipid, and glucose changes between risperidone- and olanzapine-treated inpatients: Metabolic outcomes after 1 year. *J Clin Psychiatry.* 2002;63:425–433.

Motsinger CD, Perron GA, Lacy TJ. Use of antipsychotic drugs in patients with dementia. *Am Fam Physician.* 2003;67 (11):2335–40.

Mullen J, Jibson M, Sweitzer D. A comparison of the relative safety, efficacy, and tolerability of quetiapine and risperidone in outpatients with schizophrenia and other psychotic disorders: The quetiapine experience with safety and tolerability (QUEST) study. *Clin Ther.* 2001;23:1839–1854.

Quraishi S, David A. Depot haloperidol decanoate for schizophrenia. *Cochrane Database of Systematic Reviews.* 2002;1.

Rafal S, Tsuang M, Carpenter W. A dilemma born of progress: Switching from clozapine to a newer antipsychotic. *Am J Psychiatry.* 1999;156:1086–1090.

Ritchie CW, Chiu E, Harrigan S, Hall K, Hassett A, Macfarlane S, Mastwyk M, O'Connor DW, Opie J, Ames D. The impact upon extra-pyramidal side effects, clinical symptoms and quality of life of a switch from conventional to atypical antipsychotics (risperidone or olanzapine) in elderly patients with schizophrenia. *Int J Geriatr Psychiatry.* 2003;18 (5):432–40.

Sernyak M, Leslie D, Alarcon R, Losonczy M, Rosenheck R. Association of diabetes mellitus with use of atypical neuroleptics in the treatment of schizophrenia. *Am J Psychiatry.* 2002;159:561–566.

Sussman N. Review of atypical antipsychotics and weight gain. *J Clin Psychiatry.* 2001;62 (Suppl 23):5–12.

Tarsy D, Baldessarini R, Tarazi F. Effects of newer antipsychotics on extrapyramidal function. *CNS Drugs.* 2002;16:23–45.

Tracy J, Monaco C, Abraham G, Josiassen R, Pollock B. Relation of serum anticholinergicity to cognitive status in schizophrenia patients taking clozapine or risperidone. *J Clin Psychiatry.* 1998;59:184–188.

Van Putten T, Marder S, Wirshing W, Aravagiri M, Chabert N. Neuroleptic plasma levels. *Schizophr Bull.* 1991;17:197–216.

Aripiprazole

De Deyn P, Jeste D, Auby P, Goyvaerts H, Breder C, Schneider L, Mintzer J. *Aripiprazole for psychosis of Alzheimer's disease.* Poster. 11th Congress, International Psychogeriatric Association, Chicago, Aug. 2003.

McGavin J, Goa K. Aripiprazole. *CNS Drugs.* 2002;16:779–786.

REFERENCES

Clozapine

Alvir J, Lieberman J. Agranulocytosis: Incidence and risk factors. *J Clin Psychiatry.* 1994;55 (Suppl B):137–138.

Baker R, Chengappa R, Baird J, Steingard S, Christ M, Schooler N. Emergence of obsessive-compulsive symptoms during treatment with clozapine. *J Clin Psychiatry.* 1992;53:439–442.

Ball C. The use of clozapine in older people [letter]. *Int J Geriatr Psychiatry.* 1992;7:689–692.

Barak Y, Wittenberg N, Naor S, Kutzuk D, Weizman A. Clozapine in elderly psychiatric patients: Tolerability, safety, and efficacy. *Compr Psychiatry.* 1999;40:320–325.

Beale M, Pritchett J, Kellner C. Supraventricular tachycardia in a patient receiving ECT, clozapine, and caffeine. *Convulsive Therapy.* 1994;10:228–231.

Bennett J, Landow E, Schuh L. Suppression of dyskinesias in advanced Parkinson's disease. *Neurol.* 1993;43:1551–1555.

Bonuccelli U, Ceravolo R, Salvetti S, et al. Clozapine in Parkinson's disease tremor. *Neurol.* 1997;49:1587–1590.

Briffa D, Meehan T. Weight changes during clozapine treatment. *Aust N Z J Psychiatry.* 1998;32:718–721.

Calabrese J, Kimmel S, Woyshville M, et al. Clozapine for treatment-refractory mania. *Am J Psychiatry.* 1996;153:759–764.

Centorrino F, Baldessarini R, Frankenburg F, Kando J, Volpicella S, Flood J. Serum, levels of clozapine and norclozapine in patients treated with selective serotonin reuptake inhibitors. *Am J Psychiatry.* 1996;153:820–822.

Chae B, Kang B. The effect of clozapine on blood glucose metabolism. *Human Psychopharmacol.* 2001;16:265–271.

Chatterton R. Eosinophilia after commencement of clozapine treatment. *Aust N Z J Psychiatry.* 1997;31:874–876.

Chengappa K, Baker R, Kreinbrook S, Adair D. Clozapine use in female geriatric patients with psychosis. *J Geriatr Psychiatry Neurol.* 1995;8:12–15.

Duffy J, Kant R. Clinical utility of clozapine in 16 patients with neurological disease. *J Neuropsychiatry.* 1996;8:92–96.

Factor S, Brown D. Clozapine prevents recurrence of psychosis in Parkinson's disease. *Mov Disord.* 1992;7:125–131.

Factor S, Brown D, Molho E, Podskalny G. Clozapine: A 2-year open trial in Parkinson's disease patients with psychosis. *Neurol.* 1994;44:544–546.

Fernandez H, Durso R. Clozapine for dopaminergic-induced paraphilias in Parkinson's disease. *Mov Disord.* 1998;13:597–598.

Frankenburg F, Kalunian D. Clozapine in the elderly. *J Geriatr Psychiatry Neurol.* 1994;7:131–134.

Frankenburg F, Suppes T, McLean P. Combined clozapine and electroconvulsive therapy. *Convulsive Therapy.* 1993;9:176–180.

Fraser D, Jibani M. An unexpected and serious complication of treatment with the atypical antipsychotic drug clozapine. *Clin Nephrology.* 2000;54:78–80.

Friedman J, Koller W, Lannon M, Busenbark K, Swanson-Hyland E, Smith D. Benztropine versus clozapine for the treatment of tremor in Parkinson's disease. *Neurol.* 1997;48:1077–1081.

Friedman J, Lannon M. Clozapine-responsive tremor in Parkinson's disease. *Mov Disord.* 1990;3:225–229.

Gupta S, Sonnenberg S, Frank B. Olanzapine augmentation of clozapine. *Ann Clin Psychiatry.* 1998;10:113–115.

Hagg S, Joelsson L, Mjorndal T, Spigset O, Oja G, Dahlqvist R. Prevalence of diabetes and impaired glucose tolerance in patients treated with clozapine compared with patients treated with conventional depot neuroleptic medications. *J Clin Psychiatry.* 1998;59:294–299.

Hagg S, Spigset O, Bate A, Soderstrom T. Myocarditis related to clozapine therapy. *J Clin Psychopharmacol.* 2001;21:382–388.

Hagg S, Spigset O, Soderstrom T. Association of venous thromboembolism and clozapine. *Lancet.* 2000;355:1155–1156.

Herst L, Powell G. Is clozapine safe in the elderly? *Aust N Z J Psychiatry.* 1997;31:411–417.

Howanitz E, Pardo M, Melson D, Engelhart C, Eisenstein N, Losonczy M. The efficacy and safety of clozapine versus chlorpromazine in geriatric schizophrenia. *J Clin Psychiatry.* 1999;60:41–44.

Hummer M, Kemmler G, Kurz M, Kurtzhaler I, Oberbauer H, Fleischhacker W. Weight gain induced by clozapine. *Eur Neuropsychopharmacol.* 1995; 5 (4)437–440.

Jansen E. Clozapine in the treatment of tremor in Parkinson's disease. *Acta Neurol Scand.* 1993;89:262–265.

Kahn N, Freeman A, Juncos J, Manning D, Watts R. Clozapine is beneficial for psychosis in Parkinson's disease. *Neurol.* 1991;41:1699–1700.

Kando J, Tohen M, Castillo J, Centorrino F. Concurrent use of clozapine and valproate in affective and psychotic disorders. *J Clin Psychiatry.* 1994;55:255–257.

Klein C, Gordon J, Pollak L, Rabey JM. Clozapine in Parkinson's disease psychosis: 5-year follow-up review. *Clin Neuropharmacol.* 2003;26 (1): 8–11.

Lieberman J, Safferman A. Clinical profile of clozapine: Adverse reactions and agranulocytosis. *Psychiatr Quy.* 1992;63:51–70.

Littrell K, Johnson C, Hilligos N, Peabody C, Littrell S. Switching clozapine responders to olanzapine. *J Clin Psychiatry.* 2000;61:912–915.

Mahmood T, Devlin M, Silverstone T. Clozapine in the management of bipolar and schizoaffective manic episodes resistant to standard treatment. *Aust N Z J Psychiatry.* 1997;31:424–426.

Meltzer H. Clozapine withdrawal: serotonergic or dopaminergic mechanism [letter]. *Arch Gen Psychiatry.* 1997;54:760–761.

Naber D, Holzbach R, Perro C, Hippius H. Clinical management of clozapine patients in relation to efficacy and side effects. *Br J Psychiatry.* 1992;160 (Suppl 17):54–59.

Nacasch N, Dolberg O, Hirschmann S, Dannon P, Grunhaus L. Clozapine for the treatment of agitated-depressed patients with cognitive impairment: A report of three cases. *Clin Neuropharmacol.* 1998;21:132–134.

Nitensen N, Kando J, Frankenburg F, Zanarini M. Fever associated with clozapine administration [letter]. *Am J Psychiatry.* 1995;152:1102.

Oberholzer A, Hendriksen C, Monsch A, Heierli B, Stahelin H. Safety and effectiveness of low-dose clozapine in psychogeriatric patients: A preliminary study. *Int Psychogeriatrics.* 1992;4:187–195.

Pacia S, Devinsky O. Clozapine: Related seizures. *Neurol.* 1994;44:2247–2249.

Pallanti S, Quercioli L, Rossi A, Pazzagli A. The emergence of social phobia during clozapine treatment and its response to fluoxetine augmentation. *J Clin Psychiatry.* 1999;60:819–823.

Peacock L, Solgaard T, Lublin H, Gerlach J. Clozapine versus typical antipsychotics. *Psychopharmacol.* 1996;124:188–196.

Pitner J, Mintzer J, Pennypacker L, Jackson C. Efficacy and adverse effects of clozapine in four elderly psychotic patients. *J Clin Psychiatry.* 1995;56:180–185.

Pollak P, French Clozapine Parkinson Study Group. Clozapine in drug-induced psychosis in Parkinson's disease. *Lancet.* 1999;353:2041–2042.

Popli A, Konicki E, Jurjus G, Fuller M, Jaskiw G. Clozapine and associated diabetes mellitus. *J Clin Psychiatry.* 1997;58:108–111.

Rabinowitz J, Avnon, Rosenberg V. Effect of Clozapine on physical and verbal aggression. *Schizophrenia Res.* 1996;22:249–255.

Reznik I, Volchek L, Mester R, et al. Myotoxicity and neurotoxicity during clozapine treatment. *Clin Neuropharmacol.* 2000;5:276–280.

Sajatovic M. Clozapine for elderly patients. *Psychiatric Annals.* 2000;30:170–174.

Sajatovic M, Ramirez L, Garver D, Thompson P, Ripper G, Lehmann L. Clozapine therapy for older veterans. *Psychiatr Serv.* 1998;49:340–344.

Satajovic M, Jaskiw G, Konicki P, Jurjus G, Kwon K, Ramirez L. Outcome of clozapine therapy for elderly patients with refractory primary psychosis. *Int J Geriat Psychiatry.* 1997;12:553–558.

Schuld A, Kuhn M, Haack M, et al. A comparison of the effects of clozapine and olanzapine on the EEG in patients with schizophrenia. *Pharmacopsychiatry.* 2000;33:109–111.

Shulman R, Singh A, Shulman K. Treatment of elderly institutionalized bipolar patients with clozapine. *Psychopharmacology Bull.* 1997;33:113–118.

The French Clozapine Parkinson Study Group. Clozapine in drug-induced psychosis in Parkinson's disease. *Lancet.* 1999;353:2041–2042.

Wahlbeck K, Cheine M, Essali M. Clozapine versus typical neuroleptic medication for schizophrenia. *Cochrane Database of Systematic Reviews* 2002; 1.

Wetzel H, Anghelescu I, Szegedi A, et al. Pharmacokinetic interactions of clozapine with selective serotonin reuptake inhibitors: Differential effects of fluvoxamine and paroxetine in a prospective study. *J Clin Psychopharmacol.* 1998;18:2–9.

Zimbroff. Switching patients from clozapine to risperidone therapy [letter]. *Am J Psychiatry.* 1995;152:1102.

Haloperidol

Andrews E, Bellard J, Walter-Ryan W. Monosymptomatic hypochondriacal psychosis manifesting as delusions of infestation: Case studies of treatment with haloperidol. *J Clin Psychiatry.* 1986;47:188–190.

Bird H, Le Gallez, Wright V. Drowsiness due to haloperidol/indomethacin in combination [letter]. *Lancet.* 1983; April 9;830–831.

Chang W, Jann M, Chiang T, Lin H, Hu W, Chien C. Plasma haloperidol and reduced haloperidol concentrations in a geriatric population. *Neuropsychobiol.* 1996;33:12–16.

Cohen-Mansfield J, Taylor L, Woosley R, Lipson S, Werner P, Billig N. Relationships between psychotropic drug dosage, plasma drug concentration, and prolactin levels in nursing home residents. *Ther Drug Monit.* 2000;22:688–694.

Darby J, Pasta D, Dabiri L, Clark L, Mosbacher D. Haloperidol dose and blood level variability: Toxicity and interindividual and intraindividual variability in the nonresponder patient in the clinical practice setting. *J Clin Psychopharmacol.* 1995;15:334–340.

DeCuyper H, Bollen J, van Praag H, Verstraeten D. Pharmacokinetics and therapeutic efficacy of haloperidol decanoate after loading dose administration. *Br J Psychiatry.* 1986;148:560–566.

Denker S, Gios I, Martensson E, et al. A long-term cross-over pharmacokinetic study comparing perphenazine decanoate and haloperidol decanoate in schizophrenic patients. *Psychopharmacol.* 1994;114:24–30.

Devanand D, Cooper T, Sackeim H, Taurke E, Mayeux R. Low dose oral haloperidol and blood levels in Alzheimer's disease: A preliminary study. *Psychopharmacology Bull.* 1992;28:169–173.

Devanand D, Marder K, Michaels K, et al. A randomized, placebo-controlled dose-comparison trial of haloperidol for psychosis and disruptive behaviors in Alzheimer's disease. *Am J Psychiatry.* 1998;155:1512–1520.

Di Salvo T, O'Gara P. Torsades de Pointes caused by high-dose intravenous haloperidol in cardiac patients. *Clin Cardiol.* 1994;18:285–290.

Dysken M, Johnson S, Holden L, et al. Haloperidol concentrations in patients with Alzheimer's disease. *Am J Geriatric Psychiatry.* 1994;2:124–133.

Ereshevsky L, Toney G, Saklad S, Anderson C, Seidel D. A loading-dose strategy for converting from oral to depot haloperidol. *Hosp Community Psychiatry.* 1993;44:1155–1161.

Hagg S, Mjorndal T. Repeated episodes of hypothermia in a subject treated with haloperidol, levomepromazine, olanzepine, and thioridazine [letter]. *J Clin Psychopharmacol.* 2001;21:113–114.

Hunt N, Stern T. The association between intravenous haloperidol and torsades de pointes. *Psychosomatics.* 1995;36:541–549.

Iwahashi K. Significantly higher plasma haloperidol level during cotreatment with carbamazepine may herald cardiac change. *Clin Neuropharmacol.* 1996;19:267–270.

Kapur S, Zipursky R, Roy P, et al. The relationship between D2 receptor occupancy and plasma levels on low dose oral haloperidol: A PET study. *Psychopharmacol.* 1997;131:148–152.

Korzets Z, Zeltzer E, J Bernheim J. Acute renal failure in the setting of the neuroleptic malignant syndrome. *Nephrol Dial Transplant.* 1996;11:885–886.

Lacro J, Kuczenski R, Roznoski M, Warren K, Harris M, Jeste D. Serum haloperidol levels in older psychotic patients. *Am J Geriatr Psychiatry.* 1996;4:229–236.

Menza M, Murray G, Holmes V, Rafuls W. Controlled study of extrapyramidal reactions in the management of delirious, medically ill patients: Intravenous

haloperidol versus intravenous haloperidol plus benzodiazepines. *Heart Lung.* 1988;17:238–241.
Pelton GH, Devanand DP, Bell K, Marder K, Marston K, Liu X, Cooper TB. Usefulness of plasma haloperidol levels for monitoring clinical efficacy and side effects in Alzheimer patients with psychosis and behavioral dyscontrol. *Am J Geriatr Psychiatry.* 2003;11:186–193.
Seneff M, Mathews R. Use of Haloperidol infusions to control delirium in critically ill adults. *Ann Pharmacother.* 1995;29:690–693.
Settle E, Ayd F. Haloperidol: A quarter century of experience. *J Clin Psychiatry.* 1983;44:440–448.
Sheikh R, Yasmeen S. Haloperidol and benztropine interaction presenting as acute intestinal pseudo-obstruction [letter]. *AJG.* 2001;96:934–935.
Someya T, Shimoda K, Suzuki Y, Sato S, Kawashima Y, Hirokane G, Morita S, Yokono A, Takahashi S. Effect of CYP2D6 genotypes on the metabolism of haloperidol in a Japanese psychiatric population. *Neuropsychopharmacology.* 2003;29 (8):1501–5.
Yasui N, Kondo T, Suzuki A, et al. Lack of significant pharmacokinetic interaction between haloperidol and grapefruit juice. *Int Clin Psychopharmacol.* 1999;14:113–118.
Zhang-Wong J, Beiser M, Zipursky R, Bean G. An investigation of ethnic and gender differences in the pharmacodynamics of haloperidol. *Psychiatry Res.* 1998;81:333–339.
Ziemba C, Foster G, Neufeld R, Breuer B. Haloperidol holiday: Is it a beneficial vacation for some nursing home residents? *Clin Gerontologist.* 1997;17: 15–24.

Loxapine

Carlyle W, Ancill R, Sheldon L. Aggression in the demented patient: A double-blind study of loxapine versus haloperidol. *Int Clin Psychopharmacol.* 1993;8:103–108.
Fenton M, Murphy B, Wood J, Bagnall A, Chue P, Leitner M. Loxapine for schizophrenia. *Cochrane Database of Syst Rev.* 2000; (2): CD001943.
Kapur S, Zipursky R, Jones C, et al. The D_2 receptor occupancy profile of loxapine determined using PET. *Neuropsychopharmacol.* 1996;15:562–566.
Kapur S, Zipursky R, Remington G, Jones C, McKay G, Houle S. PET evidence that loxapine is an equipotent blocker of 5-HT_2 and D_2 receptors: Implications for the therapeutics of schizophrenia. *Am J Psychiatr.* 1997;154:1525–1529.

Olanzapine

Aarsland D, Larsen J, Lim N, Tandberg E. Olanzapine for psychosis in patients with Parkinson's disease with and without dementia. *J Neuropsychiatry Clin Neurosci.* 1999;11:392–394.
Bhana N, Foster R, Olney R, Plosker G. Olanzepine: An updated review of its use in the management of schizophrenia. *Drugs.* 2001;61:111–161.

Callaghan J, Bergstrom R, Ptak L, Beasley C. Olanzapine: Pharmacokinetic and pharmacodynamic profile. *Clin Pharmacokinet.* 1999;37:177–193.

Clarke W, Street J, Feldman P, Breier A. The effects of olanzapine in reducing the emergence of psychosis among nursing home patients with Alzheimer's disease. *J Clin Psychiatry.* 2001;62:34–40.

Cummings J, Street J, Masterman D, Clark W. Efficacy of olanzapine in the treatment of psychosis in dementia with Lewy bodies. *Dement Geriatr Cogn Disord.* 2002;13:67–73.

Czekalla J, Beasley C, Dellva M, Berg P, Grundy S. Analysis of the QTc interval during olanzapine treatment of patients with schizophrenia and related disorders. *J Clin Psychiatry.* 2001;62:191–198.

Filice G, McDougall B, Ercan-Fang N, Billington C. Neuroleptic malignant syndrome associated with olanzapine. *Ann Pharmacother.* 1998;32:1158–1159.

Fontaine CS, Hynan LS, Koch K, Martin-Cook K, Svetlik D, Weiner MF. A double-blind comparison of olanzepine versus risperidone in the acute treatment of dementia-related behavioral disturbances in extended care facilities. *J Clin Psychiatry.* 2003;64 (6):726–30.

Friedman J, Goldstein S, Jacques C. Substituting clozapine for olanzapine in psychiatrically stable Parkinson's disease patients: Results of an open label pilot study. *Clin Neuropharmacol.* 1998;5:285–288.

Goetz C, Blasucci L, Leurgans S, Pappert E. Olanzapine and clozapine comparative effects on motor function in hallucinating PD patients. *Neurol* 2000;55:789–794.

Gomberg R. Interaction between olanzapine and haloperidol [letter]. *J Clin Psychopharmacol.* 1999;19:272–273.

Graham J, Sussman J, Ford K, Sagar H. Olanzapine in the treatment of hallucinosis in idiopathic parkinson's disease: A cautionary note. *J Neurol Neurosurg Psychiatry.* 1998;65:774–777.

Granger A, Hanger H. Olanzapine: Extrapyramidal side effects in the elderly [letter]. *Aust N Z J Med.* 1999;29:371–372.

Hwang JP, Yang CH, Lee TW, Tsai SJ. The efficacy and safety of olanzapine for the treatment of geriatric psychosis. *J Clin Psychopharmacol.* 2003;23 (2):113–8.

Johnson V, Bruxner G. Neuroleptic malignant syndrome associated with olanzapine. *Aust N Z J Psychiatry.* 1998;32:884–886.

Koch HJ, Szecsey A, Vogel M, Fischer-Barnicol D. Successful therapy of tardive dyskinesia in a 71-year-old woman with a combination of tetrabenazine, olanzapine and tiapride. *Int J Clin Pract.* 2003;57 (2):147–9.

Konig F, van Hippel C, Petersdorff T, Neuhoffer-Weiss M, Wolfersdorf M, Kaschka W. First experiences in combination therapy using olanzapine with SSRIs (citalopram, paroretine) in delusional depression. *Neuropsychobiol.* 2001;43:170–174.

Madhusoodanan S, Brenner R, Suresh P, et al. Efficacy and tolerability of olanzapine in elderly patients with psychotic disorders: A prospective study. *Ann Clin Psychiatry.* 2000;12:11–18.

Madhusoodanan S, Suresh P, Brenner R, Pillai R. Experience with the

atypical antipsychotics: risperidone and olanzapine in the elderly. *Ann Clin Psychiatry.* 1999;11:113–118.
Manson A, Schrag A, Lees A. Low-dose olanzapine for levodopa induced dyskinesias. *Neurol.* 2000;55:795–799.
Marsh L, Lyketsos C, Reich S. Olanzapine for the treatment of psychosis in patients with Parkinson's disease and dementia. *Psychosomatics.* 2001;42:477–481.
Meehan K, Wang H, David S, et al. Comparison of rapidly acting intramuscular olanzapine, lorazepam, and placebo: A double-blind, randomized study in acutely agitated patients with dementia. *Neuropsychopharmacol.* 2002;26:494–504.
Molho E, Factor S. Worsening of motor features of Parkinsonism with olanzapine. *Mov Disord.* 1999;14:1014–1016.
Oyewumi L, Al-Semaan Y. Olanzepine: Safe during clozapine-induced agranulocytosis [letter]. *J Clin Psychopharmacol.* 2000;20:279–280.
Sajatovic M, Perez D, Brescan D, Ramirez L. Olanzapine therapy in elderly patients with schizophrenia. *Psychopharmacology Bull.* 1998;34:819–823.
Solomons K, Geiger O. Olanzapine use in the elderly: A retrospective analysis. *Can J Psychiatry.* 2000;45:151–155.
Street J, Clark W, Gannon K, et al. Olanzapine treatment of psychotic and behavioral symptoms in patients with Alzheimer disease in nursing care facilities: A double-blind, randomized, placebo-controlled trial. *Arch Gen Psychiatry.* 2000;57:968–976.
Street J, Tollefson G, Tohen M, et al. Olanzapine for psychotic conditions in the elderly. *Psychiatric Annals.* 2000;30:191–196.
Tohen M, Sanger T, McElvoy S, et al. Olanzapine versus placebo in the treatment of acute mania. *Am J Psychiatry.* 1999;156:702–709.
Verma S, Orengo C, Kunik M, Hale D, Molinari V. Tolerability and effectiveness of atypical antipsychotics in male geriatric inpatients. *Int J Geriat Psychiatry.* 2001;16:223–227.
Weigmann H, Gerek S, Zeiseg A, Muller M, Hartter S, Hiemke C. Fluvoxamine but not sertraline inhibits the metabolism of olanzapine: From a therapeutic drug monitoring service. *Therap Drug Monit.* 2001;23:410–413.
Weintraub E, Robinson C. A case of Monosymptomatic hypochondriacal psychosis treated with olanzapine. *Ann Clin Psychiatry.* 2000;12:247–249.

Perphenazine

Hansen L, Larsen N. Therapeutic advantages of monitoring concentrations of perphenazine in clinical practice. *Psychopharmacology.* 1985;87:16–19.
Mazure C, Nelson C, Jatlow P, Bowers M. Acute neuroleptic treatment in elderly patients without dementia. *Am J Geriatr Psychiatry.* 1998;6:221–229.
Sweet R, Pollock B, Mulsant B, et al. Pharmacologic profile of perphenazine's metabolites. *J Clin Psychopharmacol.* 2000;20:181–187.

Quetiapine

Arvanitis L, Miller B, Seroquel Trial Group. Multiple fixed doses of "Seroquel" (quetiapine) in patients with acute exacerbation of schizophrenia: A comparison with haloperidol and placebo. *Biol Psychiatry.* 1997;42:233–246.

Dev V, Raniwalla J. Quetiapine: A review of its safety in the management of schizophrenia. *Drug Saf.* 2000;23:295–307.

Dogu O, Sevim S, Kaleagasi HS. Seizures associated with quetiapine treatment. *Ann Pharmacother.* 2003;39 (9):1224–7.

Fernandez H, Friedman J, Jacques C, Rosenfeld M. Quetiapine in the treatment of drug-induced psychosis in Parkinson's disease. *Mov Disord.* 1999;14:484–487.

Fernandez H, Lannon M, Friedman J, Abbott B. Clozapine replacement by quetiapine for the treatment of drug-induced psychosis in Parkinson's disease. *Mov Disord.* 2000;15:579–586.

Garver D. Review of Quetiapine side effects. *J Clin Psychiatry.* 2000;61 (Suppl 8):31–33.

Green B. Focus on quetiapine. *Curr Med Res Opinion.* 1999;15:145–151.

Kim K, Bader G, Kotlyar V, Gropper D. Treatment of delirium in old adults with quetiapine. *J. Geriatr Psychiatry Neurol.* 2003;16:29–31.

Madhusoodanan S, Brenner R, Alcantra A. Clinical experience with quetiapine in elderly patients with psychotic disorders. *J Geriatr Psychiatry Neurol.* 2000;13:28–32.

McManus D, Arvanitis L, Kowalcyk B. Quetiapine, a novel antipsychotic: Experience in elderly patients with psychotic disorders. *J Clin Psychiatry.* 1999;60:292–298.

Raymund D, Fernandez H. Quetiapine for hypnogogic musical release hallucinations. *J Geriatr Psychiatry Neurol.* 2000;13:210–211.

Tariot P, Salzman C, Yeung P, Pultz J, Rak I. Long-term use of quetiapine in elderly patients with psychiatric disorders. *Clin Ther.* 2000;22:1068–1084.

Yeung P, Tariot P, Schneider L, Salzman C, Rak W. Quetiapine for elderly patients with psychotic disorders. *Psychiatric Annals.* 2000;30:197–201.

Risperidone

Almond D, Rhodes L, Pirmohamed M. Risperidone-induced photosensitivity. *Postgrad Med J.* 1998;74:252–253.

Aronson S. Cost-effectiveness and quality of life in psychosis: The pharmacoeconomics of risperidone. *Clin Therapeutics.* 1997;19:139–147.

Bahro M, Kampf C, Strand J. Catatonia under medication with risperidone in a 61-year-old patient. *Acta Psychiatr Scand.* 1999;99:223–226.

Berman I, Merson A, Rachov-Pavlov J, Allan E, Davidson M, Losonczy M. Risperidone in elderly schizophrenics. *Am J Geriatr Psychiatry.* 1996;4:173–179.

Bhana N, Spencer C. Risperidone: A review of its use in the management of the behavioral and psychological symptoms of dementia. *Drugs Aging.* 2000;16:451–471.

Bonwick R, Hopwood M, Morris P. Neuroleptic malignant syndrome and risperidone: A case report. *Aust N Z J Psychiatry.* 1996;30:419–421.

Brodaty H, Ames D, Snowdon J, Woodward M, Kirwan J, Clarnette R, Lee E, Lyons B, Grossman F. A randomized placebo-controlled trial of risperidone for the treatment of aggression, agitation, and psychosis of dementia. *J Clin Psychiatry.* 2003;64 (2):134–43.

Cates M, Collins R, Woolley T. Antiparkinsonian drug prescribing in elderly inpatients receiving risperidone therapy. *Am J Health System Pharmacy.* 1999;56:2139–2140.

Chengappa K, Levine J, Ulrich R, et al. Impact of risperidone on seclusion and restraint at a state psychiatric hospital. *Can J Psychiatry.* 2000;45:827–832.

Coley K, Carter C, DaPos S, Maxwell R, Wilson J, Branch R. Effectiveness of antipsychotic therapy in a naturalistic setting: A comparison between risperidone, perphenazine, and haloperidol. *J Clin Psychiatry.* 1999;60:850–856.

Collins A, Anderson J. SIADH induced by two atypical antipsychotics. *Int J Geriatric Psychiatry.* 2000;15:282–285.

Davidson M, Harvey P, Vervarcke J, et al. A long-term, multicenter, open-label study of risperidone in elderly patients with psychosis. *Int J Geriat Psychiatry.* 2000;15:506–514.

De Deyn P, Katz I. Control of aggression and agitation in patients with dementia: Efficacy and safety of risperidone. *Int J Geriatr Psychiatry.* 2000;15:S14–S22.

De Deyn P, Rabheru K, Rasmussen A, et al. A randomized trial of risperidone, placebo, and haloperidol for behavioral symptoms of dementia. *Neurol.* 1999;53:946–955.

De Deyn P. Risperidone in the treatment of behavioral and psychological symptoms of dementia. *Int Psychogeriatrics.* 2000;12 (Suppl 1):263–269.

De Leon J, Bork J. Risperidone and cytochrome P450 3A [letter]. *J Clin Psychiatry.* 1997;58:450.

Durrenberger S, De Leon J. Acute dystonic reaction to lithium and risperidone. *J Neuropsychiatry Clin Neurosci.* 1999;11:518–519.

Edwards J. Risperidone for schizophrenia. *BMJ.* 1994;308:1311–1312.

Emes C, Millson R. Risperidone-induced priapism [letter]. *Can J Psychiatry.* 1994;39:315–316.

Falsetti A. Risperidone for control of agitation in dementia patients. *Am J Health System Pharmacy.* 2000;57:862–870.

Gallucci G, Beard G. Risperidone and the treatment of delusions of parasitosis in an elderly patient. *Psychosomatics.* 1995;36:578–580.

Glick I, Lemmens P, Vester-Blokland E. Treatment of the symptoms of schizophrenia: A combined analysis of double-blind studies comparing risperidone with haloperidol and other antipsychotic agents. *Int Clin Psychopharmacol.* 2001;16:265–274.

Goldberg R, Goldberg J. Risperidone for dementia-related disturbed behavior in nursing home residents: A clinical experience. *Int Psychogeriatrics.* 1997;9:65–68.

Grant S, Fitton A. Risperidone: A review of its pharmacology and therapeutic potential in the treatment of schizophrenia. *Drugs.* 1994;48:253–273.

Green B. Focus on risperidone. *Curr Med Res Opin.* 2000;16:57–65.

Heimberg C, Yearian A. Risperidone-associated burning paresthesia. *J Clin Psychopharmacol.* 1996;16:446–448.

Herrmann N, Rivard M, Flynn M, Ward C, Rabheru K, Campbell B. Risperidone for the treatment of behavioral disturbances in dementia: A case series. *J Neuropsychiatry Clin Neurosci.* 1998;10:220–223.

Hesslinger B, Walden J, Normann C. Acute and long-term treatment of catatonia with risperidone. *Pharmacopsychiatry.* 2001;34:25–26.

Heykants J, Huang M, Mannens G, et al. The pharmacokinetics of risperidone in humans: A summary. *J Clin Psychiatry.* 1994;55 (Suppl 5):13–17.

Hwang J, Yang C, Yu H, et al. The efficacy and safety of risperidone for the treatment of geriatric psychosis. *J Clin Psychopharmacol.* 2001;21:583–587.

Irizarry M, Ghaemi S, Lee-Cherry E, et al. Risperidone treatment of behavioral disturbances in outpatients with dementia. *J Neuropsychiatry Clin Neurosci.* 1999;11:336–342.

Jeste D, Lacro J, Bailey A, Rockwell E, Harris J, Caligiuri M. Lower incidence of tardive dyskinesia with risperidone compared with haloperidol in older patients. *JAGS.* 1999;47:716–719.

Jeste D, Okamoto A, Napolitano J, Kane J, Martinez R. Low incidence of persistent tardive dyskinesia in elderly patients with dementia treated with risperidone. *Am J Psychiatry.* 2000;157:1150–1155.

Karki SD, Masood GR. Combination risperidone and SSRI-indiced serotonin syndrome. *Ann Pharmacother.* 2003;37 (3):388–91.

Katz I, Jeste D, Mintzer J, Clyde C, Napolitano J, Brecher M. Comparison of risperidone and placebo for psychosis and behavioral disturbances associated with dementia: A randomized double-blind trial. *J Clin Psychiatry.* 1999;60:107–115.

Keegan D. Risperidone: Neurochemical pharmacologic and clinical properties of a new antipsychotic drug. *Can J Psychiatry.* 1994;39 (Suppl 2):S46–S52.

Kiraly S, Gibson R, Ancill R, Holliday S. Risperidone: Treatment response in adult and geriatric patients. *Int J Psychiatry Med.* 1998;28:255–263.

Kopala L, Honer W. The use of risperidone in severely demented patients with persistent vocalizations. *Int J Geriatr Psychiatry.* 1997;12:73–77.

Lane H, Chang W, Chou J. Seizure during risperidone treatment on an elderly woman treated with concomitant medications [letter]. *J Clin Psychiatry.* 1998;59:81–82.

Lane H, Chang Y, Su M, Chiu C, Huang M, Chang W. Shifting from haloperidol to risperidone for behavioral disturbances in dementia: Safety, response predictors, and mood effects. *J Clin Psychopharmacol.* 2002;22:4–10.

Lavretsky H, Sultzer D. A structured trial of risperidone for the treatment of agitation in dementia. *Am J Geriatr Psychiatry.* 1998;6:127–135.

Lemmens P, Brecher M, Van Baelen B. A combined analysis of double-blind studies with risperidone vs. placebo and other antipsychotic agents: Factors associated with extrapyramidal symptoms. *Acta Psychiatr Scand.* 1999;99:160–170.

Leopold N. Risperidone treatment of drug-related psychosis in patients with parkinsonism. *Mov Disord.* 2000;15:301–304.

Madhusoodanan S, Brenner R, Araujo L, Abaza A. Efficacy of risperidone treatment for psychoses associated with schizophrenia, schizoaffective disorder, bipolar disorder, or senile dementia in 11 geriatric patients: A case series. *J Clin Psychiatry.* 1995;56:514–518.

Madhusoodanan S, Brenner R, Cohen C. Risperidone for elderly patients with schizophrenia or schizoaffective disorder. *Psychiatric Annals.* 2000;30:175–180.

Martin H, Slyk MP, Deymann S, Cornacchione MJ. Safety profile assessment of risperidone and olanzapine in long-term care patients with dementia. *J Am Med Dir Assoc.* 2003;4 (4):183–8.

McKeith I, Ballard C, Harrison R. Neuroleptic sensitivity to risperidone in Lewy Body dementia [letter]. *Lancet.* 1995;346:699.

Mintzer J, Madhusoodanan S, Brenner R. Risperidone in dementia. *Psychiatric Annals.* 2000;30:181–187.

Nair N, Risperidone Study Group. Therapeutic equivalence of risperidone given once daily and twice daily in patients with schizophrenia. *J Clin Psychopharmacol.* 1988;18:103–110.

Nyberg S, Eriksson B, Oxenstierna G, Halldin C, Farde L. Suggested minimal effective dose of risperidone based on PET-measured D_2 and 5-HT_{2A} receptor occupancy in schizophrenic patients. *Am J Psychiatry.* 1999;156:869–875.

Ostroff R, Nelson J. Risperidone augmentation of selective serotonin reuptake inhibitors in major depression. *J Clin Psychiatry.* 1999;60:256–259.

Peuskens J, Van Baelen B, De Smedt C, Lemmens P. Effects of risperidone on affective symptoms in patients with schizophrenia. *Int Clin Psychopharmacol.* 2000;15:343–349.

Phillips E, Liu B, Knowles S. Rapid onset of risperidone-induced hepatotoxicity [letter]. *Ann Pharmacother.* 1998;32:843.

Practice. Risperidone (risperidal): Increased rate of cerebrovascular events in dementia. *CMAJ.* 2002;167:1269–1270.

Ragwani S, Gupta S, Burke W, Potter J. Improvement of debilitating tardive dyskinesia with risperidone. *Ann Clin Psychiatry.* 1996;8:27–29.

Raheja R, Bharwani I, Penetrante A. Efficacy of risperidone for behavioral disorders in the elderly: A clinical observation. *Psychiatry Neurol.* 1995;8:159–161.

Rainer M, Masching A, Ertl M, Kraxberger E, Haushofer M. Effect of risperidone on behavioral and psychological symptoms and cognitive function in dementia. *J Clin Psychiatry.* 2001;62:894–900.

Ravona-Springer R, Dolberg O, Hirschmann S, Grunhaus L. Delirium in elderly patients treated with risperidone: A report of three cases [letter]. *J Clin Psychopharmacol.* 1998;18:171–172.

Reyntjens A, Heylen S, Gelders Y, et al. Risperidone in the treatment of behavioral symptoms in psychogeriatric patients: A pilot clinical investigation. *Psychopharmacol.* 1988;96 (Suppl):335.

Risperidal (risperidone) and cerebrovascular adverse events in placebo-controlled dementia trials [dear health professional letter] (2002). Toronto: Janssen-Ortho, Inc: Oct 11.

Rosebush P, Kennedy K, Dalton B, Mazurek M. Protracted akathisia after risperidone withdrawal [letter]. *Am J Psychiatry.* 1997;154:437–438.

Shigenobu K, Ikeda M, Fukuhara R, Komori K, Tanabe H. A structured, open trial of risperidone therapy for delusions of theft in Alzheimer disease. *Am J Geriatr Psychiatry.* 2003;11 (2):256–7.

Sajatovic M, Ramirez L, Vernon L, Brescan D, Simon M, Jurjus G. Outcome of risperidone therapy in elderly patients with chronic psychosis. *Int J Psychiatry Med.* 1996;26:309–317.

Snoeck E, Van Peer A, Sack M, et al. Influence of age, renal, and liver impairment on the pharmacokinetics of risperidone in man. *Psychopharmacol.* 1995;122:223–229.

Tune L. Risperidone for the treatment of behavioral and psychological symptoms of dementia. *J Clin Psychiatry.* 2001;62 (Suppl 21):29–32.

Williams R. Optimal dosing with risperidone: Updated recommendations. *J Clin Psychiatry.* 2001;62:282–289.

Workman R, Orengo C, Bakey A, Molinari V, Kunik M. The use of risperidone for psychosis and agitation in demented patients with Parkinson's disease. *J Neuropsychiatry.* 1997;9:594–597.

Zarate C, Baldessarini R, Siegel R, et al. Risperidone in the elderly: A pharmacoepidemiologic study. *J Clin Psychiatry.* 1997;58:311–317.

Zaudig M. A risk-benefit assessment of risperidone for the treatment of behavioral and psychological symptoms in dementia. *Drug Saf.* 2000;23:183–195.

Thioridazine

Ather S, Shaw S, Stoker M. A comparison of chlormethiazole and thioridazine in agitated confusional states of the elderly. *Acta Psychiatr Scand.* 1986;73 (Suppl 329):81–91.

Carrillo J, Ramos S, Herraiz A, et al. Pharmacokinetic interaction of fluvoxamine and thioridazine in schizophrenic patients. *J Clin Psychopharmacol.* 1999;19:494–499.

Cohen B, Sommer B. Metabolism of thioridazine in the elderly. *J Clin Psychiatry.* 1988;8:336–339.

Kirchner V, Kelly C, Harvey R. Thioridazine for dementia. Cochrane library, *Cochrane database of systematic studies*, 2002 (1).

Liberatore M, Robinson D. Torsades de Pointes: A mechanism for sudden death associated with neuroleptic drug therapy. *J Clin Psychopharmacol.* 1984;4:143–146.

Liu Y, Stagni G, Walden J, Shepherd A, Lichtenstein M. Thioridazine dose-related effects on biomechanical force platform measures of sway in young and old men. *JAGS.* 1998;46:431–437.

Phanjoo A, Link C. Remoxipride versus thioridazine in elderly psychotic patients. *Acta Psychiatr Scand.* 1990;82 (Suppl 358):181–185.

Steele C, Lucas M, Tune L. Haloperidol versus thioridazine in the treatment of behavioral symptoms in senile dementia of the Alzheimer's type: Preliminary findings. *J Clin Psychiatry.* 1986;47:310–312.

Sultana A, Reilly J, Fenton M. Thioridazine for schizophrenia. *Cochrane Database Syst Rev.* 2000; (3):CD001944. Review.

Timell A. Thioridazine: Reevaluating the risk/benefit equation. *Ann Clin Psychiatry.* 2000;12:147–151.

Thiothixene

Scuderi S, Gift T. Thiothixene-induced edema. *Psychiatric Med.* 1987;4:249–251.

Ziprasidone

Bagnall A, Lewis R, Leitner M. Ziprasidone for schizophrenia and severe mental illness. *Cochrane Database Syst Rev.* 2000; (4):CD001945. Review.

Brook S, Lucey J, Gunn K. Intramuscular ziprasidone compared with intramuscular haloperidol in the treatment of acute psychosis. *J Clin Psychiatry.* 2000;61:933–941.

Carnahan R, Lund B, Perry P. Ziprasidone: A new atypical antipsychotic drug. *Pharmacother.* 2001;21:717–730.

Keck P, Reeves K, Harrigan E. Ziprasidone in the short-term treatment of patients with schizoaffective disorder: Results from two double-blind, placebo- controlled, multicenter studies. *J Clin Psychopharmacol.* 2001;21: 27–35.

Lesem M, Zajecka J, Swift R, Reeves K, Harrigan E. Intramuscular ziprasidone, 2 mg versus 10 mg, in the short-term management of agitated psychotic patients. *J Clin Psychiatry.* 2001;62:12–18.

Schmidt A, Lebel L, Howard H, Zorn S. Ziprasidone: a novel antipsychotic agent with a unique human receptor binding profile. *Europ J Pharmacol.* 2001;425:197–201.

Stimmel G, Gutierrez M, Lee V. Ziprasidone: An atypical antipsychotic drug for the treatment of schizophrenia. *Clin Therpeutics.* 2002;24:21–37.

ANTIANXIETY DRUGS AND SEDATIVE/HYPNOTICS

Agostini J, Leo-Summers L, Inouye S. Cognitive and other adverse effects of diphenhydramine use in hospitalized older patients. *Arch Intern Med.* 2001;161:2091–2097.

Albeck J. Withdrawal and detoxification form benzodiazepine dependence: A potential role for clonazepam. *J Clin Psychiatry.* 1987;48 (Suppl 10):43–48.

Ankier S, Goa K. Quazepam: A preliminary review of its pharmacodynamic and pharmacokinetic properties and therapeutic efficacy in insomnia. *Drugs.* 35:42–62.

Arnold J. Determinants of pharmacologic effects and toxicity of benzodiazepine hypnotics: Role of lipophilicity and plasma elimination rates. *J Clin Psychiatry.* 1991;52 (Suppl 9):11–14.

Ashton H. Guidelines for the rational use of benzodiazepines. *Drugs.* 1994;48:25–40.

Asplund R. Sleep and hypnotics among the elderly in relation to body weight and somatic disease. *J Intern Med.* 1995;238:65–70.

Baker M, Olen M. The use of benzodiazepine hypnotics in the elderly. *Pharmacotherapy.* 1988;8:241–247.

Ballenger J, Burrows G, DuPont R, et al. Alprazolam in panic disorder and agoraphobia: Results from a multicenter trial. *Arch General Psychiatry.* 1988;45:413–422.

Bandera R, Bollini P, Garatini S. Long-acting and short acting benzodiazepines in the elderly: Kinetic differences and clinical relevance. *Curr Med Res Opin.* 1984;8 (Suppl 4):94–107.

Barclay A. Psychotropic drugs in the elderly. *Postgrad Med.* 1985;77:153–163.

Baumgartner G, Rowen R. Clonidine vs. chlordiazepoxide in the management of acute alcohol withdrawal syndrome. *Ach Intern Med.* 1987;147:1223–1226.

Beaumont G. Clobazam in the treatment of anxiety. *Human Psychopharmacol.* 1995;10:S27–S41.

Beitman B, Mukerji V, Alpert M, Peters J. Panic disorder in cardiology patients. *Psychiatric Med.* 1990;8:67–81.

Bertz R, Kroboth P, Kroboth F et al. Alprazolam in young and elderly men: Sensitivity and tolerance to psychomotor, sedative, and memory effects. *J Pharmacol Experimental Therapeutics.* 1997;281:1317–1329.

Bocca M, Le Doze F, Etard O, Pottier M, L'Hoste J, Denise P. Residual effects of zolpidem 10 mg and zopiclone 7.5 mg versus flunitrazepam 1 mg and placebo on driving performance and ocular saccades. *Psychopharmacol.* 1999;143:373–379.

Brower K, Mudd S, Blow F, Young J, Hill E. Severity and treatment of alcohol withdrawal in elderly versus younger patients. *Alcohol Clin Exp Res.* 1994;18:196–201.

Carlsten A, Waern M, Holmgren P, Allbeck P. The role of benzodiazepines in elderly suicides. *Scand J Public Health.* 2003;31 (3):224–8.

Carskadon M, Seidel W, Greenblatt D, Dement W. Daytime carryover of triazolam and flurazepam in elderly insomniacs. *Sleep.* 1982;5:361–371.

Cohen-Mansfield J, Taylor L, Woosley R, Lipson S, Werner P, Billig N. Relationship between psychotropic drug dosage, plasma drug concentration, and prolactin levels in nursing home residents. *Therapeutic Drug Monitoring.* 2000;22;688–694.

Comella C, Nardine T, Diederich N, Stebbins G. Sleep-related violence, injury, and REM sleep behavior disorder in Parkinson's disease. *Neurol.* 1998;51:526–529.

Cook P. Benzodiazepine hypnotics on the elderly. *Acta Psychiatr Scand.* 1986;74 (Suppl 332):149–158.

Curran H, Schiwy W, Lader M. Differential amnesic properties of benzodiazepines: A dose-response comparison of two drugs with similar elimination half-lives. *Psychopharmacol.* 1987;92:358–396.

Cutson T, Gray S, Hughes M, Carson S, Hanlon J. Effect of a single dose of diazepam on balance measures in older people. *JAGS.* 1997;45:435–440.

Dent L, Orrock M. Warfarin-fluoxetine and diazepam-fluoxetine interaction. *Pharmacotherapy.* 1997;17:170–172.

Deuschle M, Lederbogen F. Benzodiazepine withdrawal-induced catatonia. *Pharmacopsychiatry.* 2001;34:41–42.

Doraiswamy P. Contemporary management of comorbid anxiety and depression in geriatric patients. *J Clin Psychiatry.* 2001;62 (Suppl 12):30–35.

Feinsilver S, Hertz G. Sleep in the elderly patient. *Clin Chest Med.* 1993;14:405–411.

Fichten C, Creti L, Amsel R, Brender W, Weinstein N, Libman E. Poor sleepers who do not complain of insomnia: Myths and realities about psychological and lifestyle characteristics of older good and poor sleepers. *J Behav Med.* 1995;18:189–223.

Flamer H. Sleep problems. *Med J Aust.* 1995;162:603–607.

Floyd J. Another look at napping in older adults. *Geriatr Nurs.* 1995;16:136–138.

Foley D, Monjan A, Brown S, Simonsick E, Wallace R, Blazer D. Sleep complaints among elderly persons: An epidemiologic study of three communities. *Sleep.* 1995;18:425–432.

Fontaine R, Chouinard G, Annable L. Rebound anxiety in anxious patients after abrupt withdrawal of benzodiazepine treatment. *Am J Psychiatry.* 1984;141:848–852.

Fox G. Restless leg syndrome. *AFP.* 1986;33:147–152.

Foy A, O'Connell D, Henry D, Kelly J, Cocking S, Halliday J. Benzodiazepine use as a cause of cognitive impairment in elderly hospital inpatients. *J Gerontol: Med Sciences.* 1995;2:M99–M106.

Gales B, Menard S. Relationship between the administration of selected medications and falls in hospitalized elderly patients. *Ann Pharmacother.* 1995;29:354–358.

Gilleard C, Smits C, Morgan K. Changes in hypnotic usage in residential homes for the elderly: A longitudinal study. *Arch Gerontol Geriatr.* 1984;3:223–228.

Goldstein M, Pataki A, Webb M. Alcoholism among elderly persons. *Psychiatric Services.* 1996;47:941–943.

Gorman J. Generalized anxiety disorders. *Mod Probl Pharmacopsychiat.* 1987;22:127–140.

Grad R. Benzodiazepines for insomnia in community-dwelling elderly: A review of benefit and risk. *J Fam Pract.* 1995;41:473–481.

Greenblatt D, Abernathy D, Lacnisker A, Ochs H, Harmatz J, Shader R. Age, sex, and nitrazepam kinetics: Relation to antipyrine disposition. *Pharmacol Ther.* 1985;38:697–703.

Greenblatt D. Benzodiazepine hypnotics: Sorting the pharmacokinetic facts. *J Clin Psychiatry.* 1991;52 (9, Suppl):4–10.

Greenblatt D, Divoll M, Abernathy D, Moschitto L, Smith R, Shader R. Alprazolam kinetics in the elderly. *Arch Gen Psychiatry.* 1983;40:287–290.

Greenblatt D, Harmatz J, Shader R. Clinical pharmacokinetics of anxiolytics and hypnotics in the elderly: Therapeutic considerations (Part I). *Clin Pharmacokinet.* 1991;21:165–177.

Guglielminotti J, Maury E, Alzieu M, et al. Prolonged sedation requiring mechanical ventilation and continuous flumazenil infusion after routine doses of clorazepam for alcohol withdrawal syndrome [letter]. *Intensive Care Med.* 1999;25:1435–1436.

Guthrie. S, Sung J, Goodson J, Grunhaus L, Tandon R. Triazolam and diphenhydramine effects on seizure duration in depressed patients receiving ECT [letter]. *Convulsive Ther.* 1996;12:261–265.

Hart R, Colenda C, Hamer R. Effects of buspirone and alprazolam on the cognitive performance of normal elderly subjects. *Am J Psychiatry.* 1991;148:73–77.

Hassan R, Pollard A. Late-life-onset panic disorder: Clinical and demographic characteristics of a patient sample. *J Geriatr Psychiatry Neurology.* 1994;7:86–90.

Henderson S, Jorm A, Scott R, Mackinnon A, Christensen H, Korten A. Insomnia in the elderly: Its prevalence and correlates in the general population. *Med J Aust.* 1995;162:22–24.

Hilbert J, Chung M, Radwanski E, Gural R, Symchowicz S, Zampaglione N. Quazepam kinetics in the elderly. *Clin Pharmacol Ther.* 1984;36:566–569.

Hogan DB, Maxwell CJ, Fung TS, Ebly EM, Canadian Study of Health and Aging. Prevalence and potential consequences of benzodiazepine use in senior citizens: results from the Canadian Study of Health and Aging. *Can J Clin Pharmacol.* 2003;10 (2):72–77.

Holbrook A, Crowther R, Lotter A, Cheng C, King D. Meta-analysis of benzodiazepine use in the treatment of insomnia. *CMAJ.* 2000;162:225–233.

Jochemsen R, Breimer D. Pharmacokinetics of benzodiazepines: Metabolic pathways and plasma levels. *Curr Med Res Opin.* 1984;8 (Suppl 4):60– 79.

Jochemsen R, Van Beusekom B, Spoelstra P, Janssens A, Breimer D. Effect of age and liver cirrhosis on the pharmacokinetics of nitrazepam. *Br J Clin Pharmac.* 1983;15:295–302.

Kahn R, McNair D, Lipman R, et al. Imipramine and chlordiazepoxide in depressive and anxiety disorders. *Arch Gen Psychiatry.* 1986;43:79–85.

Kales A. Quazepam: Hypnotic efficacy and side effects. *Pharmacother.* 1990;10:1–12.

Kenny R, Kafetz K, Impallomeni M. Impaired nitrazepam metabolism in hypothyroidism. *Postgrad Med J.* 1984;60:296–297.

Kramer M, Schoen L. Problems in the use of long-acting hypnotics in older patients. *J Clin Psychiatry.* 1984;45:176–177.

Kripke d, Klauber M, Wingard D, Fell R, Assmus J, Garfinkel L. Mortality hazard associated with prescription hypnotics. *Biol Psychiatry.* 1998;43:687–693.

Kumar R, Mac D, Gabrielli W, Goodwin D. Anxiolytics and memory: A comparison of lorazepam and alprazolam. *J Clin Psychiatry.* 1987;48:158–160.

Lader M. Benzodiazepine dependence. *Prog Neuro-Psychopharmacol & Biol Psychiatr.* 1984;8:85–95.

Lader M. Implications of hypnotic flexibility on patterns of clinical use. *IJCP supp.* 2001;116:14–19.

Lader M. Rebound insomnia and newer hypnotics. *Psychopharmacology.* 1992;108:248–255.

Lechin F, van der Dijs B, Benaim M. Benzodiazepines: Tolerability in elders. *Psychotherap Psychosom.* 1996;65:171–182.

Leger D, Scheuermaier K, Roger M. The relationship between alertness and sleep in a population of 769 elderly insomniacs with and without treatment with zolpidem. *Arch Gerontol Geriatr.* 1999;29:165–173.

Lesser I, Rubin R, Refkin A, et al. Secondary depression in panic disorder and agoraphobia II. Dimensions of depressive symptomatology and their response to treatment. *J Affective Dis.* 1989;16:49–58.

Lindsay W, Gamsu C, McLaughlin E, Hood E, Espie C. A controlled trial of treatment for generalized anxiety. *Br J Clin Psychology.* 1987;26:3–15.

Londborg P, Smith W, Glaudin V, Painter J. Short-term cotherapy with clonazepam and fluoxetine: Anxiety, sleep disturbance, and core symptoms of depression. *J Affective Disorders.* 2000;61:73–79.

Lucki I, Rickels K, Geller A. Chronic use of benzodiazepines and psychomotor and cognitive test performance. *Psychopharmacol.* 1986;88:426–433.

Mah l, Upshur R. Long term benzodiazepine use for insomnia in patients over the age of 60: Discordance of patient and physician perceptions. *BMC Family practice.* 2002;3:9.

Maletta G, Mattox K, Dysken M. Guidelines for prescribing psychoactive drugs in the elderly: Part 2. *Geriatrics.* 1991;46:52–60.

Maletta G. Use of benzodiazepines in elderly patients [letter]. *Mayo Clin Proc.* 1996;71:1124–1125.

Mamelak M, Csima A, Buck L, Price V. A comparative study on the effects of brotizolam and flurazepam of sleep and performance in the elderly. *J Clin Psychopharmacol.* 1989;9:260–267.

Markovitz P. Treatment of anxiety in the elderly. *J Clin Psychiatry.* 1993;54 (5 Suppl):64–68.

Martinez-Cano H, Vela-Bueno A, de Iceta M, Pomalima R, Martinez-Gras I. Benzodiazepine withdrawal syndrome seizures. *Pharmacopsychiat.* 1995;28:257–262.

Martinez H, Serna C. Short-term treatment with quazepam of insomnia in geriatric patients. *Clin therapeutics.* 1982;5:174–178.

McCall W. A psychiatric perspective on insomnia. *J Clin Psychiatry.* 2001;62 (Suppl 10):27–32.

Mitler M. Nonselective and selective benzodiazepine receptor agonists: Where are we today? *Sleep.* 2000;23:S39–S47.

Monane M, Glynn R, Avorn J. The impact of sedative-hypnotic use on sleep in elderly nursing home residents. *Clin Pharmacol Ther.* 1996;59:83–92.

Montagna P, Provini F, Plazzi G, Liguori R, Lugaresi E. Propriospinal myoclonus upon relaxation and drowsiness: A cause of severe insomnia. *Movement Disorders.* 1997;12:66–72.

Morgan K. Effect of repeated doses of nitrazepam and lormetazepam on psychomotor performance in the elderly. *Psychopharmacol.* 1985;86:209–211.

Neutel C, Hirdes J, Maxwell C, Patten S. New evidence on benzodiazepine use and falls: The time factor. *Age Ageing.* 1996;25:273–278.

Neutel I. Benzodiazepine-related traffic accidents in young and elderly drivers. *Hum Psychopharmacol Clin Exp.* 1998;13:S115–S123.

Newman J, Terris D, Moore M. Trends in the management of alcohol withdrawal syndrome. *Laryngoscope.* 1995;105:1–7.

Nikaido A, Ellinwood E, Heatherly D, Gupta S. Age-related increased CNS sensitivity to benzodiazepines as assessed by task difficulty. *Psychopharmacol.* 1990;100:90–97.

Nofzinger E, Reynolds C. Sleep impairment and daytime sleepiness in later life. *Am J Psychiatry.* 1996;153:941–943.

Ochs H, Miller L, Greenblatt D, Shader R. Actual versus reported benzodiazepine usage by medical outpatients. *Eur J Clin Pharmacol.* 1987;32:383–388.

Ochs H, Oberem U, Greenblatt D. Nitrazepam clearance unimpaired in patients with renal insufficiency. *J Clin Psychopharmacol.* 1992;12:183–185.

Olajide D, Lader M. Depression following withdrawal from long-term benzodiazepine use: A report of four cases. *Psychological Medicine.* 1984;14:937–940.

Oswald K. Can a rapidly-eliminated hypnotic cause daytime anxiety? *Pharmacopsychiatr.* 1989;22:115–119.

Ozdemir V, Fourie J, Busto U, Naranjo C. Pharmacokinetic changes in the elderly. *Clin Pharmacokinet.* 1996;31:372–385.

Pat McAndrews M, Weiss RTm Sandor P, Taylor A, Carlen PL, Shapiro CM.

Cognitive effects of long-term benzodiazepine use in older adults. *Hum Psychopharmacol.* 2003;18 (1):51–7.

Paterniti S, Dufouil C, Alperovitch A. Long-term benzodiazepine use and cognitive decline in the elderly: The epidemiology of vascular aging study. *J Clin Psychopharmacol.* 2002;22:285–293.

Peppers M. Benzodiazepines for alcohol withdrawal in the elderly and in patients with liver disease. *Pharmacotherapy.* 1996;16:49–58.

Petrovic M, Mariman A, Warie H, Afschrift M, Pevernagie D. Is there a rationale for prescription of benzodiazepines in the elderly? Review of the literature. *Acta Clin Belg.* 2003;58 (1):27–36.

Pollak C, Perlick D, Linsner J. Sleep and motor activity of community elderly who frequently use bedtime medications. *Biol Psychiatry.* 1994;35: 73–75.

Pomara N, Tun H, DaSilva D, Hernando R, Deptula D, Greenblatt D. The acute and chronic performance effects of alprazolam and lorazepam in the elderly: Relation to duration of treatment and self-rated sedation. *Psychopharmacol Bull.* 1998;34:139–153.

Rapport D, Covington E. Motor phenomena in benzodiazepine withdrawal. *Hosp Community Psychiatry.* 1989;40:1277–1279.

Ray W, Fought R, Decker M. Psychoactive drugs and the risk of injurious motor vehicle crashes in elderly drivers. *Am J Epidemiol.* 1992;136:873–883.

Ray W, Thapa P, Gideon P. Benzodiazepines and the risk of falls in nursing home residents. *JAGS.* 2000;48:682–685.

Reich J, Yates W. A pilot study of social phobia with alprazolam. *Am J Psychiatry.* 1988;145:590–594.

Richards H, Valle-Jones C. A double-blind comparison of two lormetazepam doses in elderly insomniacs. *Curr Med Res Opinion.* 1988;11:48–55.

Rickels K, DeMartinis N, Garcia-Espana F, Greenblatt D, Mandos L, Rynn M. Imipramine and buspirone in treatment of patients with generalized anxiety disorder who are discontinuing long-term benzodiazepine therapy. *Am J Psychiatry.* 2000;157:1973–1979.

Rickels K, Fox I, Greenblatt D, Sandler K, Schless A. Clorazepate and lorazepam: Clinical improvement and rebound anxiety. *Am J Psychiatry.* 1988;145:312–317.

Robinson, D, Rickels K, Feighner J, et al. Clinical effects of the 5-HTIA partial agonists in depression: a composite analysis of buspirone in the treatment of depression. *J Clin Psychopharmacol.* 1990;10 (3 Suppl):67S–76S.

Rosebush P, Mazurek M. Catatonia after benzodiazepine withdrawal. *J Clin Psychopharmacol.* 1996;16:315–319.

Roth T, Roehrs T. A review of the safety profiles of benzodiazepine hypnotics. *J Clin Psychiatry.* 1991;52 (Suppl 9):38–41.

Roth T, Roehrs T, Koshorek G, Greenblatt D, Rosenthal L. Hypnotic effects of low doses of quazepam in older insomniacs. *J Clin Psychopharmacol.* 1997;17:401–406.

Sadavoy J. The effect of personality disorder on Axis I disorders in the elderly. In M Duffy (ed), *Handbook of Counseling and Psychotherapy with Older Adults.* New York: Wiley; 1999; pp 397–413.

Salzman C. Anxiety in the elderly: treatment strategies. *J Clin Psychiatry.* 1990;51 (Suppl 10):18–21.

Salzman C, Shader R, Greenblatt D, Harmatz D. Long v. short half-life benzodiazepines in the elderly. *Arch General adult data Psychiatry.* 1983;40:293–297.

Sanger D, Benavides J, Perrault G, et al. Recent developments in the behavioral pharmacology of benzodiazepine (ω) receptors: Evidence for the functional significance of receptor subtypes. *Neurosci Biobehavioral Rev.* 18;355–372.

Scharf M, Hirschowitz J, Woods M, Scharf S. Lack of amnesic effects of Clorazepate on geriatric recall. *J Clin Psychiatry.* 1985;46:518–520.

Scharf M. Individualizing therapy for early, middle-of-the-night and late-night insomnia. *IJCP. suppl.* 2001;116:20–24.

Schenck C, Bundlie S, Ettinger M, Mahowald M. Chronic behavioral disorders of human REM sleep: A new category of parasomnia. *Sleep.* 1986;9:293–308.

Schmidt U, Brendemuhl D, Ruther E. Aspects of driving after hypnotic therapy with particular reference to temazepam. *Acta Psychiatr Scand.* 1986;74 (Suppl 332):112–118.

Schneider L. Overview of generalized anxiety disorder in the elderly. *J Clin Psychiatry.* 1996;57 (Suppl 7):34–45.

Sevransky JE, Haponik EF. Respiratory failure in elderly patients. *Clin Geriatr Med.* 2003;19 (1):205–24.

Sheikh J. Anxiety disorders and their treatment. *Clinics Geriatr Medicine.* 1992;8:411–426.

Sheikh J, Salzman C. Anxiety in the elderly. *Psychiatric Clin North Am.* 1995;18:871–883.

Sheikh J, Swales P. Treatment of panic disorder in older adults: A pilot study comparison of alprazolam, imipramine, and placebo. *Intl J Psychiatry Med.* 1999;29:107–117.

Shorr R, Bauwens S. Effects of patient age and physician training on choice and dose of benzodiazepine hypnotic drugs. *Arch Intern Med.* 1990;150:293–295.

Shorr R, Bauwens S, Landefeld C. Failure to limit quantities of benzodiazepine hypnotic drugs for outpatients: Placing the elderly at risk. *Am J Med.* 1990;89:725–732.

Small G. Recognizing and treating anxiety in the elderly. *J Clin psychiatry.* 1997;58 (suppl 3):41–47.

Smith M, Perlis M, Park A, et al. Comparative meta-analysis of pharmacotherapy and behavior therapy for persistent insomnia. *Am J Psychiatry.* 2002;159:5–11.

Smith W, Londborg P, Glaudin V, Painter J. Short-term augmentation of fluoxetine with clonazepam in the treatment of depression: A double-blind study. *Am J Psychiatry.* 1998;155:1339–1345.

Soldatos C, Dikeos D, Whitehead A. Tolerance and rebound insomnia with rapidly eliminated hypnotics: A meta-analysis of sleep laboratory studies. *Int Clin Psychopharmacol.* 1999;14:287–303.

Stewart R, Marks R, Padgett P, Hale W. Benzodiazepine use in an ambulatory elderly population: A 14-year overview. *Clin Therapeutics.* 1994;16:118–124.

Stoudemire A. Epidemiology and psychopharmacology of anxiety in medical patients. *J Clin Psychiatry.* 1996;57 (Suppl 7):64–72.

Stoudemire A, Moran M. Psychopharmacologic treatment of anxiety in the medically ll elderly patient: Special considerations. *J Clin Psychiatry.* 1993;54 (Suppl 5):27–33.

Sussman N. Treating anxiety while minimizing abuse and dependence. *J Clin Psychiatry.* 1993;54 (Suppl 5):44–51.

Sweden B, Hoste S. Are complex partial seizures an uncommon withdrawal sign in the elderly? *Eur Neurol.* 1987;27:239–244

Swift C, Swift M, Hamley J, Stevenson I, Crooks J. Side effect "tolerance" in elderly long-term recipients of benzodiazepine hypnotics. *Age Ageing.* 1984;13:335–343.

Teboul E, Chouinard G. A guide to benzodiazepine selection. Part II: Clinical aspects. *Can J Psychiatry.* 1991;36:62–73.

Thoman E, Acebo C, Lamm S. Stability and instability of sleep in older persons recorded in the home. *Sleep.* 1993;16:578–585.

Trewin V, Lawrence C, Veltch G. An investigation of the association of benzodiazepines and other hypnotics with the incidence of falls in the elderly. *J Clin Pharmacy Therapeutics.* 1992;17:129–133.

Trullen J, Pardo P, Andre M, Lozano J. Bromazepam-induced dystonia [letter]. *Biomed Pharmacother.* 1992;46:375–376.

Ungvari G, Leung C, Wong M, Lau J. Benzodiazepines in the treatment of catatonic syndrome. *Acta Psychiatr Scand.* 1994;89:285–288.

Vanakoski J, Mattila M, Seppala T. Driving under light and dark conditions: Effects of alcohol and diazepam in young and older subjects. *Eur J Clin Pharmacol.* 2000;56:453–458.

Vidailhet P, Danion J, Kauffmann-Muller F, et al. Lorazepam and diazepam effects on memory acquisition in priming tasks. *Psychopharmacol.* 1994;115:397–406.

Vogel G. Clinical use and advantages of low doses of benzodiazepine hypnotics. *J Clin Psychiatry.* 1992;53 (Suppl 6):19–22.

Walsh J, Mahowald M. Avoiding the blanket approach to insomnia. *Postgrad Med.* 1991;90:211–224.

Wang P, Bohn R, Glynn R, Mogun H, Avorn J. Hazardous benzodiazepine regimens in the elderly: Effects of half-life, dosage, and duration on risk of hip fracture. *Am J Psychiatry.* 2001;158:892–898.

Weinbroum A, Rudick V, Sorkine P, Fleishon R, Geller E. Long-term intravenous and oral flumazenil treatment of acute diazepam overdose in an older woman [letter]. *JAGS.* 1996;44:737–738.

Wengel S, Burke W, Ranno A, Roccaforte W. Use of benzodiazepines in the elderly. *Psychiatric Ann.* 1993;23:325–331.

Wheatley D. Insomnia in general practice: The role of temazepam and a comparison with zopiclone. *Acta Psychiatr Scand.* 1986;74 (Suppl 332):142–148.

Wheatley D. Prescribing short-acting hypnosedatives. *Drug Safety.* 1992;7:106–115.

Winsauer H, O'Hair D. Quazepam short-term treatment of insomnia in geriatric outpatients. *Curr Therapeutic Res.* 1984;35:228–234.

Wise M, Griffies W. A combined treatment approach to anxiety in the medically ill. *J Clin Psychiatry.* 1995;56 (suppl 2):14–19.

Woo E, Proulx S, Greenblatt D. Differential side effect profile of triazolam versus flurazepam in elderly patients undergoing rehabilitation therapy. *J Clin Pharmacol.* 1991;31:168–173.

Wooten V. Sleep disorders in geriatric patients. *Clin Geriatr Med.* 1992;8:427–439.

Alprazolam

Busto U, Kaplan H, Wright E, et al. A comparative pharmacokinetic and dynamic evaluation of alprazolam sustained-release, bromazepam, and lorazepam. *J Clin Psychopharmacol.* 2000;20:628–635.

Cassano G, Toni C, Petracca A, et al. Adverse effects associated with the short-term treatment of panic disorder with imipramine, alprazolam, or placebo. *Eur Neuropsychopharmacol.* 1994;4:47–53.

Chouinard G. Antimanic effects of clonazepam. *Psychosomatics.* 1985;26 (Suppl 12):7–12.

Christensen D, Benfield W. Alprazolam as an alternative to low-dose haloperidol in older, cognitively-impaired nursing facility patients. *J Am Geriatr Soc.* 1998;46:620–625.

Dehlin O, Kullingsjo H, Liden A, Agrell A, Moser G, Olsen I. Pharmacokinetics of alprazolam in geriatric patients with neurotic depression. *Pharmacol Toxicol.* 1991;68:121–124.

Freda J, Bush H, Barie P. Alprazolam withdrawal in a critically ill patient. *Critical Care Med.* 1992;20:545–546.

Fyer A, Liebowitz M, Gorman J, et al. Discontinuation of alprazolam treatment in panic patients. *Am J Psychiatry.* 1987;144:303–308.

Guven H, Tunock Y, Guneri S, Cavdar C, Fowler J. Age-related digoxin-alprazolam interaction. *Clin Pharmacol Ther.* 1993;54:42–44.

Holland J, Morrow G, Schmale A, et al. A randomized clinical trial of alprazolam versus progressive muscle relaxation in cancer patients with anxiety and depressive symptoms. *J Clin Oncology.* 1991;9:1004–1011.

Kaplan G, Greenblatt D, Ehrenberg B, Goddard J, Harmatz J, Shader R. Single-dose pharmacokinetics and pharmacodynamics of alprazolam in elderly and young subjects. *J Clin Pharmacol.* 1997;38:14–21.

Kravitz H, Fawcett J, Newman A. Alprazolam and depression: A review of risks and benefits. *J Clin Psychiatry.* 1993;54 (Suppl 10):78–84.

Kroboth P, McAuley J, Smith R. Alprazolam in the elderly: Pharmacokinetics and pharmacodynamics during multiple dosing. *Psychopharmacol.* 1990;100:477–484.

Levy A. Delirium and seizures due to abrupt alprazolam withdrawal: Case report. *J Clin Psychiatry.* 1984;45:38–39.

Lydiard B, Lesser I, Ballenger J, Rubin R, Laraia M, DuPont R. A fixed-dose study of alprazolam 2 mg, alprazolam 6 mg, and placebo in panic disorder. *J Clin Psychopharmacol.* 1992;12:96–103.

McCormick S, Nielsen J, Jatlow P. Alprazolam overdose: Clinical findings and serum concentrations in two cases. *J Clin Psychiatry.* 1985;46:247–248.

Mendels J, Chernoff R, Blatt M. Alprazolam as an adjunct to propranolol in anxious outpatients with stable angina. *J Clin Psychiatry.* 1986;47:8–11.

Muhlberg W, Rieck W, Arnold E, Ott G, Lungershausen E. Pharmacokinetics of alprazolam in elderly patients with multiple diseases. *Arch Gerontol Geriatr.* 1997;25:91–100.

Ochs H, Greenblatt D, Labedzki L, Smith R. Alprazolam kinetics in patients with renal insufficiency. *J Clin Psychopharmacol.* 1986;6:292–294.

Penati G, Panza G, Mantero M, Mauri M. Paranoid ideation in geriatric depressed patients treated with alprazolam [letter]. *J Clin Psychopharmacol.* 1991;11:70–71.

Pitts W, Fann W, Sajadi C, Snyder S. Alprazolam in older depressed inpatients. *J Clin Psychiatry.* 1983;44:213–215.

Rothschild A, Shindul-Rothschild, Viguera A, Murray M, Brewster S. Comparison of the frequency of behavioral disinhibition on alprazolam, clonazepam, or no benzodiazepine in hospitalized psychiatric patients. *J Clin Psychopharmacol.* 2000;20:7–11.

Sachs G, Weilburg J, Rosenbaum J. Clonazepam vs. neuroleptics as adjuncts to lithium maintenance. *Psychopharmacol Bull.* 1990;26:137–143.

Swantek S, Grossberg G, Neppe V, Doubek W, Martin T, Bender J. The use of carbamazepine to treat benzodiazepine withdrawal in a geriatric population. *J Geriatr Psychiatry Neurol.* 1991;4:106–109.

Tollefson G. Alprazolam in the treatment of obsessive symptoms. *J Clin Psychopharmacol.* 1985;5:39–42.

Tollefson G, Lesar T, Grothe D, Garvey M. Alprazolam –related digoxin toxicity. *Am J Psychiatry.* 1984;141:1612–1614.

Udelman H, Udelman D. Concurrent use of buspirone in anxious patients during withdrawal from alprazolam therapy. *J Clin Psychiatry.* 1990;51;(Suppl 9):46–51.

Warner M, Peabody C, Boutros N, Whiteford H. Alprazolam and withdrawal seizures [letter]. *J Nerv Ment Disease.* 1990;178:208–209.

Weissman M, Prusoff B, Sholomskas A, Greenwald S. A double-blind clinical trial of alprazolam, imipramine, or placebo in the depressed elderly. *J Clin Psychopharmacol.* 1992;12:175–182.

Zalsman G, Hermesh H, Munitz H. Alprazolam withdrawal delirium: A case report. *Clin Neuropharmacol.* 1998;3:201–202.

Zipursky R, Baker R, Zimmer B. Alprazolam withdrawal delirium unresponsive to diazepam: Case report. *J Clin Psychiatry.* 1985;46:344–345.

Buspirone

Alderman C, Frith P, Ben-Tovim D. Buspirone for the treatment of anxiety in patients with chronic obstructive airways disease. *J Clin Psychopharmacol.* 1996;16:410–411.

Allmann B, Domantay A, Schoeman H. Antidepressant activity of buspirone in anxiety. *Curr Therapeutic Res.* 1992;52:406–411.

Ansseau M, Papart P, Gerard M, Frenckell R, Franck G. Controlled comparison of buspirone and oxazepam in generalized anxiety. *Neuropsychobiol.* 1990;24:74–78.

Bhandary A, Masand P. Buspirone in the management of disruptive behaviors due to Huntington's disease and other neurological disorders. *Psychosomatics.* 1997;38:389–391.

Bonifati V, Fabrizio E, Cipriani R, Vanacore N, Mecco G. Buspirone in levodopa-induced dyskinesia. *Clin Neuropharmacol.* 1994;17:73–82.

Cadieux R. Azapirones: An alternative to benzodiazepines for anxiety 1996;53:2349–2353.

Cantillon M, Brunswick R, Molina D, Bahro M. Buspirone vs. haloperidol: A double-blind trial for agitation in a nursing home population with Alzheimer's disease. *AM J Geriatr Psychiatry.* 1996;4:263–267.

Cohn J, Bowden C, Fisher J, Rodos J. Double-blind comparison of buspirone and clorazepate in anxious outpatients. *Am J Med.* 1986;80 (Suppl 3B): 10–16.

Cohn J, Rickels K, Steege J. A pooled, double-blind comparison of the effects of buspirone, diazepam, and placebo in women with chronic anxiety. *Curr Med Res Opinion.* 1989;11:304–320.

Feighner J. Buspirone in the long-term treatment of generalized anxiety disorder. *J Clin Psychiatry.* 1987;48 (Suppl 12):3–6.

Gammans R, Hvizdos A, Cohn J, et al. Use of buspirone in patients with generalized anxiety disorder and coexisiting depressive symptoms. *Neuropsychobiol.* 1992;25:193–201.

Gammans R, Westrick M, Shea J, Mayol R, LaBudde J. Pharmacokinetics of buspirone in elderly subjects. *J Clin Pharmacol.* 1989;29:72–78.

Goldberg R, Huk M. Serotonin syndrome for trazadone and buspirone [letter]. *Psychosomatics.* 1992;33:235.

Greenberg D. Buspirone for myoclonus, obsessive fears, and confusion. *Psychosomatics.* 1993;34:270–272.

Hargrave R. Serotonergic agents in the management of dementia and posttraumatic stress disorder [letter]. *Psychosomatics.* 1993:5:461–462.

Hart R, Colenda C, Hamer R. Effects of buspirone and alprazolam on the cognitive performance of normal elderly subjects. *Am J Psychiatry.* 1991;148: 73–77.

Herrmann N, Eryavec G. Buspirone in the management of agitation and aggression associated with dementia. *Am J Geriat Psychiatry.* 1993;1:249–253.

Joffe R, Schuller D. An open study of buspirone augmentation of serotonin reuptake inhibitors in refractory depression. *J Clin Psychiatry.* 1993;54:269–271.

Lawlor B, Hill J, Radcliffe J, Minichiello M, Molchan S, Sunderland T. A single oral dose challenge of buspirone dose not affect memory processes in older volunteers. *Biol Psychiatry.* 1992;32:101–103.

Lebert F, Pasquier F, Goudemand M, Petit H. Euphoria with buspirone after fluoxetine treatment [letter]. *Am J Psychiatry.* 1993;150:167.

Levine S, Napoliello M, Domantay A. An open study of buspirone in octogenarians with anxiety. *Human Psychopharmacol.* 1989;4:51–53.

Liegghio N, Yeragani V, Moore N. Buspirone-induced jitteriness in three patients with panic disorder and one patient with generalized anxiety disorder. *J Clin Psychiatry.* 1988;49:165–166.

Mahmood I, Sahajwalla C. Clinical pharmacokinetics and pharmacodynamics of buspirone, an anxiolytic drug. *Clin Pharmacokinet.* 1999;36:277–287.

Manfredi R, Kales A, Vgontzas A, Bixler E, Isaac M, Falcone C. Buspirone: Sedative or stimulant effect? *Am J Psychiatry.* 1991;148:1213–1217.

Martensson B, Murray V, Arbin V, Asberg M, Bartfai A, Malm K. Alternative treatment for poststroke depression [letter]. *Am J Psychiatry.* 1997; 154:583–584.

Moss L, Neppe V, Drevets W. Buspirone in the treatment of tardive dyskinesia *J Clin Psychopharmacol.* 1993;13:204–209.

Newton R, Marunycz J, Alderdice M, Napoliello M. Review of the side-effect profile of buspirone. 1986;80 (Suppl 3B):17–21.

Pecknold J, Matas M, Howarth B, ross C, Swinson R, Vezeau C, Ungar W. Evaluation of buspirone as an antianxiety agent: Buspirone and diazepam versus placebo. *Can J Psychiatry.* 1989;34:766–771.

Rickels K, Amsterdam J, Clary C, Puzzuoli G, Schweizer E. Buspirone in major depression: A controlled study. *J Clin Psychiatry.* 1991;52:34–38.

Rickels K, DeMartinis N, Garcia-Espana F, Greenblatt D, Mandos L, Rynn M. Imipramine and buspirone in treatment of patients with generalized anxiety disorder who are discontinuing long-term benzodiazepine therapy. *Am J Psychiatry.* 2000;157:1973–1979.

Robillard M, Lieff S. Augmentation of antidepressant therapy by buspirone: Three geriatric case histories [letter]. *Can J Psychiatry.* 1995;40:639–640.

Robinson D, Napoliello M, Schenk J. The safety and usefulness of buspirone as an anxiolytic drug in elderly versus young patients. *Clin Therapeutics.* 1988;6:740–746.

Rocco P, Giavedoni A, Pacella G. Withdrawal of benzodiazepines in a hospital setting: An open trial with buspirone. *Cur Therapeutic Res.* 1992;52:386–389.

Strand M, Hetta J, Rosen A, et al. A double-blind, controlled trial in primary care patients with generalized anxiety: A comparison between buspirone and oxazepam. *J C Psychiatry.* 1990;51 (Suppl 9):40–45.

Strauss A. Oral dyskinesia associated with buspirone use in an elderly woman. *J Clin Psychiatry.* 1988;49:322–323.

Van Laar M, Volkerts E, van Willigenburg A. Therapeutic effects and effects on actual driving performance of chronically administered buspirone and diazepam in anxious outpatients. *J Clin Psychopharmacol.* 1992;12:86–95.

Young A, McShane R, Park S, Cowen P. Buspirone-induced hypothermia in normal male volunteers. *Biol Psychiatry.* 1993;34:665–666.

Clonazepam

Bradwejn J, Shriqui C, Koszycki D, Meterissian G. Double-blind comparison of the effects of clonazepam and lorazepam in acute mania. *J Clin Psychopharmacol.* 1990;10:403–408.

Freinhar J, Alvarez W. Clonazepam treatment of organic brain syndromes in three elderly patients. *J Clin Psychiatry.* 1986;47:525–526.

Gates P, Thyagarajan D. Orthostatic tremor: A cause of postural instability in the elderly. *Med J Australia.* 1990;152:373.

Gerding L, Labbate L. Use of clonazepam in an elderly bipolar patient with tardive dyskinesia: A case report. *Ann Clin Psychiatry.* 1999;11:87–89.

Ginsburg M. Clonazepam for agitated patients with Alzheimer's disease. *Can J Psychiatry.* 1991;36:237–238.

Heilman K. Orthostatic tremor. *Arch Neurol.* 1984;41:880–881.
Kuniyoshi M, Katsuyoshi A, Miura C, Inanaga K. Effect of clonazepam on tardive dyskinesia. *Human Psychopharmacol.* 1991;6:39–42.
Morishita S, Aoki S. Clonazepam in the treatment of prolonged depression. *J Affect Disorder.* 1999;53:275–278.
Moroz G, Rosenbaum J. Efficacy, safety, and gradual discontinuation of clonazepam in panic disorder: A placebo-controlled, multicenter study using optimized dosages. *J Clin Psychiatry.* 1999;60:604–612.
Obeso J, Artieda J, Rothwell J, Day B, Thompson P, Marsden C K. The treatment of severe action myoclonus. *Brain.* 1989;112:765–777.

Diazepam

Dent L, Orrock M. Warfarin-fluoxetine and diazepam–fluoxetine interaction. *Pharmacotherapy.* 1997;17:170–172.
Herman R, Wilkinson G. Disposition of diazepam in young and elderly subjects fter acute and chronic dosing. *Br J Clin Pharmacol.* 1996;42:147–155.

Estazolam

Vogel G, Morris D. The effects of estazolam on sleep, performance, and memory: A long-term sleep laboratory study of elderly insomniacs. *J Clin Pharmacol.* 1992;32:647-651.

Herbal Remedies: KAVA

Health Canada Advisory. Health Canada is advising consumers not to use any products containing kava January 16, 2002; *www.hc-sc.gc.ca/english/protection/warnings/2002/2002_02e.htm.*

Lorazepam

Blin O, Simon N, Jouve E, et al. Pharmacokinetic and pharmacodynamic analysis of sedative and amnesic effects of lorazepam in healthy volunteers. *Clin Neuropharmacol.* 2001;24:71–81.
Bonnet M, Arand D. The use of lorazepam TID for chronic insomnia. *Int Clin Psychopharmacol.* 1999;14:81–89.
Buysse D, Reynolds C, Houck P, Perel J, Frank E, Begley A, Mazumdar S, Kupfer D. Does lorazepam impair the antidepressant response to nortriptyline and psychotherapy? *J Clin Psychiatry.* 1997;58:426–432.
Carroll B. Catatonia on the consultation–liaison service. *Psychosomatics.* 1992;33:310–315.
Ceraianu A, Delrossi A, Flum D, et al. Lorazepam and midazolam in the intensive care unit: A randomized, prospective, multicenter study of hemodynamics, oxygen transport, efficacy, and cost. *Crit Care Med.* 1996;24:222–228.
Foulhoux A. Effect on body sway of various benzodiazepine tranquillizers. *Br J Clin Pharmacol.* 1985;20:9–16.
Gram-Hansen P, Schultz A. Plasma concentrations following oral and sublingual administration of lorazepam. *Int J Clin Pharmacol, Therapy, Toxicol.* 1988;26:323–324.
Lenox R, Newhouse P, Creelman W, Whitaker T. Adjunctive treatment of

manic agitation with lorazepam versus haloperidol: A double-blind study. *J Clin Psychiatry.* 1992;53:47–52.

Morrison G, Chiang S, Koepke H, Walker B. Effect of renal impairment and hemodialysis on lorazepam kinetics. *Clin Pharmacol Ther.* 1984;35:646–652.

Satzger W, Engel R, Ferguson E, Kapfhammer H, Eich F, Hippius H. Effects of single doses of alpidem, lorazepam, and placebo on memory and attention in healthy young and elderly volunteers. *Pharmacopsychiatry.* 1990;23:114–119.

Scharf M, Khosla N, Brocker N, Goff P. Differential amnestic properties of short- and long-acting benzodiazepines. *J Clin Psychiatry.* 1984;45:51–53.

Van Laar M, Volkerts E, Verbaten M. Subchronic effects of the GABA-agonist lorazepam and the 5-$HT_{2A/2C}$ antagonist ritanserin on driving performance, slow wave sleep, and daytime sleepiness in healthy volunteers. *Psychopharmacol.* 2001;154:189–197.

van Steveninck A, Wallnofer A, Schoemaker R, et al. A study of the effects of long-term use on individual sensitivity to temazepam and lorazepam in a clinical population. *Br J Clin Pharmacol.* 1997;44:267–275.

Midazolam

Albrecht S, Ihmsen H, Hering W, et al. The effect of age on the pharmacokinetics and pharmacodynamics of midazolam. *Clin Pharmacol Ther.* 1999;65:630–639.

Beck H, Saloma M, Holzer J. Midazolam dosage studies in institutionalized geriatric patients. *Br J Clin Pharmac.* 1983;16:133S–137S.

Castleden C, Allen J, Altman J, St. John-Smith P. A comparison of oral midazolam, nitrazepam, and placebo in young and elderly subjects. *Eur J Pharmacol.* 1987;32:353–357.

Holazo A, Winkler M, Patel I. Effects of age, gender, and oral contraceptives on intramuscular midazolam pharmacokinetics. *J Clin Pharmacol.* 1988;28:1040–1045.

Oldenhhof H, de Jong M, Steenhoek A, Janknegt R. Clinical pharmacokinetics of midazolam in intensive care patients, a wide interpatient variability. *Clin Pharmacol Ther.* 1988;43:263–269.

Platten H, Schweizer E, Dilger K, Mikus G, Klotz U. Pharmacokinetics and the pharmacodynamic action of midazolam in young and elderly patients undergoing tooth extraction. *Clin Pharmacol Therap.* 1998;63:552–560.

Smith M, Heazlewood V, Eadie M, Brophy T, Tyrer J. Pharmacokinetics of midazolam in the elderly. *Eur J Clin Pharmacol.* 1984;26:381–388.

Wandel C, Bocker R, Bohrer H, et al. Relationship between hepatic cytochrome P450 3A content and activity and the disposition of midazolam administered orally. *Drug Metab Distribution.* 1998;26:110–114.

Oxazepam

Dreyfuss D, Shader R, Harmatz J, Greenblatt D. Kinetics and dynamics of single doses of oxazepam in the elderly: Implications of absorption rate. *J Clin Psychiatry.* 1986;47:511–514.

Hersch E, Billings R. Acute confusional state with status petit mal as a withdrawal syndrome and five year follow-up. *Can J Psychiatry.* 1988;33:157–159.

Temazepam

Archer c, English J. Extensive fixed drug reaction induced by temazepam. *Clin Exp Dermatology.* 1988;13:336–338.

Begg A, Drummond G, Tiplady B. Effects of temazepam on memory and psychomotor performance: A dose-response study. *Hum Psychopharmacol Clin Exp.* 2001;16:475–480.

Clark G, Erwin D, Yate P, Burt D, Major E. Temazepam as premedication in elderly patients. *Anaesthesia.* 1982;37:421–425.

Cook P, Huggett A, Graham-Pole R, Savage I, James I. Hypnotic accumulation and hangover in elderly inpatients: A controlled double-blind study of temazepam and nitrazepam. *BMJ.* 1983;286:100–102.

Cumming R, Klineberg R. Psychotropics, thiazide diuretics, and hip fractures in the elderly. *Med J Aust.* 1993;158:414–417.

Ford G, Hoffman B, Blaschke T. Effect of temazepam on blood pressure regulation in healthy elderly subjects. *Br J Clin Pharmac.* 1990;29:61–67.

Ghabrial H, Desmond P, Watson K, et al. The effects of age and chronic liver disease on the elimination of temazepam. *Eur J Clin Pharmacol.* 1986;30:93–97.

Jochemsen R, Breimer D. Pharmacokinetics of temazepam compared with other benzodiazepine hypnotics: Some clinical consequences. *Acta Psychiatrica Scand.* 1986;74 (Suppl 332):20–21.

Kales A, Bixler E, Soldatos C, Vela-Bueno A, Jacoby J, Kales. Quazepam and temazepam: Effects of short- and intermediate-term use and withdrawal. *Clin Pharmacol Ther.* 1986;39:345–352.

Kamali F, Herd B, Edwards C, Nicholson E, Wynne H. The influence of ciprofloxacin on the pharmacokinetics and pharmacodyamics of a single dose of temazepam in the young and elderly. *J Clin Pharmacy Therap.* 1994;19:105–109.

Klem K, Murray G, Laake K. Pharmacokinetics of temazepam in geriatric patients. *Eur J Clin Pharmacol.* 1986;30:745–747.

Meuleman J, Nelson R. Evaluation of temazepam and diphenhydramine as hypnotics in a nursing-home population. *Drug Intel Clin Pharm.* 1987;21:716–720.

Morin CM, Basstien CH, Brink D, Brown TR. Adverse effects of temazepam in older adults with chronic insomnia. *Hum Psychopharmacol.* 2003; 19 (1):75–82.

Nakra B, Gfeller J, Hassan R. A double-blind comparison of the effects of temazepam and triazolam on residual, daytime performance in elderly insomniacs. *Internat Psychogeriatr.* 1992;4:45–53.

Tham T, Brown H, Taggart M. Temazepam withdrawal in elderly hospitalized patients: A double-blind randomized trial comparing abrupt versus gradual withdrawal. *IJMS.* 1989;158:294–296.

van Steveninck, Wallnofer A, Schoemaker R, et al. A study of the effects of long-term use on individual sensitivity to temazepam and lorazepam in a clinical population. *Br J Clin Pharmacol.* 1997;44:267–275.

Vgontzas A, Kales A, Bixler E, Myers D. Temazepam 7.5mg: Effects of sleep in elderly insomniacs. *Eur J Clin Pharmacol.* 1994;46:209–213.

Triazolam

Bayer A, Bayer E, Pathy M, Stoker M. A double-blind controlled study of chlormethiazole and triazolam as hypnotics in the elderly. *Acta Psychiatr Scand.* 1986;73 (Suppl 329):104–111.

Bixler E, Kales A, Brubaker B, Kales J. Adverse reactions to benzodiazepine hypnotics: Spontaneous reporting system. *Pharmacol.* 1987;35:286–300.

Bonnet M, Arand D. The use of triazolam in older patients with periodic leg movements, fragmented sleep, and daytime sleepiness. *J Gerontol.* 1990:45:M139–144.

Dchlin O, Bjornson G, Borjesson L, Abrahamsson L, Smith R. Pharmacokinetics of triazolam in geriatric patients. *Eur J Clin Pharmacol.* 1983;25:91–94.

Dehlin O, Bjornson G. Triazolam as a hypnotic for geriatric patients. *Acta Psychiatr Scand.* 1983;67:290–296.

Fisch H, Baktir G, Karlaganis G, Minder C, Bircher J. Excessive motor impairment two hours after triazolam in the elderly. *Eur J Clin Pharmacol.* 1990;38:229–232.

Greenblatt D, Divoll M, Abernathy D, Moschitto L, Smith R, Shader R. Reduced clearance of triazolam in old age: Relation to antipyrine oxidizing capacity. *Br J Clin Pharmacol.* 1983;15:303–309.

Greenblatt D, Harmatz J, Shapiro L, Engelhardt N, Gouthro T, Shader R. Sensitivity to triazolam in the elderly. *N Eng J Med.* 1991;324:1691–1698.

Kales A, Bixler E, Vela-Bueno A, Soldatos C, Niklaus D, Manfredi R. Comparison of short and long half-life benzodiazepine hypnotics: Triazolam and quazepam. *Clin Pharmacol Ther.* 1986;40:378–386.

Kanba S, Miyaoka H, Terada H, et al. Triazolam accumulation in the elderly after prolonged use [letter]. *Am J Psychiatry.* 1991;148:1265–1266.

McCarten J, Kovera C, Maddox M, Cleary J. Triazolam in Alzheimer's disease: Pilot study on sleep and memory effects. *Pharmacol Biochem Behavior.* 1995;52:447–452.

Murphy P, Hindmarch I, Hyland C. Aspects of short-term use of two benzodiazepine hypnotics in the elderly. *Age Ageing.* 1982;11:222–228.

Parker W, MacLachlan R. Prolonged hypnotic response to triazolam-cimetidine combination in an elderly patient. *Drug Intell Clin Pharm.* 1984;18:980–981.

Patterson J. Triazolam syndrome in the elderly. *Southern Med J.* 1987;80:1425–1426d.

Regestein Q, Reich P. Agitation observed during treatment with newer hypnotic drugs. *J Clin Psychiatry.* 1985;46:280–283.

Robin D, Hasan S, Edeki T, Lichtenstein M, Shiavi R, Wood A. Increased baseline sway contributes to increased losses of balance in older people following triazolam. *JAGS.* 1996;44:300–304.

Roehrs T, Zorick F, Wittig R, Roth T. Efficacy of a reduced triazolam dose in elderly insomniacs. *Neurobiol Aging.* 1985;6:293–296.

Smith R, Divoll M, Gillespie W, Greenblatt D. Effect of subject age and gender on the pharmacokinetics of oral triazolam and temazepam. *J Clin Psychopharmacol.* 1983;3:172–176.

Takami N, Okada A. Triazolam and nitrazepam use in elderly outpatients. *Ann Psychopharmacol.* 1993;27:506–509.

Wysowski D, Barash D. Adverse behavioral reactions attributable to triazolam in the Food and Drug Administration's spontaneous reporting system. *Arch Intern Med.* 1991;151:2003–2008.

Zaleplon

Doghramji P. Treatment of insomnia with zaleplon, a novel sleep medication. *IJCP.* 2001;55:329–334.

Dooley M, Plosker G. Zaleplon: A review of its use in the treatment of insomnia. *Drugs.* 2000;60:413–435.

Drover D, Lemmens H, Naidu S, Cevallos W, Darwish M, Stanski D. Pharmacokinetics, pharmacodynamics, and relative pharmacokinetic/pharmacodynamic profiles of zaleplon and zolpidem. *Clin Ther.* 2000;22: 1443–1461.

Mangano R. Efficacy and safety of zaleplon at peak plasma levels. *IJCP suppl.* 2001;116:9–13.

Renwick A, Mistry H, Ball S, Walters D, Kao J, Lake B. Metabolism of zaleplon by human hepatic microsomal cytochrome P450 isoforms. *Xenobiotica.* 1998;28:337–348.

Stone B, Turner C, Mills S, et al. Noise-induced sleep maintenance insomnia: Hypnotic and residual effects of zaleplon. *Br J Clin Pharmacol.* 2002; 53:196–202.

Weitzel K, Wickman J, Augustin S, Strom J. Zaleplon: A pyrazolopyrimidine sedative-hypnotic agent for the treatment of insomnia. *Clin therapeutics.* 2000;22:1254–1265.

Zolpidem

Allain H, Le Coz F, Borderies P, et al. Use of zolpidem 10 mg as a benzodiazepine substitute in 84 patients with insomnia. *Hum Psychopharmacol Clin Exp.* 1998;13:551–559.

Ancoli-Israel S, Walsh J, Mangano R, et al. Zaleplon, a novel nonbenzodiazepine hypnotic, effectively treats insomnia in elderly patients without causing rebound effects. *Primary Care Companion, J Clin Psychiatry.* 1999;1:114–120.

Aragona M. Abuse, dependence, and epileptic seizures after zolpidem withdrawal: Review and case report. *Clin Neuropharmacol.* 2000;23:281–283.

Asnis G, Chakraburtty A, DuBoff E, et al. Zolpidem for persistent insomnia in SSRI-treated depressed patients. *J Clin Psychiatry.* 1999;60:668–676.

Berlin, I, Warot D, Hergueta T, Molinier P, Bagot C, Puech A. Comparison of the effects of zolpidem and triazolam on memory functions, psychomotor performances, and postural sway in healthy subjects. *J Clin Psychopharmacol.* 1992;13:100–106.

Declerck A, Smits M. Zolpidem: A valuable alternative to benzodiazepine hypnotics for chronic insomnia? *J International Med Res.* 1999;27:253–263.

Fairweather D, Kerr J, Hindmarch I. The effect of acute and repeated doses of zolpidem on subjective sleep, psychomotor performance, and cognitive function in elderly volunteers. *Eur J Clin Pharmacol.* 1992;43:597–601.

Garnier R, Guerault E, Muzard D, Azoyan P, Chaumet-Riffaud A, Efthymiou M. Acute zolpidem poisoning-analysis of 344 cases. *Clin Toxicology.* 1994;32: 391–404.

Girault C, Muir F, Mihaltan F, et al. Effects of repeated administration of zolpidem on sleep, diurnal and nocturnal respiratory function, vigilance, and physical performance in patients with COPD. *Chest.* 1993;110:1203–1211.

Herrmann W, Kubicki S, Boden S, Eich F, Attali P, Coquelin J. Pilot-controlled double-blind study of the hypnotic effects of zolpidem in patients with chronic "learned" insomnia: Psychometric and polysomnographic evaluation. *J Internat Med Res.* 1993;21:306–322.

Holm K, Goa K. Zolpidem: An update of its pharmacology, therapeutic efficacy, and tolerability in the treatment of insomnia. *Drugs.* 2000;59:865–889.

Jackson C, PitneerJ, Mintzer J. Zolpidem for the treatment of agitation in elderly demented patients [letter]. *J Clin Psychiatry.* 1996;57:372–373.

Kummer J, Guendel L, Linden J, et al. Lang-term polysomnographic study of the efficacy and safety of zolpidem in elderly psychiatric in-patients with insomnia. *J Int Med Res.* 1993;21:171–184.

Lewohl J, Crane D, Dodd P. Zolpidem binding sites on the $GABA_A$ receptor in brain from human cirrhotic and non-cirrhotic alcoholics. *Eur J Pharmacol.* 1997;326:265–272.

Liappas IA, Malitas PN, Dimopoulos NP, Gitsa OE, Liappas AI, Nikolaou ChK, Christodoulou GN. Zolpidem dependence case series: possible neurobiological mechanisms and clinical management. *J Psychopharmacol.* 2003; 19 (1):131–5.

Lichtenwalner M, Tully R. A fatality involving zolpidem. *J Analytical Toxicol.* 1997;21:567–569.

Madrak L, Rosenberg M. Zolpidem abuse [letter]. *Am J Psychiatry.* 2001;158: 1330–1331.

Mattila M, Vanakoski J, Kalska H, Seppala T. Effects of alcohol, zolpidem, and some other sedatives and hypnotics on human performance and memory. *Pharmacol Biochem Behav.* 1998;59:917–923.

Rhodes S, Parry P, Hanning C. A comparison of the effects of zolpidem and placebo on respiration and oxygen saturation during sleep in the healthy elderly. *Br J Clin Pharmacol.* 1990;30:817–824.

Roger M, Attali P, Coquelin J. Multi-center, double-blind controlled comparison of zolpidem and triazolam in elderly patients with insomnia. *Clin Therapeutics.* 1993;15:127–136.

Rush C, Baker R, Wright K. Acute behavioral effects and abuse potential of trazadone, zolpidem, and triazolam in humans. *Psychopharmacol.* 1999; 144:220–233.

Rush C, Griffiths R. Zolpidem, triazolam, and temazepam: Behavioral and subject-rated effects in normal volunteers. *J Clin Psychopharmacol.* 1996;16:146–157.

Salva P, Costa J. Clinical pharmacokinetics and pharmacodynamics of zolpidem. *Clin Pharmacokinet.* 1995;29:142–153.

Sanger D, Perrault G, Joly D, Zivkovic B. The behavioral profile of zolpidem, a novel hypnotic drug of imidazopyridine structure. *Physiology Behav.* 1987;41:235–240.

Scharf M, Mayleben D, Kaffeman M, Kralliu R, Ochs R. Dose response effects of zolpidem in normal geriatric subjects. *J Clin Psychiatry.* 1991;52: 77–83.

Scharf M, Roth T, Vogel G, Walsh J. A multi-center, placebo-controlled study evaluating zolpidem in the treatment of chronic insomnia. *J Clin Psychiatry.* 1994;55:192–199.

Schlich D, Heritier C, Coquelin J, Attali P. Long-term treatment of insomnia with zolpidem: A multi-center general practitioner study of 107 patients. *J Internat Med Res.* 1991;19:271–279.

Shaw S, Curson H, Coquelin J. A double-blind, comparative study of zolpidem and placebo in the treatment of insomnia in elderly psychiatric in-patients. *Internat Med Res.* 1992;20:150–161.

Soyka M, Bottlender R, Moller H. Epidemiological evidence for a low abuse potential of zolpidem. *Pharmacopsychiatry.* 2000;33:138–141.

Tsutsui S, Zolpidem Study Group. A double-blind comparative study of zolpidem versus zopiclone in the treatment of chronic primary insomnia. *J Int Med Res.* 2001;29:163–177.

Voderholzer U, Reimann D, Hornyak M, et al. A double-blind, randomized and placebo-controlled study on the polysomnographic withdrawal effects of zopiclone, zolpidem, and triazolam in healthy subjects. *Eur Arch Psychiatry Neurosci.* 2001;251:117–123.

Ware J, Walsh J, Scharf M, Roehrs T, Roth T, Vogel G. Minimal rebound insomnia after treatment with 10-mg zolpidem. *Clin Neuropharmacol.* 1997;20:116–125.

Zopiclone

Alderman C, Gebauer M, Gilbert A, Condon J. Possible interaction of zopiclone and nefazodone. *Ann Pharmacother.* 2001;35:1378–1380.

Becquemont L, Mouajjah S, Escaffre O, Beaune P, Funck-Bretano C, Jaillon P. Cytochrome P_450 3A4 and 2C8 are involved in zopiclone metabolism. *Drug Metab Disposition.* 1999;27:1068–1073.

Begg E, Robson R, Frampton C, Campbell J. A comparison of efficacy and tolerance of the short acting sedatives midazolam and zopiclone. *NZ Med J.* 1992;28:428–429.

Boniface P, Russell S. Two cases of fatal zopiclone overdose. *J Analytical Toxicol.* 1996;20:131–133.

Bramness J, Arnestad M, Karinen R, Hilberg T. Fatal overdose of zopiclone in an elderly woman with bronchogenic carcinoma. *J Forensic Sci.* 2001;46:1247–1249.

Dehlin O, Rubin B, Rundgren A. Double-blind comparison of zopiclone and flunitrazepam in elderly insomniacs with special focus on residual effects. *Curr Med Res Opinion.* 1995;13:317–324.

Elie R, Frenay M, Le Morvan P, et al. Efficacy and safety of zopiclone and triazolam in the treatment of geriatric insomniacs, 1990. *Int Clin Psychopharacol.* 1990; 5(suppl 2):39–46.

Fava G. Amnestic syndrome induced by zopiclone [letter]. *Eur J Clin Pharmacol.* 1966;50:509.

Hajak G, Clarenbach P, Fischer W, Haase W, Ruther E. Zopiclone improves sleep quality and daytime well-being in insomniac patients: Comparison with triazolam, flunitrazepam, and placebo. *Int Clin Psychopharmacol.* 1994;9:251–261.

Hemmeter U, Muller M, Bischof R, Annen B, Holsboer-Trachsler E. Effect of zopiclone and temazepam on sleep EEG parameters, psychomotor, and memory functions in healthy elderly volunteers. *Psychopharmacol.* 2000;147:384–396.

Jones I, Sullivan G. Physical dependence on zopiclone: Case reports. *BMJ* 1998;316:117.

Kliejn B. Effects of zopiclone and temazepam on sleep, behaviour, and mood during the day. *Eur J Clin Pharmacol.* 1989;36:247–251.

Klimm H, Dreyfus J, Delmonte M. Zopiclone versus nitrazepam: A double-blind comparative study of efficacy and tolerance in elderly patients with chronic insomnia. *Sleep.* 1987;10 (Suppl 1):73–78.

Lemoine P, Ohayon M. Is hypnotic withdrawal facilitated by the transitory use of a substitute drug. *Prog Neuropsychopharmacol & Biol Psychiat.* 1997;21:111–121.

Noble S, Langtry H, Lamb H. Zopiclone: An update of its pharmacology, clinical efficacy, and tolerability in the treatment of insomnia. *Drugs.* 1998;55:277–302.

Pat-Horenczyk R, Hacohen D, Herer P, Lavie P. The effects of substituting zopiclone in withdrawal from chronic use of benzodiazepine hypnotics. *Psychopharmacol.* 1998;140:450–457.

Shapiro C, MacFarlane J, MacLean A. Alleviating sleep-related discontinuance symptoms associated with benzodiazepine withdrawal: A new approach. *J Psychosom Res.* 1993;37:55–57.

Singh A, Bourgouin J. Comparison of zopiclone and flurazepam treatments in insomnia. *Hum Psychopharmacol.* 1990;5:217–221.

Stip E, Furlan M, Lussier I, Bourgouin P, Elie R. Double-blind, placebo-controlled study comparing effects of zopiclone and temazepam on cognitive functioning of insomniacs. *Hum Psychopharmacol Clin Exp.* 1999;14:253–261.

Tada K, Sato Y, Sakai T, Ueda N, Kasamo K, Kojima T. Effects of zopiclone, triazolam, and nitrazepam on standing steadiness. *Neuropsychobiol.* 1994;29:17–22.

Villikka K, Kivisto K, Lamberg T, Kantola T, Neuvonen P. Concentrations and effects of zopiclone are greatly reduced by rifampicin. *Br J Clin Pharmacol.* 1997;43:471–474.

MOOD STABILIZERS

Abou-Saleh M, Coppen A. Prognosis of depression in old age: The case for lithium therapy. *Br J Psychiatry.* 1983;143:527–528.

Bauer M, Whybrow P, Winokur A. Rapid cycling bipolar affective disorder. *Arch Gen Psychiatry.* 1990;47:427–492.

Berk M, Segal J, Janet L, Vorster M. Emerging options in the treatment of bipolar disorders. *Drugs.* 2001;61:1407–1414.

Bottlender R, Rudolf D, Straub A, Moller H. Mood-stabilizers reduce the risk of developing antidepressant-induced maniform states in acute treatment of bipolar I depressed patients. *J Affective Disord.* 2001;63:79–83.

Bradwejn J, Shriqui C, Koszycki D, Meterissian G. Double-blind comparison of the effects of clonazepam and lorazepam in acute mania. *J Clin Psychopharmacol.* 1990;10:403–408.

Casey D. Mania and Pseudodementia. *J Clin Psychiatry.* 1988;49:73–74.

Charron M, Fortin L, Paquette I. De Novo mania among elderly people. *Acta Psychiatr Scand.* 1991;84:503–507.

Chen S, Altshuler L, Melnyk K, Erhart S, Miller E, Mintz J. Efficacy of lithium versus valproate in the treatment of mania in the elderly: A retrospective study. *J Clin Psychiatry.* 1999;60:181–186.

Colenda C. Mania in late life: the challenges of treating older adults. *Geriatrics.* 2002;57:50–54.

Cowdry R, Goodwin F. Dementia of bipolar illness: Diagnosis and response to lithium. *Am J Psychiatry.* 1981;138:1118–1119.

Evans D. Bipolar disorder: diagnostic challenges and treatment considerations. *J Clin Psychiatry.* 2000;61 (Suppl 13):26–31.

Evans D, Byerly M, Greer R. Secondary mania: Diagnosis and treatment. *J Clin Psychiatry.* 1995;56 (Suppl 3):S31–S37.

Gnam W, Flint A. New onset rapid cycling bipolar disorder in an 87-year-old woman. *Can J Psychiatry.* 1993;38:324–326.

Hardy B, Shulman K, Mackenzie S, Kutcher S, Silverberg J. Pharmacokinetics of lithium in the elderly. *J Clin Psychopharmacol.* 1987;7:153–158.

Hussein Z, Posner J. Population pharmacokinetics of lamotrigine monotherapy in patients with epilepsy: Retrospective analysis of routine monitoring data. *Br J Clin Pharmacol.* 1997;43:457–465.

Joyce E, Levy R. Treatment of mood disorder associated with Binswanger's disease [letter]. *Br J Psychiatry.* 1989;154:261.

Keck P, Nelson E, McElroy S. Update on bipolar disorder: How to better predict response to maintenance treatment. *Curr Psychiatry.* 2002;1:40–47.

Leppik I. Metabolism of antiepileptic medication: Newborn to elderly. *Epilepsia.* 1992;33 (Suppl 4):S32–S40.

Loranger A, Levine P. Age at onset of bipolar affective illness. *Arch Gen Psychiatry.* 1978;35:1345–1348.

McDonald W, Nemeroff C. The diagnosis and treatment of mania in the elderly. *Bull Menninger Clin.* 1996;60:174–196.

Meyers B, Young R. Psychopharmacology. In J Sadavoy, L Jarvik, G Grossberg, B Meyers (eds). *Comprehensive Textbook of Geriatric Psychiatry.* New York: Norton, in press.

Mirchandani I, Young R. Management of mania in the elderly: An update. *Ann Clin Psychiatry.* 1993;5:67–77.

Nath J, Sagar N. Late-onset bipolar disorder due to hyperthyroidism. *Acta Psychiatrica Scand.* 2001;104:72–75.

Okuma T. Effects of carbamazepine and lithium on affective disorders. *Neuropsychobiol.* 1993;27:138–145.

Roose S, Bone S, Haidorfer C. Lithium treatment in older patients. *Am J Psychiatry.* 1979;136:843–844.

Sajatovic M, Brescan D, Perez D, et al. Quetiapine alone and added to a mood stabilizer for serious mood disorders. *J Clin Psychiatry.* 2001;62:728–732.

Sajatovic M. Treatment of bipolar disorder in older adults. *Int J Geriatr Psychiatry.* 2002;17:865–873.

Schaffer C, Garvey M. Use of lithium in acutely manic elderly patients. *Clin Gerontol.* 1984;3:58–60.

Shulman K, Herrmann N. Bipolar disorder in old age. *Can Fam Physician.* 1999;45:1229–1237.

Shulman K, Post F. Bipolar affective disorder in old age. *Br J Psychiatry.* 1980;136:26–32.

Smith R Helms P. Adverse effects of lithium therapy in the acutely ill elderly patient. *J Clin Psychiatry.* 1982;43:94–99.

Snowdon J. The relevance of guidelines for treatment of mania in old age. *Int J Geriatr Psychiatry.* 2000;15:779–783.

Solomon D, Ryan C. Keitner G, et al. A pilot study of lithium carbonate plus divalproex sodium for the continuation and maintenance treatment of patients with bipolar I disorder. *J Clin Psychiatry.* 1997;58:95–99.

Stone K. Mania in the elderly. *Br J Psychiatry.* 1989;155:220–224.

Taylor M, Abrams R. Manic states: A genetic study of early and late onset affective disorders. *Arch Gen Psychiatry.* 1973;28:656–658.

Wylie M, Mulsant B, Pollock B, et al. Age at onset in geriatric bipolar disorder. *Am J Geriatric Psychiatry.* 1999;7:77–83.

Yassa R, Nair V, Nastase C, et al. Prevalence of bipolar disorder in a psychogeriatric population. *J Affect Disord.* 1988;14:197–201.

Young R, Falk J. Age, manic pathology, and treatment response. *Int J Geriatr Psychiatry.* 1989;4:73–78.

Young R. Geriatric mania. *Clin Ger Med.* 1992;8:387–399.

Young R, Klerman G. Mania in late life: Focus on age at onset. *Am J Psychiatry.* 1992;149:867–876.

Carbamazepine

De Vriese A, Philippe J, Renterghem D, et al. Carbamazepine hypersensitivity syndrome: Report of 4 cases and review of the literature. *Medicine.* 1995;74:144–151.

Grossman F. A review of anticonvulsants in treating agitated demented elderly patients. *Pharmacother.* 1998;18:600–606.

Iwahashi K. Significantly higher plasma haloperidol level during cotreatment with carbamazepine may herald cardiac change. *Clin Neuropharmacol.* 1996;19:267–270.

Lemke M. Effect of carbamazepine on agitation in Alzheimer's inpatients refractory to neuroleptics. *J Clin Psychiatry.* 1995;354–357.

Rittmannsberger H. Asterixis induced by psychotropic drug treatment. *Clin Neuropharmacol.* 1996;19:349–355.

Steckler T. Lithium- and carbamazepine-associated sinus node dysfunction: Nine-year experience in a psychiatric hospital. *J Clin Psychopharmcol.* 1994;14:336–339.

Takayanagi K, Watanabe J, Fujito T, et al. Carbamazepine-induced sinus node dysfunction and atrioventricular block in elderly women. *Jpn Heart J.* 1998;39:469–479.

Tariot P, Erb R, Podgorski C, et al. Efficacy and tolerability of carbamazepine for agitation and aggression in dementia. *Am J Psychiatry.* 1998;155: 54–61.

Gabapentin

Boyd R, Turck D, Abel R, Sedman A, Bockbrader H. Effects of age and gender on single-dose pharmacokinetics of gabapentin. *Epilepsia.* 1999;40:474–479.

Evidente V, Adler C, Caviness J, Gwinn K. Effective treatment of orthostatic tremor with gabapentin. *Movement disorders.* 1998;13:829–831.

Ghaemi S, Katzow J, Desai S, Goodwin F. Gabapentin treatment of mood disorders: A preliminary study. *J Clin Psychiatry.* 1998;59:426–429.

Herrmann N, Lanctot K, Myszak M. Effectiveness of gabapentin for the treatment of behavioral disorders in dementia. *J Clin Psychopharmacol.* 2000;20:90–93.

Martin R, Meador K, Turrentine L, et al. Comparative cognitive effects of carbamazepine and gabapentin in healthy senior adults. *Epilepsia.* 2001;42:764–771.

Olson W, Gruenthal M, Mueller M, Olson W. Gabapentin for parkinsonism: A double-blind, placebo-controlled, crossover trial. *Am J Med.* 1997;102:60–66.

Sethi M, Mehta R, Devanand D. Gabapentin in geriatric mania. *J. Geriatr Psychiatry Neurol.* 2003;16 (2):117–20.

Lamotrigine

Barbosa L, Berk M, Vorster M. A double-blind, randomized, placebo-controlled trial of augmentation with lamotrigine or placebo in patients concomitantly treated with fluoxetine for resistant major depressive episodes. *J Clin Psychiatry.* 2003;64 (4):403–7.

Bowden C, Calabrese J, Sachs G, et al. A randomized placebo-controlled 18-month trial of lamotrigine and lithium maintenance treatment in recently manic or hypomanic patients with bipolar I disorder [abstract]. *Arch Gen Psychiatry.* 2003;60:392–400.

Calabrese J, Bowden C, McElroy S, et al. Spectrum of activity of lamotrigine in treatment-refractory bipolar disorder. *Am J Psychiatry.* 1999;156:1019–1023.

Calabrese J, Bowden C, Sachs G, Ascher J, Monaghan E, Rudd G. A double-blind placebo-controlled study of lamotrigine monotherapy in outpatients with bipolar I depression. *J Clin Psychiatry.* 1999;60:79–88.

Calabrese J, Suppes T, Bowden C, et al. A double-blind, placebo-controlled, prophylaxis study of lamotrigine in rapid-cycling bipolar disorder. *J Clin Psychiatry.* 2000;61:841–850.

Chaffin J, Davis S. Suspected lamotrigine-induced toxic epidermal necrolysis. *Ann Pharmacother.* 1997;31:720–723.

Chan V, Morris R, Ilett K, Tett S. Population pharmacokinetics of lamotrigine. *Therap Drug Monit.* 2001;23:630–635.

Kotler M, Matar M. Lamotrigine in the treatment of resistant bipolar disorder. *Clin Neuropharmacol.* 1998;21:65–67.

Tekin S, Aykut-Bingol C, Tanridag T, Aktan S. Antiglutamatergic therapy in Alzheimer's disease: Effects of lamotrigine. *J Neural Transm.* 1998;105:295–303.

Lithium

Amdisen A, Andersen C. Lithium treatment and thyroid function: A survey of 237 patients in long-term lithium treatment. *Pharmacopsychiatr.* 1982;15:149–155.

Austin L, Arana G, Melvin J. Toxicity resulting from lithium augmentation of antidepressant treatment in elderly patients. *J Clin Psychiatry.* 1990;51:344–345.

Bell A, Cole A, Eccleston D, et al. Lithium neurotoxicity at normal therapeutic levels. *Br J Psychiatry.* 1993;162:689–692.

Bendz H, Aurell M, Balldin J, Mathe A, Sjodin L. Kidney damage in long-term lithium patients: A cross-sectional study of patients with 15 years or more on lithium. *Nephrol Dial Transplant.* 1994;9:1250–1254.

Bendz H, Sjodin L, Aurell M. Renal function on and off lithium in patients treated with lithium for 15 years or more. A controlled, prospective lithium-withdrawal study. *Nephrol Dial Transplant.* 1996;11:457–460.

Burgess S, Geddes J, Hawton K, Townsend E, Jamison K, Goodwin G. Lithium for maintenance of mood disorders. *Cochrane Database of Systematic Reviews.* 1, 2002; 1.

Cervantes P, Ghadirian A, Vida S. Vitamin B12 and folate levels and lithium administration in patients with affective disorders. *Biol Psychiatry.* 1999;45:214–221.

Chen S, Altshuler L, Melnyk, initial et al. Efficacy of lithium versus valproate in the treatment of mania in the elderly. *J Clin Psychiatry.* 1999;60:181–185.

Coppen A, Abou-Saleh M. Lithium therapy: From clinical trials to practical management. *Acta Psychiatr Scand.* 1988;78:754–762.

De Angelis L. Lithium treatment and the geriatric population. *J Clin Pharmacol Therapeutic Toxicol.* 1990;28:194–198.

De Maio D, Laviani M. Lithium-TCA–induced malignant syndrome. *Prog Neuro Psychopharmacol.* 1991;15:427–431.

Deodhar S, Singh B, Pathak C, Sharan P, Kulhara P. Thyroid functions in lithium treated psychiatric patients. *Biol Trace Element Res.* 1999;67:151–163.

El-Mallakh R, Kantesaria A, Chaikovsky L. Lithium toxicity presenting as mania. *Drug Intell Clin Pharm.* 1987;21:979–981.

Fein S, Paz V, Rao N, LaGrassa J. The combination of lithium carbonate and an MAOI in refractory depressions. *Am J Psychiatry.* 1988;145:249–250.

Ghadirian A, Annable L, Belanger. Lithium, benzodiazepines, and sexual function in bipolar patients. *Am J Psychiatry.* 1992;149:801–805.

Ghadirian A, Annable L, Belanger M, Chouinard G. A cross-sectional study of parkinsonism and tardive dyskinesia in lithium-treated affective-disordered patients. *J Clin Psychiatry.* 1996;57:22–28.

Head L, Dening T. Lithium in the over 65: Who is taking it and who is monitoring it? A survey of older adults on lithium in the Cambridge mental health services catchment area. *Int J Geriatric Psychiatry.* 1998;13:164–171.

Hetmar O, Brun C, Clemmensen L, Ladefoged J, Larsen S, Rafaelsen O. Lithium: Long-term effects on the kidney—II. Structural changes. *J Psychiatr Res.* 1987;21:279–288.

Himmelhoch J, Neil J, May S, et al. Age, dementia dyskinesias, and lithium response. *Am J Psychiatry.* 1980;137:941–945.

Hoencamp E, Haffmans J, Dijken W, Huijbrechts I. Lithium augmentation of venlafaxine: An open-label trial. *J Clin Psychopharmacol.* 2000;20:538–543.

Jainer AK, Soni N, Onalaja D. Re: Prophylactic therapy with lithium in elderly patients with Unipolar Major Depression. *Int J Geriatr Psychiatry.* 2003; 19 (4):353–354; (author reply 354).

Johnson G, Hunt G, Lewis J, St. George B. Pharmacokinetics of standard (Lithicarb) and sustained-release (Priadel) lithium carbonate preparations in patients. *Austr N Z J Psychiatry.* 1982;16:64–68.

Jorkasky D, Amsterdam J, Oler J, et al. Lithium-induced renal disease: A prospective study. *Clin Nephrology.* 1988;30:293–302.

Kelwala S, Pomara N, Stanley M, Sitaram N, Gershon S. Lithium-induced accentuation of extrapyramidal symptoms in individuals with Alzheimer's disease. *J Clin Psychiatry.* 1984;45:342–344.

Kores B, Lader M. Irreversible lithium neurotoxicity: An overview. *Clin Neuropharmacol.* 1997;20:283–299.

Kushnir S. Lithium-antidepressant combinations in the treatment of depressed, physically ill geriatric patients. *Am J Psychiatry.* 1986;143:378–379.

Lehmann K, Ritz E. Angiotensin-converting enzyme inhibitors may cause renal dysfunction inpatients on long-term lithium treatment. *Am J Kidney Disorder.* 196;25:82–87.

Miller F, Menninger J, Whitcup S. Lithium-neuroleptic neurotoxicity in the elderly bipolar patient. *J Clin Psychopharmacol.* 1986;6:176–178.

Mukhopadhyay D, Gokulkrishnan L, Mohanaruban K. Lithium-induced nephrogenic diabetes insipidus in older people. *Age Ageing.* 2001;30:347–350.

Murray N, Hopwood S, Balfour D, Ogston S, Hewick D. The influence of age on lithium efficacy and side-effects in out-patients. *Psychological Med.* 1983;13:53–60.

Nambudrini D, Meyers B, Young R. Delayed recovery from lithium neurotoxicity. *J Geriatr Psychiatry Neurol.* 1991;4:40–43.

Ong A, Handler C. Sinus arrest and asystole due to severe lithium intoxication. *Int J Cardiol.* 1991;30:364–366.

Plenge P, Mellerup E, Bolwig T, et al. Lithium treatment: Does the kidney prefer one daily dose instead of two? *Acta Psychiatr Scand.* 1982;66:121–128.

Pomara N, Banay-Schwartz M, Block R, Stanley M, Gershon S. Elevation of RBC glycine and choline levels in geriatric patients treated with lithium. *Am J Psychiatry.* 1983; 40 (7):911–918.

Price L, Charney D, Heninger G. Variability of response to lithium augmentation in refractory depression. *Am J Psychiatry.* 1986;143:1387–1392.

Ramchandani D, Schindler B. The lithium toxic patient in the general hospital: Diagnostic and management dilemmas. *Int J Psychiatry Med.* 1993;23:55–62.

Rendell JM, Geddes JR, Ostacher MJ. Older patients are eligible for trial of lithium and valproate. *BMJ.* 2003;327 (7411):395-6.

Roose S, Bone S, Haidorfer C, et al. Lithium treatment in older patients. *Am J Psychiatry.* 136:843–844.

Rosenqvist M, Bergfeldt L, Aili H, Mathe A. Sinus node dysfunction during long-term lithium treatment. *Br Heart J.* 1993;70:371–375.

Rouillon F, Gorwood P. The use of lithium to augment antidepressant medication. *J Clin Psychiatry.* 1998;59 (Suppl 5):32–39.

Santiago R, Rashkin M. Lithium toxicity and myxedema coma in an elderly woman. *J Emerg Med.* 1990;8:63–66.

Sashidharan S, McGuire R. Recurrence of affective illness after withdrawal of long-term lithium treatment. *Acta Psychiatr Scand.* 1983;68:126–133.

Shulman K, Mackenzie S, Hardy B. The clinical use of lithium carbonate in old age: A review. *Prog Neuro-Psychopharmacol Biol Psychiatr.* 1987;11:159–164.

Smith R, Helms P. Adverse effects of lithium therapy in the acutely ill elderly patient. *J Clin Psychiatry.* 1982;43:94–99.

Stancer H, Forbath N. Hyperparathyroidism, hypothyroidism, and impaired renal function after 10–20 years of lithium treatment. *Arch Intern Med.* 1989; 149:1042–1045.

Stolzenburg W, Mairhofer M, Haag M. Lithium dosage in the elderly. *J Affect Dis.* 1985;9:1–4.

Stoudemire A, Hill C, Lewison B, Marquardt M, Dalton S. Lithium intolerance in a medical-psychiatric population. *Gen Hosp Psychiatry.* 1998;20:85–90.

Tueth M, Murphy T, Evans D. Special considerations: Use of lithium in children, adolescents, and elderly populations. *J Clin Psychiatry.* 1998;59 (Suppl 6): 66–73.

Van Marwijk H, Bekker F, Nolen W, Jansen P, Nieuwkerk J, Hop W. Lithium augmentation in geriatric depression. *J Affect Dis.* 1990;20:217–223.

Vestergaard P, Schou M. The effect of age on lithium dosage requirements. *Pharmacopsychiatr.* 1984;17:199–201.

Wilson K, Scott M, Abou-Saleh M, Burns R, Copeland J. Long-term effects of cognitive-behavioural therapy and lithium therapy on depression in the elderly. *Br J Psychiatry.* 1995;167:653–658.

Yassa R, Saunders A, Nastase C, Camille Y. Lithium-induced thyroid disorder: A prevalence study. *J Clin Psychiatry.* 1988;49:14–16.

Young R, Kalayam B, Tsuboyama G, et al. Mania: Response to lithium across the age spectrum. *Soc Neurosci.* 1992;18:669.

Topiramate

Marcotte D. Use of topiramate, a new anti-epileptic as a mood stabilizer. *J Affect Disord.* 1998;50:245–251.

Valproic Acid, Valproate, Divalproex

Armon C, Shin C, Miller P, et al. Reversible parkinsonism and cognitive impairment with chronic valproate use. *Neurol.* 1996;47:626–635.

Buchalter E, Lantz M. Treatment of impulsivity and aggression in a patient with vascular dementia. *Geriatrics.* 2001;56:53–54.

Connacher A, Borsey D, Browning M, Davidson D, Jung R. The effective evaluation of thyroid status in patients on phenytoin, carbamazepine, or sodium valproate attending an epilepsy clinic. *Postgrad Med J.* 1987;63:841–845.

Craig I, Tallis R. Impact of valproate and phenytoin on cognitive function in elderly patients: Results of a single-blind randomized comparative study. *Epilepsia.* 1994;35:381–390.

Gyulai L, Bowden CL, McElroy SL, Calabrese JR, Petty F, Swann AC, Chou JC, Wassef A, Risch CS, Hirschhfeld RM, Nemeroff CB, Keck PE Jr, Evans DL, Wozniak PJ. Maintenance efficacy of divalproex in the prevention of bipolar depression. *Neuropsychopharmacology.* 2003;28 (7):1374–82.

Haas S, Vincent K, Holt J, Lippman S. Divalproex: A possible treatment alternative for demented, elderly aggressive patients. *Ann Clin Psychiatry.* 1997;9: 145–147.

Herrmann N. Valproate treatment of agitation in dementia. *Can J Psychiatry.* 1988;43:69–72.

Hori H, Terao T, Shiraishi Y, Nakamura J. Treatment of Charles Bonnet syndrome with valproate. *Int J Psychopharmacol.* 2000;15:117–119.

Kando J, Tohen M, Castillo J, Zarate C. The use of valproate in an elderly population with affective symptoms. *J Clin Psychiatry.* 1996;57:238–240.

Lott A, McElroy S, Keys M. Valproate in the treatment of behavioral agitation in elderly patients with dementia. *J Neuropsychiatry Clin Neurosci.* 1995; 7:314–319.

McFarland B, Miller M, Straumfjord A. Valproate use in the older manic patient. *J Clin Psychiatry.* 1990;51:479–481.

Mellow A, Solano-Lopez C, Davis S. Sodium valproate in the treatment of behavioral disturbance in dementia. *J Geriatr Psychiatry Neurol.* 1993;6:205–209.

Norton J, Quarles E. Intravenous valproate in neuropsychiatry. *Pharmacother.* 2000;20:88–92.

Perucca E, Grimaldi R, Gatti G, Pirrachio S, Crema F, Frigo G. Pharmacokinetics of valproate in the elderly. *Br J Clin Pharmacol.* 1984;17:665–669.

Peryear L, Kunik M, Workman R. Tolerability of divalproex sodium in elderly psychiatric patients with mixed diagnoses. *J Geriatr Psychiatry.* 1995;8: 234–237.

Risinger R, Risby E, Risch S. Safety and efficacy of divalproex sodium in elderly bipolar patients. *J Clin Psychiatry.* 1994;55:215.

Schaff M, Fawcett J, Zajecka J. Divalproex sodium in the treatment of refractory affective disorders. *J Clin Psychiatry.* 1993;54:380–384.

Schneider A, Wilcox C. Divalproate augmentation in lithium-resistant rapid cycling mania in four geriatric patients. *J Affect Disorder.* 1998;47:201–205.

Shulman KI, Rochon P, Sykora K, Anderson G, Mamdani M, Bronskill S, Tran CT. Changing prescription patterns for lithium and valproic acid in old age: shifting practice without evidence. *BMJ*. 2003;326 (7396):960–1.

Spiller H, Krenzelok E, Klein-Schwartz W, et al. Multi-center case series of valproic acid ingestion: Serum concentrations and toxicity. *Clin Toxicol*. 2000; 38:755–760.

Stephen LJ. Drug treatment of epilepsy in elderly people: focus on valproic Acid. *Drugs Aging*. 2003;20 (2):141–52.

Trannel T, Ahmed I, Goebert D. Occurrence of thrombocytopenia in psychiatric patients taking valproate. *Am J Psychiatry*. 2001;158:128–130.

Zaccara G, Messori A, Moroni F. Clinical pharmacokinetics of valproic acid, 1988. *Clin pharmacokinetics*. 1988;15:367–389.

COGNITIVE ENHANCERS

American Psychiatric Association. Practice guidelines for the treatment of patients with Alzheimer's disease and other dementias of late life. *Am J Psychiatry*. 1997;154 (5, Suppl):1–38.

Auriacombe S, Pere J, et al. Efficacy and safety of rivastigmine in patients with Alzheimers disease who failed to benefit from treatment with donepezil. *Curr Med Res Opinion*. 2002;18:129–138.

Borroni B, Colciaghi F, et al. Amyloid precursor protein in platelets of patients with Alzheimer disease: Effect of acetylcholin esterase inhibitors treatment. *Arch Neurology*. 2001;58:442–446.

Bullock R, Connolly C. Switching cholinesterase inhibitor therapy in Alzheirmer's disease-Donepezil to rivastigmine: Is it worth it? *Int J Geriatr Psychiatry*. 2002;17:288–289.

Coelho, Filho C, Birks J. Physostigmine for Alzheimer's disease. *Cochrane Database of Systematic Reviews*. 2002; 1.

De Deyn P, Jeste D, Goyvaerts H, Breder C, Schneider L, Mintzer J. Aripiprazole for psychosis of Alzheimer's disease [abstract]. *Int Psychogeriatrics*. 2003; 15 (suppl 2): 227.

Erkinjuntti T, et al. Efficacy of galantamine in probable vascular dementia and Alzheimer's disease combined with cerebrovascular disease: a randomised trial. *Lancet*. 2002;359.

Feldman Y, et al. A 24-week randomised, double-blind study of donepezil in moderate to severe Alzheimer's disease. *Neurology*. 2001;57:613–620.

Giacobini E. Cholinesterase inhibitors stabilize Alzheimer disease. *Neurochem Res*. 2000;25:1185–1190.

Hanyu H, Tanaka Y, Sakurai H, et al. Atrophy of the substantia innominata on magnetic resonance imaging and response to donepezil treatment in Alzheimer's disease. *Neuroscience letters*. 2002;319:33–36.

Hauber A, Gnanasakthy A, Snyder E, Bala M, Richter A, Mauskopf A. Potential savings in the cost of caring for Alzheimer's disease. *Pharmacoeconomics*. 2000;17:351–360.

Hill J, Futterman R, Mastey V, et al. The effect of donepezil therapy on health costs in a Medicare managed care plan. *Managed Care Interface*. 2002;15:63–70.

Hopper P, Trotter C. Assessing the efficacy of cholinesterase inhibitor drugs. *Int J Periatr Psychiatry.* 2003;18 (1):86–7.

Kim JM, Lyons D, Shin IS, Yoon JS. Differences in the behavioral and psychological symptoms between Alzheimer's disease and vascular dementia: are the different pharmacologic treatment strategies justifiable? *Hum Psychopharmacol.* 2003;19 (3):215–20.

Krall W, Sramek J, Cutler N. Cholinesterase inhibitors: A therapeutic strategy for Alzheimer disease. *Ann Pharmacother.* 1999;33:441–450.

Mayeux R, Sano M. Treatment of Alzheimer's disease. *NEJM* 1999;341:1670–1679.

McGavin J, Goa K. Aripiprazole. *CNS Drugs.* 2002;16:779–786.

McKeith I, et al. Efficacy of rivastigmine in dementia with Lewy bodies: A randomised, double-blind, placebo controlled international study. *Lancet.* 2000;356:203–2036.

Taylor A, Hoehns J, Anderson D, Tobert D. Fatal aspiration pneumonia during transition from donepezil to rivastigmine. *Annals Pharmacotherapy.* 2002;36:1550–1553.

Winblad B, Wimo A. Assessing the societal impact of acetylcholinesterase inhibitor therapies. *Alz Dis Associated Disord.* 1999;13 (Suppl 2):S9–S19.

Donepezil

Babic T, Zurak N. Convulsions induced by donepezil [letter]. *J Neurol Neurosurg Psychiatry.* 1999;66:410.

Ballard C, Neill D, O'Brien J, McKeith I, Ince P, Perry R. Anxiety, depression, and psychosis in vascular dementia: Prevalence and associations. *J Affective Disorders.* 2000;59:97–106.

Barner EJ, Gray SL. Donepezil use in Alzheimer's disease. *Ann. Pharmacotherapy.* 1998;32:70–77.

Benazzi F. Mania associated with donepezil. *Int J Geriatr Psychiatry.* 1998;13:814–15.

Bergman J, Brettholz I, Shneidman M, Lerner V. Donepezil as add-on treatment of psychotic symptoms in patients with dementia of Alzheimer's type. *Clin Neuropharmacol.* 2003:26:88–92.

Bergman J, Brettholz I, Shneidman M, Lerner V. Donepezil as add-on treatment of psychotic symptoms in patients with dementia of the Alzheimer's type. *Clin Neuropharmacol.* 2003;26 (2):88–92.

Berthier ML, Hinojosa J, Martin Mdel C, Fernandez I. Open-label study of donepezil in chronic poststroke aphasia. *Neurology.* 2003;60 (7);1218–9.

Birks JS, Melzer D, Beppu H. Donepezil for mild and moderate Alzheimer's disease. *The Cochrane Library.* 2000; 4.

Brodaty H. Realistic expectations for the management of Alzheimer's disease. *Eur Neuropsychopharmacol.* 1999;9:S43–S52.

Bureau of Drug Surveilance (Canada). Donepezil: Suspected adverse reactions. *CMAJ.* 1998;159:81.

Burns A, Rossor M, Hecker J, et al. The effects of donepezil in Alzheimer's disease: Results from a multinational study. *Dementia Geriatr Cogn Disord.* 1999;10:237–244.

Burns A, Russell E, Page S. New drugs for Alzheimer's disease [editorial]. *BMJ*. 1999;174:476–479.

Carrier L. Donepezil and paroxetine: Possible drug interaction [letter]. *JAGS*. 1999;47:1037.

Cummings J. L. Cholinesterase inhibitors: A new class of psychotropic compounds. *Am J Psychiatry*. 2000;157:4–15.

Cummings J, Donohue J, Brooks R. The relationship between donepezil and behavioral disturbances in patients with Alzheimer's disease. *Am J Geriatr Psychiatry*. 2000;8:134–140.

Dallocchio C, Buffa C, Ligure N, Mazzarello P. Combination of donepezil and gabapentin for behavioural disorders in Alzheimer's disease [letter]. *J Clin Psychiatry*. 2000;61:64.

Delagarza V. W. New Drugs for Alzheimer's disease. *Am Family Physician*. 1998;58:1775–1782.

Doody RS, Geldmacher DS, Pratt RD, Perdomo CA. Optimal donepezil efficacy in Alzheimer's disease is dependant on continued administration. Poster presented at the 9th meeting of the European Neurological Society, June 5–9 1999, Milan, Italy.

Doody RS. Clinical profile of donepezil in the treatment of Alzheimer's disease. *Gerontology*. 1999;45 (Suppl 1):23–32.

Farlow M R, Evans R M. Pharmacologic treatment of cognition in Alzheimer's dementia. *Neurology*. 1998;51 (Suppl 1):S36–S44.

Farlow M. Pharmacokinetic profiles of current therapies for Alzheimer's disease: Implications for switching to galantamine. *Clin Therapeutics*. 2001;23 (Suppl):A13–A23.

Feldman H, Gauthier S, Hecker J, Vellas B, Emir B, Mastey V, Subbiah P, Donepezil MSAD Study Investigators Group. *Am Geriatr Soc*. 2003;51 (6): 737–44.

Ferris S. Switching previous therapies for Alzheimer's disease to galantamine. *Clin Therapeutics*. 2001;23 (Suppl):A3–A7.

Greenberg SM, Tennis MK, Brown LB, et al. Donepezil therapy in clinical practice. *Arch Neurology*. 2000;57:94–99.

Greene Y M, Tariot P N, Wishart H, et al. A 12-week open trial of donepezil hydrochloride in patients with multiple sclerosis and associated cognitive impairments. *J Clin Psychopharm*. 2000;20:350–356.

Hashimoto M, Imamura T, Tanimukai H, Mori E. Urinary incontinence: An unrecognized adverse effect with donepezil. *Lancet*. 2000;356:568.

Jacobsen FM, Comas-Diaz l. Donepezil for psychotropic-induced memory loss. *J Clin Psychiatry*. 1999;60:698–704.

Jonsson L, Lindgren P, Wimo A, Jonsson B, Winblad B. The cost effectiveness of donepezil therapy in Swedish patients with Alzheimer's disease: A Markov model. *Clinical Therapeutics*. 1999;21:1230–1240.

Kaufer DI, Catt KE, Lopez OL, DeKosky ST. Dementia with Lewy Bodies: Response of delirium like features to donepezil [letter]. *Neurol*. 1998;51: 1512.

Kawashima T, Yamada S. Delirium caused by donepezil: A case study. *J Clin Psychiatry*. 2002;63:250–251.

Krall W, Sramek J, Cutler N. Cholinesterase inhibitors a therapeutic strategy for Alzheimer's disease. *Ann Pharmacotherapy*. 1999;33:441–450.

REFERENCES

Kwak Y, Han I, Baik J, Koo M. Relation between cholinesterase inhibitor and Pisa syndrome [letter]. *Lancet.* 2000;355:2222.

Lanctot K, Herrmann N. Donepezil for behavioural disorders associated with Lewy Bodies: A case series. *Int J Geriatr Psychiatry.* 2000;15:338–345.

Lemiere J, Van Gool D, Dom R. Treatment of Alzheimer's disease: An evaluation of the cholinergic approach. *Acta Neurol Belg.* 1999;99:96–106.

Levy M l, Cummings JL, Kahn-Rose R. Neuropsychiatric symptoms and cholinergic therapy for Alzheimer's Disease. *Gerontology.* 1999;45 (Suppl 1): 15–25.

Lopez-Arrieta J, Rodriguez J, Sanz F. Efficacy and safety of nicotine on Alzheimer's disease patients. Cochrane Library, *Cochrane Review of Systematic Studies.* 2002; 1.

Maelicke A. Pharmacokinetic rationale for switching from donepezil to galantamine. *Clin Therapeutics.* 2001;23 (Suppl A):A8–A11.

Magnuson TM, Keller BK, Burke W J. Extrapyramidal side effects in a patient treated with riperidone plus donepezil [letter]. *Am J Psychiatry.* 1998; 155:1458–1459.

Meadows M, Sperling R, Growdon J, et al. Donepezil therapy in clinical practice: A randomized cross-over study. *Arch Neurol.* 2000;57:94–99.

Mega MS, Masterman DM, O'Connor SM, Barclay TR, Cummings JL. The spectrum of behavioral responses to cholinesterase inhibitor therapy in Alzheimer's disease. *Arch Neurol.* 1999;56:1388–1393.

Mohs R, Doody R, Morris J, et al. A 1-year placebo-controlled preservation of function survival study of donepezil AD patients: *Neurol.* 2001;57:481–488.

Morris J. Overview. *Clin Therapeutics.* 2001;23 (Suppl):A1–A2.

Nordberg A, Svensson A. Cholinesterase inhibitors in the treatment of Alzheimer's disease. *Drugs Ageing.* 1998;19:465–480.

Patterson CJ., Gauthier S., Bergman H., et al. The recognition assessment and management of dementing disorders: Conclusions from the Canadian Concensus Conference on Dementing Disorders. *CMAJ.* 1999;160:12 (Suppl):S1–S15.

Rojas-Fernandez C. Successful use of donepezil for the treatment of dementia with Lewy Bodies. *Ann Pharmacotherapy.* 2001;35:202–205.

Rogers SL, Doody RS, Mohs RC, Friedhoff LT. Donepezil improves cognition and Global Function in Alzheimer's disease : A 15-week double-blind placebo–controlled study. *Arch Int Med.* 1998;158:1021–1031.

Rogers SL, Doody RS, Pratt RD, Ieni JR. Long-term efficacy and safety of donepezil in the treatment of Alzheimer's disease: Final analysis of a US multi-center open-label study. *European Neuropsychopharmacology.* 2000; 10:195–203.

Rogers SL, Farlow MR, Doody RS, Mohs R, Friedhoff LT. A 24-week double blind placebo-controlled trial of Aricept in patients with Alzheimer's disease. *Neurol.* 1998;50:136–145.

Roth M Huppert FA, Tym E, Mountjoy CQ. CAMDEX: The Cambridge Examination for Mental Disorders of the Elderly. Cambridge, U.K.: Cambridge University Press, 1988.

Singh S, Dudley C. Discontinuation syndrome following donepezil cessation. *Int J Geriatr Psychiatry.* 2003;18 (4):282–4.

Stryjer R, Strous RD, Bar F, Werber E, Shaked G, Buhiri Y, Kotler M, Weizman A, Rabey JM. Beneficial effect of donepezil augmentation for the management of comorbid schizophrenia and dementia. *Clin Neuropharmacol.* 2003; 26 (1):12–7.

Tanaka M, Yokode M, Kita T, Matsubayashi K. Donepezil and athetoosis in an elderly patient with Alzheimer's disease. *J Am Ger Soc.* 2003;51 (6):889–890.

Tariot P, Cummings J, Katz I, et al. A randomized, double-blind, placebo-controlled study of the efficacy and safety of donepezil in patients with Alzheimer's disease in the nursing home setting. *JAGS.* 2001;49:1590–1599.

Tariot P, Perdomo C, Whalen E, Sovel M, Scham E. Age is not a barrier to donepezil treatment of Alzheimer's disease in the long-term care setting. *Int Psychogeriatr.* 1999;11:134.

Tariot PN, Jakimoovich L. Donepezil use for advanced Alzheimer's disease—a case study from a long-term care facility. *J Am Med Dir Assoc.* 2003; 4 (4):216–9.

Wengel SP, Roccaforte WH, Burke WJ. Donepezil improves symptoms of delirium in dementia: Implications for future research. *J Geriatr Psychiatry Neurol.* 1998;11:159–161.

Wengle SP, Roccaforte W H, Burke W J, et al. Behavioural complications associated with donepezil. *Am J Psychiatry.* 1998;155:1632–1633.

Winblad B, Engedal K, Soininen H, et al. A 1-year, randomized placebo-controlled study of donepezil in patients with mild to moderate AD. *Neurol.* 2001;57:489–495.

Winblad B, Engedal K, Soininen H, et al. Donepezil enhances global function, cognition, and activities of daily living compared with placebo in a one-year, double-blind trial in patients with mild to moderate Alzheimer's disease. *Int Psychogeriatrics.* 1999;11 (Suppl 1):138.

Zhao Q, Xie C, Pesco-Koplowitz L, Jia X, Parier JL. Pharmacokinetic and safety assessments of concurrent administration of risperidone and donepezil. *J Clin Pharmacol.* 2003;43 (2):180–6.

Galantamine

Bachus R, Bickel U, Thomsen T, Roots I, Kewitz H. The O-demethylation of the antidementia drug galantamine is catalysed by cytochrome P450 2D6. *Pharmacogenetics.* 1999;9:661–668.

Blesa R. Galantamine: Therapeutic effects beyond cognition. *Dement Geriatr Cogn Disord.* 2000;11 (Suppl 1):28–34.

Blesa R, Davidson M, Kurz A, Reichman W, van Baelen B, Schwalen S. Galantamine provides sustained benefits in patients with 'advanced moderate' Alzheimer's disease for at least 12 months. *Dement Geriatr Cogn Disord.* 2003;15 (2):79–87.

Erkinjuntti T, Kurz A, S Gauthier S, et al. Efficacy of galantamine in probable vascular dementia and Alzheimer's disease combined with cerebrovascular disease: A randomized trial. *Lancet.* 2002;359:1283–1290.

Fulton B, Benfield P. Galantamine. *Drugs Ageing.* 1996;9:60–65.

Lilienfeld S, Parys W. Galantamine: Additional benefits to patients with Alzheimer's disease. *Dement Geriatr Cogn Disord.* 2000;11 (Suppl 1):19–27.

Macgowan S, Wilcock G, Scott M. Effect of gender and apolipoprotein E genotype on response to anticholinesterase therapy in Alzheimer's disease. *Int J Geriatr Psychiatry.* 1998;13:625–630.

Mintzer JE, Kershaw P. The efficacy of galantamine in the treatment of Alzheimer's disease: comparison of patients previously treated with acetylcholinesterase inhibitors to patients with no prior exposure. *Int J Geriatr Psychiatry.* 2003;18 (4):292–7.

Olin J, Schneider L. Galantamine for Alzheimer's disease. *Cochrane Database of Systematic Reviews.* 2002; 1.

Raskind M A, Peskind E R, Wessel T, Parys W, Ding C. Galantamine in AD: A 6-month randomized placebo–controlled trial with a 6-month extension. *Neurol.* 2000;54 (12):2261–2268.

Rasmusen L, Yan B, Robillard A, et al. Effects of washout and dose escalation periods on the efficacy, safety, and tolerability of galantamine in patients previously treated with donepezil: Ongoing clinical trials. *Clin Therapeutics.* 2001;23 (Suppl A):A25–A30.

Riemann D, Gann H, Dressing H, Muller W, Aldenhoff J. Influence of the cholinesterase inhibitor galantamine hydrobromide on normal sleep. *Psychiatry Res.* 1994;51:253–267.

Rosler M, Anand R, Cicin-Sain A, et al. Efficacy and safety of rivastigmine in patients with Alzheimer's disease: International randomized controlled study. *BMJ.* 1999;318:633–638.

Scott LJ, Goa KL. Galantamine: A review of its use in Alzheimer's disease. *Drugs.* 2000;60:1095–1122.

Tariot PN, Solomon PR, Morris JC, et al. A 5-month randomized placebo–controlled trial of galantamine in AD. *Neurol.* 2000;54 (12):2269–2276.

Wilcock G K, LilienfeldS, Gaens E. Efficacy and safety of galantamine in patients with mild to moderate Alzheimer's disease: Multi-center randomized controlled trial. *BMJ.* 2000;321:1–7.

Wilcock G, Howe I, Coles H, Lilienfelds, Trugen L, ZhuY, Bullock R, et al. A long-term comparison of galantamine and donepezil in the treatment of Alzheimer's Disease. *Drugs Aging.* 2003;20: 777–789.

Rivastigmine

Birks J, Grimley Evans J, Iakovidou V, Tsolaki M. Rivastigmine for Alzheimer's disease. *Cochrane Database of Systematic Reviews.* 2000; 1.

Corey-Bloom J. et al. A randomized trial evaluating the efficacy and safety of ENA-713 (rivastigmine tartrate), a new acytylcholinesterase inhibitor, in patients with mild to moderately severe Alzheimer disease. *Int J Geriatric Psychopharm.* 1998;1:55–65.

Krall WJ, et al. Cholinesterase inhibitors: A therapeutic strategy for Alzheimer disease. *Annals of Pharmacotherapy.* 1999;33:441–450.

Krishnan K et al. Rivastigmine in the treatment of moderately severe to severe Alzheimer's disease. Industry-sponsored symposium report. Barcelona, March 1999;25–27.

Maclean L, Collins C, Byrne E. Dementia with Lewy Bodies treated with rivastigmine: Effects on cognition, neuropsychiatric symptoms, and sleep. *Int Psychogeriatrics*. 2001;13:277–288.

McKeith I, Del Ser T, Spano P, et al. Efficacy of rivastigmine in dementia with Lewy Bodies: A randomized double-blind, placebo-controlled international study. *Lancet*. 2000;356:2031–2036.

Rosler M, Anand R, Cicin-Sain A, et al. Efficacy and safety of rivastigmine in patients with Alzheimer's disease: International randomized controlled trial. *BMJ*. 1999;318:633–638.

Spencer C, Noble S. Rivastigmine: A review of its use in Alzheimer's disease. *Drugs Ageing*. 1998;13:391–411.

Index

absorption, drug, 15
acetazolamide, 540
acetylcholine, 17, 18
acetylcholinesterase inhibitors, 43, 44, 573
  caregiver considerations in therapy with, 573
  contraindications, 571
  cost-effectiveness, 572–73
  dementia therapy, 554, 565–70
  discontinuing, 571–72
  efficacy, 567
  mechanism of action, 553
  predictors of nonresponse, 566
  side effects, 570–71
  switching, 568–70
activities of daily living, grief reactions and, 33
affective functioning
  apathetic and avolitional states, 44
  in BPSD, 239
  citalopram effects, 144
  pathologic emotionalism, 41–42
age, drug metabolism and, 12–16
aggressive behavior, 43
  anticonvulsant drug therapy, 541
  antidepressant drug therapy, 144, 145
  antipsychotic drug therapy, 342
  in BPSD, 236, 239
agoraphobia, 40, 395–96
agranulocytosis, as antipsychotic drug side effect, 298, 313, 317
akathisia, as antipsychotic drug side effects, 285–86, 293
albumin, 16
alcohol abuse
  antidepressant drug therapy, 42, 144, 145
  definition, 423
  epidemiology, 423
  mood disorders and, 487
  risk factors, 423
  SSRI therapy, 128
  withdrawal management, 423–26, 441, 447, 450, 455
alcohol consumption
  assessment, 424
  bupropion and, 141
  drug interactions, 349, 362, 369, 469, 473, 512
  MAOI interaction, 119
  nefazodone and, 184
  see also alcohol abuse
alpha-a acid glycoprotein metabolism, 16
alprazolam
  advantages/disadvantages, 431
  anxiety therapy, 389, 392
  classification, 430*t*
  contraindications, 434–35
  depression therapy, 62
  dosing, 431
  drug–illness interactions, 434–35
  drug interactions, 165, 184, 434
  indications, 430
  mechanism of action, 431
  overdose, 435
  panic disorder management, 395
  patient education, 435
  pharmacokinetics, 430
  precautions, 435–36
  side effects, 432–34
  sleep disorder management, 420
  treatment monitoring, 389, 434
  withdrawal, 432
  see also benzodiazepines
alternative therapies
  depression treatment, 64
  drug interactions, 149, 155
  kava, 474–76
  valerian, 476–77

INDEX

Alzheimer's disease, 513
  clinical features, 561–62
  cognitive enhancer therapy, 551, 552, 565, 566, 575, 582, 587, 592
  dementia in, 557
  diagnosis, 564
  pathology, 563–64
  severity classification, 562
amantadine
  drug interactions, 141
  sexual dysfunction treatment, 88
  side effects, 306*t*
amiloride, 532
amitryptyline
  cytochrome P450 metabolism and, 21
  depression treatment, 48
  drug interactions, 149
  side effects, 103
  toxicity, 51
  see also antidepressant drugs
amoxapine, 103
anesthesia, 400
angiotensin converting enzyme inhibitors, 533
antacids, drug interactions, 362, 512
antiarrhythmia drugs, 362, 369
anticholinergic drugs, 71–73, 306*t*
  drug interactions, 154, 284, 319, 362, 580, 586, 591
anticholinergic side effects, 71–76
  antipsychotic drug therapy, 284–85
anticonvulsant drugs
  mood disorder therapy, 495–96, 502
  see also specific drug
antidepressant drugs
  anticholinergic, 71–76
  for anxiety disorders, 40–41
  augmentation and combination strategies, 60–65, 68–69
  bipolar disorder treatment, 37–38
  chronic pain management, 42
  classification, 23–24*t*
  compliance issues, 47
  cost considerations, 53
  discontinuing or switching, 67–68, 80
  doses, 23–24, 48, 52–53, 67
  drug interactions, 52, 90–96, 532, 533
  dysthymia treatment, 34–35
  effectiveness, 49
  elder-specific concerns, 45–46
  enzyme interactions, 92–93*t*, 95–96*t*
  mood disorder therapy, 480
  for nondepressive disorders, 38–44, 45*t*
  nonresponse, 58–65, 65–66
  overdose risk, 51
  panic disorder treatment, 39–40
  personality disorder management, 43
  pharmacokinetics, 20, 90*t*, 91*t*
  phases of depression treatment, 53–55
  prescribing patterns, 3, 4, 10
  for psychotic depression, 35–36
  selection, 49–51, 52*t*
  for severe depression, 31
  side effects, 11, 70
    anticholinergic, 71–76
    breast cancer risk, 84–85
    cardiovascular, 77–78
    cognitive, 88*t*
    drug selection, 89–90*t*
    extrapyramidal, 76
    fall risk, 78
    neuroreceptor action in, 89*t*
    safety concerns, 70–71
    seizure potential, 76–77
    serotonin syndrome, 79–82
    sexual functioning, 85–88
    SIADH, 82–83
    weight change, 83–84
  time to onset of action, 49–50, 66
  treatment algorithms, 66–70
  treatment outcomes, 55–58
  treatment planning, 46–49
  uses, 44–45*t*, 371
  see also specific drug; specific drug type
antidiuretic hormone secretion, syndrome of inappropriate (SIADH), 82–83, 301
antifungal agents, 283
antihistamines
  adverse effects, 372
  drug interactions, 362, 464
  side effects, 11, 421
  uses, 371
antihypertensive drugs, 215
antimalarial drugs, 282
antiparkinsonian drugs, 303–4, 305–6*t*
antipsychotic drugs
  administration, 273–74
  agents and characteristics, 229–30*t*
  antiparkinsonian agents, 303–4, 305–6*t*
  atypical, 229, 231–32, 233*t*, 279–81
  bipolar disorder treatment, 496–97
  BPSD therapy, 242–44, 309, 325, 327, 334, 350, 351
  choosing, 266–73
  classification, 229
  combination therapies, 277
  contraindications, 263–64
  cost-effectiveness, 280–81
  delirium management, 255–56
  depot forms, 235, 272–73

discontinuing, 247, 276
drug interactions, 140, 154, 164, 306–7*t*, 464, 533
indications, 229, 230
maintenance phase of treatment, 275–76
management of psychosis in diffuse lewy body disease, 251
management of psychosis in Parkinson's disease/parkinsonism, 247–49
mood disorder therapy, 479–80, 497
neuropharmacology, 266
overdose, 307–8
pharmacokinetics, 20, 232–36
prescribing patterns, 3, 4, 10
pretreatment evaluation, 264–65
principles of treatment, 262–64
for psychotic depression, 36, 64
schizophrenia management, 260
side effects, 11, 268–71*t*, 279
anticholinergic, 284–85
atypicals, 279–81
catatonia, 293
cognitive, 300
edema, 303
endocrinologic, 299
extrapyramidal, 285–93
glycemic metabolism, 301–2
hematologic, 298
hepatic, 302
jaundice, 298
neuroleptic malignant syndrome, 294–97
ophthalmologic, 297–98
postural hypotension, 283–84
sedation, 281
seizure potential, 297
sexual functioning, 285
SIADH, 301
skin manifestations, 300
sudden death, 303
temperature dyscontrol, 302–3
weight gain, 298–99
symptom specificity, 278*t*
treatment monitoring, 274–76
treatment resistance, 277–78
typical, 229, 232–36
see also specific drug; specific drug type
anxiety/anxiety disorders
antidepressant drug therapy, 41, 192, 217
assessment and diagnosis, 387–88
benzodiazepine therapy, 386, 389–91, 391*t*, 392
clinical features, 40
comorbid depression, 54
due to medical condition, 398
generalized (GAD), 40–41, 397–98
presentation, 394
secondary, 398–400*t*
SSRI therapy, 127
substance-induced, 398
see also anxiolytics and sedative/hypnotics
anxiolytics and sedative/hypnotics
agents and characteristics, 371–72, 372–75*t*, 389
alcohol withdrawal management, 423, 424–26
dependence, 403
depression threatment, 62, 69
drug interactions, 410–11*t*
fall risk, 404
for GAD, 41, 397–98
hangover effects, 403
herbal remedies, 474–77
incontinence risk, 405
indications, 371, 394, 400
motor vehicle operation and, 404–5
nonbenzodiazepine, 371
overdose, 429
pharmacokinetics, 377–84*t*
rebound insomnia, 402–3
respiration effects, 403–4
side effects, 11, 401, 405–9*t*, 422–23
sleep disorder therapy, 400, 415–16, 418–23
tolerance, 401–2
toxicity, 401
withdrawal, 426–29
see also specific drug
aphasia, primary progressive, 560
aripiprazole, 223*t*, 243*t*, 308, 597–99
aspirin, 546
assessment
alcohol use, 424
Alzheimer's disease, 562
Alzheimer's disease treatment outcomes, 567–68
anxiety, 387–88
bipolar disorder, 489–90
delirium, 254
depressive disorders, 28–38
MAOI therapy, 115
monoamine oxidase inhibitor therapy, 112–13
neuroleptic pretreatment evaluation, 264–65
polypharmacy, 52
sleep behavior, 416, 417
valproate therapy, 543
see also monitoring

INDEX

astemizole
drug interactions, 165, 185, 362, 369
side effects, 282
atorvastatin, 185
atropine, 473
augmentation and combination strategies
antiparkinsonian drugs, 304
antipsychotic drug therapy, 277
benzodiazepines, 395
bipolar disorder therapy, 479, 497–98
bupropion, 138–39
citalopram, 147
clonazepam, 446
clozapine, 312
depression treatment, 60–65, 68–69
donepezil, 577–78
fluoxetine, 161
lithium therapy, 521
mirtazapine, 170
moclobemide, 175, 178
MAOIs, 113, 114–15
nortriptyline, 188
SSRIs, 395
venlafaxine, 221

Balint's syndrome, 258
barbiturates
adverse effects, 371
drug interactions, 141, 164, 199, 331, 349, 362, 439, 464
behavioral and psychological symptoms of dementia (BPSD)
aggression in, 239
anticonvulsant drug therapy, 510, 541
antipsychotic drug therapy, 242–44, 309, 325, 327, 334, 350, 351
anxiolytic therapy, 436
associated affective states, 239
clinical features, 236–38
cognitive enhancer therapy, 574, 587
epidemiology, 236
management, 231–32, 240–47
mood stabilizer therapy, 485
pharmacotherapy, 561
psychotic symptoms, 238–39
benzodiazepines
advantages, 389
alcohol withdrawal management, 423, 425–26
anxiety disorder therapy, 397–98
chemical classification, 372, 375
clinical characteristics, 386
combination therapies, 395
compliance, 393
delirium management, 256
depression threatment, 62
dosing, 391
drug interactions, 172, 319, 339, 362, 464, 473, 533, 546
duration of treatment, 390–91
efficacy, 386, 392
geriatric utilization, 386–87
indications, 371
mechanism of action, 376
mood disorder therapy, 480, 497
panic disorder therapy, 394–95
patient education, 391*t*
pharmacokinetics, 376, 385–86
PTSD management, 397
respiration effects, 404
risks for elders, 392–93
side effects, 11, 376, 401
sleep disorder therapy, 415, 418
sleep effects, 418–19
tolerability, 392–93, 401–2
toxicity, 401
treatment guidelines, 391*t*
withdrawal, 426–29
see also anxiolytics and sedative/hypnotics; *specific drug*
beta-2 agonists, 155
beta blockers
anxiety therapy, 389–90
drug–illness interactions, 390
drug interactions, 141, 362, 369
uses, 371
bethanechol, 72
drug interactions, 580
sexual dysfunction treatment, 87
bethanidine, 155
bipolar disorder
acute mania, 493–95
anticonvulsant drug therapy, 502, 510, 513, 538–39
antidepressant therapy, 37–38, 135
antipsychotic drug therapy, 231, 309, 334, 350, 351
classification, 485–86
clinical characteristics, 486–88
combination pharmacotherapy, 497–98
comorbidities, 489
diagnosis, 489–92, 493*t*
discontinuation of therapy, 501–2
epidemiology, 488–89
mood stabilizer therapy, 485
nonresponse to treatment, 498–500
pharmacotherapy, 495–502
relapse prevention, 500–501, 517
treatment challenges, 492–93
treatment strategies, 479–81
BPSD. *see* behavioral and psychological symptoms of dementia

breast cancer, antidepressant drug therapy and, 84–85
budenoside, 362, 369
bupropion
advantages, 137
bipolar disorder treatment, 38, 135
classification, 135*t*
combination therapies, 114, 138–39, 221
contraindications, 142
depression therapy, 31, 65, 66
dosing, 137–38
drug interactions, 140–41, 199, 469
indications, 135
laboratory tests affected by, 142
for managing apathetic and avolitional states, 44
mechanism of action, 135
mood disorder therapy, 480–81
overdose, 142–43
pharmacokinetics, 135, 136*t*
seizure precautions, 142
sexual dysfunction treatment, 87
side effects, 139–40
treatment monitoring, 143
buspirone
advantages/disadvantages, 389, 437
anxiety disorder therapy, 397–98
classification, 436*t*
depression therapy, 61, 62
discontinuing, 438
dosing, 438
drug–illness interactions, 439–40
drug interactions, 61, 198, 207, 439
for generalized anxiety disorder, 41
indications, 371, 436
laboratory tests affected by, 440
mechanism of action, 437
overdose, 440
panic disorder management, 395
pharmacokinetics, 436
phobia management, 396
precautions, 440–41
sexual dysfunction treatment, 87
side effects, 438–39
see also anxiolytics and sedative/hypnotics

caffeine, 534
calcium channel blockers
drug interactions, 497, 533
mood disorder therapy, 480, 497
carbachol, 580
carbamazepine
advantages/disadvantages, 503
benzodiazepine withdrawal management, 429
classification, 502*t*
depression therapy, 63
dosing, 503
drug–illness interactions, 508
drug interactions, 83, 141, 149, 165, 184, 331, 349, 357, 434, 439, 464, 473, 497, 506*t*, 507, 515, 533, 546
indications, 502*t*
laboratory tests affected by, 508
mechanism of action, 503
mood disorder therapy, 479, 497
overdose, 508–9
pharmacology, 502
precautions, 509
side effects, 504–6*t*
treatment monitoring, 507–8
cardiovascular functioning
antidepressant drug side effects, 77–78, 102–3
antipsychotic drug side effects, 281–83
beta blocker therapy and, 390
clozapine side effects, 314–15
depression treatment considerations, 46
lithium side effects, 523
nortriptyline effects, 187, 188, 190, 191
pharmacotherapy precautions, 185
propranolol therapy and, 376
caregivers
depression in, 34
depression therapy role, 96–97
treatment compliance role, 49
catatonia
antipsychotic drug side effects, 293
antipsychotic drug therapy, 350
anxiolytic therapy, 450
cerivastatin, 185
certizine, 362
Charles Bonnet syndrome, 257, 541
cheese, 118
chloral hydrate, 371
advantages/disadvantages, 441
classification, 441*t*
contraindications, 443
discontinuing, 441
dosing, 441
drug–illness interactions, 443
drug interactions, 442
indications, 441
laboratory tests affected by, 442
overdose, 443
pharmacokinetics, 441
precautions, 443–44
side effects, 442
see also anxiolytics and sedative/hypnotics

chlordiazepoxide, 371
chlorpromazine
  drug interactions, 546
  pharmacokinetics, 16
  side effects, 298
  see also antipsychotic drugs
choline bitartrate, 481
cimetidine, drug interactions, 141, 149, 165, 178, 190, 198, 199, 206, 225, 349, 369, 434, 439, 546, 594
cirrhosis, pharmacotherapy precautions, 185
cisapride, 154, 185
citalopram, 130
  classification, 144*t*
  combination therapies, 147
  contraindications, 149
  cytochrome P450 metabolism and, 20
  discontinuation and switching, 147, 151
  dosing, 146–47
  drug–illness interactions, 149
  drug interactions, 148–49, 164
  efficacy, 145–46
  indications, 144–45
  mechanism of action, 145
  OCD treatment, 39
  overdose, 149–50
  pharmacokinetics, 145
  side effects, 147–48
  treatment monitoring, 150, 151
  see also selective serotonin reuptake inhibitors
clarithromycin, 184
clearance, drug, 16
clomipramine
  classification, 151*t*
  combination therapies, 114
  contraindications, 155
  cytochrome P450 metabolism and, 20, 21
  depression therapy, 50, 63
  discontinuing or switching, 80
  dosing, 152–53
  drug interactions, 20, 154–55, 178
  indications, 151
  mechanism of action, 152
  OCD treatment, 39
  panic disorder treatment, 40
  pharmacokinetics, 152
  side effects, 104, 152, 153–54, 155
  withdrawal, 154
  see also antidepressant drugs
clonazepam
  advantages/disadvantages, 445
  anxiety disorder therapy, 397–98
  classification, 444*t*
  combination therapy, 446
  depression therapy, 62
  discontinuing, 445
  dosing, 445, 446
  drug interactions, 446
  indications, 400, 444
  laboratory tests affected by, 446
  mechanism of action, 444
  panic disorder management, 395
  pharmacology, 444
  phobia management, 396
  for restless leg syndrome, 416
  side effects, 445–46*t*
  treatment monitoring, 446
  see also benzodiazepines
clonidine
  alcohol withdrawal management, 426
  drug interactions, 155, 215, 362
clozapine
  advantages/disadvantages, 310–11
  bipolar disorder treatment, 497
  classification, 308*t*
  combination therapies, 312
  contraindications, 320
  cost effectiveness, 232
  discontinuing, 312–13
  dosing, 311–12
  drug–illness interactions, 320
  drug interactions, 149, 164, 199, 207, 319, 507
  indications, 308–9, 310
  mechanism of action, 309–10
  mood disorder therapy, 497
  overdose, 320
  pharmacokinetics, 309
  precautions, 321–22
  side effects, 279, 280, 283, 298, 299, 313–18, 321
  switching to/from, 350
  treatment monitoring, 318–19
  see also antipsychotic drugs
codeine, 164, 198, 207
cognitive enhancers
  agents, 551–52*t*
  dementia therapy, 565–70
  indications, 552–53
  mechanism of action, 553
  see also specific drug
cognitive functioning
  anticholinergic drug side effects, 76
  antidepressant drug side effects, 88*t*, 107
  antipsychotic drug side effects, 300
  anxiolytic and sedative/hypnotic drug side effects, 405–9*t*
  benzodiazepine effects, 376, 393
  delirium, 252–56

delusional disorder, 256–57
depression and, 26, 32–33, 48
lithium side effects, 524
parkinsonism-associated psychosis, 247–49
paroxetine effects, 200
schizophrenia symptoms, 258–59
visual hallucinations, 257–58
see also cognitive enhancers; dementia
combination therapy. *see* augmentation and combination strategies
Compendium of Pharmaceutical Specialties, 6
compliance
antipsychotic drug therapy, 277–78
benzodiazepine therapy, 393
depression treatment considerations, 47
lithium therapy, 538
conjugation, 16
contraindications, generally, 11
cost and cost-effectiveness, 5
acetylcholinesterase inhibitors, 572–73
antidepressant drug therapy, 53
antipsychotic drugs, 280–81, 335
risperidone, 351
Creutzfelt-Jacob disease, 560
cyclobenzaprine, 362
cyclophosphamide, 141
cyclosporine, 185
cyclothymic disorder, 488
CYP1A, 21
CYP3A4, 20, 180, 348
CYP2B6, 141
CYP2C19, 19, 20
CYP2D6, 19, 20, 140–41, 180
citalopram interaction, 148–49
sertraline action, 203
cyproheptadine, 88
cytochrome P-450
inhibition, 19–20
isoenzyme activity, 20–21
isoenzyme system, 18–19
metabolism, 16

data sources, 6–8
delirium
antipsychotic drug therapy, 325, 334
assessment, 254
causes, 252*t*
clinical features, 253–54
definition, 252
epidemiology, 252
lithium side effects, 524
management, 254–56
predisposing factors, 253
delusional disorder, 256–57
dementia
in Alzheimer's disease, 557, 575
anticonvulsant drug therapy, 502
antidepressant drug therapy, 144
antipsychotic drug therapy, 352
clinical features, 554
cognitive enhancer therapy, 551, 552, 583
definition, 554
depression and, 32–33
differential diagnosis, 557–61
in diffuse lewy body disease, 249, 250, 557, 558–59, 575–76
epidemiology, 554–57
fronto temporal, 44, 559–60, 576
medical condition-associated, 561
pharmacotherapy agents, 554, 565–70, 574
in Pick's disease, 559–60
primary progressive aphasia, 560
SSRI therapy, 128
subcortical, 560
treatment strategies, 558, 564–65
vascular, 557–58, 576, 582, 587
see also Alzheimer's disease; behavioral and psychological symptoms of dementia (BPSD)
dental problems, as antidepressant drug side effect, 106
depressive disorders
aberrant grief reactions, 33
acute intervention, 53–54
age-specific features, 29–30*t*, 45–46
agitation in, 43
anticonvulsant drug therapy, 541
antipsychotic drug therapy, 359
anxiolytic therapy, 436
assessment and diagnosis, 28–30
associated medical conditions, 33
bipolar disorder, 37–38
caregiver role, 96–97
in caregivers, 34
classification, 25
clinical features, 25–26
with dementia, 32–33
dysthymia, 34
epidemiology, 27*t*
late-onset, 32
lithium therapy, 517, 518
mood stabilizer therapy, 485
phases of treatment, 53–55
poststroke, 35
prognosis, 55–58
psychotic, 35–36, 64, 261
relapse prevention, 54–55, 56–58, 127, 191
secondary, 33–34

depressive disorders (*cont.*)
severe, 30–31
treatment, 24
see also antidepressant drugs
desipramine
advantages/disadvantages, 156
classification, 155*t*
combination therapies, 114, 161
depression therapy, 50, 65
dosing, 156–57
drug interactions, 20, 149, 154, 157, 225, 434, 469
indications, 156
overdose, 157
pharmacokinetics, 16, 156
side effects, 157
toxicity, 51
treatment monitoring, 157
see also antidepressant drugs
dexamethasone, 439
dextroamphetamine, 62–63
dextromethorphan, 164, 178
diabetes
antipsychotic drug-induced, 280, 301–2
beta blocker therapy and, 390
neuropathy, 42
nortriptyline effects, 190
diazepam
classification, 446*t*
clinical characteristics, 447
dosing, 447–48
drug interactions, 185, 207, 448
indications, 447
overdose, 448
pharmacology, 447
side effects, 448
sleep disorder therapy, 420–21
withdrawal, 426–27
see also anxiolytics and sedative/hypnotics
diffuse lewy body disease, 249–51
antipsychotic drug therapy, 334, 350
clinical features, 558–59
cognitive enhancer therapy, 552, 575–76, 583, 587
dementia in, 557
digoxin, 165, 185, 198, 216, 362, 369, 434
diltiazem, 439, 497, 580
discontinuing drug therapy
acetylcholinesterase inhibitors, 571–73
antidepressants, 67–68
antipsychotic drugs, 276
bipolar disorder treatment, 501–2
buspirone, 438
chloral hydrate, 441
citalopram, 147, 151
clonazepam, 445
clozapine, 312–13
duloxetine, 158
fluoxetine, 161
gabapentin, 511
haloperidol, 328–29
lithium, 522
mirtazapine, 170
MAOIs, 114, 115
paroxetine, 193, 195
phenelzine, 201
risperidone, 355
SSRIs, 132–34
venlafaxine, 222
zaleplon, 463
zopiclone, 472
see also washout period; withdrawal
distribution, drug, 15
diuretics, 362, 369, 532–33
divalproex/valproate/valproic acid
advantages/disadvantages, 542–43
bipolar disorder treatment, 495–96
classification, 541*t*
depression therapy, 63
dosing, 543–44
drug–illness interactions, 547
drug interactions, 497, 515, 516, 546–47
indications, 541–42
laboratory tests affected by, 547
mechanism of action, 542
mood disorder therapy, 479, 495–96, 496, 497
overdose, 547–48
patient/caregiver education, 548–49
pharmacokinetics, 542
precautions, 549
pretreatment assessment, 543
side effects, 544–46
treatment monitoring, 546
treatment response indicators, 543
donepezil
advantages/disadvantages, 576–77
Alzheimer's disease therapy, 575
classification, 574*t*
combination therapies, 577–78
diffuse lewy body disease therapy, 575–76
dosing, 577
drug–illness interactions, 581
drug interactions, 357, 580
mechanism of action, 574–75
mood disorder therapy, 481
overdose, 581

pharmacokinetics, 574
precautions, 582
side effects, 578–79
treatment monitoring, 579, 582
dosage forms, 5
dose, 5
alprazolam, 431
antidepressant drugs, 23–24, 48, 52–53, 67
antipsychotic drugs, 273–75
benzodiazepines, 391
bupropion, 137–38
buspirone, 438
carbamazepine, 503
chloral hydrate, 441
citalopram, 146–47
clomipramine, 152–53
clonazepam, 445, 446
clozapine, 311–12
desipramine, 156–57
diazepam, 447–48
divalproex/valproate/valproic acid, 543–44
donepezil, 577
duloxetine, 158
estazolam, 449
fluoxetine, 160–61
fluphenazine, 323–24
gabapentin, 510–11
galantamine, 584–85
haloperidol, 327–28
heterocyclic antidepressant drug therapy, 109–10
kava, 475
knowledge base, 8
lamotrigine, 514
lithium, 519–22
lorazepam, 451
loxapine, 333
midazolam, 454
mirtazapine, 169–70
moclobemide, 175
MAOIs, 112
nefazodone, 182–83
nortriptyline, 187–88
olanzapine, 336–37
oxazepam, 456
paroxetine, 193, 194
perphenazine, 342
phenelzine, 201
physiology of aging and, 21
quetiapine, 346–47
recommended practice, 8–9
risperidone, 353–54
rivastigmine, 589
SSRIs, 130, 131–32
sertraline, 204–5
St. John's wort, 210
tacrine, 593
temazepam, 458
thioridazine, 360
thiothixene, 364
topiramate, 539
trazadone, 213–14
triazolam, 460–61
venlafaxine, 220–21
zaleplon, 463
ziprasidone, 367–68
zolpidem, 467
zopiclone, 472
doxepin
depression treatment, 48, 69
side effects, 103
toxicity, 51
see also antidepressant drugs
dronabinol, 464
droperidol, 464
drug–drug interactions, 5, 9, 11
alprazolam, 434
antidepressant drug therapy, 52, 90–96
antiparkinsonian drugs, 304
antipsychotic drugs, 306–7*t*
anxiolytics and sedative/hypnotics, 410–11*t*
avoiding, 10
bupropion, 140–41
buspirone, 61, 439
carbamazepine, 506*t*, 507
chloral hydrate, 442
citalopram, 148–49
clomipramine, 154–55
clonazepam, 446
clozapine, 319
cytochrome P-450 metabolism in, 19–20
desipramine, 157
diazepam, 448
divalproex/valproate/valproic acid, 546–47
donepezil, 580
estazolam, 449
fluoxetine, 164–65
fluphenazine, 324–25
gabapentin, 512
galantamine, 586
haloperidol, 330–31
kava, 476
lamotrigine, 515–16
lithium, 532–34
lorazepam, 452
loxapine, 334
midazolam, 455
mirtazapine, 172

drug–drug interactions (*cont.*)
moclobemide, 178
MAOIs, 114–15, 119–20, 121–22*t*
nefazodone, 61, 184–85
nortriptyline, 190
olanzapine, 339–40
oxazepam, 456
paroxetine, 198–99
perphenazine, 343
pharmacodynamic, 90
pharmacokinetic, 90
physiologic mechanisms, 21
polypharmacy assessment, 52
quetiapine, 348–49
risperidone, 357
rivastigmine, 591
SSRIs, 65
sertraline, 206–7
tacrine, 594
temazepam, 459
thioridazine, 362
thiothixene, 365
topiramate, 540, 541
trazodone, 215–16
tricyclic antidepressants, 65
venlafaxine, 224–25
zaleplon, 464
ziprasidone, 369
zolpidem, 468–69
zopiclone, 473
drug–illness interactions, 9, 11
alprazolam, 434–35
beta blockers, 390
buspirone, 439–40
carbamazepine, 508
chloral hydrate, 443
citalopram, 149
clozapine, 320
divalproex/valproate/valproic acid, 547
donepezil, 581
estazolam, 449
gabapentin, 512
galantamine, 586
kava, 476
lithium, 534–35*t*
mirtazapine, 172–73
moclobemide, 178–79
MAOIs, 122
nefazodone, 185
nortriptyline, 190
olanzapine, 340
oxazepam, 456
paroxetine, 199
physiologic mechanisms, 21
propranolol, 376
risperidone, 358
sertraline, 208
tacrine, 594–95
thioridazine, 363
venlafaxine, 225
zaleplon, 465
ziprasidone, 369–70
zolpidem, 469
zopiclone, 473
duloxetine
classification, 157*t*
discontinuation, 158
dosing, 158
efficacy, 158
indications, 158
mechanism of action, 158
side effects, 158
see also serotonin noradrenaline reuptake inhibitors
dysphagia, antipsychotic drug-related, 289
dysthymia, 34
dystonia, antipsychotic drug-related, 279, 288–89, 292–93

efavirenz, 141
electroconvulsive therapy, 249
depression relapse prevention, 55
depression treatment, 68
lithium therapy and, 538
mood disorder therapy, 481, 500
obsessive–compulsive disorder treatment, 396
for psychotic depression, 36–37
elimination of drug, age-related changes in, 12–15
endocrine disorders, 486–87
lithium side effects, 526–27
ephedrine-MAOI interaction, 119
epinephrine, 120
drug interactions, 339
erythromycin, 184, 349, 439, 473, 546, 586
escitalopram, 23*t*, 81*t*, 90*t*, 92*t*, 124*t*, 158, 599–603
estazolam
advantages/disadvantages, 448–49
classification, 448*t*
dosing, 449
drug–illness interactions, 449
drug interactions, 449
overdose, 449
pharmacology, 448
side effects, 449
sleep disorder therapy, 420
see also benzodiazepines
estrogen supplementation, 63
ethanol, 464, 540
ethosuximide, 515
extrapyramidal symptoms

antidepressant drug side effects, 76, 104–5
antiparkinsonian drug therapy, 303–4
antipsychotic drug side effects, 279, 285–93
anxiolytic therapy for, 400, 444
haloperidol side effects, 329
thiothixene side effects, 363, 364

falls/falling
antidepressant drug side effects, 78
anxiolytics and sedative/hypnotic side effects, 404
felbamate, 546
fever, as clozapine side effect, 313–14, 322
flecainide, 198, 199
fluconazole, 349, 439
fludrocortisone, 102
flumazenil, 469
fluoxetine, 130, 131, 165–66
advantages/disadvantages, 160
classsification, 158*t*
combination therapies, 63, 138, 161
depression therapy, 63, 65
discontinuation, 132–33, 161–62
dosing, 160–61
drug interactions, 20, 141, 154, 164–65, 185, 190, 215, 225, 439, 469, 546, 580
efficacy, 159
indications, 158
mechanism of action, 159
OCD treatment, 39
overdose, 165
pharmacokinetics, 158–59
posttraumatic stress disorder treatment, 41
for psychotic depression, 64
side effects, 160, 162–64, 166
switching to/from, 185
treatment monitoring, 164, 166
see also selective serotonin reuptake inhibitors
fluphenazine
classification, 322*t*
delusional disorder therapy, 257
dosing, 323–24
drug interactions, 324–25
indications, 322
overdose, 325
pharmacokinetics, 322–23
precautions, 324, 325
side effects, 324
see also antipsychotic drugs
fluvoxamine, 130, 131
augmentation, 63
depression therapy, 63, 65
discontinuation, 132–33, 151
drug interactions, 154, 319, 330, 362, 439, 594
obsessive–compulsive disorder treatment, 39
see also selective serotonin reuptake inhibitors
food-MAOI interactions, 118–19
furosemide, 532

GABA, 17, 18
alcohol effects, 424
benzodiazepine action, 376
gabapentin
advantages/disadvantages, 510
anxiety disorder therapy, 398
benzodiazepine withdrawal management, 429
classification, 509*t*
combination therapies, 577
discontinuing, 511
dosing, 510–11
drug–illness interactions, 512
drug interactions, 512
indications, 510
mechanism of action, 510
mood disorder therapy, 479
overdose, 512–13
pharmacokinetics, 510
side effects, 511–12
GAD. *see under* anxiety/anxiety disorders
galantamine, 586
advantages/disadvantages, 584
classification, 582*t*
dosing, 584–85
drug–illness interactions, 586
drug interactions, 207, 586
indications, 582–84
mechanism of action, 553, 583
pharmacokinetics, 583
side effects, 585
gastrointestinal problems
antidepressant drug side effects, 103–4
clozapine side effects, 316–17
lithium side effects, 527
gender, 3
metabolic differences, 20
glucocorticoids, 349
glucuronidation, 16
glycemic metabolism
antidepressant drug side effects, 105
antipsychotic drug side effects, 301–2
grapefruit juice, 206, 434
grieving, 33
guanethidine, 155

hallucinations, 257–58
  antipsychotic drug therapy for, 350
haloperidol
  advantages/disadvantages, 326–27, 331, 332
  classification, 325*t*
  contraindications, 331
  delirium management, 255
  discontinuing, 328–29
  dosing, 327–28
  drug interactions, 164, 185, 198, 207, 330–31, 339, 439
  indications, 325
  mechanism of action, 326
  overdose, 331
  pharmacokinetics, 16, 325–26, 327
  precautions, 331–32
  side effects, 283, 298, 329–30
  treatment monitoring, 330
  see also antipsychotic drugs
hepatic clearance, 16
heterocyclic antidepressants
  combination therapies, 114–15
  contraindications, 106–7
  depression treatment, 31
  for depression with dementia, 32–33
  dosing, 109–10
  drug interactions, 19, 107
  mechanism of action, 97
  panic disorder treatment, 40
  pharmacokinetics, 98*t*, 99–101
  for psychotic depression, 35–36
  side effects, 71, 78, 79, 84, 101–6
  toxicity, 51, 107–8
  treatment monitoring, 108–9
  washout period, 110
  withdrawal, 110–11
  see also specific drug
HRT, 63
5-HT agonists, 198, 206
5-HT2/3 receptor antagonists, 88
Huntington's disease, 262
hydroxybupropion, 140
hyperthermia, 302, 303
hyperthyroidism, a nortriptyline interaction, 190
hypnotics. *see* anxiolytics and sedative/hypnotics
hypomania, 488
hypotension
  antipsychotic drug side effects, 283–84
  heterocyclic antidepressant side effects, 101–2
  management, 102
  MAOI side effects, 116
  nortriptyline effects, 191
hypothermia, as antipsychotic drug side effect, 302, 303

ifosfamide, 141
imipramine
  combination therapies, 114
  cytochrome P450 metabolism and, 21
  depression treatment, 48
  drug interactions, 154, 225, 434
  side effects, 103, 104
  see also antidepressant drugs
inappropriate prescribing, 3–4
indications for use, 10–11
indomethacin, 330
inositol, 481
integrated treatment approach, 10
itraconazole, 185, 349, 439, 473

jaundice, as antipsychotic drug side effect, 298

kava, 474–76
ketoconazole, 185, 349, 369, 439, 469, 580, 586

lamotrigine
  advantages/disadvantages, 514
  bipolar disorder treatment, 496
  classification, 513*t*
  depression therapy, 63
  dosing, 514
  drug interactions, 497, 507, 515–16, 546
  indications, 513
  mechanism of action, 513–14
  mood disorder therapy, 479, 497, 498
  overdose, 516
  pharmacokinetics, 513
  side effects, 514, 515*t*
levodopa
  drug interactions, 141, 172
  for restless leg syndrome, 416
lidocaine, 165
lithium
  advantages/disadvantages, 518
  classification, 516*t*
  combination therapies, 175, 221, 521
  compliance, 538
  controlled-release, 518–19
  depression treatment, 61, 69
  discontinuing, 522
  dosing, 519–22
  drug–illness interactions, 534–35*t*
  drug interactions, 165, 198, 207, 357, 497, 507, 532–34, 546
  electroconvulsive therapy and, 538
  indications, 517, 518
  laboratory tests affected by, 535–36
  mechanism of action, 517
  mood disorder therapy, 479, 495, 496, 497, 498

overdose, 536–37
patient/caregiver education, 537
pharmacokinetics, 517
precautions, 537–38
side effects, 522–29
treatment monitoring, 530–32
treatment response predictors, 519
lopinavir, 515
lorazepam
advantages/disadvantages, 450–51
alcohol withdrawal management, 425
anxiety disorder therapy, 389, 397–98
classification, 449*t*
dosing, 451
drug interactions, 190, 349, 452
indications, 400, 450
mechanism of action, 450
overdose, 452
parenteral, 389
pharmacokinetics, 21, 450
precautions, 452–53
side effects, 451–52
sleep disorder therapy, 420
treatment monitoring, 452
see also benzodiazepines
lovastatin, 185
loxapine
advantages/disadvantages, 333
classification, 332*t*
dosing, 333
drug interactions, 334, 452
indications, 333
mechanism of action, 333
overdose, 334
side effects, 333, 334*t*
see also antipsychotic drugs

mania
anticonvulsant therapy, 541
anxiolytic therapy, 400, 444, 450
in bipolar disorder, 486–87, 493–95
lithium therapy, 517, 518
mood stabilizer therapy, 485
organic pathology, 486–87
secondary, pharmacotherapy for, 496
MAOIs. *see* monoamine oxidase inhibitors
maprotiline
side effects, 103, 106
toxicity, 51
see also antidepressant drugs
marketing studies, 7
medical conditions
anxiety related to, 398
dementia associated with, 561
depression treatment considerations, 46
mania induced by, 486–87
mood disorders and, 33
with psychosis, 262*t*
see also drug–illness interactions
mefloquin, 154
melatonin, 421
meperidine, 149, 199, 207
mephenytoin, 515
meprobamate, 371
metabolism of medication
clinical significance, 10, 12, 21
definition, 11
determinants of, 15, 16
phase II processes, 16
phase I processes, 16
phenotypes, 19
see also pharmacokinetics
methotrexate, 516
methsuximide, 515
methyldopa, 215, 330, 362, 534
methylphenidate
combination therapies, 221
depression therapy, 62–63
for managing apathetic and avolitional states, 44
sexual dysfunction treatment, 87
metoclopramide, 464, 473
metoprolol, 178, 198
midazolam
advantages/disadvantages, 453–54
classification, 453*t*
dosing, 454
drug interactions, 185, 455
indications, 400, 453
parenteral, 389
pharmacokinetics, 453
side effects, 454–55*t*
see also benzodiazepines
migraine headaches, 541
mirtazapine, 54
anxiety disorder therapy, 398
classification, 166*t*
combination therapies, 114, 170
contraindications, 173
depression therapy, 49, 65
discontinuation, 67, 170
dosing, 169–70
drug–illness interactions, 172–73
drug interactions, 172, 199, 207
efficacy, 169
indications, 166–68
laboratory tests affected by, 173
mechanism of action, 167
overdose, 173
pharmacokinetics, 167, 168*t*
PTSD treatment, 41
sexual dysfunction treatment, 87
side effects, 170–72
treatment monitoring, 172, 173–74

moclobemide, 65
advantages/disadvantages, 174–75
combination therapies, 175, 178
discontinuation, 151
dosing, 175
drug interactions, 178, 199, 207
indications, 174
laboratory tests affected by, 178
mechanism of action, 174
overdose, 179
pharmacokinetics, 174, 176*t*
precautions, 178–79
side effects, 177, 179
switching to/from, 178
modafinil, 63
molindone, 298
monitoring
for adverse drug effects, 9–10
alprazolam therapy, 434
antidepressant drug therapy, 48, 108–9
antipsychotic drug therapy, 274–76
carbamazepine therapy, 507–8
clonazepam therapy, 446
clozapine therapy, 318–19
divalproex/valproate/valproic acid therapy, 546
donepezil therapy, 579, 582
fluoxetine therapy, 164, 166
haloperidol therapy, 330
lithium therapy, 530–32
lorazepam therapy, 452
mirtazapine therapy, 172, 173–74
nefazodone therapy, 184
nortriptyline therapy, 188, 190
olanzapine therapy, 339
paroxetine therapy, 198, 200
propranolol therapy, 376
quetiapine therapy, 348
risperidone therapy, 357
sertraline therapy, 206
thioridazine therapy, 361
venlafaxine therapy, 224
ziprasidone therapy, 369, 370
zolpidem therapy, 468
monoamine oxidase inhibitors
augmentation and combination, 63, 69, 113, 114–15
bipolar disorder treatment, 38
contraindications, 122
depression treatment, 50–51
discontinuing or switching, 80, 114, 115
dosing, 113*t*
drug–illness interactions, 122
drug interactions, 140, 149, 164–65, 172, 185, 199, 207, 215, 225, 439
efficacy, 112
hypertensive crisis, 118–21
indications, 111–12
irreversible class, 111
mechanism of action, 111
overdose, 122–23
personality disorder management, 43
pharmacokinetics, 113*t*
phobia management, 396
pre-treatment evaluation, 112–13
reversible inhibitors, 80
side effects, 79, 83, 112, 116–17
switching to/from SSRIs, 132
tolerance, 114
toxicity, 51
treatment monitoring, 115
mood disorders
psychosis in, 261–62
secondary, in elders, 487
substance-induced, 487
mood stabilizing drugs, 63
dementia therapy, 554
indications, 479, 485
pharmacology, 482–84*t*
see also specific drug
motor vehicle operation, 404–5
lorazepam therapy and, 452–53
movement disorders. *see* extrapyramidal symptoms
moxifloxacin, 362, 369
multiple sclerosis, 262

nefazodone
advantages/disadvantages, 182
classification, 179*t*
combination therapies, 114
cytochrome P450 metabolism and, 20
discontinuing or switching, 80
dosing, 182–83
drug interactions, 61, 184–85, 199, 207, 349, 439, 473, 580
indications, 179–80
mechanism of action, 180–82
overdose, 186
pharmacokinetics, 180, 181*t*
precautions, 185, 186
side effects, 183
treatment monitoring, 184
see also antidepressant drugs
nelfinavir, 141
neuroleptic malignant syndrome, 294–97, 314
neuroleptics. *see* antipsychotics
neurophysiology
age-related changes, 12
antidepressant drug side effects, 89*t*
heterocyclic antidepressant action, 97

mania induced by organic pathology, 486
presynaptic activity, 17
principles of, 17–21
nimodipine, 64
nonsteroidal antiinflammatory drugs, 534, 580, 586, 591, 594
noradrenergic and specific serotonergic antidepressant, 51
depression therapy, 66
nortriptyline
advantages/disadvantages, 187
chronic pain management, 42
classification, 186*t*
combination therapies, 138, 188
contraindications, 190
depression treatment, 50, 54, 55, 65
dosing, 187–88
drug interactions, 149, 190, 207
for GAD, 41
indications, 186, 394
mechanism of action, 187
overdose, 190
for pathologic emotionalism, 42
pharmacokinetics, 186–87
precautions, 191
side effects, 101, 103, 189–90
toxicity, 51
treatment monitoring, 188, 190
see also antidepressant drugs; heterocyclic antidepressants
nursing homes
polypharmacy in, 52
prescribing patterns, 3, 230

obsessive–compulsive disorder (OCD)
antidepressant drug therapy, 39, 144, 147, 151, 192, 202
antipsychotic drug therapy, 334
anxiolytic therapy, 436
clinical features, 38–39
comorbidities, 396
epidemiology, 396
management, 396
SSRI therapy, 127
off-label drug use, 10–11
olanzapine
advantages/disadvantages, 335–36, 341
bipolar disorder treatment, 496–97
classification, 334*t*
cost effectiveness, 232, 335
delirium management, 255–56
dosing, 336–37
drug–illness interactions, 340
drug interactions, 339–40
indications, 334
laboratory tests affected by, 340
mechanism of action, 335
mood disorder therapy, 479–80
overdose, 340–41
pharmacokinetics, 335
precautions, 341
for psychotic depression, 64
side effects, 279, 280, 298, 337–39
treatment monitoring, 339
see also antipsychotic drugs
omega-3 fatty acids, 64, 481
Omnibus Budget Reconciliation Act, 263–64
opioids
drug interactions, 362, 464
side effects, 11
orphenadrine, 141
overdose
alprazolam, 435
antidepressant drugs, 51
antipsychotic drugs, 307–8
anxiolytics and sedative/hypnotics, 429
bupropion, 142–43
buspirone, 440
carbamazepine, 508–9
chloral hydrate, 443
citalopram, 149–50
clozapine, 320
desipramine, 157
diazepam, 448
divalproex/valproate/valproic acid, 547–48
donepezil, 581
estazolam, 449
fluoxetine, 165
fluphenazine, 325
gabapentin, 512–13
haloperidol, 331
heterocyclic antidepressants, 107
lamotrigine, 516
lithium, 536–37
lorazepam, 452
loxapine, 334
mirtazapine, 173
moclobemide, 179
MAOIs, 122–23
nefazodone, 186
nortriptyline, 190
olanzapine, 340–41
oxazepam, 456
paroxetine, 199–200
perphenazine, 344
quetiapine, 349–50
risperidone, 358
SSRI, 129–30
sertraline, 208
tacrine, 595

overdose (*cont.*)
temazepam, 459
thioridazine, 363
thiothixene, 365–66
trazodone, 216
triazolam, 461
venlafaxine, 226
zaleplon, 465
ziprasidone, 370
zolpidem, 469–70
zopiclone, 473–74
over-the-counter drugs, 149, 155, 199, 207
oxazepam
advantages/disadvantages, 455
alcohol withdrawal management, 425
classification, 455*t*
dosing, 456
drug–illness interactions, 456
drug interactions, 456
overdose, 456
pharmacokinetics, 455
precautions, 456
side effects, 456
see also benzodiazepines
oxcarbazine, 516
oxybutynin, 439

pain
antidepressant drug therapy, 42, 151, 180, 217
chronic, 42
pancuronium, 455
panic disorder
antidepressant drug therapy, 39–40, 144, 147, 151, 166, 174, 192, 202
anxiolytic therapy, 430, 444
associated disorders, 394
benzodiazepine therapy, 375, 392, 394–95
clinical features, 39
epidemiology, 394
SSRI therapy, 40, 389, 394
treatment, 394–95
Parkinson's disease/parkinsonism
antipsychotic drug-induced, 279, 286–88
antipsychotic drug therapy, 309, 350, 352
cognitive enhancer therapy, 553
in diffuse lewy body disease, 250–51
management of psychosis in, 247–49, 309, 350
paroxetine, 131
advantages/disadvantages, 193–94
anxiety disorder therapy, 398
classification, 191*t*
combination therapies, 138
cytochrome P450 metabolism and, 20, 21
depression therapy, 65
discontinuation, 132–33, 193, 195
dosing, 193, 194
drug interactions, 20, 164, 198–99, 469, 580, 586
indications, 192–93
mechanism of action, 192
OCD treatment, 39
overdose, 199–200
pharmacokinetics, 192
PTSD treatment, 41
precautions, 199, 200
side effects, 194–98, 200
treatment monitoring, 198, 200
see also antidepressant drugs; selective serotonin reuptake inhibitors
pathologic emotionalism, 41–42
pemoline, 63
pergolide, 416
perphenazine
advantages/disadvantages, 342
classification, 342
dosing, 342
drug interactions, 190, 343
indications, 342
mechanism of action, 342
overdose, 344
pharmacokinetics, 342
precautions, 343–44
side effects, 343
see also antipsychotic drugs
personality disorders
antidepressant drug therapy, 43
mood stabilizer therapy, 485
SSRI therapy, 128
pethidine, 120
phantom limb pain, 400
pharmacodynamics, 11
pharmacokinetics
age-related effects, 12–16
alprazolam, 430
antianxiety agents, 377–84*t*
antidepressant drugs, 20, 90*t*
antipsychotic drugs, 232–36
benzodiazepines, 376, 385–86
bupropion, 135, 136*t*
buspirone, 436
carbamazepine, 502
chloral hydrate, 441
citalopram, 145
clomipramine, 152
clonazepam, 444
clozapine, 309

definition, 11
desipramine, 156
diazepam, 447
divalproex/valproate/valproic acid, 542
donepezil, 574
estazolam, 448
fluoxetine, 158–59
gabapentin, 510
galantamine, 583
haloperidol, 325–26
heterocyclic antidepressants, 98*t*, 99–101
lamotrigine, 513–14
lithium, 517
lorazepam, 450
midazolam, 453
mirtazapine, 167, 168*t*
moclobemide, 174, 176*t*
monitoring antidepressant drug therapy, 108–9
mood stabilizing srugs, 482–84*t*
nefazodone, 180, 181*t*
nonlinear, 15, 90*t*
olanzapine, 335
oxazepam, 455
perphenazine, 342
principles of neurotransmission in, 17–21
protein binding, 16
quetiapine, 345
risperidone, 351
rivastigmine, 587
sedative/hypnotic agents, 377–84*t*
sertraline, 203
SSRIs, 123–27
St. John's wort, 210
tacrine, 592–93
temazepam, 457
terminology, 13*t*
topiramate, 539
trazodone, 211, 212*t*
triazolam, 459–60
venlafaxine, 217, 218*t*
zaleplon, 462
ziprasidone, 366
zolpidem, 465–66
zopiclone, 471–72
see also metabolism of medication
phenelzine, 112
advantages/disadvantages, 201
classification, 200*t*
depression treatment, 54, 69
dosing, 113, 201
indications, 200–201
side effects, 112, 201, 202*t*
withdrawal, 201
phenobarbitol, 198, 464, 515, 546
phenylpropanolamine, 362
phenytoin, drug interactions, 141, 164, 198, 199, 207, 216, 331, 349, 434, 439, 464, 515, 534, 540, 546
pheochromocytoma, 179
phobias
antidepressant drug therapy, 40, 146
epidemiology, 395
presentation, 395
see also agoraphobia; social phobia
Physicians' Desk Reference (PDR), 6
physostigmine, 256
Pick's disease, 559–60
pilocarpine, 580
pimozide
delusional disorder therapy, 257
drug interactions, 362, 369
side effects, 283
see also antipsychotic drugs
pindolol, 62
Pisa syndrome, 293
posttraumatic stress disorder (PTSD)
antidepressant drug therapy, 41, 135, 180, 192, 202
mood stabilizer therapy, 485
pharmacotherapy options, 397
presentation, 397
potassium channel blockers, 362, 369
pramipexole, 88
premenstrual dysphoric disorder, 202
prescribing patterns, 3–4, 7
variation by treatment setting, 9–10
primidone, 516
probenicid, 452
procyclidine, 198
propafenone, 198
propoxyphene, 362, 369, 464
propranolol
benzodiazepine withdrawal management, 429
cytochrome P450 metabolism and, 21
drug–illness interactions, 376
drug interactions, 185
indications, 375
phobia management, 396
side effects, 376
treatment monitoring, 376
propoxyphene, 362
protein binding, 16, 99
protriptyline, 103
pseudodementia, 33
psychosis
antipsychotic drug therapy, 309, 322, 325, 326, 350, 359
in BPSD, 236–37, 238–39
in mood disorders, 261–62

psychotherapy, 10
  antidepressant therapy with, 188
  anxiety disorder therapy, 398
  anxiety management, 388
  with cognitive enhancer therapy, 578
  depression treatment, 64
psychotic depression, 35–36, 64, 261
  antidepressant drug therapy, 145
  antipsychotic drug therapy, 335
PTSD. *see* posttraumatic stress disorder
pyrimethamine, 516

quazepam, 421
quetiapine
  advantages/disadvantages, 346
  classification, 345*t*
  dosing, 346–47
  drug interactions, 348–49
  indications, 345
  laboratory tests affected by, 349
  mechanism of action, 345
  mood disorder therapy, 480
  overdose, 349–50
  pharmacokinetics, 345
  precautions, 349, 350
  side effects, 279, 280, 299, 347–48
  switching to/from, 350
  see also antipsychotic drugs
quinidine
  cytochrome P450 metabolism and, 20
  drug interactions, 165, 199, 362, 580
  side effects, 282
quinolone drugs
  drug interactions, 154
  see also specific drug

rabbit syndrome, 293
race/ethnicity, 3, 10
  haloperidol pharmacokinetics, 327
  metabolic differences, 19*t*
  risperidone pharmacokinetics, 353
relapse prevention
  bipolar disorder, 500–501, 517
  depression, 54–55, 56–58, 127, 191
  schizophrenia, 261*t*
renal clearance, 16, 21
reserpine, 155
restless leg syndrome, 400, 415–16, 444, 459
rifampicin, 469
rifampin, 141, 349, 439, 464, 473, 516
risperidone
  bipolar disorder treatment, 496–97
  classification, 350*t*
  cost effectiveness, 232, 351
  delirium management, 255–56
  discontinuing, 355
  dosing, 353–54
  drug–illness interactions, 358
  drug interactions, 198, 225, 357, 580
  efficacy, 353, 359
  indications, 350–51, 352
  mechanism of action, 351–52
  mood disorder therapy, 480
  overdose, 358
  pharmacokinetics, 351
  precautions, 358, 359
  for psychotic depression, 64
  safety, 352–53
  side effects, 279, 355–57
  see also antipsychotic drugs
ritonavir, 141, 439
rivastigmine
  classification, 587*t*
  clinical practice, 591–92
  dosing, 589
  drug interactions, 591
  efficacy, 588–89
  indications, 587
  mechanism of action, 553, 588
  pharmacokinetics, 587
  side effects, 589–91

SAM-E, 64, 207
schizoaffective disorder
  anticonvulsant drug therapy, 513, 542
  lithium therapy, 517
  mood stabilizer therapy, 485
schizophrenia
  aggression in, 43
  antidepressant drug therapy, 104, 144, 145
  antipsychotic drug therapy, 308, 333, 334, 342, 345, 350, 352, 363, 366
  clinical features, 258–59
  early onset, 258–59
  epidemiology, 258
  late onset, 258*t*, 259
  management, 260
  pharmacotherapy, 231
  relapse prevention, 261*t*
  vs. bipolar disorder, 491
sedative/hypnotics. *see* anxiolytics and sedative/hypnotics
sedative side effects, 11
seizure disorders
  anticonvulsant drug therapy, 513, 541
  anxiolytic therapy, 444, 447, 450
seizures, drug-induced
  antidepressant drug side effects, 76–77, 105
  antipsychotic drug side effects, 297
  bupropion effects, 142
  nortriptyline effects, 190

serotonin noradrenaline reuptake inhibitors (SNRIs)
chronic pain management, 42
depression therapy, 66
discontinuing or switching, 80
panic disorder treatment, 40
toxicity, 51
see also specific drug
selective serotonin reuptake inhibitors (SSRIs)
augmentation, 61, 62, 69
benzodiazepine withdrawal management, 428–29
bipolar disorder treatment, 38
cardiovascular health and, 32
chronic pain management, 42
combination therapies, 65, 114, 175, 178, 395, 578
cost-effectiveness, 53
cytochrome P450 metabolism and, 20
depression therapy, 50, 65, 66
discontinuing or switching, 67, 80, 132–34
dosing, 130, 131–32
drug interactions, 19, 65, 83, 107, 140, 154, 199, 357, 533
dysthymia treatment, 34–35
indications, 127–28
for managing aggressive behavior, 43
nonresponse, 60
OCD treatment, 39, 396
overdose, 129–30
panic disorder treatment, 40, 389, 394
personality disorder management, 43
pharmacokinetics, 123–27
phobia management, 396
PTSD treatment, 41
for psychotic depression, 36–37
selection of, 130–31
for severe depression, 31
side effects, 71, 76, 77–78, 79, 83, 84–85, 129
toxicity, 51
see also specific drug
serotonin syndrome, 79–82
combination therapy risks, 149
sertraline, 131
advantages/disadvantages, 204
clinical characteristics, 208–9
combination therapies, 138
discontinuation, 132–33
dosing, 204–5
drug interactions, 20, 206–7, 469, 580
indications, 202–4
mechanism of action, 203
OCD treatment, 39
overdose, 208
pharmacokinetics, 203
PTSD treatment, 41
precautions, 208
side effects, 205–6
treatment monitoring, 206
sexual functioning
antidepressant drug side effects, 85–88
antipsychotic drug side effects, 285
clozapine side effects, 318
mirtazapine therapy, 166
SIADH. *see* syndrome of inappropriate antidiuretic hormone secretion
sibutramine, 199, 207
side effects, 5, 6
acetylcholinesterase inhibitors, 570–71
alprazolam, 432–34
antidepressant drugs. *see* antidepressant drugs, side effects
antipsychotic drugs. *see* antipsychotic drugs, side effects
anxiolytics and sedative/hypnotics, 422–23
avoiding, 10
benzodiazepines, 401
bupropion, 139–40
buspirone, 438–39
carbamazepine, 504–6*t*
chloral hydrate, 442
citalopram, 147–48
clinical response, 12
clomipramine, 152, 153–54, 155
clonazepam, 445–46*t*
clozapine, 313–18, 321
contraindications to use, 11
depressive symptoms as, 33–34
desipramine, 157
diazepam, 448
divalproex/valproate/valproic acid, 544–46
donepezil, 578–79
duloxetine, 158
estazolam, 449
fluoxetine, 160, 162–64, 166
fluphenazine, 324
gabapentin, 511–12
galantamine, 585
haloperidol, 329–30
heterocyclic antidepressants, 101–6
initial dose selection, 8–9
kava, 475–76*t*
lamotrigine, 514, 515*t*
lithium, 522–29
lorazepam, 451–52
loxapine, 333, 334*t*
midazolam, 454–55*t*
mirtazapine, 170–72

side effects (*cont.*)
moclobemide, 177
monitoring for, 9
monoamine oxidase inhibitors, 112, 116–17
nefazodone, 183–84
nortriptyline, 189–90
olanzapine, 337–39
oxazepam, 456
paroxetine, 194–98
perphenazine, 343
phenelzine, 201, 202*t*
propranolol, 376
quetiapine, 347–48
risk, 11–12
risperidone, 355–57
rivastigmine, 589–91
selective serotonin reuptake inhibitors, 129
sertraline, 205–6*t*
tacrine, 593–94
temazepam, 458–59
thioridazine, 360, 361*t*
thiothixene, 364
topiramate, 540
trazodone, 214–15
triazolam, 461
tricyclic antidepressants, 129*t*
valerian, 477
venlafaxine, 222–24
zaleplon, 463–64*t*
ziprasidone, 368
zolpidem, 467, 468*t*
zopiclone, 472, 473*t*
sildenafil, 87
simvastatin, 185
skin problems
antidepressant drug side effects, 105–6
antipsychotic drug side effects, 300
lithium side effects, 528
sleep behavior
age-related changes, 412
antidepressant drug side effects, 88*t*, 105
anxiolytic and sedative/hypnotic effects, 402–3
assessment, 416, 417
in diffuse lewy body disease, 250
MAOI side effects, 116
see also sleep disorders
sleep deprivation therapy, 65
sleep disorders
antidepressant drug therapy, 167
anxiolytic therapy, 400, 444
causes, 413–14*t*
classification, 411
epidemiology, 411–12
management, 416–20
pharmacotherapy agents for, 371–72
sedative/hypnotic therapy, 415–16, 418–23, 441, 448, 449, 459, 465
side effects, 416
smoking cessation therapy, 135
SNRIs. *see* serotonin noradrenaline reuptake inhibitors
social phobia
antidepressant drug therapy, 40, 128, 144, 146, 151, 180, 396
benzodiazepine therapy, 375, 392
treatment options, 396
sodium, dietary, 534
sparfloxacin, 154, 362, 369
SSRIs. *see* selective serotonin reuptake inhibitors
St. John's wort, 64, 209
drug interactions, 207, 210, 439
side effects, 210*t*
stimulants, 62–63
stroke
poststroke depression, 35, 144, 146
prevention in dementia, 558
SSRI prophylaxis, 128
visual hallucinations related to, 258
substance-induced disorders
anxiety, 398
mood disorders, 487
succinylcholine, 580, 586, 591, 594
suicidal behavior/ideation
citalopram use and, 150
depression and, 26
SSRI therapy and, 133
sympathomimetic drugs, 119–20
syndrome of inappropriate antidiuretic hormone secretion (SIADH), 82–83, 301

tacrine, 573
classification, 592*t*
disadvantages, 593
dosing, 593
drug–illness interactions, 594–95
drug interactions, 594
indications, 592
mechanism of action, 553
overdose, 595
pharmacokinetics, 592–93
side effects, 593–94
tardive dyskinesia
antipsychotic drug side effects, 279, 289–92
anxiolytic therapy, 444
tartrazine, 106
taste, antidepressant drug side effects, 106

temazepam
  advantages/disadvantages, 457–58
  anxiety therapy, 389
  classification, 457*t*
  dosing, 458
  drug interactions, 459
  overdose, 459
  pharmacokinetics, 457
  side effects, 458–59
  sleep disorder therapy, 420
  withdrawal, 458
  see also benzodiazepines
temperature dyscontrol, as antipsychotic drug side effect, 302–3
terfenadine
  drug interactions, 165, 185
  side effects, 282
theophyllines, 198, 594
thiazides, 533
thioridazine
  advantages/disadvantages, 360
  classification, 359*t*
  dosing, 360
  drug–illness interactions, 363
  drug interactions, 140, 198, 362, 369
  indications, 359
  mechanism of action, 360
  overdose, 363
  pharmacokinetics, 359
  side effects, 282, 360, 361*t*
  treatment monitoring, 361
  see also antipsychotic drugs
thiothixene
  advantages/disadvantages, 363–64
  classification, 363*t*
  dosing, 364
  drug interactions, 365
  overdose, 365–66
  pharmacology, 363
  precautions, 365
  side effects, 364
  see also antipsychotic drugs
thyroid hormone replacement, 61
tinnitus, 400
tolbutamide, 207
tolerance
  benzodiazepines, 392–93, 401–2
  MAOIs, 114
topiramate
  advantages/disadvantages, 539
  classification, 538*t*
  dosing, 539
  drug interactions, 540
  indications, 538–39
  mechanism of action, 539
  mood disorder therapy, 479
  pharmacokinetics, 539
  precautions, 541
  side effects, 540
Tourette's disorder, 293
  antipsychotic drug therapy, 325
tramadol, 199, 207, 225, 362, 464
transcranial magnetic stimulation, 38
  mood disorder therapy, 481
tranylcypromine, 112
  combination therapy, 114
  discontinuation, 115
  dosing, 113
  food interactions, 118
  side effects, 112
trazodone, 42
  advantages/disadvantages, 213
  classification, 210*t*
  combination therapies, 175, 578
  dosing, 213–14
  drug interactions, 199, 207, 215–16, 439
  indications, 210–13
  mechanism of action, 211
  overdose, 216
  pharmacokinetics, 211, 212*t*
  precautions, 216
  side effects, 214–15, 216–17
  sleep disorder therapy, 421
  see also antidepressant drugs
treatment settings, prescribing patterns in, 3, 9–10
triazolam
  advantages/disadvantages, 460
  classification, 459*t*
  dosing, 460–61
  drug interactions, 185
  indications, 459
  overdose, 461
  pharmacokinetics, 459–60
  precautions, 462
  side effects, 461
  see also benzodiazepines
triazolobenzodiazepines, 62
tricyclic antidepressants
  augmentation, 61, 63, 69
  bipolar disorder treatment, 38
  chronic pain management, 42
  combination therapies, 65, 114, 175
  depression therapy, 50, 61, 65
  drug interactions, 65, 140, 149, 164, 178, 198, 362, 369, 533, 547
  nonresponse, 60
  OCD treatment, 396
  for pathologic emotionalism, 41–42
  psychotic depression treatment, 35
  side effects, 76, 77, 83, 84, 107, 129*t*
  switching to/from, 67, 80, 132, 178
trihexyphenidyl, 331
trimethoprim, 516

trimetrexate, 516
trimipramine
  side effects, 103
  toxicity, 51
  see also antidepressant drugs
tryptophans, 165, 421
tyramine-containing foods
  MAOI interaction, 118
  moclobemide precautions, 179

urinary problems, as lithium side effect, 528–29

vagus nerve stimulation, 481
valerian, 476–77
valproate. *see* divalproex/valproate/valproic acid
valproic acid. *see* divalproex/valproate/valproic acid
vascular dementia, 557–58, 576, 582, 587
venlafaxine, 42
  advantages/disadvantages, 219–20
  bipolar disorder treatment, 38
  classification, 217*t*
  combination therapies, 114, 138, 221
  contraindications, 226
  depression treatment, 49, 65
  discontinuing, 67, 222
  dosing, 220–21
  drug–illness interactions, 225
  drug interactions, 164, 199, 207, 224–25, 469
  efficacy, 219
  indications, 217
  laboratory tests affected by, 225
  mechanism of action, 217–19
  OCD treatment, 396
  overdose, 226
  panic disorder treatment, 40
  pharmacokinetics, 217, 218*t*
  PTSD treatment, 41
  precautions, 225–27
  psychotic depression treatment, 35
  side effects, 83, 222–24
  treatment monitoring, 224
  see also antidepressant drugs
verapamil
  drug interactions, 164, 439, 497
  mood disorder therapy, 480
vinblastine, 185
vision problems
  antipsychotic drug side effects, 297–98
  clozapine side effects, 316
  hallucinations, 257–58
  lithium side effects, 527
warfarin, 141, 165, 172, 198, 207, 215, 469, 547
washout period
  antidepressants, 67, 68, 80, 110
  citalopram, 151
  moclebamide, 178
  MAOIs, 114
  SSRIs, 132–34
weight changes
  antidepressant drug side effects, 83–84, 103
  antipsychotic drug side effects, 298–99
  clozapine side effects, 314
  lithium side effects, 522
  topiramate effects, 539
withdrawal
  alcohol, 423–26, 441, 447, 450, 455
  alprazolam, 432
  antidepressants, 67, 110–11
  antiparkinsonian drugs, 304
  antipsychotic drugs, 247
  anxiolytics and sedative/hypnotics, 403, 426–29
  chloral hydrate, 441
  citalopram, 147
  clomipramine, 154
  fluoxetine, 162
  paroxetine, 193, 195
  phenelzine, 201
  SSRIs, 132–33
  temazepam, 458
  venlafaxine, 222
  zolpidem, 467

yellow dye. *see* tartrazine
yohimbine, 88

zaleplon
  advantages/disadvantages, 462–63
  classification, 462*t*
  discontinuing, 463
  dosing, 463
  drug–illness interactions, 465
  drug interactions, 464
  indications, 462
  mechanism of action, 462
  overdose, 465
  pharmacokinetics, 462
  precautions, 465
  side effects, 463–64*t*
  sleep disorder therapy, 420
  see also anxiolytics and sedative/hypnotics
zidovudine, 547
ziprasidone
  advantages/disadvantages, 366–67
  classification, 366*t*

dosing, 367–68
drug–illness interactions, 369–70
drug interactions, 369
indications, 366
mechanism of action, 366
mood disorder therapy, 480
overdose, 370
pharmacokinetics, 366
precautions, 370
side effects, 244*t*, 279, 280, 283, 298, 368
treatment monitoring, 369, 370
see also antipsychotic drugs
zolpidem
advantages/disadvantages, 466–67
classification, 465*t*
dosage, 467
drug–illness interactions, 469
drug interactions, 468–69
indications, 465, 466
mechanism of action, 466
overdose, 469–70
pharmacokinetics, 465–66
precautions, 470–71
side effects, 467, 468*t*
sleep disorder therapy, 420
treatment monitoring, 468
withdrawal, 467
see also anxiolytics and sedative/hypnotics
zopiclone
advantages/disadvantages, 472
benzodiazepine withdrawal management, 428
classification, 471*t*
discontinuing, 472
dosing, 472
drug–illness interactions, 473
drug interactions, 473
indications, 471, 472
mechanism of action, 472
overdose, 473–74
pharmacokinetics, 471–72
precautions, 405, 474
side effects, 472, 473*t*
sleep disorder therapy, 420
see also anxiolytics and sedative/hypnotics

INDEX